Contemporary Immunology: B Cells and T Cells

Contemporary Immunology: B Cells and T Cells

Editor: Josiah Robinson

MURPHY & MOORE
www.murphy-moorepublishing.com

www.murphy-moorepublishing.com

MURPHY & MOORE

Cataloging-in-Publication Data

Contemporary immunology : B cells and T cells / edited by Josiah Robinson.
p. cm.
Includes bibliographical references and index.
ISBN 978-1-63987-134-6
1. Immunology. 2. B cells. 3. T cells. 4. Lymphocytes. I. Robinson, Josiah.
QR181 .C66 2022
616.079--dc23

Murphy & Moore Publishing,
1 Rockefeller Plaza,
New York City, NY 10020, USA

ISBN 978-1-63987-134-6 (Hardback)

Contents

Preface

B and T cells are significant parts of the adaptive immune response which is also antigen specific immune response. These are the only cells in the body that are able to recognize the epitopes of the antigen and can respond specifically to each antigenic epitope. The B cells are responsible for the production of antibodies; therefore, the humoral immunity depends on the B cells. Cell immunity depends on the T cells. B cells are also known as antigen presenting cells because they present antigens and secrete cytokines. Immune-mediated cell death is carried out by two major subtypes of T cells: CD8+ "killer T cells" and CD4+ "helper" T cells. The aim of this book is to present researches that have transformed this discipline and aided its advancement. It explores all the important aspects of B and T cells. A number of latest researches have been included in this book to keep the readers up-to-date with the global concepts in this area of study.

The researches compiled throughout the book are authentic and of high quality, combining several disciplines and from very diverse regions from around the world. Drawing on the contributions of many researchers from diverse countries, the book's objective is to provide the readers with the latest achievements in the area of research. This book will surely be a source of knowledge to all interested and researching the field.

In the end, I would like to express my deep sense of gratitude to all the authors for meeting the set deadlines in completing and submitting their research chapters. I would also like to thank the publisher for the support offered to us throughout the course of the book. Finally, I extend my sincere thanks to my family for being a constant source of inspiration and encouragement.

Editor

1

Regulation of B cell differentiation by intracellular membrane-associated proteins and microRNAs: role in the antibody response

*Zheng Lou, Paolo Casali and Zhenming Xu**

Department of Microbiology and Immunology, School of Medicine, The University of Texas Health Science Center, San Antonio, TX, USA

Edited by:
George C. Tsokos, Harvard Medical School, USA

Reviewed by:
To-Ha Thai, Harvard Medical School, USA
Nina Papavasiliou, The Rockefeller University, USA

***Correspondence:**
Zhenming Xu
xuz3@uthscsa.edu

B cells are central to adaptive immunity and their functions in antibody responses are exquisitely regulated. As suggested by recent findings, B cell differentiation is mediated by intracellular membrane structures (including endosomes, lysosomes, and autophagosomes) and protein factors specifically associated with these membranes, including Rab7, Atg5, and Atg7. These factors participate in vesicle formation/trafficking, signal transduction and induction of gene expression to promote antigen presentation, class switch DNA recombination (CSR)/somatic hypermutation (SHM), and generation/maintenance of plasma cells and memory B cells. Their expression is induced in B cells activated to differentiate and further fine-tuned by immune-modulating microRNAs, which coordinates CSR/SHM, plasma cell differentiation, and memory B cell differentiation. These short non-coding RNAs would individually target multiple factors associated with the same intracellular membrane compartments and collaboratively target a single factor in addition to regulating AID and Blimp-1. These, together with regulation of microRNA biogenesis and activities by endosomes and autophagosomes, show that intracellular membranes and microRNAs, two broadly relevant cell constituents, play important roles in balancing gene expression to specify B cell differentiation processes for optimal antibody responses.

Keywords: B cell activation and differentiation, plasma cell, memory B cell, intracellular membrane associated proteins, endosome, lysosome, autophagosome, microRNA

Abbreviations: Ago, argonaute; AID, activation-induced cytidine deaminase; Atg, autophagy-related gene; BCR, B cell receptor; Blimp-1, B lymphocyte-induced maturation protein-1; CSR, class switch DNA recombination; ER, endoplasmic reticulum; GAP, GTPase activating protein; HDI, histone deacetylase inhibitors; Ig, immunoglobulin; KO, knockout; MHC II, major histocompatibility complex II; PI-3K, class III phosphatidylinositol 3-kinase; RA, rheumatoid arthritis; Rab, Ras-related in brain; RISC, RNA-induced silencing complex; SHM, somatic hypermutation; TCR, T cell receptor; TLR, toll-like receptor; VPS, vacuolar protein sorting.

INTRODUCTION

B lymphocytes are critical to immunity by mediating production of neutralization antibodies to infectious pathogens and tumor cells (1). They develop through several highly regulated steps, first as pro-B cells and then pre-B cells in the bone marrow, in which immunoglobulin (Ig) V(D)J DNA recombination occurs, and subsequently as immature B cell stages and then mature B cells in the periphery. V(D)J recombination gives rise to a highly diverse repertoire of the B cell receptor (BCR) for antigens. Unlike immature B cells, which express predominantly IgM-containing BCRs, mature naïve B cells express high levels of IgD on their surface. In secondary lymphoid organs (e.g., spleen and lymph nodes), B cells are organized into the follicular or marginal zone areas (2), in part due to their BCR signaling differences.

Upon antigen encounter, B cells are activated in a T cell-independent or T cell-dependent manner. In T-independent antibody responses and the early T-independent phase of T-dependent antibody responses, B cells differentiate upon dual engagement of BCR (e.g., by repetitive antigenic ligands) and an innate immune receptor, such as a toll-like receptor (TLR) (3). In T-dependent antibody responses, specific B cells are induced through cognate interaction, and engagement of CD40, which is constitutively expressed on B cells, by trimeric CD154 expressed by specific T helper (T_H) cells (4). Activated B cells differentiate in germinal centers, the newly formed specialized microenvironment within secondary lymphoid organs (5). They undergo class switch DNA recombination (CSR) in the Ig heavy chain (IgH) locus to switch their BCR from IgM or IgD to, depending on eliciting stimuli, IgG, IgE, or IgA, which endows an antibody with different biological effector functions without changing antigen specificity (4). B cells also undergo somatic hypermutation (SHM). This inserts point-mutations into Ig V region DNA, thereby providing the substrate for positive selection of antibody mutants with higher affinity to the antigen (6). Finally, B cells differentiate into plasma cells, which secrete large amounts of antibodies, or memory B cells, which can be re-activated for amnestic antibody responses upon second challenge by the same antigen (7–10). Memory B cells and plasma cells are long-lived and play an important role in the protection against re-exposure to microbial and other antigens.

B cell CSR/SHM and differentiation into plasma cells and memory B cells are tightly regulated. Dysregulation of these processes can lead to immune deficiencies, autoimmunity, or B lymphomagenesis. In this review, we will focus on how B cell differentiation is regulated for effective antibody responses by intracellular membranes, particularly the emerging functions of endosomes and autophagosomes. We will also emphasize the induction of proteins associated with these intracellular membranes and the role of these proteins in signaling and induction of gene expression. Furthermore, we will summarize the evidence of the epigenetic modulation of expression of these proteins by microRNAs and the consequence to B cell differentiation – readers are referred to other articles that have extensively reviewed the regulation/dysregulation of immune functions by microRNAs (11–15). Finally, we will discuss the notion that microRNA activities are reciprocally regulated by intracellular membranes, as part of the controlling mechanisms that fine-tune gene expression and buffer molecular aberrancies to ensure the specificity of B cell differentiation and functions.

B CELL REGULATION BY INTRACELLULAR MEMBRANE-ASSOCIATED PROTEINS

Intracellular Membrane Structures and Associated Proteins

Endosomes are internalized lipid vesicles containing extracellular molecules and cell surface components, including fluid, solutes and their carriers, lipids, membrane proteins, and receptor–ligand complexes (16). They regulate various cellular processes by sorting, processing, recycling, storing, and degrading these cargos. Early endosomes, which have tubular and vacuolar domains, are the main sorting station of internalized cargos, most of which are recycled back to the plasma membrane directly or through recycling endosomes (**Figure 1**). Late endosomes form from the vacuolar domains of early endosomes, with many changes in the lipid and protein contents. They mature upon moving from the peripheral cytoplasm to the perinuclear area, where mature late endosomes fuse with each other and eventually fuse with lysosomes or pre-existing hybrid organelle endolysosomes (**Figure 1**). Endosome maturation is regulated by a group of Rab (Ras-related in brain) small GTPases (17). Rab5 is a defining component of early endosomes through various stages, and regulates the conversion of early endosomes to late endosomes (17). The GTP-bound form of Rab5 (Rab5-GTP) recruits Rab7 and is then converted to Rab5-GDP, which dissociates from the membrane (18, 19). Rab7, upon recruitment, can auto-activate to bind GTP and suppress Rab5 binding to GTP (20). Rab7-GTP recruits its own effectors, including RILP, which connects late endosomes to dynein motors for trafficking, and components of the HOPS complex, which promotes late endosome fusion with lysosomes (21, 22). Lysosomes are the terminal degradative compartments. These have a luminal pH of 4.6–5.0 and contain hydrolases that digest the cargo (17). They can also fuse with autophagosomes to form autolysosomes, which carries out degradation of extracellular and intracellular components.

Macroautophagy (referred here as autophagy) is a process that degrades cytoplasmic compartments and organelles and is underpinned by the formation of autophagosomes, which are enclosed double-membrane structures (23). Autophagy was first characterized as a cellular process to counter stress, e.g., by mediating degradation of cytoplasmic organelles/proteins in starved cells for the generation of energy and macromolecules to maintain cell viability (24). Autophagosomes, however, can be induced under physiological stress-free conditions, likely through slightly different pathways, and play important roles in immunity (25, 26). Their induction starts from activation of a protein complex containing ULK1 and the autophagy-related gene (Atg) 13, and formation of a phagophore, a double-membrane structure (**Figure 1**). The nucleation of phagophores requires activation of the class III phosphatidylinositol 3-kinase (PI-3K) complex consisting of the VPS34 (vacuolar protein sorting 34), which is activated by a complex containing Beclin 1, VPS15, and Atg14

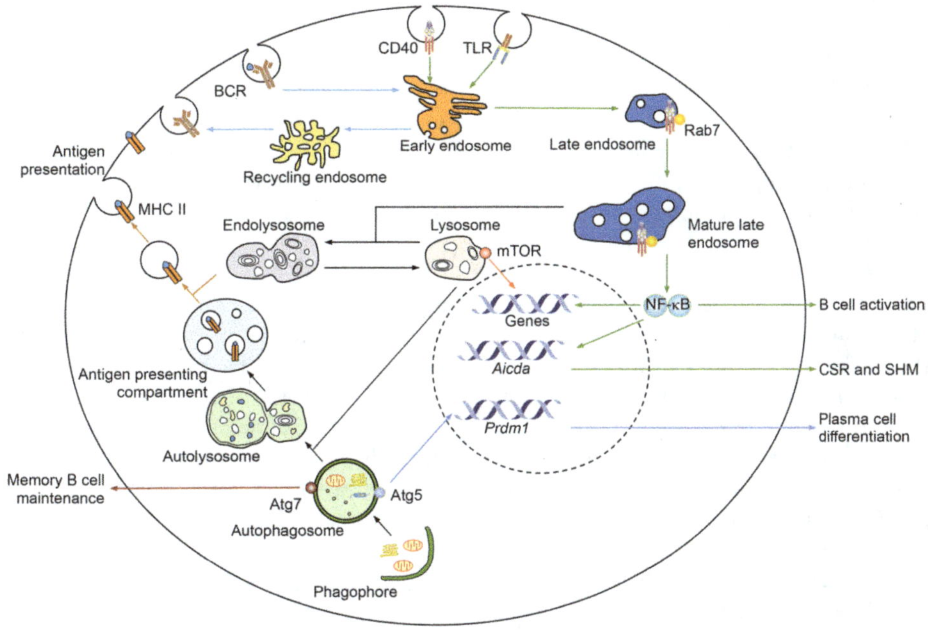

FIGURE 1 | Regulation of B cell differentiation and functions by intracellular membranes and associated proteins. Several B cell processes are regulated by endosomes, lysosomes, and autophagosomes. Upon antigen-triggered internalization, BCR is sorted by early endosomes to either recycle back onto the cell surface or go through antigen processing, which are mediated by endolysosomes, for the MHC II-dependent antigen presentation. Signaling receptors, such as CD40 (as depicted) and TLRs (both surface TLRs and intracellular TLRs), can be internalized and/or sorted by early endosomes to localize to mature late endosomes, as marked by Rab7. A Rab7-dependent process would stabilize the interaction of such receptors and their adaptors (e.g., CD40 and TRAF6), thereby promoting sustained signaling, such as NF-κB activation, for induction of genes important for B cell activation and CSR/SHM, e.g., AID. Lysosomes, as transformed from and maintained by mature late endosomes, can recruit mTOR, which plays an important role in B cell activation. Autophagosomes are important for memory B cell maintenance, i.e., through Atg7, and plasma cell differentiation and survival, e.g., through Atg5. They can also fuse with lysosomes to become autolysosomes, which then transform into a specialized compartment for antigen presentation.

(24). Phosphorylation of ULK1 and Atg13 by the mTOR kinase, which regulates B cell differentiation and CSR (27, 28), inhibits autophagy activation. Inhibition of mTOR, e.g., by rapamycin, promotes autophagosome formation (29). Autophagosomes form after the expansion and final closure of phagophores, and then fuse with either mature endosomes to form amphisomes or lysosomes to form autolysosomes, in which luminal cargos and the inner membrane are degraded (**Figure 1**) – amphisomes can also fuse with lysosomes to form autolysosomes.

Antigen Presentation

In T-dependent antibody responses, B cells uptake antigens through the BCR, process it, and present it through the major histocompatibility complex II (MHCII) to cognate CD4$^+$ T_H cell TCR to prime T_H cells. These, in turn, will prime B cells for full activation, proliferation, and differentiation. It has been long known that antigen processing for MHC II-dependent presentation is mediated by endosomes/lysosomes (30), while MHC I-dependent antigen presentation is mediated by endoplasmic reticulum (ER). Autophagy also plays an important role in MHC II-dependent antigen presentation in B cells and dendritic cells, in which autophagosomes continuously merge with multi-vesicular compartments loaded with MHC II (**Figure 1**). Targeting of the influenza virus matrix protein-1 to autophagosomes by fusion of this protein with LC3, a marker of growing autophagosomes, strongly enhances the presentation of this protein to CD4$^+$ T cells (31). Mice with conditional knockout (KO) of autophagosome-associated protein Atg5 in dendritic cells fail to mount sufficient CD4$^+$ T cell priming after herpes simplex virus infection (32). Conditional KO mice lacking Atg5 in B cells have not been analyzed in this context, but would likely display a similar phenotype.

Protein citrullination is highly relevant to rheumatoid arthritis (RA), as RA patients display high levels of autoantibodies to citrullinated self-proteins (33). Citrullinated peptides, but not unmodified peptides, are presented to T cells by dendritic cells and macrophages through autophagy. In B cells, citrullinated peptides are also presented in a manner dependent on BCR engagement (e.g., triggered by anti-IgM) and autophagosome formation (which can be blocked by 3-methyladenine, an inhibitor of PI-3K and autophagy). Upon brief serum starvation, B lymphoma cells can also present citrullinated peptides through an Atg5- and autophagosome-dependent pathway (34).

B Cell Activation and CSR/SHM

Intracellular membrane-associated proteins regulate activation and differentiation of B cells, in addition to their development and survival – pre-B cell development in the bone marrow and B-1 cell survival in the periphery are defective in mice with B cell conditional KO (*Cd19-cre*) of *Atg5* (35). Upon BCR engagement by antigen, the fast and extensive induction of autophagosomes, in which the antigen would be rapidly processed, can cause cell death (36). Autophagy-dependent cell death can be overcome by CD40 engagement for full B cell activation (36), suggesting a role of autophagy in controlling self-reactive B cell activation and autoimmunity.

In B cells activated by CD40 engagement or dual TLR/BCR engagement (37), Rab7 is upregulated, suggesting a role of Rab7 and Rab7⁺ late endosomes in peripheral antigen-dependent B cell differentiation. In conditional KO $Igh^{+/C\gamma 1\text{-}cre}Rab7^{fl/fl}$ mice, *Rab7* is ablated only in B cells undergoing $Igh^{C\gamma 1\text{-}cre}$ Iγ1-Sγ1-Cγ1-*cre* transcription, as induced – like *Igh* germline Iγ1-Sγ1-Cγ1 transcription – by IL-4 in conjunction with CD40 or dual TLR/BCR engagement (38). These mice are normal in B and T cell development, but cannot mount T-independent or T-dependent class-switched IgG1 responses, while maintaining normal IgM levels. $Igh^{+/C\gamma 1\text{-}cre}Rab7^{fl/fl}$ B cells are normal in proliferation, survival, and plasma cell differentiation, as well as activation of the p38 kinase and ERK1/2 kinase pathways, but show defective CSR (38). This defect can be rescued by enforced expression of activation-induced cytidine deaminase (AID), which is essential for CSR and SHM. In addition, inhibition of Rab7 activity by a small molecule compound, CID 1067700 (39), reduces CSR and antibody responses in normal B cells/mice as well as autoantibody response and disease symptoms in lupus-prone MRL/$Fas^{lpr/lpr}$ mice (40). These findings, together with our demonstration that Rab7 mediates canonical NF-κB activation, as critical to AID induction, outline a novel role of Rab7 in signaling pathways that lead to AID expression and CSR, likely by promoting assembly of signaling complexes along mature endosomes. Such a role of Rab7 is consistent with the proximity of Rab7-containing mature late endosomes to the nucleus (**Figure 1**), as activated NF-κB would have a short path to reach genes, an advantage shared by ER membrane-mediated NF-κB activation, as occurring in BL41 B cells upon CD40 engagement and in Jurkat T cells upon TCR engagement (41). It would also be irrespective of the initial location of engaged immune receptors, e.g., on the plasma membrane (such as CD40, TLR1/2, and TLR4) or in endosomes (TLR7 and TLR9), and their trafficking pattern.

Lysosomes have been recently implicated to regulate signal transduction, serving as the "docking station" for mTOR in various cancer cells (42–44) and likely in B cells. Knock-in mice expressing a hypomorphic mTOR mutation and conditional KO mice with B cells mTOR deficiency are defective in germinal center formation and antibody responses, in concomitant with reduced AID expression and CSR (28). Pharmacological inhibition of mTOR kinase activity results in complicated phenotypes, likely due to non-redundant functions of two mTOR-containing complexes, mTORC1 and mTOC2 (28, 45).

Plasma Cell Differentiation

The differentiation of activated B cells into antibody-secreting plasma cells is associated with changes in gene expression that lead to the loss of the B cell identity and the gain of protein secretion functions. Such changes are mediated by the master transcription factor Blimp-1 (B lymphocyte-induced maturation protein-1), as encoded by *Prdm1* (8). In plasma cells, ER membranes expand and enhance their capacity to fold nascent peptides, a process driven by X-box binding protein-1, to promote antibody secretion (46). Both differentiating plasmablasts (which still proliferate) and terminally differentiated long-lived plasma cells have high autophagic activities. In two independently generated mouse strains with conditional *Atg5* KO in B cells (both through *Cd19-cre*), antibody responses and generation of antigen-specific long-lived plasma cells are defective (47, 48), likely due to impairment in generation of plasma cells (47), plasma cell survival (48), or both – the ER-related secretion function of plasma cells, however, does not seem to be affected (48). In addition, autophagosomes have been suggested to serve as a platform in recruiting ERK and its activation (49), which plays an important role in Blimp-1 induction and plasma cell differentiation (50). Rab7 does not play a major role in the generation of plasma cells, but may help in maintaining plasma cell survival, perhaps also through NF-κB-dependent sustained expression of Blimp-1 (40). Thus, intracellular-associated proteins are important for plasma cell homeostasis and sustainable antibody production.

Memory B Cell Differentiation

As recently shown, memory B cells specifically express high levels of autophagic activities and do so over time, i.e., low/no levels of autophagosome formation (LC3⁺ puncta) in naïve B cells, germinal center B cells, and newly formed memory B cells, but high levels in memory B cells isolated much later after the primary immunization (51). Atgs, such as *Ulk1*, *Atg14*, *Becn1* (encoding Beclin 1), *Atg5*, *Atg7*, and *LC3*, display similar expression patterns. Furthermore, Atg7 is dispensable for the initial generation of memory B cells, but critical for the long-term survival of memory B cells, likely by preventing apoptosis, as mice with B cell conditional KO of Atg7 (through *Cd19-cre*) can mount normal primary antibody responses, but much reduced secondary antibody responses and SHM upon re-challenging by antigen (51, 52). Finally, memory B cells express high levels of a forkhead family transcription factor FoxO3 and, to a lesser extent, FoxO1, consistent with the important role of these two factors in autophagy gene expression (53). How Atg7 and related intracellular membranes regulate apoptosis and perhaps other metabolic processes for the maintenance of memory B cells remains to be determined. Overall, intracellular membranes play an important role in peripheral antigen-dependent B cell differentiation. And, different membrane structures, likely through their associated proteins, specify different differentiation processes, e.g., Rab7 in CSR/SHM, Atg5 in plasma cell differentiation, and Atg7 in memory B cell differentiation (**Figure 1**).

REGULATION OF B CELL DIFFERENTIATION BY INTRACELLULAR MEMBRANE-ASSOCIATED PROTEINS AND MicroRNAs

MicroRNAs Regulate Peripheral Antigen-Dependent B Cell Differentiation

MicroRNAs are endogenous small non-coding RNAs that regulate adaptive and innate immunity, including B cell differentiation (54, 55). They modulate gene expression through mainly post-transcriptional mechanisms, such as inhibiting translation of mRNAs and/or promoting their degradation after pairing with the 3′-untranslated region (3′-UTR) of the target mRNA (**Box 1**). A single microRNA can regulate multiple gene targets and, conversely, a single gene can be regulated by multiple microRNAs. Conditional KO of *Dicer*, which is essential for microRNA biogenesis, through *Cd19-cre* leads to impairment in the generation of follicular B cells with concomitant increase in marginal zone B cells (56). This, together with the higher Dicer expression in follicular B cells, supports the notion that selected microRNAs mediate this stage of B cell development. High titers of autoantibodies in female *Dicer* conditional KO mice suggest a role of microRNAs in preventing autoimmune diseases (56).

MicroRNAs regulate the germinal center reaction. As *Aicda* gene expression is restricted to B cells activated by T-independent or T-dependent stimuli, *Aicda-cre* mice have been widely used to generate activated B cell-specific KO of genes. Conditional KO of *Dicer* through *Aicda-cre* dampens germinal center formation, likely through elevated expression of Bim, a pro-apoptotic protein (57). *Dicer* KO B cells are also defective in proliferation and survival, leading to impairment in production of high-affinity class-switched antibodies and generation of plasma cells or memory B cells. The relevant microRNAs missing in these KO B cells would include miR-155, as this microRNA is highly expressed in germinal center B cells and miR-155 KO leads to defective germinal centers (58, 59).

MicroRNAs play vital roles in CSR and SHM. MiR-155 targets the *Aicda* 3′-UTR, as knock-in or transgenic mice with the miR-155-binding site mutated in *Aicda* 3′-UTR show higher level of AID expression with upregulation of CSR and SHM (60). MiR-181b can also target *Aicda* 3′-UTR to regulate AID expression and CSR. Accordingly, miR-181b expression is downregulated in activated B cells, thereby allowing accumulation of AID (61). MiR-210 has been shown to be upregulated in activated B cells and inhibit CSR, likely by downregulating CSR factors – miR-210-deficient mice produce high levels of autoantibodies (62). B cell differentiation into plasma cells is also regulated by microRNAs. Overexpression of miR-125b, which is expressed in centroblasts (activated germinal center B cells that are enlarged and proliferating), represses plasma cell differentiation and Ig secretion by targeting *Prdm1* (63). Finally, histone deacetylase inhibitors (HDI) upregulate miR-155, miR-181b, and miR-361 to silence *AICDA/Aicda*, as well as miR-23b, miR-30a, and miR-125b to silence *PRDM1/Prdm1* in human and mouse B cells (64), but not other CSR/SHM-related genes or microRNAs that are not known to regulate *AICDA/Aicda* or *PRDM1/Prdm1* (65). Importantly, HDI also abolish CSR/SHM and impair the class-switched high-affinity antibody responses in normal mice and pathogenic autoantibody response in lupus-prone mice (64).

MicroRNAs Regulate Intracellular Membrane Functions

MicroRNAs regulate virtually all cellular pathways, including intracellular membrane functions, such as endocytosis (66), lysosome degradation (67), and autophagy (68). They would do so in cancer cells, stem cells, and B cells, which express relevant intracellular membrane structures. For instance, miR-509 can bind to the transcripts encoding Rab5C, one of the three Rab5 isoforms, thereby inhibiting Rab5C expression in pre-B acute lymphoblastic leukemia cells and resulting in a growth defect that can be rescued by Rab5C overexpression (69). Targeting

BOX 1 | MicroRNAs biogenesis and function.

MicroRNAs are a class of endogenous small non-coding RNAs, usually 19-23 nucleotide in length, that regulate gene expression through mainly post-transcriptional mechanisms. In microRNA biogenesis, a microRNA host gene is first transcribed by RNA polymerase II, giving rise to primary microRNA (pri-microRNA) transcripts. These are then processed by a complex composed of Drosha, an RNase III enzyme, and Pasha, a double-stranded RNA binding protein, to precursor microRNAs (pre-microRNAs), a stem-loop structure of 70-100 nucleotides. Pre-microRNAs are transported into the cytoplasm and cleaved by the Dicer RNase III. Resulting microRNA duplexes are incorporated into a RISC complex that also contains Ago. The "lead" functioning strand is guided to match the 3′-UTR of the mRNA target, while the "passenger" strand is degraded. A functional microRNA can pair perfectly or imperfectly with the microRNA recognition sites within mRNA 3′-UTR, leading to transcript degradation and translation inhibition, respectively.

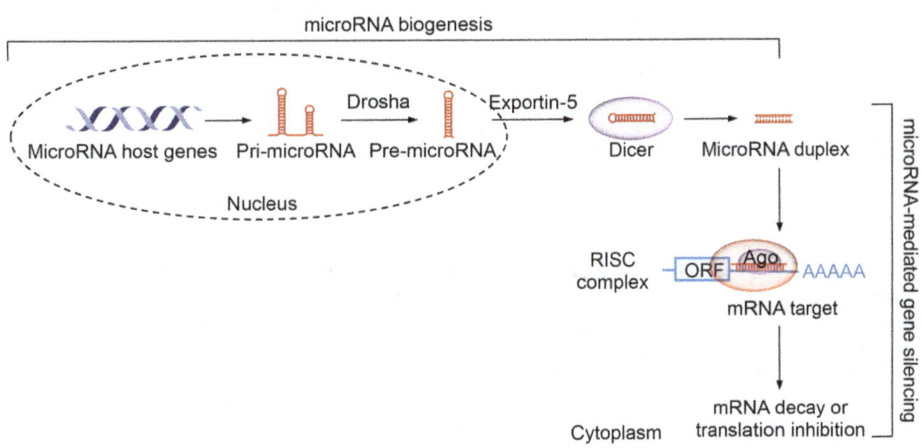

of SUMF1, a cellular sulfatase activator, by miR-95 disrupts sulfatase activities, resulting in an accumulation of sulfated substrates in lysosomes that, in turn, impairs lysosome-mediated cargo degradation – miR-95-mediated lysosome dysfunction also results in defects in autophagy-mediated cargo degradation (67). Knocking down of miR-95 in cells isolated from patients with a severe lysosomal storage disorder called multiple sulfatase deficiency due to hypomorphic *SUMF1* mutations can increase SUMF1 protein levels, suggesting a potential therapeutic intervention for this disease (67). MiR-376b directly targets the 3′UTR of *ATG4C* and *BECN1* mRNA, thereby inhibiting Atg4C- and Beclin 1-dependent autophagy induced by starvation or rapamycin, and an antagomir of miR-376b increases Atg4C- and Beclin 1 expression and autophagy (70). Likewise, miR-20a and miR-106b suppresses ULK1 expression and autophagy, a process that can be de-repressed by nutrient (leucine) deprivation (71). Finally, systems biology approaches have led to the identification of several microRNAs (e.g., miR-130, miR-98, miR-124, miR-204, and miR-142) that can target lysosome-related proteins to modulate the autophagy–lysosomal pathways (72).

MicroRNAs Regulate Intracellular Membrane-Associated Proteins Involved in B Cell Differentiation

The miR-17–92 locus encodes a cluster of microRNAs (miR-17, miR-18a, miR-19a, miR-19b, miR-20a, and miR-92a) that play important roles in regulating immune functions (73). These microRNAs are essential for B cell development (74), but dispensable for mature B cell survival (75). Mature B cell-specific miR-17-92 KO mice are defective in producing class-switching IgG2c antibodies (75). Lymphocyte-specific overexpression of miR-17-92 increases proliferation and survival of B cells and germinal center B cell differentiation, eventually leading to lymphomagenesis (76). Among microRNAs in the miR-17-92 cluster, miR-17 targets transcripts encoding TBC1D2, which acts as a GTPase activating protein (GAP) of Rab7 to downregulates Rab7 activity (66) – TBC1D2 is also an effector of Rab7-GTP and would participate in the negative feedback-loop that controls Rab7 activities. MiR-17-dependent upregulation of Rab7 activities may explain, at least in part, the role of miR-17-92 in class-switched antibody responses. MiR-17 also targets Atg7 (77), suggesting a role of miR-17-92 in memory B cell differentiation, in addition to its inhibition of plasma cell homing to the bone marrow (75).

As we have recently reported (64), both miR-23b and miR-30a are upregulated by HDI in B cells to target the *Prdm1* 3′-UTR, thereby playing a role in mediating HDI repression of B cell differentiation into plasma cells (**Figure 2**). These microRNAs would also modulate plasma cell differentiation and/or functions by downregulating autophagic proteins, such as Atg5, Atg12, Beclin 1, and others factors (78–80) (**Table 1**). Another member of the miR-30 family, miR-30c, is predicted to target both Rab7 and AID, consistent with the notion that one microRNA can target multiple factors in the same pathway to maximize its influence on the outcome of that pathway (**Figure 2**, a). Other examples supporting this notion include miR-302b, which can target IRAK4 and likely Rab7, both of which are important for TLR-induced NF-κB activation (38, 81). In addition, miR-155 and miR-181b downregulate CSR by targeting AID. They may also inhibit plasma cell differentiation by virtue of their ability to target the 3′-UTR of transcripts encoding autophagic proteins, such as Atg5 and possibly Rheb and Rictor. MiR-93 targets the *AICDA* 3′-UTR and would regulate AID expression in activated B cells, as it does in the MCF7 breast cancer cell line (82), which, like several cancer cell lines, expresses elevated levels of AID, a potent DNA mutator and tumorigenesis factor (83). MiR-93 would also downregulate plasma cell differentiation by inhibiting autophagy and likely do so by targeting Atg16L1 (82), SQSTM1 (84), and possibly a battery of other autophagic proteins, such as ULK1, ATG14 and RB1CC1 (**Table 1**). Finally, consistent with the notion that a single factor can be regulated by multiple microRNAs, Rab7 would be regulated by both miR-30c

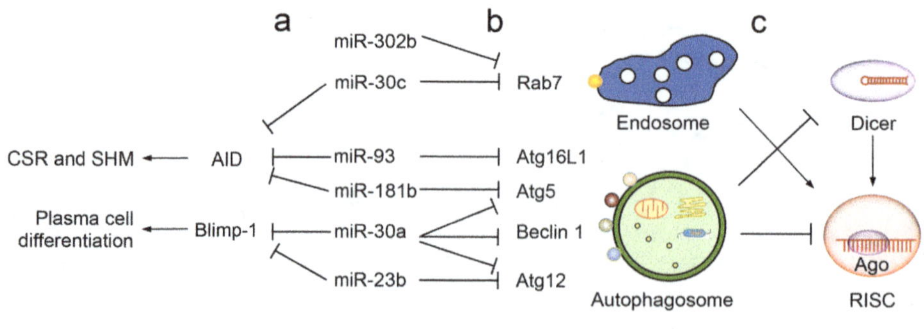

FIGURE 2 | Cross-regulation of intracellular membrane-associated proteins and microRNAs in B cell differentiation. (a) Regulation of multiple intracellular membrane-associated proteins as well as AID (critical for CSR/SHM) and Blimp-1 (driving plasma cell differentiation) by a single microRNA. For example, miR-30a regulates Atg5, Beclin 1 and Atg12 in autophagy and Blimp-1, miR-30c regulates Rab7 (in the endosome pathway) and AID, as well, miR-93 and miR-181b regulate AID as well as Atg16L1 and Atg5, respectively. (b) Regulation of one intracellular membrane-associated protein by several microRNAs. For example, Rab7 is regulated by both miR-30c and miR-302b, and Atg12 is regulated by both miR-30a and miR-23b. (c) Regulation of microRNA activities by endosomes and autophagosomes. Endosomes provide a structure to support the assembly of RISC in microRNA-mediated gene silencing. Autophagosomes promote degradation of Dicer and Ago, thereby downregulating microRNA biogenesis and functions, respectively.

TABLE 1 | MicroRNAs target intracellular membrane-associated proteins and factors critical for B cell differentiation and functions.

MicroRNAs	Intracellular membrane-associated protein target	Specific factor target	Relevant B cell function	Reference
miR-17-92	TBC1D2, Atg7	Bim, Pten	B cell development, Germinal center reaction	(66, 73, 76, 84)
miR-23b	Atg12, Atg2B[a], RAB11FIP2[a]	Blimp-1	Plasma cell differentiation	(64, 85)
miR-30[b]	Rab7[a]	AID[a]	CSR	(64, 79, 80)
	Atg5, Beclin 1, Atg12[a]	Blimp-1	Plasma cell differentiation	
miR-155	Rheb, Rictor	AID SHIP-1	CSR, SHM, Germinal center reaction	(60, 86, 87)
miR-181b	Atg5	AID	CSR	(61, 88)
miR-93	Atg16L1, SQSTM1, Atg14[a], RB1CC1[a], ULK1[a]	AID	CSR	(82, 84, 89)
miR-302b	Rab7[a], RABGAP1[a], Rab9A[a]	IRAK4	NF-κB activation	(81)
miR-9	Atg14[a], ULK2[a]	NF-κB	CSR	(90)
miR-10a	RB1CC1	BCL6	Germinal center reaction	(91, 92)
miR-146a	SQSTM1[a]	TRAF6	NF-κB activation	(93)

[a]*High confident targets predicted by miRDB (www.miRDB.org) (94).*
[b]*Rab7 and AID are predicted to be targeted by miR-30c, with others being targets of miR-30a.*

and miR-302b (**Figure 2**, b), suggesting an (indirect) regulation of NF-κB induction and AID activation by these microRNAs.

As suggested by a recent study (95), intracellular membrane proteins would evade microRNA regulation by using mRNA transcripts with short 3′-UTRs for their production. Proteins can be encoded by mRNAs with alternative 3′-UTRs, the longer ones of which function as scaffold to interact with the RNA-binding proteins HuR and SET and facilitate the plasma membrane localization of membrane-associated proteins (95, 96) – HuR plays an important role in germinal center formation, CSR, and antibody responses, possibly though facilitating protein localization to the plasma membrane (97). When encoded by transcripts with shorter 3′-UTRs, which contain much fewer microRNA targeting sites and are less susceptible to microRNA-mediated silencing, these membrane-associated proteins would display a different subcellular localization, shifting from the plasma membrane to intracellular membrane structures.

Overall, the regulation of B cell differentiation and intracellular membrane-associated proteins by microRNAs would be deeply intertwined to achieve highly fine-tuned antibody responses.

CONCLUSION AND PERSPECTIVES

Intracellular membrane structures regulate, in addition to cellular homeostasis and basic metabolic processes, B cell differentiation in antibody responses and likely other cell type-specific functions. Different intracellular membranes are responsible primarily for distinct B cell differentiation processes, such as Rab7$^+$ mature late endosomes in AID induction and CSR/SHM, Atg5$^+$ autophagosomes in plasma cell differentiation and survival, and Atg7$^+$ autophagosomes for memory B cell maintenance. Nevertheless, these lipid-containing micro-domains would also cross-talk, e.g., through their partially shared biogenesis pathways, thereby regulating multiple processes. Indeed, Rab7 would regulate plasma cell survival, in addition to its major role in CSR/SHM, and the collaboration of different membranes in regulating B cell differentiation is suggested by the role of ER in endosome biogenesis (98).

Specific functions of selected intracellular membrane-associated proteins would reflect their induction in differentiating B cells, as epitomized by the upregulation of Rab7 in activated B cells and elevated levels of Atg7 as memory B cells survive over the time. This notion emphasizes the importance of the profiling of expression of intracellular membrane-associated proteins and biogenesis of intracellular membrane structures in B cells toward our full understanding of B cell differentiation fate decision. As such, a comprehensive analysis of the role of intracellular membranes in signal transduction, which is ultimately responsible for gene regulation, is intriguing, as it would not only support the emerging paradigm that membrane organization specifies the signal output, but also reveal feedback-loop regulation mechanisms that contribute to the tight regulation of B cell differentiation.

As suggested by the critical dependence of endosomes on Rab5 expression levels (99), intracellular membranes are sensitive for their maintenance to the depletion of relevant factors, making microRNA, powerful regulators of intracellular membrane functions and, therefore, B cell differentiation. Interestingly, intracellular membranes would regulate B cell differentiation in part by modulating microRNA activities, as suggested by an important role of endosomes in promoting formation of an RNA-induced silencing complex (RISC) and downregulation of Dicer and Ago by autophagy (**Figure 2**, c). Ago2, a component of RISC, localizes to mature endosomes and RISC-bound mRNAs accumulate in GW bodies, which are discrete cytoplasmic foci associated with mature endosomes (100). Blocking endosomes maturation (by deletion of ESCRT complexes) results in loss of GW bodies and impairment in microRNA-mediated gene silencing, while accumulation of mature endosomes (through depletion of a tethering factor HPS4) enhances microRNA-mediated silencing (101, 102), all pointing to a positive role of endosomes in microRNA functions. By contrast, the autophagic pathway degrades Dicer and Ago that are not bound with any pre-microRNA and microRNA, respectively, in a manner dependent on the autophagy receptor NDP2, which interacts with LC3 (103). Dicer accumulates in cells deficient of the critical autophagy components Atg5, Atg6, or Atg7 (104), suggesting that B cell-specific conditional KO of *Atg5* and *Atg7* may display elevated levels of microRNAs that would, in turn, downregulate factors important for plasma cell differentiation (e.g., Blimp-1) and memory B cell maintenance.

Collectively, intracellular membrane structures and microRNAs would regulate important B cell processes. The reciprocal regulation of intracellular membranes and microRNAs would fine-tune at any time the gene expression necessary to achieve the specificity of B cell differentiation processes. Intracellular membranes can quickly regenerate upon replenishment of important relevant factors that were previously downregulated by microRNAs. This buffers the effect of a broad spectrum of aberrant molecular events, which frequently occur in highly proliferating B cells, and would play an important role in preventing disastrous overexpression of proto-oncogenes (such as Myc and BCL6) and the DNA mutator AID and, therefore, B cell lymphomagenesis (105–107).

ACKNOWLEDGMENTS

We apologize that owing to space limitations only a fraction of the relevant literature was cited in this review article. We thank Dr. Hong Zan for sharing data presented in a manuscript in press on the effect of HDI on gene expression in B cells. This work was supported by National Institutes of Health (NIH) grants AI 079705, AI 105813 and the Alliance for Lupus Research Target Identification in Lupus Grant ALR 295955 (to PC).

REFERENCES

1. Li G, Zan H, Xu Z, Casali P. Epigenetics of the antibody response. *Trends Immunol* (2013) **34**(9):460–70. doi:10.1016/j.it.2013.03.006
2. Cerutti A, Cols M, Puga I. Marginal zone B cells: virtues of innate-like antibody-producing lymphocytes. *Nat Rev Immunol* (2013) **13**(2):118–32. doi:10.1038/nri3383
3. Pone EJ, Zan H, Zhang J, Al-Qahtani A, Xu Z, Casali P. Toll-like receptors and B-cell receptors synergize to induce immunoglobulin class-switch DNA recombination: relevance to microbial antibody responses. *Crit Rev Immunol* (2010) **30**(1):1–29. doi:10.1615/CritRevImmunol.v30.i1.10
4. Xu Z, Zan H, Pone EJ, Mai T, Casali P. Immunoglobulin class-switch DNA recombination: induction, targeting and beyond. *Nat Rev Immunol* (2012) **12**(7):517–31. doi:10.1038/nri3216
5. Victora GD, Nussenzweig MC. Germinal centers. *Annu Rev Immunol* (2012) **30**:429–57. doi:10.1146/annurev-immunol-020711-075032
6. Casali P. Somatic recombination and hypermutation in the immune system. In: Krebs JE, Goldstein ES, Kilpatrick ST, editors. *Lewin's Genes XI*. Sudbury, MA: Jones & Bartlett (2014). p. 459–507.
7. Shapiro-Shelef M, Calame K. Regulation of plasma-cell development. *Nat Rev Immunol* (2005) **5**(3):230–42. doi:10.1038/nri1572
8. Nutt SL, Taubenheim N, Hasbold J, Corcoran LM, Hodgkin PD. The genetic network controlling plasma cell differentiation. *Semin Immunol* (2011) **23**(5):341–9. doi:10.1016/j.smim.2011.08.010
9. McHeyzer-Williams M, Okitsu S, Wang N, McHeyzer-Williams L. Molecular programming of B cell memory. *Nat Rev Immunol* (2011) **12**(1):24–34. doi:10.1038/nri3128
10. Kurosaki T, Kometani K, Ise W. Memory B cells. *Nat Rev Immunol* (2015) **15**(3):149–59. doi:10.1038/nri3802
11. Xiao C, Rajewsky K. MicroRNA control in the immune system: basic principles. *Cell* (2009) **136**(1):26–36. doi:10.1016/j.cell.2008.12.027
12. Thai TH, Christiansen PA, Tsokos GC. Is there a link between dysregulated miRNA expression and disease? *Discov Med* (2010) **10**(52):184–94.
13. de Yebenes VG, Bartolome-Izquierdo N, Ramiro AR. Regulation of B-cell development and function by microRNAs. *Immunol Rev* (2013) **253**(1):25–39. doi:10.1111/imr.12046
14. Danger R, Braza F, Giral M, Soulillou JP, Brouard S. MicroRNAs, major players in B cells homeostasis and function. *Front Immunol* (2014) **5**:98. doi:10.3389/fimmu.2014.00098
15. Zan H, Tat C, Casali P. MicroRNAs in lupus. *Autoimmunity* (2014) **47**(4):272–85. doi:10.3109/08916934.2014.915955
16. Choi AM, Ryter SW, Levine B. Autophagy in human health and disease. *N Engl J Med* (2013) **368**(7):651–62. doi:10.1056/NEJMra1205406
17. Huotari J, Helenius A. Endosome maturation. *EMBO J* (2011) **30**(17):3481–500. doi:10.1038/emboj.2011.286
18. Rink J, Ghigo E, Kalaidzidis Y, Zerial M. Rab conversion as a mechanism of progression from early to late endosomes. *Cell* (2005) **122**(5):735–49. doi:10.1016/j.cell.2005.06.043
19. Poteryaev D, Datta S, Ackema K, Zerial M, Spang A. Identification of the switch in ear*ly-to*-late endosome transition. *Cell* (2010) **141**(3):497–508. doi:10.1016/j.cell.2010.03.011
20. Del Conte-Zerial P, Brusch L, Rink JC, Collinet C, Kalaidzidis Y, Zerial M, et al. Membrane identity and GTPase cascades regulated by toggle and cut-out switches. *Mol Syst Biol* (2008) **4**:206. doi:10.1038/msb.2008.45
21. Johansson M, Rocha N, Zwart W, Jordens I, Janssen L, Kuijl C, et al. Activation of endosomal dynein motors by stepwise assembly of Rab7-RILP-p150Glued, ORP1L, and the receptor betalll spectrin. *J Cell Biol* (2007) **176**(4):459–71. doi:10.1083/jcb.200606077
22. Nickerson DP, Brett CL, Merz AJ. Vps-C complexes: gatekeepers of endolysosomal traffic. *Curr Opin Cell Biol* (2009) **21**(4):543–51. doi:10.1016/j.ceb.2009.05.007
23. Klionsky DJ, Baehrecke EH, Brumell JH, Chu CT, Codogno P, Cuervo AM, et al. A comprehensive glossary of autophagy-related molecules and processes (2nd edition). *Autophagy* (2011) **7**(11):1273–94. doi:10.4161/auto.7.11.17661
24. Feng Y, He D, Yao Z, Klionsky DJ. The machinery of macroautophagy. *Cell Res* (2014) **24**(1):24–41. doi:10.1038/cr.2013.168
25. Deretic V. Autophagy in immunity and cell-autonomous defense against intracellular microbes. *Immunol Rev* (2011) **240**(1):92–104. doi:10.1111/j.1600-065X.2010.00995.x
26. Levine B, Mizushima N, Virgin HW. Autophagy in immunity and inflammation. *Nature* (2011) **469**(7330):323–35. doi:10.1038/nature09782
27. Limon JJ, Fruman DA. Akt and mTOR in B cell activation and differentiation. *Front Immunol* (2012) **3**:228. doi:10.3389/fimmu.2012.00228
28. Zhang S, Pruitt M, Tran D, Du Bois W, Zhang K, Patel R, et al. B cell-specific deficiencies in mTOR limit humoral immune responses. *J Immunol* (2013) **191**(4):1692–703. doi:10.4049/jimmunol.1201767
29. Hosokawa N, Hara T, Kaizuka T, Kishi C, Takamura A, Miura Y, et al. Nutrient-dependent mTORC1 association with the ULK1-Atg13-FIP200 complex required for autophagy. *Mol Biol Cell* (2009) **20**(7):1981–91. doi:10.1091/mbc.E08-12-1248
30. Dani A, Chaudhry A, Mukherjee P, Rajagopal D, Bhatia S, George A, et al. The pathway for MHCII-mediated presentation of endogenous proteins involves peptide transport to the endo-lysosomal compartment. *J Cell Sci* (2004) **117**(Pt 18):4219–30. doi:10.1242/jcs.01288
31. Schmid D, Pypaert M, Munz C. Antigen-loading compartments for major histocompatibility complex class II molecules continuously receive input from autophagosomes. *Immunity* (2007) **26**(1):79–92. doi:10.1016/j.immuni.2006.10.018
32. Lee HK, Mattei LM, Steinberg BE, Alberts P, Lee YH, Chervonsky A, et al. In vivo requirement for Atg5 in antigen presentation by dendritic cells. *Immunity* (2010) **32**(2):227–39. doi:10.1016/j.immuni.2009.12.006
33. Mastrangelo A, Colasanti T, Barbati C, Pecani A, Sabatinelli D, Pendolino M, et al. The role of posttranslational protein modifications in rheumatological diseases: focus on rheumatoid arthritis. *J Immunol Res* (2015) **2015**:712490. doi:10.1155/2015/712490
34. Ireland JM, Unanue ER. Autophagy in antigen-presenting cells results in presentation of citrullinated peptides to CD4 T cells. *J Exp Med* (2011) **208**(13):2625–32. doi:10.1084/jem.20110640
35. Miller BC, Zhao Z, Stephenson LM, Cadwell K, Pua HH, Lee HK, et al. The autophagy gene ATG5 plays an essential role in B lymphocyte development. *Autophagy* (2008) **4**(3):309–14. doi:10.4161/auto.5474
36. Watanabe K, Tsubata T. Autophagy connects antigen receptor signaling to costimulatory signaling in B lymphocytes. *Autophagy* (2009) **5**(1):108–10. doi:10.4161/auto.5.1.7278
37. Pone EJ, Zhang J, Mai T, White CA, Li G, Sakakura JK, et al. BCR-signalling synergizes with TLR-signalling for induction of AID and immunoglobulin class-switching through the non-canonical NF-kappaB pathway. *Nat Commun* (2012) **3**:767. doi:10.1038/ncomms1769

38. Pone EJ, Lam T, Lou Z, Wang R, Chen Y, Liu D, et al. B cell Rab7 mediates induction of activation-induced cytidine deaminase expression and class-switching in T-dependent and T-independent antibody responses. *J Immunol* (2015) **194**(7):3065–78. doi:10.4049/jimmunol.1401896
39. Agola JO, Hong L, Surviladze Z, Ursu O, Waller A, Strouse JJ, et al. A competitive nucleotide binding inhibitor: in vitro characterization of Rab7 GTPase inhibition. *ACS Chem Biol* (2012) **7**(6):1095–108. doi:10.1021/cb3001099
40. Lam T, Lou Z, Kulp VD, Wang R, Lafleur C, Taylor J, et al. *Inhibition of Class-Switching and Plasma Cell Survival in Lupus Autoantibody Responses by a Small Molecule Compound that Targets Rab7* (2015).
41. Alexia C, Poalas K, Carvalho G, Zemirli N, Dwyer J, Dubois SM, et al. The endoplasmic reticulum acts as a platform for ubiquitylated components of nuclear factor kappaB signaling. *Sci Signal* (2013) **6**(291):ra79. doi:10.1126/scisignal.2004496
42. Settembre C, Zoncu R, Medina DL, Vetrini F, Erdin S, Erdin S, et al. A lysosome-to-nucleus signalling mechanism senses and regulates the lysosome via mTOR and TFEB. *EMBO J* (2012) **31**(5):1095–108. doi:10.1038/emboj.2012.32
43. Efeyan A, Zoncu R, Sabatini DM. Amino acids and mTORC1: from lysosomes to disease. *Trends Mol Med* (2012) **18**(9):524–33. doi:10.1016/j.molmed.2012.05.007
44. Laplante M, Sabatini DM. mTOR signaling in growth control and disease. *Cell* (2012) **149**(2):274–93. doi:10.1016/j.cell.2012.03.017
45. Limon JJ, So L, Jellbauer S, Chiu H, Corado J, Sykes SM, et al. mTOR kinase inhibitors promote antibody class switching via mTORC2 inhibition. *Proc Natl Acad Sci U S A* (2014) **111**(47):E5076–85. doi:10.1073/pnas.1407104111
46. Ron D, Walter P. Signal integration in the endoplasmic reticulum unfolded protein response. *Nat Rev Mol Cell Biol* (2007) **8**(7):519–29. doi:10.1038/nrm2199
47. Conway KL, Kuballa P, Khor B, Zhang M, Shi HN, Virgin HW, et al. ATG5 regulates plasma cell differentiation. *Autophagy* (2013) **9**(4):528–37. doi:10.4161/auto.23484
48. Pengo N, Scolari M, Oliva L, Milan E, Mainoldi F, Raimondi A, et al. Plasma cells require autophagy for sustainable immunoglobulin production. *Nat Immunol* (2013) **14**(3):298–305. doi:10.1038/ni.2524
49. Martinez-Lopez N, Athonvarangkul D, Mishall P, Sahu S, Singh R. Autophagy proteins regulate ERK phosphorylation. *Nat Commun* (2013) **4**:2799. doi:10.1038/ncomms3799
50. Yasuda T, Kometani K, Takahashi N, Imai Y, Aiba Y, Kurosaki T. ERKs induce expression of the transcriptional repressor Blimp-1 and subsequent plasma cell differentiation. *Sci Signal* (2011) **4**(169):ra25. doi:10.1126/scisignal.2001592
51. Chen M, Kodali S, Jang A, Kuai L, Wang J. Requirement for autophagy in the long-term persistence but not initial formation of memory B cells. *J Immunol* (2015) **194**(6):2607–15. doi:10.4049/jimmunol.1403001
52. Chen M, Hong MJ, Sun H, Wang L, Shi X, Gilbert BE, et al. Essential role for autophagy in the maintenance of immunological memory against influenza infection. *Nat Med* (2014) **20**(5):503–10. doi:10.1038/nm.3521
53. Zhou J, Liao W, Yang J, Ma K, Li X, Wang Y, et al. FOXO3 induces FOXO1-dependent autophagy by activating the AKT1 signaling pathway. *Autophagy* (2012) **8**(12):1712–23. doi:10.4161/auto.21830
54. Lu LF, Liston A. MicroRNA in the immune system, microRNA as an immune system. *Immunology* (2009) **127**(3):291–8. doi:10.1111/j.1365-2567.2009.03092.x
55. Zan H, Casali P. Epigenetic modulation of class switch DNA recombination, somatic hypermutation, as well as plasma cell and memory B cell differentiation: shaping of the antibody response. *Front Immunol* (2015).
56. Belver L, de Yebenes VG, Ramiro AR. MicroRNAs prevent the generation of autoreactive antibodies. *Immunity* (2010) **33**(5):713–22. doi:10.1016/j.immuni.2010.11.010
57. Xu S, Guo K, Zeng Q, Huo J, Lam KP. The RNase III enzyme dicer is essential for germinal center B-cell formation. *Blood* (2012) **119**(3):767–76. doi:10.1182/blood-2011-05-355412
58. Thai TH, Calado DP, Casola S, Ansel KM, Xiao C, Xue Y, et al. Regulation of the germinal center response by microRNA-155. *Science* (2007) **316**(5824):604–8. doi:10.1126/science.1141229
59. Rodriguez A, Vigorito E, Clare S, Warren MV, Couttet P, Soond DR, et al. Requirement of bic/microRNA-155 for normal immune function. *Science* (2007) **316**(5824):608–11. doi:10.1126/science.1139253
60. Teng G, Hakimpour P, Landgraf P, Rice A, Tuschl T, Casellas R, et al. MicroRNA-155 is a negative regulator of activation-induced cytidine deaminase. *Immunity* (2008) **28**(5):621–9. doi:10.1016/j.immuni.2008.03.015
61. de Yebenes VG, Belver L, Pisano DG, Gonzalez S, Villasante A, Croce C, et al. miR-181b negatively regulates activation-induced cytidine deaminase in B cells. *J Exp Med* (2008) **205**(10):2199–206. doi:10.1084/jem.20080579
62. Mok Y, Schwierzeck V, Thomas DC, Vigorito E, Rayner TF, Jarvis LB, et al. MiR-210 is induced by Oct-2, regulates B cells, and inhibits autoantibody production. *J Immunol* (2013) **191**(6):3037–48. doi:10.4049/jimmunol.1301289
63. Gururajan M, Haga CL, Das S, Leu CM, Hodson D, Josson S, et al. MicroRNA 125b inhibition of B cell differentiation in germinal centers. *Int Immunol* (2010) **22**(7):583–92. doi:10.1093/intimm/dxq042
64. White CA, Pone EJ, Lam T, Tat C, Hayama KL, Li G, et al. Histone deacetylase inhibitors upregulate B cell microRNAs that silence AID and Blimp-1 expression for epigenetic modulation of antibody and autoantibody responses. *J Immunol* (2014) **193**(12):5933–50. doi:10.4049/jimmunol.1401702
65. Shen T, Sanchez H, Zan H, Casali P. Genome-wide analysis reveals selective modulation of microRNAs and mRNAs by histone deacetylase inhibitor in B cells induced to undergo class switch DNA recombination and plasma cell differentiation. *Front Immunol* (2015).
66. Serva A, Knapp B, Tsai YT, Claas C, Lisauskas T, Matula P, et al. miR-17-5p regulates endocytic trafficking through targeting TBC1D2/Armus. *PLoS One* (2012) **7**(12):e52555. doi:10.1371/journal.pone.0052555
67. Frankel LB, Di Malta C, Wen J, Eskelinen EL, Ballabio A, Lund AH. A non-conserved miRNA regulates lysosomal function and impacts on a human lysosomal storage disorder. *Nat Commun* (2014) **5**:5840. doi:10.1038/ncomms6840
68. Fullgrabe J, Klionsky DJ, Joseph B. The return of the nucleus: transcriptional and epigenetic control of autophagy. *Nat Rev Mol Cell Biol* (2014) **15**(1):65–74. doi:10.1038/nrm3716
69. Tan YS, Kim M, Kingsbury TJ, Civin CI, Cheng WC. Regulation of RAB5C is important for the growth inhibitory effects of MiR-509 in human precursor-B acute lymphoblastic leukemia. *PLoS One* (2014) **9**(11):e111777. doi:10.1371/journal.pone.0111777
70. Korkmaz G, le Sage C, Tekirdag KA, Agami R, Gozuacik D. miR-376b controls starvation and mTOR inhibition-related autophagy by targeting ATG4C and BECN1. *Autophagy* (2012) **8**(2):165–76. doi:10.4161/auto.8.2.18351
71. Wu H, Wang F, Hu S, Yin C, Li X, Zhao S, et al. MiR-20a and miR-106b negatively regulate autophagy induced by leucine deprivation via suppression of ULK1 expression in C2C12 myoblasts. *Cell Signal* (2012) **24**(11):2179–86. doi:10.1016/j.cellsig.2012.07.001
72. Jegga AG, Schneider L, Ouyang X, Zhang J. Systems biology of the autophagy-lysosomal pathway. *Autophagy* (2011) **7**(5):477–89. doi:10.4161/auto.7.5.14811
73. Mogilyansky E, Rigoutsos I. The miR-17/92 cluster: a comprehensive update on its genomics, genetics, functions and increasingly important and numerous roles in health and disease. *Cell Death Differ* (2013) **20**(12):1603–14. doi:10.1038/cdd.2013.125
74. Ventura A, Young AG, Winslow MM, Lintault L, Meissner A, Erkeland SJ, et al. Targeted deletion reveals essential and overlapping functions of the miR-17 through 92 family of miRNA clusters. *Cell* (2008) **132**(5):875–86. doi:10.1016/j.cell.2008.02.019
75. Xu S, Ou X, Huo J, Lim K, Huang Y, Chee S, et al. Mir-17-92 regulates bone marrow homing of plasma cells and production of immunoglobulin G2c. *Nat Commun* (2015) **6**:6764. doi:10.1038/ncomms7764
76. Xiao C, Srinivasan L, Calado DP, Patterson HC, Zhang B, Wang J, et al. Lymphoproliferative disease and autoimmunity in mice with increased miR-17-92 expression in lymphocytes. *Nat Immunol* (2008) **9**(4):405–14. doi:10.1038/ni1575
77. Comincini S, Allavena G, Palumbo S, Morini M, Durando F, Angeletti F, et al. microRNA-17 regulates the expression of ATG7 and modulates the autophagy process, improving the sensitivity to temozolomide and low-dose ionizing radiation treatments in human glioblastoma cells. *Cancer Biol Ther* (2013) **14**(7):574–86. doi:10.4161/cbt.24597

78. Huang Y, Guerrero-Preston R, Ratovitski EA. Phospho-DeltaNp63alpha-dependent regulation of autophagic signaling through transcription and micro-RNA modulation. *Cell Cycle* (2012) **11**(6):1247–59. doi:10.4161/cc.11.6.19670
79. Zhu H, Wu H, Liu X, Li B, Chen Y, Ren X, et al. Regulation of autophagy by a beclin 1-targeted microRNA, miR-30a, in cancer cells. *Autophagy* (2009) **5**(6):816–23. doi:10.4161/auto.9064
80. Yu Y, Yang L, Zhao M, Zhu S, Kang R, Vernon P, et al. Targeting microRNA-30a-mediated autophagy enhances imatinib activity against human chronic myeloid leukemia cells. *Leukemia* (2012) **26**(8):1752–60. doi:10.1038/leu.2012.65
81. Zhou X, Li X, Ye Y, Zhao K, Zhuang Y, Li Y, et al. MicroRNA-302b augments host defense to bacteria by regulating inflammatory responses via feedback to TLR/IRAK4 circuits. *Nat Commun* (2014) **5**:3619. doi:10.1038/ncomms4619
82. Lu C, Chen J, Xu HG, Zhou X, He Q, Li YL, et al. MIR106B and MIR93 prevent removal of bacteria from epithelial cells by disrupting ATG16L1-mediated autophagy. *Gastroenterology* (2014) **146**(1):188–99. doi:10.1053/j.gastro.2013.09.006
83. Babbage G, Ottensmeier CH, Blaydes J, Stevenson FK, Sahota SS. Immunoglobulin heavy chain locus events and expression of activation-induced cytidine deaminase in epithelial breast cancer cell lines. *Cancer Res* (2006) **66**(8):3996–4000. doi:10.1158/0008-5472.CAN-05-3704
84. Meenhuis A, van Veelen PA, de Looper H, van Boxtel N, van den Berge IJ, Sun SM, et al. MiR-17/20/93/106 promote hematopoietic cell expansion by targeting sequestosome 1-regulated pathways in mice. *Blood* (2011) **118**(4):916–25. doi:10.1182/blood-2011-02-336487
85. Wang P, Zhang J, Zhang L, Zhu Z, Fan J, Chen L, et al. MicroRNA 23b regulates autophagy associated with radioresistance of pancreatic cancer cells. *Gastroenterology* (2013) **145**(5): 1133–43.e12. doi:10.1053/j.gastro.2013.07.048
86. Wan G, Xie W, Liu Z, Xu W, Lao Y, Huang N, et al. Hypoxia-induced MIR155 is a potent autophagy inducer by targeting multiple players in the MTOR pathway. *Autophagy* (2014) **10**(1):70–9. doi:10.4161/auto.26534
87. O'Connell RM, Chaudhuri AA, Rao DS, Baltimore D. Inositol phosphatase SHIP1 is a primary target of miR-155. *Proc Natl Acad Sci U S A* (2009) **106**(17):7113–8. doi:10.1073/pnas.0902636106
88. Tekirdag KA, Korkmaz G, Ozturk DG, Agami R, Gozuacik D. MIR181A regulates starvation- and rapamycin-induced autophagy through targeting of ATG5. *Autophagy* (2013) **9**(3):374–85. doi:10.4161/auto.23117
89. Zan H, Casali P. Regulation of Aicda expression and AID activity. *Autoimmunity* (2013) **46**(2):83–101. doi:10.3109/08916934.2012.749244
90. Bazzoni F, Rossato M, Fabbri M, Gaudiosi D, Mirolo M, Mori L, et al. Induction and regulatory function of miR-9 in human monocytes and neutrophils exposed to proinflammatory signals. *Proc Natl Acad Sci U S A* (2009) **106**(13):5282–7. doi:10.1073/pnas.0810909106
91. Takahashi H, Kanno T, Nakayamada S, Hirahara K, Sciume G, Muljo SA, et al. TGF-beta and retinoic acid induce the microRNA miR-10a, which targets Bcl-6 and constrains the plasticity of helper T cells. *Nat Immunol* (2012) **13**(6):587–95. doi:10.1038/ni.2286
92. Bryant A, Palma CA, Jayaswal V, Yang YW, Lutherborrow M, Ma DD. miR-10a is aberrantly overexpressed in Nucleophosmin1 mutated acute myeloid leukaemia and its suppression induces cell death. *Mol Cancer* (2012) **11**:8. doi:10.1186/1476-4598-11-8
93. Stickel N, Prinz G, Pfeifer D, Hasselblatt P, Schmitt-Graeff A, Follo M, et al. MiR-146a regulates the TRAF6/TNF-axis in donor T cells during GVHD. *Blood* (2014) **124**(16):2586–95. doi:10.1182/blood-2014-04-569046
94. Wong N, Wang X. miRDB: an online resource for microRNA target prediction and functional annotations. *Nucleic Acids Res* (2015) **43**(Database issue):D146–52. doi:10.1093/nar/gku1104
95. Berkovits BD, Mayr C. Alternative 3' UTRs act as scaffolds to regulate membrane protein localization. *Nature* (2015) **522**(7556):363–7. doi:10.1038/nature14321
96. Sandberg R, Neilson JR, Sarma A, Sharp PA, Burge CB. Proliferating cells express mRNAs with shortened 3' untranslated regions and fewer microRNA target sites. *Science* (2008) **320**(5883):1643–7. doi:10.1126/science.1155390
97. Diaz-Munoz MD, Bell SE, Fairfax K, Monzon-Casanova E, Cunningham AF, Gonzalez-Porta M, et al. The RNA-binding protein HuR is essential for the B cell antibody response. *Nat Immunol* (2015) **16**(4):415–25. doi:10.1038/ni.3115
98. Rowland AA, Chitwood PJ, Phillips MJ, Voeltz GK. ER contact sites define the position and timing of endosome fission. *Cell* (2014) **159**(5):1027–41. doi:10.1016/j.cell.2014.10.023
99. Zeigerer A, Gilleron J, Bogorad RL, Marsico G, Nonaka H, Seifert S, et al. Rab5 is necessary for the biogenesis of the endolysosomal system in vivo. *Nature* (2012) **485**(7399):465–70. doi:10.1038/nature11133
100. Gibbings DJ, Ciaudo C, Erhardt M, Voinnet O. Multivesicular bodies associate with components of miRNA effector complexes and modulate miRNA activity. *Nat Cell Biol* (2009) **11**(9):1143–9. doi:10.1038/ncb1929
101. Lee YS, Pressman S, Andress AP, Kim K, White JL, Cassidy JJ, et al. Silencing by small RNAs is linked to endosomal trafficking. *Nat Cell Biol* (2009) **11**(9):1150–6. doi:10.1038/ncb1930
102. Li W, Rusiniak ME, Chintala S, Gautam R, Novak EK, Swank RT. Murine Hermansky-Pudlak syndrome genes: regulators of lysosome-related organelles. *Bioessays* (2004) **26**(6):616–28. doi:10.1002/bies.20042
103. Gibbings D, Mostowy S, Jay F, Schwab Y, Cossart P, Voinnet O. Selective autophagy degrades DICER and AGO2 and regulates miRNA activity. *Nat Cell Biol* (2012) **14**(12):1314–21. doi:10.1038/ncb2611
104. Gibbings D, Mostowy S, Voinnet O. Autophagy selectively regulates miRNA homeostasis. *Autophagy* (2013) **9**(5):781–3. doi:10.4161/auto.23694
105. Kovalchuk AL, Qi CF, Torrey TA, Taddesse-Heath L, Feigenbaum L, Park SS, et al. Burkitt lymphoma in the mouse. *J Exp Med* (2000) **192**(8):1183–90. doi:10.1084/jem.192.8.1183
106. Cattoretti G, Pasqualucci L, Ballon G, Tam W, Nandula SV, Shen Q, et al. Deregulated BCL6 expression recapitulates the pathogenesis of human diffuse large B cell lymphomas in mice. *Cancer Cell* (2005) **7**(5):445–55. doi:10.1016/j.ccr.2005.03.037
107. Dominguez PM, Shaknovich R. Epigenetic function of activation-induced cytidine deaminase and its link to lymphomagenesis. *Front Immunol* (2014) **5**:642. doi:10.3389/fimmu.2014.00642

2

The role of invariant natural killer T cells in dendritic cell licensing, cross-priming, and memory CD8$^+$ T cell generation

*Catherine Gottschalk, Elisabeth Mettke and Christian Kurts**

Institute of Experimental Immunology, Rheinische Friedrich-Wilhelms-University of Bonn, Bonn, Germany

Edited by:
Elisabetta Padovan, Basel University Hospital and University of Basel, Switzerland

Reviewed by:
Francesca Di Rosa, National Research Council, Italy
Alena Donda, University of Lausanne, Switzerland
Paolo Dellabona, San Raffaele Scientific Institute, Italy

***Correspondence:**
Christian Kurts, Institute of Experimental Immunology, Rheinische Friedrich-Wilhelms-University of Bonn, Sigmund-Freud-Str. 25, Bonn D-53127, Germany
ckurts@uni-bonn.de

New vaccination strategies focus on achieving CD8$^+$ T cell (CTL) immunity rather than on induction of protective antibody responses. While the requirement of CD4$^+$ T (Th) cell help in dendritic cell (DC) activation and licensing, and in CTL memory induction has been described in several disease models, CTL responses may occur in a Th cell help-independent manner. Invariant natural killer T cells (iNKT cells) can substitute for Th cell help and license DC as well. iNKT cells produce a broad spectrum of Th1 and Th2 cytokines, thereby inducing a similar set of costimulatory molecules and cytokines in DC. This form of licensing differs from Th cell help by inducing other chemokines, while Th cell-licensed DCs produce CCR5 ligands, iNKT cell-licensed DCs produce CCL17, which attracts CCR4$^+$ CD8$^+$ T cells for subsequent activation. It has recently been shown that iNKT cells do not only enhance immune responses against bacterial pathogens or parasites but also play a role in viral infections. The inclusion of iNKT cell ligands in influenza virus vaccines enhanced memory CTL generation and protective immunity in a mouse model. This review will focus on the role of iNKT cells in the cross-talk with cross-priming DC and memory CD8$^+$ T cell formation.

Keywords: natural killer T cells, dendritic cells, licensing, memory, CD8 T cells, cross-presentation

Classification of Natural Killer T Cells

Natural killer T cells (NKT cells) are a subset of lymphocytes with innate and adaptive immune functions, for example, in tumor and anti-infectious defense (1). Their TCR can be either semi-invariant and encoded by a germline Valpha gene [type I invariant natural killer T cells (iNKT cells)] or may react against the self-antigen sulphatide using an oligoclonal TCR (type II NKT cells) (2–4). This review focusses on iNKT cells in dendritic cell (DC) licensing and T cell activation leading to a sustained memory response.

Invariant natural killer T cells respond to the marine sponge (*Agelas mauritianus*)-derived glycolipid alpha-galactosylceramide (αGalCer) presented by the non-polymorphic CD1d molecule and respond by rapidly producing various cytokines (5, 6). Mostly studied in mice, they represent about 0.5% of T cells in the blood, 2% in secondary lymphatic organs, and over 30% of T cells in the liver. During inflammation and infection, iNKT cell numbers can strongly increase in numerous organs, e.g., the pancreas in type I diabetes or the lung in asthma (7, 8). In human blood, only 0.1–0.2% of T cells are iNKT cells, with 5× lower numbers than in mice (9). Recently, iNKT cells came into focus as promising targets for the development of vaccine adjuvants and immunotherapies, mostly

TABLE 1 | Summary of iNKT cell activation studies in treatment of different diseases.

Therapeutic target	Species studied	Outcome	Reference, remarks
Viral and bacterial infections	Human, mouse	Effective vaccination in mice; oral and nasal route possible; no clear effect on chronic viral infections in clinical trials shown	(12–21)
Parasites and fungi	Mouse	Enhanced vaccine effects in mice	(10, 22–24) αGalCer analogs were used in Ref. (10) (7DW8–5) and Ref. (20) (α-C-GalCer) for NKT cell activation
Tumors	Human, mouse	Enhanced tumor protection and rejection in mice; clinical trials show only moderate effects in humans	(11, 14, 24–39) Antigen-pulsed DC were transferred in Ref. (32), no αGalCer or analog was added. αGalCer and α-C-GalCer were tested for tumor therapy in Ref. (34)
Autoimmune diseases	Mouse	αGalCer dose-dependent amelioration or aggravation of autoimmune diseases; NKT cell hypo-responsiveness involved in some cases	(8, 40–52) Ref. (43) used OCH, a sphingosine-truncated analog of αGalCer for NKT cell activation

iNKT cells were activated by αGalCer treatment if not indicated otherwise.

in the field of cancer treatment and in autoimmune and inflammatory diseases (**Table 1**). Preclinical studies using αGalCer demonstrated moderate therapeutic activity by activating DCs and providing Th-like functions, generating $CD8^+$ cytotoxic T cell (CTL) and antibody responses. Currently, more potent αGalCer analogs for iNKT cell activation are under investigation (10–13). Applying NKT cell immunization schemes in clinical settings is a promising therapeutic opportunity, but requires detailed knowledge on how iNKT cells activate DCs.

iNKT Cell Activation, Subsets, and Cytokine Production

Most knowledge on NKT cell activation came from the use of αGalCer, a strong and prototypical CD1-restricted agonist. In the last years, additional microbial-derived glycolipid ligands were identified, including α-glucuronosylceramides (from *Sphingomonas*), cholesteryl α-glucoside (from *Helicobacter*), or diacylglycerol-containing glycolipids (from *Borrelia*) (53, 54). These lead to sustained iNKT cell activation with inflammatory cytokine production that is independent of TLR stimulation, IL-12, or the recognition of endogenous antigens, hence relying only on engaging the invariant TCR. α-glucuronosylceramide induces IFNγ and IL-4 release similar to αGalCer (55–57). Both glycolipid antigens are structurally similar and can be recognized by the majority of mouse and human iNKT cells (58). Synthetic iNKT cell antigens have been and continue to be studied extensively for potential therapeutic application (59). However, iNKT cell activation may also promote allergic airway inflammation, and their overstimulation can induce iNKT cell anergy (1, 60).

Most microorganisms lack cognate iNKT cell antigens, hence activation of these cells relies on cytokines, such as IL-12 or IL-18, in conjunction with endogenous antigens. Even in the absence of TCR stimulation, some bacterial and viral infections induce a robust IL-12 response by DCs thereby activating iNKT cells *in vivo* (61, 62). Indirect iNKT cell activation results in the release of IFNγ but usually not IL-4 and is not restricted to TLR (62–65).

Analogous to Th cells subsets, different NKT cell subsets termed NKT1, NKT2, NKT17, NKT_{FH}, and NKT10 subsets were described with corresponding functionalities (66, 67). NKT17 cells produce the cytokines, IL-17 and IL-22, and are abundant in the lymph nodes, lungs, and skin of mice with airway neutrophilia induced by αGalCer (68). Recently, it was shown that iNKT17 cells are enriched in NOD mice, a mouse model for type I diabetes, which hint toward a possible role of those cells in disease development (69). iNKT17 cells rely on IL-7 for homeostasis and survival (70) and seem to require activation in the presence of TGF-β and IL-1β (71). The recently described NKT10 subset can dampen inflammatory responses by IL-10 production and is enriched in adipose tissue, providing protection in obesity-induced inflammation (72).

Dendritic Cell Maturation and $CD8^+$ T Cell Cross-Priming

Dendritic cells classically gather antigens in tissues and transport them into lymphatic organs, where they orchestrate the activation and differentiation of naïve $CD8^+$ T cells into CTL. Recent work showed that some DCs remain in tissues in order to regulate immigrating effector T cell responses, which is important in the defense against infections and may also promote the progression of many immune-mediated diseases. The cross-talk of myeloid cells with other immune cells, such as T cells and innate lymphocytes, is especially important in this context. Cellular encounters are orchestrated by chemokines, cytokines, and cell surface molecules. Some DCs, especially the $XCR1^+$ DC subset, are specialized in cross-presentation, which allows the presentation of extracellular antigens to activate CTL, a process important for immunity against tumors, viruses, and intracellular bacteria and for vaccination (73–76). Immunogenic cross-presentation, also referred to as cross-priming, requires the presence of pathogen-derived molecules (PAMPs) and/or of specific Th cells or NKT cells that mature the cross-presenting DC (77). This process is called "licensing," a term introduced by Lanzavecchia (78), and it aims at preventing unwanted immune answers against innocuous or self antigens. Licensing was first described by Matzinger, Heath, and Melief (79–81), and classically is mediated by CD40 ligand provided by specific $CD4^+$ helper T cells (Th). In addition to licensing, immunogenic T cell priming requires the DCs to mature, a process that results from sensing various PAMPs, including ligands for TLR, lectins, intracellular nucleotide-binding oligomerization domain receptors, or retinoic acid-induced genes (82–85). Major consequences of DC maturation are the upregulation of costimulatory molecules like CD80 and CD86, CD40, of MHC II and the production of pro-inflammatory cytokines, especially IL-12p70 and TNF. These consequences partially can result also from CD40–CD40L interactions, but it is not clearly defined how much DC licensing and maturation functionally overlap. CD40–CD40L interactions are not only crucial for upregulation of costimulatory molecules but also for DC survival (86). Additionally, mature DCs produce chemokines to attract other immune cells and to orchestrate the ongoing immune response. In contrast to maturation-induced upregulation of MHC II, CD1 trafficking is differentially regulated during DC maturation, and CD1 molecules are already expressed on immature DCs. While human DCs express all classes of CD1 molecules, murine DCs express only CD1d (87), which is crucial for DC–iNKT cell interactions. Trafficking studies showed that antigen presentation by CD1d to iNKT cells might already occur before DC maturation and MHC II presentation (88). This notion hinted to a possible role of iNKT cells as immunological helper cells.

iNKT Cells as Immunological Helper Cells

αGalCer was found to mediate CD40-dependent activation of CTL by NKT cell-helped DC (89), directing attention to the adjuvant activity for this agent. Furthermore, αGalCer also induced resistance to tumors and intracellular pathogens (25). Compared to CD40 ligation, LPS, and CpG, αGalCer induced equally high levels of CD40, CD80, CD86, MHC II, and DEC205 in $CD11c^+$ $CD8a^+$ and $CD11c^+$ $CD8a^-$ DCs, but was unable to induce DC maturation from bone marrow progenitors. Rather than acting directly on DCs, αGalCer mediated DC maturation through iNKT cells in a MyD88-independent manner. Combining αGalCer with CD40 stimulation caused DC to produce high amounts of IL12p70, while LPS and CD40 stimulation showed no such effect. IL12p70 production might explain the results of another study (90), where the simultaneous administration of OVA and αGalCer enhanced Th and CTL responses in an iNKT cell-dependent manner. A close temporal association between αGalCer and OVA-derived peptides and additional experiments with antigen-loaded DCs led to the conclusion that αGalCer and peptides must reach the same DC. Formal *in vivo* evidence for such a tripartite cellular interaction was provided with the use of bm1/CD1d bone marrow chimeras (91). In addition, there was synergy when Th and iNKT help were combined. The means by which iNKT cells license DCs are not fully understood but in addition to providing CD40L to DCs, iNKT cells may act by promoting cross-talk of $XCR1^+$ DCs and plasmacytoid DC (92) or by abundant cytokine production upon activation. Whether iNKT cells play a role as helper cells when activated by less potent ligands remains to be elucidated.

iNKT Cells Help in CTL and $CD8^+$ Memory T Cell Formation

The knowledge on mechanisms iNKT cells use to substitute $CD4^+$ T cell help for antibody production, CTL generation, or memory formation is central for developing new vaccination strategies. An unresolved question is why some groups observed NKT cell-dependent reduction of CTL-mediated autoimmune diseases, whereas NKT cell-licensed DC induced strong CTL responses against tumors and viruses in other studies. The most obvious difference is the use of a single low dose of αGalCer for induction of protective CTL responses and the use of multiple doses or high single doses of αGalCer to inhibit unwanted T cell responses (93). In some clinical trials, αGalCer was used to treat cancer, and human $CD4^+$ iNKT cells expanded predominantly during early stages (26). $CD4^+$ iNKT cells can induce IL12p70 production by DC and thereby Th1 polarization (93). Double negative (DN) iNKT cells expanded later after αGalCer treatment and can induce apoptosis in αGalCer-loaded DC, thereby limiting the immune response (26). Functional differences between iNKT cell subsets in regards to cytokine production are evident both in mice and humans (94), but the effects on DC maturation, apoptosis, and CTL generation remain to be elucidated (**Figure 1**). A high frequency of a DN iNKT cell subset and their potential to lyse DCs may impair treatment of cancer patients and vaccination strategies. The role of iNKT cells during viral infections and the use of αGalCer as vaccine adjuvant in the context of influenza infections have been reviewed recently in Ref. (14, 95). αGalCer increased the levels of influenza-specific systemic IgG and mucosal IgA antibodies, even in the absence of Th cells and antigen-specific CTL responses (14, 95). In contrast, after combined iNKT cell activation and influenza virus vaccination, an impaired CTL response but enhanced memory CTL generation was seen (96). In line with this, enhanced CTL memory differentiation during viral infection was also shown previously (97). Another study showed that iNKT cell enrichment in the CNS during Theiler's murine encephalomyelitis virus (TEMV) infection inhibited the antiviral CTL response and delayed the accumulation of TEMV-specific CTL. Also, the magnitude of the TEMV-specific CTL response was impaired (98). CTL memory formation was not assessed in that study. Co-administration of αGalCer with suboptimal doses of irradiated sporozoites or recombinant viruses expressing a malaria antigen enhanced protective anti-malaria immunity in mice, and co-administration of αGalCer with various immunogens enhanced antigen-specific CTL responses and Th1 responses (99). In conclusion, vaccination with αGalCer as adjuvant induced iNKT cell help for DCs, which promoted CTL memory formation but impaired primary antigen-specific CTL responses.

Before we can fully understand the mechanisms of iNKT cell help in CTL formation and memory generation, it is crucial to know how "help" influences CTL responses in general. Many reports about Th help are available and most of them show a diverse picture of the requirement for $CD4^+$ T cell help in primary and/or secondary infections. Th help seems to be crucial for the clearance of some primary virus infections like HSV or influenza that do not affect DCs directly (100, 101), while in some viral

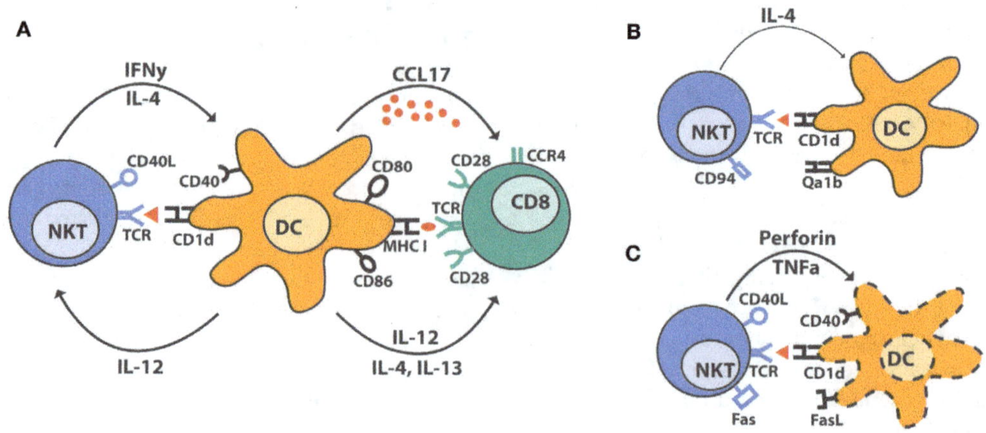

FIGURE 1 | iNKT cell–DC interactions after stimulation with αGalCer. (A) Under optimal stimulatory conditions, iNKT cells produce IL-4, large amounts of IFNγ and upregulate CD40L, thereby inducing maturation in DC. DC maturation leads to increased costimulatory capacity through upregulation of CD80 and CD86, of MHC molecules, and by producing the pro-inflammatory cytokine, IL-12, and the chemokine, CCL17. CCL17 attracts CCR4$^+$ cells, including CD8$^+$ T cells, which can be activated by the licensed DC. **(B)** Overstimulated iNKT cells upregulate inhibitory receptors like CD94 and are incapable of producing IFNγ. DC interacing with hyporesponsive iNKT cells cannot be activated and do not induce CD8$^+$ T cell activation. **(C)** Some activated iNKT cells induce DC lysis rather than maturation by yet unknown mechanisms. Proposed mechanisms suggest a role for TNFα, perforin, Fas–FasL interactions, and even CD40–CD40L.

infections, Th help can be overcome (102). Additionally, CTL responses against minor H antigens, soluble proteins, tumors, and peptide-pulsed DC require Th help for the induction of optimal primary responses (79, 103, 104). Some groups disagreed whether Th help was needed during secondary responses for proper re-expansion of CTL (105, 106) or whether Th help was merely a prerequisite during primary infections for CTL memory formation (107). Additionally, Th help was dispensable for the expansion, but not for the cytotoxic capacity of CTL in tuberculosis (108).

These differential observations may be explained not only by the variance of pathogens and model antigens used but also by different experimental setups. Moreover, Th dependency was studied by using CD4$^{-/-}$ mice, MHC II$^{-/-}$ mice, or CD4-depleting antibodies, which are not biologically equivalent (109). For example, CD4-depleting antibodies also deplete regulatory T cells, CD4$^+$ NKT cells, and CD4$^+$ DCs. However, most older studies agreed that the requirement for Th help is not a CTL-intrinsic property but dependent on the infectious agent and DC maturation. Given the huge discrepancies in studies on Th help requirements, observations in a single model do not permit general conclusions on how CD4$^+$ help may be substituted by iNKT cells. A deeper insight into CTL generation and memory formation is required to allow predictions for the role of iNKT cell help in CTL responses.

As reviewed previously in Ref.(110), CTL in primary responses can be divided into short-lived effector cells (SLEC) that mostly die off during the contraction phase and memory precursor cells (MPEC) that received less stimulation but more survival signals (111, 112). Even a single naive CTL can differentiate into a diverse population of effector and memory cells (113, 114) by multiple mechanisms, which have been reviewed in detail by Kaech and Cui (115). Prolonged antigen exposure and pro-inflammatory cytokines like IL-12 and IL-2 promote terminal differentiation of CTL and induce superior cytotoxic capacities (116–118). NKT cells may affect CTL differentiation other than Th cells, but this hypothesis requires further experimental exploration.

iNKT Cells and Chemokines in CTL and CD8$^+$ T Cell Memory Formation

Chemokines play a major role in orchestrating primary and memory CTL responses. During infections, CTL upregulated CXCR3, which allowed them to enter peripheral tissues (119). Th help was required for enhanced recruitment of CTL to the site of infection in some situations (120) by promoting CXCL9 and CXCL10 production, with CXCL9 being especially important for rapid memory responses in the lymph node (121). Infections of the lung and intestine showed no requirement of Th help for migration as lung infections, e.g., by influenza induce on-site proliferation of CTL rather than recruitment (122, 123) but Th cells promoted development of lung-resident memory cells (124).

CXCR3 also drove CTL toward an effector fate rather than memory fate (125). In line with this, CXCR3 × CCR5 double-deficient mice showed a decreased contraction phase and harbored more memory CTL, which were unable to migrate into tissues and to clear infections (126). In humans, CCR5 expression was associated with effector memory T cells, whereas CCR7 was predominantly expressed on naïve and central memory T cells and CCR6 expression was found on early effector memory T cells (127–129).

iNKT cell-helped DCs produced high amounts of CCL17, thereby attracting CCR4$^+$ lymphocytes (91). This contrasts the situation in classical Th cell-dependent cross-priming, where DCs produced CCR5 ligands to attract CTL for cross-priming. These chemokines synergically guided CTL toward those DCs that have presented relevant antigen to helper T cell subsets, and thereby facilitated the ensuing CTL response. Thus, CCR4- and CCR5-binding chemokines have been described as a new signal in T cell activation, distinct from signal 1, antigen, and signal 2, costimulation (130).

CCR4 is traditionally considered to be associated with skin homing Th2 and memory $CD4^+$ T cells (131–134), but also with the recruitment of Treg to the inflamed liver (135). Several studies in humans showed increased CCR4 expression also on CTL in cutaneous diseases (136–138). A $CCR4^+$ $CD8^+$ central memory subset has been described that was generated in the presence of IL-4 and produced IL4 and IL-13 upon restimulation (139). These cells were not cytotoxic and produced little IFNγ, features associated with a so-called Tc2 subset (139, 140). Kondo and Takiguchi showed that human $CCR4^+$ $CD8^+$ T cells expressed less effector molecules like perforin or granzymes compared to $CCR6^+$ early effector memory T cells, but produced more TNFα and IL-4 than $CCR7^+$ naïve or central memory $CD8^+$ T cells. They concluded that $CCR4^+CD8^+$ T cells are a "little more differentiated than $CCR7^+$ central memory ones and less differentiated than $CCR6^+$ early effector memory ones" and that they can migrate into secondary lymphoid organs where they mature after interacting with DCs expressing CCR4 ligand (141). Since iNKT cells produce IL-4 upon activation and induce CCL17 production by helped DC, they might play a role in the development or restimulation of $CCR4^+$ $CD8^+$ T cells. The physiological role of this subset in viral infections and tumors remains to be elucidated.

Concluding Remarks

CD4-helped DCs and NKT cell-helped DCs provide various costimulatory signals and cytokines deciding the fate of $CD8^+$ T cells toward effector or memory. However, the set of chemokines produced by NKT cell-helped DCs attract different subsets of naïve or memory $CD8^+$ T cells compared to chemokines produced by Th-helped DCs. Dissecting the role of those $CD8^+$ T cells subsets in effector and memory responses directed against tumors and viral infections may facilitate developing effective NKT cell-based vaccines.

Acknowledgments

We thank Dr. Kristina Koch for help with artwork. This work was supported by the Deutsche Forschungsgemeinschaft (grants SFB704 and 645). EM is supported by the German National Academic Foundation. CK is a member of the Excellence-Cluster ImmunoSensation.

References

1. Parekh VV, Wilson MT, Van Kaer L. iNKT-cell responses to glycolipids. *Crit Rev Immunol* (2005) **25**(3):183–213. doi:10.1615/CritRevImmunol.v25.i3.20
2. Bendelac A, Savage PB, Teyton L. The biology of NKT cells. *Annu Rev Immunol* (2007) **25**:297–336. doi:10.1146/annurev.immunol.25.022106.141711
3. Godfrey DI, Kronenberg M. Going both ways: immune regulation via CD1d-dependent NKT cells. *J Clin Invest* (2004) **114**(10):1379–88. doi:10.1172/JCI23594
4. Kumar V, Delovitch TL. Different subsets of natural killer T cells may vary in their roles in health and disease. *Immunology* (2014) **142**(3):321–36. doi:10.1111/imm.12247
5. Zeng Z, Castano AR, Segelke BW, Stura EA, Peterson PA, Wilson IA. Crystal structure of mouse CD1: an MHC-like fold with a large hydrophobic binding groove. *Science* (1997) **277**(5324):339–45. doi:10.1126/science.277.5324.339
6. Porcelli SA. The CD1 family: a third lineage of antigen-presenting molecules. *Adv Immunol* (1995) **59**:1–98. doi:10.1016/S0065-2776(08)60629-X
7. Akbari O, Stock P, Meyer E, Kronenberg M, Sidobre S, Nakayama T, et al. Essential role of NKT cells producing IL-4 and IL-13 in the development of allergen-induced airway hyperreactivity. *Nat Med* (2003) **9**(5):582–8. doi:10.1038/nm851
8. Sharif S, Arreaza GA, Zucker P, Mi QS, Sondhi J, Naidenko OV, et al. Activation of natural killer T cells by alpha-galactosylceramide treatment prevents the onset and recurrence of autoimmune Type 1 diabetes. *Nat Med* (2001) **7**(9):1057–62. doi:10.1038/nm0901-1057
9. Lee PT, Benlagha K, Teyton L, Bendelac A. Distinct functional lineages of human V(alpha)24 natural killer T cells. *J Exp Med* (2002) **195**(5):637–41. doi:10.1084/jem.20011908
10. Li X, Fujio M, Imamura M, Wu D, Vasan S, Wong CH, et al. Design of a potent CD1d-binding NKT cell ligand as a vaccine adjuvant. *Proc Natl Acad Sci U S A* (2010) **107**(29):13010–5. doi:10.1073/pnas.1006662107
11. Faveeuw C, Trottein F. Optimization of natural killer T cell-mediated immunotherapy in cancer using cell-based and nanovector vaccines. *Cancer Res* (2014) **74**(6):1632–8. doi:10.1158/0008-5472.CAN-13-3504
12. Carreno LJ, Kharkwal SS, Porcelli SA. Optimizing NKT cell ligands as vaccine adjuvants. *Immunotherapy* (2014) **6**(3):309–20. doi:10.2217/imt.13.175
13. Padte NN, Li X, Tsuji M, Vasan S. Clinical development of a novel CD1d-binding NKT cell ligand as a vaccine adjuvant. *Clin Immunol* (2011) **140**(2):142–51. doi:10.1016/j.clim.2010.11.009
14. Ko SY, Ko HJ, Chang WS, Park SH, Kweon MN, Kang CY. Alpha-galactosylceramide can act as a nasal vaccine adjuvant inducing protective immune responses against viral infection and tumor. *J Immunol* (2005) **175**(5):3309–17. doi:10.4049/jimmunol.175.5.3309
15. Chackerian A, Alt J, Perera V, Behar SM. Activation of NKT cells protects mice from tuberculosis. *Infect Immun* (2002) **70**(11):6302–9. doi:10.1128/IAI.70.11.6302-6309.2002
16. Huang Y, Chen A, Li X, Chen Z, Zhang W, Song Y, et al. Enhancement of HIV DNA vaccine immunogenicity by the NKT cell ligand, alpha-galactosylceramide. *Vaccine* (2008) **26**(15):1807–16. doi:10.1016/j.vaccine.2008.02.002
17. Kakimi K, Guidotti LG, Koezuka Y, Chisari FV. Natural killer T cell activation inhibits hepatitis B virus replication in vivo. *J Exp Med* (2000) **192**(7):921–30. doi:10.1084/jem.192.7.921
18. Kopecky-Bromberg SA, Fraser KA, Pica N, Carnero E, Moran TM, Franck RW, et al. Alpha-C-galactosylceramide as an adjuvant for a live attenuated influenza virus vaccine. *Vaccine* (2009) **27**(28):3766–74. doi:10.1016/j.vaccine.2009.03.090
19. Veldt BJ, van der Vliet HJ, von Blomberg BM, van Vlierberghe H, Gerken G, Nishi N, et al. Randomized placebo controlled phase I/II trial of alpha-galactosylceramide for the treatment of chronic hepatitis C. *J Hepatol* (2007) **47**(3):356–65. doi:10.1016/j.jhep.2007.04.018
20. Woltman AM, Ter Borg MJ, Binda RS, Sprengers D, von Blomberg BM, Scheper RJ, et al. Alpha-galactosylceramide in chronic hepatitis B infection: results from a randomized placebo-controlled phase I/II trial. *Antivir Ther* (2009) **14**(6):809–18. doi:10.3851/1295
21. Youn HJ, Ko SY, Lee KA, Ko HJ, Lee YS, Fujihashi K, et al. A single intranasal immunization with inactivated influenza virus and alpha-galactosylceramide induces long-term protective immunity without redirecting antigen to the central nervous system. *Vaccine* (2007) **25**(28):5189–98. doi:10.1016/j.vaccine.2007.04.081
22. Gonzalez-Aseguinolaza G, de Oliveira C, Tomaska M, Hong S, Bruna-Romero O, Nakayama T, et al. Alpha-galactosylceramide-activated Valpha 14 natural killer T cells mediate protection against murine malaria. *Proc Natl Acad Sci U S A* (2000) **97**(15):8461–6. doi:10.1073/pnas.97.15.8461
23. Kawakami K, Kinjo Y, Yara S, Koguchi Y, Uezu K, Nakayama T, et al. Activation of Valpha14(+) natural killer T cells by alpha-galactosylceramide results in development of Th1 response and local host resistance in mice infected with Cryptococcus neoformans. *Infect Immun* (2001) **69**(1):213–20. doi:10.1128/IAI.69.1.213-220.2001

24. Schmieg J, Yang G, Franck RW, Tsuji M. Superior protection against malaria and melanoma metastases by a C-glycoside analogue of the natural killer T cell ligand alpha-Galactosylceramide. *J Exp Med* (2003) **198**(11):1631–41. doi:10.1084/jem.20031192
25. Fujii S, Shimizu K, Smith C, Bonifaz L, Steinman RM. Activation of natural killer T cells by alpha-galactosylceramide rapidly induces the full maturation of dendritic cells in vivo and thereby acts as an adjuvant for combined CD4 and CD8 T cell immunity to a coadministered protein. *J Exp Med* (2003) **198**(2):267–79. doi:10.1084/jem.20030324
26. Chang DH, Osman K, Connolly J, Kukreja A, Krasovsky J, Pack M, et al. Sustained expansion of NKT cells and antigen-specific T cells after injection of alpha-galactosyl-ceramide loaded mature dendritic cells in cancer patients. *J Exp Med* (2005) **201**(9):1503–17. doi:10.1084/jem.20042592
27. Crowe NY, Smyth MJ, Godfrey DI. A critical role for natural killer T cells in immunosurveillance of methylcholanthrene-induced sarcomas. *J Exp Med* (2002) **196**(1):119–27. doi:10.1084/jem.20020092
28. Giaccone G, Punt CJ, Ando Y, Ruijter R, Nishi N, Peters M, et al. A phase I study of the natural killer T-cell ligand alpha-galactosylceramide (KRN7000) in patients with solid tumors. *Clin Cancer Res* (2002) **8**(12):3702–9.
29. Ishikawa A, Motohashi S, Ishikawa E, Fuchida H, Higashino K, Otsuji M, et al. A phase I study of alpha-galactosylceramide (KRN7000)-pulsed dendritic cells in patients with advanced and recurrent non-small cell lung cancer. *Clin Cancer Res* (2005) **11**(5):1910–7. doi:10.1158/1078-0432.CCR-04-1453
30. Kim D, Hung CF, Wu TC, Park YM. DNA vaccine with alpha-galactosylceramide at prime phase enhances anti-tumor immunity after boosting with antigen-expressing dendritic cells. *Vaccine* (2010) **28**(45):7297–305. doi:10.1016/j.vaccine.2010.08.079
31. Kim YJ, Ko HJ, Kim YS, Kim DH, Kang S, Kim JM, et al. Alpha-galactosylceramide-loaded, antigen-expressing B cells prime a wide spectrum of antitumor immunity. *Int J Cancer* (2008) **122**(12):2774–83. doi:10.1002/ijc.23444
32. Kobayashi E, Motoki K, Uchida T, Fukushima H, Koezuka Y. KRN7000, a novel immunomodulator, and its antitumor activities. *Oncol Res* (1995) **7**(10–11):529–34.
33. Kunii N, Horiguchi S, Motohashi S, Yamamoto H, Ueno N, Yamamoto S, et al. Combination therapy of in vitro-expanded natural killer T cells and alpha-galactosylceramide-pulsed antigen-presenting cells in patients with recurrent head and neck carcinoma. *Cancer Sci* (2009) **100**(6):1092–8. doi:10.1111/j.1349-7006.2009.01135.x
34. Motohashi S, Nagato K, Kunii N, Yamamoto H, Yamasaki K, Okita K, et al. A phase I-II study of alpha-galactosylceramide-pulsed IL-2/GM-CSF-cultured peripheral blood mononuclear cells in patients with advanced and recurrent non-small cell lung cancer. *J Immunol* (2009) **182**(4):2492–501. doi:10.4049/jimmunol.0800126
35. Nieda M, Okai M, Tazbirkova A, Lin H, Yamaura A, Ide K, et al. Therapeutic activation of Valpha24+Vbeta11+ NKT cells in human subjects results in highly coordinated secondary activation of acquired and innate immunity. *Blood* (2004) **103**(2):383–9. doi:10.1182/blood-2003-04-1155
36. Shibolet O, Alper R, Zlotogarov L, Thalenfeld B, Engelhardt D, Rabbani E, et al. NKT and CD8 lymphocytes mediate suppression of hepatocellular carcinoma growth via tumor antigen-pulsed dendritic cells. *Int J Cancer* (2003) **106**(2):236–43. doi:10.1002/ijc.11201
37. Silk JD, Hermans IF, Gileadi U, Chong TW, Shepherd D, Salio M, et al. Utilizing the adjuvant properties of CD1d-dependent NK T cells in T cell-mediated immunotherapy. *J Clin Invest* (2004) **114**(12):1800–11. doi:10.1172/JCI22046
38. Teng MW, Westwood JA, Darcy PK, Sharkey J, Tsuji M, Franck RW, et al. Combined natural killer T-cell based immunotherapy eradicates established tumors in mice. *Cancer Res* (2007) **67**(15):7495–504. doi:10.1158/0008-5472.CAN-07-0941
39. Uchida T, Horiguchi S, Tanaka Y, Yamamoto H, Kunii N, Motohashi S, et al. Phase I study of alpha-galactosylceramide-pulsed antigen presenting cells administration to the nasal submucosa in unresectable or recurrent head and neck cancer. *Cancer Immunol Immunother* (2008) **57**(3):337–45. doi:10.1007/s00262-007-0373-5
40. Hong S, Wilson MT, Serizawa I, Wu L, Singh N, Naidenko OV, et al. The natural killer T-cell ligand alpha-galactosylceramide prevents autoimmune diabetes in non-obese diabetic mice. *Nat Med* (2001) 7(9):1052–6. doi:10.1038/nm0901-1052
41. Jahng AW, Maricic I, Pedersen B, Burdin N, Naidenko O, Kronenberg M, et al. Activation of natural killer T cells potentiates or prevents experimental autoimmune encephalomyelitis. *J Exp Med* (2001) **194**(12):1789–99. doi:10.1084/jem.194.12.1789
42. Naumov YN, Bahjat KS, Gausling R, Abraham R, Exley MA, Koezuka Y, et al. Activation of CD1d-restricted T cells protects NOD mice from developing diabetes by regulating dendritic cell subsets. *Proc Natl Acad Sci U S A* (2001) **98**(24):13838–43. doi:10.1073/pnas.251531798
43. Singh AK, Wilson MT, Hong S, Olivares-Villagomez D, Du C, Stanic AK, et al. Natural killer T cell activation protects mice against experimental autoimmune encephalomyelitis. *J Exp Med* (2001) **194**(12):1801–11. doi:10.1084/jem.194.12.1801
44. Wang B, Geng YB, Wang CR. CD1-restricted NK T cells protect nonobese diabetic mice from developing diabetes. *J Exp Med* (2001) **194**(3):313–20. doi:10.1084/jem.194.3.313
45. Furlan R, Bergami A, Cantarella D, Brambilla E, Taniguchi M, Dellabona P, et al. Activation of invariant NKT cells by alphaGalCer administration protects mice from MOG35-55-induced EAE: critical roles for administration route and IFN-gamma. *Eur J Immunol* (2003) **33**(7):1830–8. doi:10.1002/eji.200323885
46. Zeng D, Liu Y, Sidobre S, Kronenberg M, Strober S. Activation of natural killer T cells in NZB/W mice induces Th1-type immune responses exacerbating lupus. *J Clin Invest* (2003) **112**(8):1211–22. doi:10.1172/JCI17165
47. Chiba A, Oki S, Miyamoto K, Hashimoto H, Yamamura T, Miyake S. Suppression of collagen-induced arthritis by natural killer T cell activation with OCH, a sphingosine-truncated analog of alpha-galactosylceramide. *Arthritis Rheum* (2004) **50**(1):305–13. doi:10.1002/art.11489
48. Chiba A, Kaieda S, Oki S, Yamamura T, Miyake S. The involvement of V(alpha)14 natural killer T cells in the pathogenesis of arthritis in murine models. *Arthritis Rheum* (2005) **52**(6):1941–8. doi:10.1002/art.21056
49. Kim HY, Kim HJ, Min HS, Kim S, Park WS, Park SH, et al. NKT cells promote antibody-induced joint inflammation by suppressing transforming growth factor beta1 production. *J Exp Med* (2005) **201**(1):41–7. doi:10.1084/jem.20041400
50. Kojo S, Seino K, Harada M, Watarai H, Wakao H, Uchida T, et al. Induction of regulatory properties in dendritic cells by Valpha14 NKT cells. *J Immunol* (2005) **175**(6):3648–55. doi:10.4049/jimmunol.175.6.3648
51. Major AS, Singh RR, Joyce S, Van Kaer L. The role of invariant natural killer T cells in lupus and atherogenesis. *Immunol Res* (2006) **34**(1):49–66. doi:10.1385/IR:34:1:49
52. Yang JQ, Wen X, Liu H, Folayan G, Dong X, Zhou M, et al. Examining the role of CD1d and natural killer T cells in the development of nephritis in a genetically susceptible lupus model. *Arthritis Rheum* (2007) **56**(4):1219–33. doi:10.1002/art.22490
53. Kinjo Y, Illarionov P, Vela JL, Pei B, Girardi E, Li X, et al. Invariant natural killer T cells recognize glycolipids from pathogenic Gram-positive bacteria. *Nat Immunol* (2011) **12**(10):966–74. doi:10.1038/ni.2096
54. Chang YJ, Kim HY, Albacker LA, Lee HH, Baumgarth N, Akira S, et al. Influenza infection in suckling mice expands an NKT cell subset that protects against airway hyperreactivity. *J Clin Invest* (2011) **121**(1):57–69. doi:10.1172/JCI44845
55. Kinjo Y, Wu D, Kim G, Xing GW, Poles MA, Ho DD, et al. Recognition of bacterial glycosphingolipids by natural killer T cells. *Nature* (2005) **434**(7032):520–5. doi:10.1038/nature03407
56. Mattner J, Debord KL, Ismail N, Goff RD, Cantu C III, Zhou D, et al. Exogenous and endogenous glycolipid antigens activate NKT cells during microbial infections. *Nature* (2005) **434**(7032):525–9. doi:10.1038/nature03408
57. Kinjo Y, Tupin E, Wu D, Fujio M, Garcia-Navarro R, Benhnia MR, et al. Natural killer T cells recognize diacylglycerol antigens from pathogenic bacteria. *Nat Immunol* (2006) 7(9):978–86. doi:10.1038/ni1380
58. Kawano T, Cui J, Koezuka Y, Toura I, Kaneko Y, Motoki K, et al. CD1d-restricted and TCR-mediated activation of valpha14 NKT cells by glycosylceramides. *Science* (1997) **278**(5343):1626–9. doi:10.1126/science.278.5343.1626
59. Mallevaey T, Selvanantham T. Strategy of lipid recognition by invariant natural killer T cells: 'one for all and all for one'. *Immunology* (2012) **136**(3):273–82. doi:10.1111/j.1365-2567.2012.03580.x
60. Oki S, Miyake S. Invariant natural killer T (iNKT) cells in asthma: a novel insight into the pathogenesis of asthma and the therapeutic implication of

glycolipid ligands for allergic diseases. *Allergol Int* (2007) **56**(1):7–14. doi:10.2332/allergolint.R-06-137

61. Brigl M, Bry L, Kent SC, Gumperz JE, Brenner MB. Mechanism of CD1d-restricted natural killer T cell activation during microbial infection. *Nat Immunol* (2003) **4**(12):1230–7. doi:10.1038/ni1002
62. Wesley JD, Tessmer MS, Chaukos D, Brossay L. NK cell-like behavior of Valpha14i NK T cells during MCMV infection. *PLoS Pathog* (2008) **4**(7):e1000106. doi:10.1371/journal.ppat.1000106
63. Tyznik AJ, Tupin E, Nagarajan NA, Her MJ, Benedict CA, Kronenberg M. Cutting edge: the mechanism of invariant NKT cell responses to viral danger signals. *J Immunol* (2008) **181**(7):4452–6. doi:10.4049/jimmunol.181.7.4452
64. Salio M, Speak AO, Shepherd D, Polzella P, Illarionov PA, Veerapen N, et al. Modulation of human natural killer T cell ligands on TLR-mediated antigen-presenting cell activation. *Proc Natl Acad Sci U S A* (2007) **104**(51):20490–5. doi:10.1073/pnas.0710145104
65. Paget C, Mallevaey T, Speak AO, Torres D, Fontaine J, Sheehan KC, et al. Activation of invariant NKT cells by toll-like receptor 9-stimulated dendritic cells requires type I interferon and charged glycosphingolipids. *Immunity* (2007) **27**(4):597–609. doi:10.1016/j.immuni.2007.08.017
66. Crowe NY, Coquet JM, Berzins SP, Kyparissoudis K, Keating R, Pellicci DG, et al. Differential antitumor immunity mediated by NKT cell subsets in vivo. *J Exp Med* (2005) **202**(9):1279–88. doi:10.1084/jem.20050953
67. Lee YJ, Holzapfel KL, Zhu J, Jameson SC, Hogquist KA. Steady-state production of IL-4 modulates immunity in mouse strains and is determined by lineage diversity of iNKT cells. *Nat Immunol* (2013) **14**(11):1146–54. doi:10.1038/ni.2731
68. Michel ML, Keller AC, Paget C, Fujio M, Trottein F, Savage PB, et al. Identification of an IL-17-producing NK1.1(neg) iNKT cell population involved in airway neutrophilia. *J Exp Med* (2007) **204**(5):995–1001. doi:10.1084/jem.20061551
69. Li S, Joseph C, Becourt C, Klibi J, Luce S, Dubois-Laforgue D, et al. Potential role of IL-17-producing iNKT cells in type 1 diabetes. *PLoS One* (2014) **9**(4):e96151. doi:10.1371/journal.pone.0096151
70. Webster KE, Kim HO, Kyparissoudis K, Corpuz TM, Pinget GV, Uldrich AP, et al. IL-17-producing NKT cells depend exclusively on IL-7 for homeostasis and survival. *Mucosal Immunol* (2014) **7**(5):1058–67. doi:10.1038/mi.2013.122
71. Monteiro M, Almeida CF, Agua-Doce A, Graca L. Induced IL-17-producing invariant NKT cells require activation in presence of TGF-beta and IL-1beta. *J Immunol* (2013) **190**(2):805–11. doi:10.4049/jimmunol.1201010
72. Lynch L, Nowak M, Varghese B, Clark J, Hogan AE, Toxavidis V, et al. Adipose tissue invariant NKT cells protect against diet-induced obesity and metabolic disorder through regulatory cytokine production. *Immunity* (2012) **37**(3):574–87. doi:10.1016/j.immuni.2012.06.016
73. Schoenberger SP, van der Voort EI, Krietemeijer GM, Offringa R, Melief CJ, Toes RE. Cross-priming of CTL responses in vivo does not require antigenic peptides in the endoplasmic reticulum of immunizing cells. *J Immunol* (1998) **161**(8):3808–12.
74. Sigal LJ, Crotty S, Andino R, Rock KL. Cytotoxic T-cell immunity to virus-infected non-haematopoietic cells requires presentation of exogenous antigen. *Nature* (1999) **398**(6722):77–80. doi:10.1038/18038
75. den Haan JM, Lehar SM, Bevan MJ. CD8(+) but not CD8(-) dendritic cells cross-prime cytotoxic T cells in vivo. *J Exp Med* (2000) **192**(12):1685–96. doi:10.1084/jem.192.12.1685
76. Kurts C, Robinson BW, Knolle PA. Cross-priming in health and disease. *Nat Rev Immunol* (2010) **10**(6):403–14. doi:10.1038/nri2780
77. Smith CM, Wilson NS, Waithman J, Villadangos JA, Carbone FR, Heath WR, et al. Cognate CD4(+) T cell licensing of dendritic cells in CD8(+) T cell immunity. *Nat Immunol* (2004) **5**(11):1143–8. doi:10.1038/ni1129
78. Lanzavecchia A. Immunology. Licence to kill. *Nature* (1998) **393**(6684):413–4. doi:10.1038/30845
79. Bennett SR, Carbone FR, Karamalis F, Miller JF, Heath WR. Induction of a CD8+ cytotoxic T lymphocyte response by cross-priming requires cognate CD4+ T cell help. *J Exp Med* (1997) **186**(1):65–70. doi:10.1084/jem.186.1.65
80. Ridge JP, Di Rosa F, Matzinger P. A conditioned dendritic cell can be a temporal bridge between a CD4+ T-helper and a T-killer cell. *Nature* (1998) **393**(6684):474–8. doi:10.1038/30989
81. Schoenberger SP, Toes RE, van der Voort EI, Offringa R, Melief CJ. T-cell help for cytotoxic T lymphocytes is mediated by CD40-CD40L interactions. *Nature* (1998) **393**(6684):480–3. doi:10.1038/31002
82. Pulendran B, Palucka K, Banchereau J. Sensing pathogens and tuning immune responses. *Science* (2001) **293**(5528):253–6. doi:10.1126/science.1062060
83. Inohara N, Nunez G. NODs: intracellular proteins involved in inflammation and apoptosis. *Nat Rev Immunol* (2003) **3**(5):371–82. doi:10.1038/nri1086
84. Geijtenbeek TB, van Vliet SJ, Engering A, t Hart BA, van Kooyk Y. Self- and nonself-recognition by C-type lectins on dendritic cells. *Annu Rev Immunol* (2004) **22**:33–54. doi:10.1146/annurev.immunol.22.012703.104558
85. Rogers NC, Slack EC, Edwards AD, Nolte MA, Schulz O, Schweighoffer E, et al. Syk-dependent cytokine induction by Dectin-1 reveals a novel pattern recognition pathway for C type lectins. *Immunity* (2005) **22**(4):507–17. doi:10.1016/j.immuni.2005.03.004
86. Miga AJ, Masters SR, Durell BG, Gonzalez M, Jenkins MK, Maliszewski C, et al. Dendritic cell longevity and T cell persistence is controlled by CD154-CD40 interactions. *Eur J Immunol* (2001) **31**(3):959–65. doi:10.1002/1521-4141(200103)31:3<959::AID-IMMU959>3.0.CO;2-A
87. Barral DC, Brenner MB. CD1 antigen presentation: how it works. *Nat Rev Immunol* (2007) **7**(12):929–41. doi:10.1038/nri2191
88. Gelin C, Sloma I, Charron D, Mooney N. Regulation of MHC II and CD1 antigen presentation: from ubiquity to security. *J Leukoc Biol* (2009) **85**(2):215–24. doi:10.1189/jlb.0308206
89. Nishimura T, Kitamura H, Iwakabe K, Yahata T, Ohta A, Sato M, et al. The interface between innate and acquired immunity: glycolipid antigen presentation by CD1d-expressing dendritic cells to NKT cells induces the differentiation of antigen-specific cytotoxic T lymphocytes. *Int Immunol* (2000) **12**(7):987–94. doi:10.1093/intimm/12.7.987
90. Hermans IF, Silk JD, Gileadi U, Salio M, Mathew B, Ritter G, et al. NKT cells enhance CD4+ and CD8+ T cell responses to soluble antigen in vivo through direct interaction with dendritic cells. *J Immunol* (2003) **171**(10):5140–7. doi:10.4049/jimmunol.171.10.5140
91. Semmling V, Lukacs-Kornek V, Thaiss CA, Quast T, Hochheiser K, Panzer U, et al. Alternative cross-priming through CCL17-CCR4-mediated attraction of CTLs toward NKT cell-licensed DCs. *Nat Immunol* (2010) **11**(4):313–20. doi:10.1038/ni.1848
92. Shimizu K, Asakura M, Shinga J, Sato Y, Kitahara S, Hoshino K, et al. Invariant NKT cells induce plasmacytoid dendritic cell (DC) cross-talk with conventional DCs for efficient memory CD8+ T cell induction. *J Immunol* (2013) **190**(11):5609–19. doi:10.4049/jimmunol.1300033
93. Liu TY, Uemura Y, Suzuki M, Narita Y, Hirata S, Ohyama H, et al. Distinct subsets of human invariant NKT cells differentially regulate T helper responses via dendritic cells. *Eur J Immunol* (2008) **38**(4):1012–23. doi:10.1002/eji.200737838
94. Coquet JM, Chakravarti S, Kyparissoudis K, McNab FW, Pitt LA, McKenzie BS, et al. Diverse cytokine production by NKT cell subsets and identification of an IL-17-producing CD4-NK1.1- NKT cell population. *Proc Natl Acad Sci U S A* (2008) **105**(32):11287–92. doi:10.1073/pnas.0801631105
95. Galli G, Pittoni P, Tonti E, Malzone C, Uematsu Y, Tortoli M, et al. Invariant NKT cells sustain specific B cell responses and memory. *Proc Natl Acad Sci U S A* (2007) **104**(10):3984–9. doi:10.1073/pnas.0700191104
96. Guillonneau C, Mintern JD, Hubert FX, Hurt AC, Besra GS, Porcelli S, et al. Combined NKT cell activation and influenza virus vaccination boosts memory CTL generation and protective immunity. *Proc Natl Acad Sci U S A* (2009) **106**(9):3330–5. doi:10.1073/pnas.0813309106
97. Reilly EC, Thompson EA, Aspeslagh S, Wands JR, Elewaut D, Brossay L. Activated iNKT cells promote memory CD8+ T cell differentiation during viral infection. *PLoS One* (2012) **7**(5):e37991. doi:10.1371/journal.pone.0037991
98. Mars LT, Mas M, Beaudoin L, Bauer J, Leite-de-Moraes M, Lehuen A, et al. Invariant NKT cells regulate the CD8 T cell response during Theiler's virus infection. *PLoS One* (2014) **9**(1):e87717. doi:10.1371/journal.pone.0087717
99. Gonzalez-Aseguinolaza G, Van Kaer L, Bergmann CC, Wilson JM, Schmieg J, Kronenberg M, et al. Natural killer T cell ligand alpha-galactosylceramide enhances protective immunity induced by malaria vaccines. *J Exp Med* (2002) **195**(5):617–24. doi:10.1084/jem.20011889
100. Jennings SR, Bonneau RH, Smith PM, Wolcott RM, Chervenak R. CD4-positive T lymphocytes are required for the generation of the primary but not the secondary CD8-positive cytolytic T lymphocyte response to herpes simplex virus in C57BL/6 mice. *Cell Immunol* (1991) **133**(1):234–52. doi:10.1016/0008-8749(91)90194-G
101. Riberdy JM, Christensen JP, Branum K, Doherty PC. Diminished primary and secondary influenza virus-specific CD8(+) T-cell responses in CD4-depleted

Ig(-/-) mice. *J Virol* (2000) **74**(20):9762–5. doi:10.1128/JVI.74.20.9762-9765.2000

102. Janssen EM, Lemmens EE, Wolfe T, Christen U, von Herrath MG, Schoenberger SP. CD4+ T cells are required for secondary expansion and memory in CD8+ T lymphocytes. *Nature* (2003) **421**(6925):852–6. doi:10.1038/nature01441
103. Husmann LA, Bevan MJ. Cooperation between helper T cells and cytotoxic T lymphocyte precursors. *Ann N Y Acad Sci* (1988) **532**:158–69. doi:10.1111/j.1749-6632.1988.tb36335.x
104. Guerder S, Matzinger P. A fail-safe mechanism for maintaining self-tolerance. *J Exp Med* (1992) **176**(2):553–64. doi:10.1084/jem.176.2.553
105. Di Rosa F, Matzinger P. Long-lasting CD8 T cell memory in the absence of CD4 T cells or B cells. *J Exp Med* (1996) **183**(5):2153–63. doi:10.1084/jem.183.5.2153
106. Bourgeois C, Veiga-Fernandes H, Joret AM, Rocha B, Tanchot C. CD8 lethargy in the absence of CD4 help. *Eur J Immunol* (2002) **32**(8):2199–207. doi:10.1002/1521-4141(200208)32:8<2199::AID-IMMU2199>3.0.CO;2-L
107. Marzo AL, Vezys V, Klonowski KD, Lee SJ, Muralimohan G, Moore M, et al. Fully functional memory CD8 T cells in the absence of CD4 T cells. *J Immunol* (2004) **173**(2):969–75. doi:10.4049/jimmunol.173.2.969
108. Serbina NV, Lazarevic V, Flynn JL. CD4(+) T cells are required for the development of cytotoxic CD8(+) T cells during *Mycobacterium tuberculosis* infection. *J Immunol* (2001) **167**(12):6991–7000. doi:10.4049/jimmunol.167.12.6991
109. Tyznik AJ, Sun JC, Bevan MJ. The CD8 population in CD4-deficient mice is heavily contaminated with MHC class II-restricted T cells. *J Exp Med* (2004) **199**(4):559–65. doi:10.1084/jem.20031961
110. Zhang N, Bevan MJ. CD8(+) T cells: foot soldiers of the immune system. *Immunity* (2011) **35**(2):161–8. doi:10.1016/j.immuni.2011.07.010
111. Mescher MF, Curtsinger JM, Agarwal P, Casey KA, Gerner M, Hammerbeck CD, et al. Signals required for programming effector and memory development by CD8+ T cells. *Immunol Rev* (2006) **211**:81–92. doi:10.1111/j.0105-2896.2006.00382.x
112. Parish IA, Kaech SM. Diversity in CD8(+) T cell differentiation. *Curr Opin Immunol* (2009) **21**(3):291–7. doi:10.1016/j.coi.2009.05.008
113. Stemberger C, Neuenhahn M, Buchholz VR, Busch DH. Origin of CD8+ effector and memory T cell subsets. *Cell Mol Immunol* (2007) **4**(6):399–405.
114. Gerlach C, van Heijst JW, Swart E, Sie D, Armstrong N, Kerkhoven RM, et al. One naive T cell, multiple fates in CD8+ T cell differentiation. *J Exp Med* (2010) **207**(6):1235–46. doi:10.1084/jem.20091175
115. Kaech SM, Cui W. Transcriptional control of effector and memory CD8+ T cell differentiation. *Nat Rev Immunol* (2012) **12**(11):749–61. doi:10.1038/nri3307
116. Curtsinger JM, Johnson CM, Mescher MF. CD8 T cell clonal expansion and development of effector function require prolonged exposure to antigen, costimulation, and signal 3 cytokine. *J Immunol* (2003) **171**(10):5165–71. doi:10.4049/jimmunol.171.10.5165
117. Pearce EL, Shen H. Generation of CD8 T cell memory is regulated by IL-12. *J Immunol* (2007) **179**(4):2074–81. doi:10.4049/jimmunol.179.4.2074
118. Pipkin ME, Sacks JA, Cruz-Guilloty F, Lichtenheld MG, Bevan MJ, Rao A. Interleukin-2 and inflammation induce distinct transcriptional programs that promote the differentiation of effector cytolytic T cells. *Immunity* (2010) **32**(1):79–90. doi:10.1016/j.immuni.2009.11.012
119. Groom JR, Luster AD. CXCR3 in T cell function. *Exp Cell Res* (2011) **317**(5):620–31. doi:10.1016/j.yexcr.2010.12.017
120. Nakanishi Y, Lu B, Gerard C, Iwasaki A. CD8(+) T lymphocyte mobilization to virus-infected tissue requires CD4(+) T-cell help. *Nature* (2009) **462**(7272):510–3. doi:10.1038/nature08511
121. Kastenmuller W, Brandes M, Wang Z, Herz J, Egen JG, Germain RN. Peripheral prepositioning and local CXCL9 chemokine-mediated guidance orchestrate rapid memory CD8+ T cell responses in the lymph node. *Immunity* (2013) **38**(3):502–13. doi:10.1016/j.immuni.2012.11.012
122. Bedoui S, Gebhardt T. Interaction between dendritic cells and T cells during peripheral virus infections: a role for antigen presentation beyond lymphoid organs? *Curr Opin Immunol* (2011) **23**(1):124–30. doi:10.1016/j.coi.2010.11.001
123. McGill J, Legge KL. Cutting edge: contribution of lung-resident T cell proliferation to the overall magnitude of the antigen-specific CD8 T cell response in the lungs following murine influenza virus infection. *J Immunol* (2009) **183**(7):4177–81. doi:10.4049/jimmunol.0901109
124. Laidlaw BJ, Zhang N, Marshall HD, Staron MM, Guan T, Hu Y, et al. CD4+ T cell help guides formation of CD103+ lung-resident memory CD8+ T cells during influenza viral infection. *Immunity* (2014) **41**(4):633–45. doi:10.1016/j.immuni.2014.09.007
125. Kurachi M, Kurachi J, Suenaga F, Tsukui T, Abe J, Ueha S, et al. Chemokine receptor CXCR3 facilitates CD8(+) T cell differentiation into short-lived effector cells leading to memory degeneration. *J Exp Med* (2011) **208**(8):1605–20. doi:10.1084/jem.20102101
126. Kohlmeier JE, Reiley WW, Perona-Wright G, Freeman ML, Yager EJ, Connor LM, et al. Inflammatory chemokine receptors regulate CD8(+) T cell contraction and memory generation following infection. *J Exp Med* (2011) **208**(8):1621–34. doi:10.1084/jem.20102110
127. Tomiyama H, Matsuda T, Takiguchi M. Differentiation of human CD8(+) T cells from a memory to memory/effector phenotype. *J Immunol* (2002) **168**(11):5538–50. doi:10.4049/jimmunol.168.11.5538
128. Sallusto F, Geginat J, Lanzavecchia A. Central memory and effector memory T cell subsets: function, generation, and maintenance. *Annu Rev Immunol* (2004) **22**:745–63. doi:10.1146/annurev.immunol.22.012703.104702
129. Tomiyama H, Takata H, Matsuda T, Takiguchi M. Phenotypic classification of human CD8+ T cells reflecting their function: inverse correlation between quantitative expression of CD27 and cytotoxic effector function. *Eur J Immunol* (2004) **34**(4):999–1010. doi:10.1002/eji.200324478
130. Bousso P, Albert ML. Signal 0 for guided priming of CTLs: NKT cells do it too. *Nat Immunol* (2010) **11**(4):284–6. doi:10.1038/ni0410-284
131. Vestergaard C, Bang K, Gesser B, Yoneyama H, Matsushima K, Larsen CGA. Th2 chemokine, TARC, produced by keratinocytes may recruit CLA+CCR4+ lymphocytes into lesional atopic dermatitis skin. *J Invest Dermatol* (2000) **115**(4):640–6. doi:10.1046/j.1523-1747.2000.00115.x
132. Nakatani T, Kaburagi Y, Shimada Y, Inaoki M, Takehara K, Mukaida N, et al. CCR4 memory CD4+ T lymphocytes are increased in peripheral blood and lesional skin from patients with atopic dermatitis. *J Allergy Clin Immunol* (2001) **107**(2):353–8. doi:10.1067/mai.2001.112601
133. Kusumoto M, Xu B, Shi M, Matsuyama T, Aoyama K, Takeuchi T. Expression of chemokine receptor CCR4 and its ligands (CCL17 and CCL22) in murine contact hypersensitivity. *J Interferon Cytokine Res* (2007) **27**(11):901–10. doi:10.1089/jir.2006.0064
134. Gehad A, Al-Banna NA, Vaci M, Issekutz AC, Mohan K, Latta M, et al. Differing requirements for CCR4, E-selectin, and alpha4beta1 for the migration of memory CD4 and activated T cells to dermal inflammation. *J Immunol* (2012) **189**(1):337–46. doi:10.4049/jimmunol.1102315
135. Oo YH, Shetty S, Adams DH. The role of chemokines in the recruitment of lymphocytes to the liver. *Dig Dis* (2010) **28**(1):31–44. doi:10.1159/000282062
136. Teraki Y, Miyake A, Takebayashi R, Shiohara T. Homing receptor and chemokine receptor on intraepidermal T cells in psoriasis vulgaris. *Clin Exp Dermatol* (2004) **29**(6):658–63. doi:10.1111/j.1365-2230.2004.01638.x
137. Wenzel J, Henze S, Worenkamper E, Basner-Tschakarjan E, Sokolowska-Wojdylo M, Steitz J, et al. Role of the chemokine receptor CCR4 and its ligand thymus- and activation-regulated chemokine/CCL17 for lymphocyte recruitment in cutaneous lupus erythematosus. *J Invest Dermatol* (2005) **124**(6):1241–8. doi:10.1111/j.0022-202X.2005.23755.x
138. Seneviratne SL, Black AP, Jones L, Bailey AS, Ogg GS. The role of skin-homing T cells in extrinsic atopic dermatitis. *QJM* (2007) **100**(1):19–27. doi:10.1093/qjmed/hcl132
139. Geginat J, Lanzavecchia A, Sallusto F. Proliferation and differentiation potential of human CD8+ memory T-cell subsets in response to antigen or homeostatic cytokines. *Blood* (2003) **101**(11):4260–6. doi:10.1182/blood-2002-11-3577
140. Le Gros G, Erard F. Non-cytotoxic, IL-4, IL-5, IL-10 producing CD8+ T cells: their activation and effector functions. *Curr Opin Immunol* (1994) **6**(3):453–7. doi:10.1016/0952-7915(94)90127-9
141. Kondo T, Takiguchi M. Human memory CCR4+CD8+ T cell subset has the ability to produce multiple cytokines. *Int Immunol* (2009) **21**(5):523–32. doi:10.1093/intimm/dxp019

3

Regulation of alloantibody responses

*Anita S. Chong[1], Peter T. Sage[2] and Maria-Luisa Alegre[3]**

[1] *Section of Transplantation, Department of Surgery, University of Chicago, Chicago, IL, United States,* [2] *Renal Division, Transplantation Research Center, Brigham and Women's Hospital, Harvard Medical School, Boston, MA, United States,* [3] *Section of Rheumatology, Department of Medicine, University of Chicago, Chicago, IL, United States*

Edited by:
Fadi Issa,
University of Oxford, United Kingdom

Reviewed by:
Alvaro De Mingo Pulido,
Moffitt Cancer Center, United States
Luis Graca,
University of Lisbon, Portugal

***Correspondence:**
Maria-Luisa Alegre
malegre@midway.uchicago.edu

The control of alloimmunity is essential to the success of organ transplantation. Upon alloantigen encounter, naïve alloreactive T cells not only differentiate into effector cells that can reject the graft, but also into T follicular helper (Tfh) cells that promote the differentiation of alloreactive B cells that produce donor-specific antibodies (DSA). B cells can exacerbate the rejection process through antibody effector functions and/or B cell antigen-presenting functions. These responses can be limited by immune suppressive mechanisms mediated by T regulatory (Treg) cells, T follicular regulatory (Tfr) cells, B regulatory (Breg) cells and a newly described tolerance-induced B (TIB) cell population that has the ability to suppress *de novo* B cells in an antigen-specific manner. Transplantation tolerance following costimulation blockade has revealed mechanisms of tolerance that control alloreactive T cells through intrinsic and extrinsic mechanisms, but also inhibit alloreactive B cells. Thus, the control of both arms of adaptive immunity might result in more robust tolerance, one that may withstand more severe inflammatory challenges. Here, we review new findings on the control of B cells and alloantibody production in the context of transplant rejection and tolerance.

Keywords: Tfh, Tfr, alloantibodies, Bregs, transplantation, tolerant B cells, transplant tolerance

INTRODUCTION

Transplantation tolerance remains an important goal to reduce side effects associated with lifelong immunosuppressive drugs and to diminish the incidence of chronic rejection that might arise from suboptimal immunosuppression. Both T cell-mediated and antibody-mediated mechanisms have been invoked in acute and chronic rejection, though some controversy exists as to whether the appearance of donor-specific antibodies (DSA) is simply a marker of incompletely suppressed T effector and T follicular helper (Tfh) cell responses, or if DSA independently cause rejection (Chong et al., 2019). Several animal models of transplantation tolerance have been developed, and proof of principle data exist that select patients can develop transplantation tolerance (Brouard et al., 2012; Morris et al., 2015; Miller et al., 2017; Savage et al., 2018). New genetic and flow cytometric tools have increased our ability to probe the mechanisms that underscore tolerance when it is successfully induced, though most of the work has focused on how alloreactive T cells are controlled. Mechanisms of T cell transplantation tolerance appear to parallel endogenous immunological mechanisms ensuring T cell self-tolerance, including clonal deletion, anergy, cell-extrinsic suppression and aborted B cell help. Whereas lack of B cell responses might result from insufficient T cell help, new studies are revealing an active tolerance crosstalk between T and B cells. Indeed, T follicular regulatory (Tfr) cells can dominantly suppress B cell responses, Bregs can inhibit T cell responses and promote Treg development, and a novel subset of tolerance-induced B (TIB) cell can infectiously inhibit the responses of naïve B cells in an antigen-specific manner. This active tolerization of the alloreactive B cell compartment may be desirable to achieve a more robust transplantation tolerance than that obtained when only the T cell compartment is regulated. This review will focus on new findings involving Tfr cells, Breg cells and alloreactive TIB cells and their roles in the control of alloimmunity and transplant rejection.

T FOLLICULAR REGULATORY (Tfr) CELLS

Tfr Cells in Antibody Regulation

Antibody responses are tightly controlled by the immune system. Tfh cells promote antibody responses by providing costimulatory and cytokine signals to promote B cell effector responses (Crotty, 2019). Humans with mutations in Tfh effector genes as well as mice with genetic deletion of the same genes have severely impaired antibody responses (Crotty, 2019). Tfr cells are a subpopulation of FoxP3$^+$ T regulatory cells that express the chemokine receptor CXCR5 and can gain access to the B cell follicle to regulate B cell responses (Fonseca et al., 2019; Sage and Sharpe, 2020; Wing et al., 2020). Although CXCR5 was originally thought to be absolutely essential for the migration of Tfr cells to the B cell follicle, newer data suggest other signals may also be involved (Vanderleyden et al., 2020). Tfr cells have a somewhat overlapping transcriptional program as Tfh and Treg cells, and follow similar differentiation cues as Tfh cells (Hou et al., 2019). The shared transcriptional program between Tfr cells and Tfh/Treg cells has hindered in-depth functional studies.

Although Tfr cells have been studied for over 10 years, the precise functions of these cells have been somewhat controversial. Human correlation studies suggest inverse correlations between Tfr cells (as well as Tfr:Tfh ratio) and antibody responses in settings of vaccination, infection and autoimmunity (Sage and Sharpe, 2016; Deng et al., 2019). In some limited settings, such as Sjogren's syndrome, the Tfr/Tfh ratio may positively correlate with ectopic lymphoid structure formation, suggesting Tfr cells may also act as biomarkers for progressive disease stages (Fonseca et al., 2018). Uncovering the precise roles for Tfr cells in murine models has also been challenging. Early studies utilized adoptive transfer techniques and *in vitro* suppression assays to demonstrate that Tfr cells inhibit antigen specific antibody responses (Wollenberg et al., 2011; Sage et al., 2013, 2016). However, these strategies have technical limitations and lack physiological complexity. Recently, two *in vivo* models have been developed to study Tfr cells: Conditional deletion of Bcl6 in Treg cells (Treg$^{\Delta Bcl6}$) and the Tfr-DTR mouse. The premise behind the Treg$^{\Delta Bcl6}$ model is that the transcription factor Bcl6 may be necessary for most Tfr cell development and eliminating Bcl6 in all Treg populations would restrain Tfr cell differentiation from Treg cells. Although the specificity and potency of Tfr depletion in this model is unclear, a number of studies have demonstrated substantial increases in autoantibodies in Treg$^{\Delta Bcl6}$ mice (Wu et al., 2016; Botta et al., 2017; Fu et al., 2018; Gonzalez-Figueroa et al., 2021). In contrast, Treg$^{\Delta Bcl6}$ mice had minor (if any) increases in foreign-antigen specific antibody responses. Moreover, in some cases such as influenza infection, Treg$^{\Delta Bcl6}$ mice have less influenza-specific antibody, suggesting Tfr cells may actually promote antibody responses in some settings (Lu et al., 2021).

As an alternative approach, we recently developed a Tfr-DTR mouse model in which Tfr cells can be deleted in an inducible manner. Using this mouse, we found that Tfr cells potently suppress germinal center formation to control both autoreactive and vaccine-specific antibody responses (Clement et al., 2019). We also found that Tfr cells potently control antigen-specific, as well as total, IgE responses. Increases in total IgE have subsequently been validated using Treg$^{\Delta Bcl6}$ models (Gonzalez-Figueroa et al., 2021). Therefore, Tfr cells seem to have potent roles in controlling autoantibody responses, and the role of Tfr cells in restraining foreign antigen-specific antibody responses may depend on experimental context.

Tfr cells utilize a number of mechanisms to control B cell responses. The coinhibitory receptor CTLA-4 seems to be a potent mediator of Tfr suppression, and both downregulation of B7-1/B7-2 on B cells, as well as prevention of Tfh-B cell interactions, have been proposed as potential mechanisms (Sage et al., 2014; Wing et al., 2014). Although Tfr cells can produce the inhibitory cytokine IL-10, studies suggest that IL-10 production by Tfr cells may actually promote, not inhibit, B cell responses in some settings (Laidlaw et al., 2017). Mechanisms of Tfr suppression that are not shared with other regulatory cell subsets are less clear. However, a new study has uncovered neuritin as a possible Tfr-specific inhibitory molecule that may restrain B cell responses, although neuritin may suppress IgE/allergic responses more potently than IgG responses (Gonzalez-Figueroa et al., 2021).

Tfr Cells in Transplantation Tolerance

The roles of follicular T cells in controlling solid organ transplant rejection are only beginning to be studied (Mohammed and Sage, 2020). In kidney transplant patients, the frequency of CXCR3$^-$ Tfh cells (including Tfh2 and Tfh17 subsets) correlated with donor-specific antibody (DSA) responses and development of antibody-mediated rejection (AMR) (Chen et al., 2017). Similarly, in cardiac transplant patients, CXCR3$^-$ Tfh cells were elevated 1 year after transplantation (Wang et al., 2020). In murine cardiac transplant models, Tfh cell expansion occurred prior to DSA responses suggesting Tfh cells may be an inducer (and biomarker) of rejection (La Muraglia et al., 2019). These studies suggest that Tfh cells may be driving AMR. Moreover, the ratio of Tfr to Tfh cells was attenuated in both kidney and cardiac transplant patients when compared to controls, and a decrease in the Tfr to Tfh ratio was associated with rejection in some transplant studies (Chen et al., 2017; Yan et al., 2019; Niu et al., 2020; Wang et al., 2020). These correlation studies suggest that Tfr cells may restrain Tfh and B cell responses to limit generation of pathogenic antibodies and prevent graft rejection, with the caveat that the ratios were quantified among circulating cells whereas regulation takes place in secondary lymphoid organs.

Elucidating the precise roles of Tfh and Tfr cells in controlling AMR after transplantation has been elusive due to a lack of tools. We recently developed a pre-clinical allogeneic kidney transplant model to assess the roles of Tfh and Tfr cells in controlling DSA and AMR. Using a Tfh-DTR model in which Tfh cells were deleted during transplantation we found that Tfh cells were essential for IgG DSA as well as AMR after kidney transplantation (Mohammed et al., 2021). We also performed allogeneic kidney transplantation in Tfr-DTR mice to assess the roles of Tfr cells in controlling AMR. Although we found that Tfr cells can limit IgG DSA using splenocyte alloantigen challenge models, we did not find substantial differences in severity of AMR during kidney transplantation when Tfr cells were deleted (Mohammed et al., 2021). However, one caveat to these experiments is that a full MHC mismatch kidney transplant model was used in which rejection rapidly occurs within 3 weeks. Therefore, it is unclear if it would be possible to detect quicker rejection by eliminating Tfr suppression. Studying the Tfr-DTR mouse in kidney transplant tolerance models will be important to determine if Tfr cells have important roles in promoting B cell tolerance during transplantation. *In vitro*, Tfr suppression of B cells results in epigenetic changes in B cells, diminishing their ability to produce class-switched antibody even after Tfr cells are no longer present (Sage et al., 2016). A somewhat similar phenotype may occur with alloreactive TIB cells acquiring a stable tolerance state during cardiac transplantation tolerance induced with costimulation blockade, although acquisition of tolerance was observed in Treg$^{\Delta Bcl6}$ recipients (Khiew et al., 2020). That Tfr cells may be able to induce a tolerant-like state in B cells is supported by a recent study where tolerance induced by specific donor-recipient MHC combinations during kidney transplantation was mediated by FoxP3$^+$ Treg cell subset(s) (Yang et al., 2020). Although the precise roles for Tfr cells in modulating transplantation tolerance are still being investigated, it is likely that Tfr cells have functional overlap with both Treg and Breg cells. Since Tfr cells differentiate mostly from Treg cells, it is possible that Treg promotion of B cell tolerance may be through a Tfr-dependent mechanism (Aloulou et al., 2016; Maceiras et al., 2017). Moreover, studies suggest that Breg cells may control Tfh cells, such that Tfr cells may synergize with Breg cells to promote tolerance by restraining Tfh-help to B cells (Lin et al., 2019).

REGULATORY B CELLS

Multiple Breg Subsets in Immunity

There is a substantial literature supporting a role for B cells in immune regulation, and numerous regulatory B cell subsets have been implicated (reviewed in Stolp et al., 2014; Alhabbab et al., 2019; Cherukuri et al., 2021a). For humans, these include the CD24^{hi}CD38^{hi} immature transitional B cells (TBs) (Blair et al., 2010), CD24^{hi}CD27$^+$ B10-like B cells (Dilillo et al., 2010), CD27$^+$CD38^{hi} plasmablast Bregs (Matsumoto et al., 2014), CD25^{hi}CD71^{hi}CD73^{lo} Br1 cells (Van De Veen et al., 2013), CD39$^+$CD73$^+$ Bregs (Saze et al., 2013), CD38$^+$CD1d$^+$IgM$^+$CD147$^+$ Bregs (Lindner et al., 2013), TIM-1$^+$ Bregs (Aravena et al., 2017), and induced Bregs (Nouel et al., 2015). Likewise multiple Breg subsets have been reported in mice, including transitional T2 (Mauri et al., 2003), marginal zone (MZ) (Lenert et al., 2005), CD5$^+$CD1d$^+$ B10 (Kalampokis et al., 2013), TIM-1$^+$ or CD9$^+$ (Ding et al., 2011; Sun et al., 2015) B cells, as well as LAG-3$^+$CD138$^+$ plasmablasts/plasma cells (Shen et al., 2014; Fillatreau, 2018; Lino et al., 2018). The numerous Breg subsets together with the absence of Breg-specific lineage markers have prevented a unifying framework for understanding the origin of these cells.

At present, it appears that Bregs may exist as two distinct subsets; natural Bregs that are similar to thymus-derived natural Tregs and driven by a yet undefined lineage-determining transcription factor instructing their development in the bone marrow; and induced Bregs generated in the periphery from distinct B cell subsets upon encounter with antigen. In support of the former subset, Fillatreau (Fillatreau, 2018, 2019) reported on a novel subset of non-dividing regulatory LAG-3$^+$CD138$^+$ plasma cells that develop at steady state, even in germ-free mice, and that require B cell receptor (BCR) signals and Bruton tyrosine kinase (Btk) for their development. Importantly, these cells produce IL-10 within hours after stimulation and are therefore classified as "natural regulatory plasma cells." In contrast, other subsets of Bregs, such as the B10 Bregs require exposure to immunizing antigen, and engagement of BCR, CD40 and/or TLR signaling (Zhang, 2013). An example are Bregs described by Rothstein and colleagues, where a 20–25-fold expansion of TIM-1$^+$ Bregs across multiple canonical B cell subsets was observed in mice receiving an islet transplant and treated with a low-affinity anti-TIM-1 antibody (Yeung et al., 2015).

Immunomodulatory Cytokines Produced by Bregs

Adding to the complexity of Breg immunobiology, each Breg subset appears capable of suppressing immune responses by shared, as well as distinct, mechanisms of action. The most widely implicated mechanism for Breg-mediated suppression is through production of the anti-inflammatory and immunomodulatory cytokine IL-10. IL-10 produced by B cells may inhibit the differentiation, or induce the apoptosis, of Th1 and Th17 cells while promoting Treg expansion, and alter DC maturation (reviewed in Stolp et al., 2014). In light of the absence of a Breg lineage marker, the expression of IL-10 has been widely used for defining Bregs. In a recent review, Cherukuri et al. (2021a) tabulated IL-10-producing cells within each mouse B cell subset upon a 5 h stimulation with LPS, PMA and ionomycin (LPIM). Only 1.7% of follicular B cells were IL-10-producing, but because they are the major B subset, they represented up to 44% of all B cells producing IL-10. A sizable 23% of MZ B cells were IL-10 producing, and represented 33% of all IL-10-producing B cells. In contrast, plasma cells by far had the highest percentage (74%) of IL-10-producing cells, but only represented 5% of all IL-10-producing B cells. Thus under *in vitro* LPIM stimulation, follicular and MZ B cells represented 77% of all IL-10-producing cells, although it remains to be determined if follicular and MZ B cells have similar dominant contribution *in vivo*.

Transitional B cells represent 4–10% of CD19$^+$ B cells in healthy adults, and 15–20% of blood B cells in mice. Transitional B cells can be further subdivided into T1, T2 and T3 subsets, and can increase in percentages upon infection and autoimmunity (Giltiay et al., 2019). There is a sizable body of literature correlating the frequency of IL-10-producing transitional (T2-MZ) B cells with transplantation tolerance (Newell et al., 2010; Pallier et al., 2010; Sagoo et al., 2010; Chesneau et al., 2014), leading to the hypothesis that Bregs were being induced and might modulate T cell responses to mediate allograft tolerance. However, a critical examination of the B cell tolerance signature when compared with cells from patients on immunosuppression and controls was subsequently conducted by Rebollo-Mesa et al. (2016). The authors found that the percentage of transitional B cells increased significantly upon steroid withdrawal. Subsequently, azathioprine as well as calcineurin inhibitors were reported to inhibit the levels of transitional IL-10-producing B cells. These findings raised concerns that transitional B cells may not predict nor mediate tolerance and that their elevated levels in tolerant recipients might be a response to the absence of immunosuppression (reviewed in Alhabbab et al., 2019). Nevertheless, the possibility remains that these IL-10-producing transitional B cells might contribute to graft survival as a consequence of their anti-inflammatory properties (reviewed in Alhabbab et al., 2019).

In addition to IL-10, IL-35-producing B cells and plasma cells have been reported to be critical regulators of immunity during autoimmune and infectious disease settings (Shen et al., 2014; Wang et al., 2014). IL-35 is a member of the IL-12 family, and is comprised of Ebi3, which is shared with IL-27, and a p35 subunit, which is shared with IL-12. As a result, the quantification of IL-35-producing B cells is challenging, and attribution of a role for IL-35 using single-chain (Ebi3)-deficient mice is complicated by concomitant loss of IL-27, a cytokine that also has anti-inflammatory and regulatory properties. Similarly, elimination of p35 not only results in loss of IL-35 but also IL-12 (Kourko et al., 2019; Mirlekar et al., 2021). Furthermore, IL-35 is produced by CD4$^+$FoxP3$^+$Tregs, CD8$^+$ Tregs, activated dendritic cells, and it signals through four receptors, IL-12Rβ2-IL-27Rα, IL-12Rβ2-IL-12Rβ2, IL-12Rβ2-GP130, and GP130-GP130 (Zhang et al., 2019). Thus, the complexity of IL-35 immunobiology requires that multiple controls be included to allow for a definitive demonstration that IL-35 is critical to the function of Bregs.

In the settings of allergy, cancer and autoimmune diseases, the regulatory function of B cells has been reported to be mediated by the potent immunoregulatory cytokine, TGFß (reviewed in Huai et al., 2021). In a model of anti-CD45RB-induced allograft tolerance, Zhao et al. (2010) reported that TGFß produced by B cells was necessary for tolerance, while IL-10 was not, and in fact appeared to promote chronic cardiac vasculopathy. Studies using a tolerance protocol of anti-CD45B and anti-TIM-1 to promote tolerance to islet allografts revealed an expansion of TIM-1$^+$LAP$^+$ B cells (Latency-associated peptide, LAP, is non-covalently associated with TGFß, and this complex is either secreted or deposited on the extracellular matrix), and TGFß was necessary for tolerance induction (Lee et al., 2012). Furthermore, TGFß, in combination with indoleamine 2,3-dioxygenase production by B cells, has been reported to regulate T cell proliferation, and promote the induction of TGFß and IL-10-producing Tregs *in vitro* (Nouel et al., 2015). Whether these TGFß-producing regulatory B cells represent a distinct phenotype and developmental lineage from the IL-10-producing Bregs requires further investigation.

Mirroring the observation that CD4$^+$ T cells have different effector and regulatory phenotypes (Hollbacher et al., 2020), B cells can also differentiate into different effector B cell subsets (Beff) producing different pro-inflammatory cytokines capable of enhancing T cell responses independently of antibody production (Lund, 2008; Shen and Fillatreau, 2015). These observations collectively raise the possibility that the ratio of Bregs to Beff may serve as a rheostat for effector T cell responses. In support of this notion, Cherukuri et al. (2014) reported that B cells co-producing TNFα and IL-10 and having a low IL-10/TNFα ratio lacked regulatory function, whereas those having a high IL-10/TNFα ratio effectively suppressed T cell production of IFNγ and TNFα. They further reported that the more immature T1 B cell subset had a significantly higher IL-10/TNFα ratio than the more mature T2 subset, and that a higher IL-10/TNFα ratio in the T1 subset best predicted an absence of T cell-mediated rejection and a better renal graft outcome (Cherukuri et al., 2017, 2021b). Despite its strong predictive value, it is nevertheless unclear whether the balance of IL10 and TNFα in the T1 B cell subset is a biomarker of tolerance or causally inhibits T cell-mediated rejection. T1 B cells are short-lived immature B cells that undergo apoptosis upon BCR engagement, and only a fraction of T1 B cells enter the B cell follicle to access appropriate survival signals and mature into naïve B cells (Chung et al., 2003; Zhou et al., 2020). Thus, where in the secondary lymphoid organs transitional B cells might gain access to T cells to suppress their activation, remains to be more fully explored. Recently, Giltiay et al. (2019) suggested a new perspective on these newly formed B cells, proposing that they function as a first line defense by producing "natural" antibodies and as antigen-presenting cells, based on their distinct BCR repertoire, high expression of activation induced cytidine deaminase (AID), high sensitivity to pathogen-associated molecular patterns (PAMPS) and their ability to produce cytokines. Thus, it is possible that B cells with a transitional phenotype may rapidly differentiate into antigen-presenting cells with the ability to regulate T cell responses through cytokine production.

Immunoregulation of T Cell Responses by Bregs Through Cognate Interactions

In addition to the production of immunomodulatory cytokines, there is accumulating evidence that cell surface molecules, such as PD-L1 and CD80/86, on Bregs, may engage coinhibitory molecules PD-1 and CTLA-4, respectively, to modulate T cell function (Blair et al., 2010; Siewe et al., 2013). Recently, Hasan et al. (2021) reported that T cell immunoreceptor with Ig and ITIM domains (TIGIT) is expressed on human memory CD19$^+$CD24$^+$CD27$^+$CD39$^+$IgD$^-$IgM$^+$CD1c$^+$ B cells that are

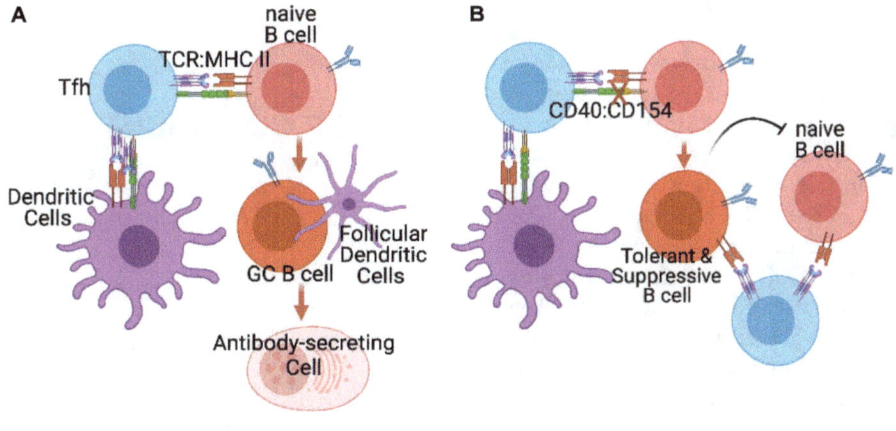

FIGURE 1 | (A) In untreated recipients of allografts, Tfh cells generated by initial encounter with recipient dendritic cells presenting alloantigen engage to provide help to naïve alloreactive B cells, and facilitate their differentiation into germinal center (GC) B cells and antibody-secreting plasmablasts and plasma cells. **(B)** In the presence of blocking anti-CD154 (X), naïve alloreactive B cells fail to receive signals from CD40 and thus differentiate into tolerance-induced B (TIB) cells incapable of differentiating into GC B cells or antibody-secreting cells. Instead these B cells acquire the ability to prevent naïve donor-specific B cells from differentiating into germinal center or antibody-secreting cells, by as yet to be defined mechanisms.

capable of mediating immune regulation *in vitro*. Although these B cells also expressed PD-L1, CD39/CD73 and TIM-1, as well as IL-10 and TGFß1, antagonism of TIGIT or granzyme B reduced their ability to suppress the production of IFNγ and IL-17 by anti-CD3/CD28-stimulated $CD4^+$ T cells. These observations suggest that the engagement of inhibitory receptors by ligands expressed on Breg cells may result in the suppression of $CD4^+$ T cell responses. Additionally, Breg cells were also able to inhibit monocyte-derived dendritic cell activation (CCR7, CD40, CD80/86, CD83, and ICOS-L) and their production of proinflammatory cytokines (IL-12A and IL-6) in response to LPS, thus highlighting a potential indirect mechanism of Breg-mediated control of T cell responses. Consistent with this possibility, Mohib et al. (2020) utilized 2-photon intravital microscopy to demonstrate cognate T:Breg cell interaction at the T:B border of spleens from immunized mice receiving antigen-pulsed Breg cells, and showed that a consequence of this T:Breg interaction is the reduced ability of the "regulated" T cells to interact with DCs. Whether Breg cells exert their regulation mainly within secondary lymphoid organs or are also able to migrate to sites of inflammation to modulate T cell responses, as has been reported for Tregs (Panduro et al., 2016; Campbell and Rudensky, 2020), remains to be clarified.

Immunoregulation of Donor-Specific B Cell Responses by TIB Cells

In models of transplantation tolerance, much of the focus has been on the ability of Bregs to control T cells responses, and indirectly, control T-dependent B cell responses. As a result, other than testing for donor-specific antibody, investigations into the fate of donor-specific B cells have been neglected. We have recently addressed this gap in knowledge by examining the fate of donor-MHC-specific B cells in a mouse model of cardiac allograft tolerance induced by anti-CD154 and donor spleen cells. We showed that donor-specific B cells become dysfunctional and are intrinsically unable to differentiate into germinal center B cells and plasma cells, even upon transfer into non-tolerant mice and exposed to donor-antigen (Khiew et al., 2020; **Figure 1**). The transferred TIB cells were able to sense antigen and respond by increasing expression of CD69 and Glut-1, and augmenting mitochondrial mass and cell size, but exhibited lower proliferation rates and expression of AID, consistent with a cell-intrinsic block after metabolic reprogramming but before entry into germinal centers.

Remarkably, when TIB cells were co-transferred with naïve B cells, they were able to inhibit the naïve B cell responses in a donor-specific manner, though it is not known whether this inhibition involves direct cognate B:B cell interaction or occurs through close by stander effects as a result of cognate interaction with a donor-specific T cell (**Figure 1**). These observations raise the novel possibility that B cells, upon encounter with alloantigen while being deprived of CD40 signals, become reprogrammed away from memory and plasma cell differentiation into B cells capable of suppressing other naïve B cells; this suppression is associated with thwarted differentiation of naïve B cells into germinal center B cells. It is notable that these TIB cells retain their ability to stimulate naïve antigen-specific T cell expansion and differentiation into Tfh cells, underscoring that such tolerant B cells were not mediating their effects though the overt suppression of T cell responses, as described for Bregs. The mechanism of donor-specific suppression of B cells responses by this unique subset of TIB cells requires further delineation.

CONCLUSION

In addition to antibody secretion, B cells can play many roles in alloimmunity, including antigen presentation to T cells, and suppression of immune responses by Breg cells or donor-specific B cells differentiating into suppressor cells when encountering alloantigens in the absence of CD40 costimulation. New results suggest that DSA production is not only regulated by the balance between Tfh and Tfr cells, but also by TIB cells that can inhibit *de novo* activation of naïve alloreactive B cells in a donor-specific manner. Moreover, Bregs may also control alloreactive T cell responses, thus potentially reinforcing transplantation tolerance. How Bregs may affect the function and ratio of Tfh and Tfr cells, and how Tfh/Tfr may impact Bregs in alloimmunity, as is being suggested in autoimmunity (reviewed in Ding et al., 2021), remains to be investigated. A better understanding of these interplays in animal models during primary alloimmune responses but also during memory alloimmune responses, as well as investigations into which of these mechanisms are conserved in humans, may help design immunosuppressive regimens that protect the transplants long term, and perhaps facilitate life-long transplantation tolerance.

AUTHOR CONTRIBUTIONS

AC, PS, and M-LA conceived and wrote the review. All authors contributed to the article and approved the submitted version.

FUNDING

AC and M-LA were funded by NIAID 2P01AI097113. AC was also funded by NIAID R01AI148705 and R01AI142747. PS was funded by NIAID P01AI56299 and R01AI153124.

REFERENCES

Alhabbab, R. Y., Nova-Lamperti, E., Aravena, O., Burton, H. M., Lechler, R. I., Dorling, A., et al. (2019). Regulatory B cells: Development, phenotypes, functions, and role in transplantation. *Immunol. Rev.* 292, 164–179. doi: 10.1111/imr.12800

Aloulou, M., Carr, E. J., Gador, M., Bignon, A., Liblau, R. S., Fazilleau, N., et al. (2016). Follicular regulatory T cells can be specific for the immunizing antigen and derive from naive T cells. *Nat. Commun.* 7:10579.

Aravena, O., Ferrier, A., Menon, M., Mauri, C., Aguillon, J. C., Soto, L., et al. (2017). TIM-1 defines a human regulatory B cell population that is altered in frequency and function in systemic sclerosis patients. *Arthritis Res. Ther.* 19:8.

Blair, P. A., Norena, L. Y., Flores-Borja, F., Rawlings, D. J., Isenberg, D. A., Ehrenstein, M. R., et al. (2010). CD19(+)CD24(hi)CD38(hi) B cells exhibit regulatory capacity in healthy individuals but are functionally impaired in systemic Lupus Erythematosus patients. *Immunity* 32, 129–140. doi: 10.1016/j.immuni.2009.11.009

Botta, D., Fuller, M. J., Marquez-Lago, T. T., Bachus, H., Bradley, J. E., Weinmann, A. S., et al. (2017). Dynamic regulation of T follicular regulatory cell responses by interleukin 2 during influenza infection. *Nat. Immunol.* 18, 1249–1260. doi: 10.1038/ni.3837

Brouard, S., Pallier, A., Renaudin, K., Foucher, Y., Danger, R., Devys, A., et al. (2012). The natural history of clinical operational tolerance after kidney transplantation through twenty-seven cases. *Am. J. Transplant.* 12, 3296–3307. doi: 10.1111/j.1600-6143.2012.04249.x

Campbell, C., and Rudensky, A. (2020). Roles of Regulatory T Cells in Tissue Pathophysiology and Metabolism. *Cell Metab.* 31, 18–25. doi: 10.1016/j.cmet.2019.09.010

Chen, W., Bai, J., Huang, H., Bi, L., Kong, X., Gao, Y., et al. (2017). Low proportion of follicular regulatory T cell in renal transplant patients with chronic antibody-mediated rejection. *Sci. Rep.* 7:1322.

Cherukuri, A., Mohib, K., and Rothstein, D. M. (2021a). Regulatory B cells: TIM-1, transplant tolerance, and rejection. *Immunol. Rev.* 299, 31–44. doi: 10.1111/imr.12933

Cherukuri, A., Rothstein, D. M., Clark, B., Carter, C. R., Davison, A., Hernandez-Fuentes, M., et al. (2014). Immunologic human renal allograft injury associates with an altered IL-10/TNF-alpha expression ratio in regulatory B cells. *J. Am. Soc. Nephrol.* 25, 1575–1585. doi: 10.1681/asn.2013080837

Cherukuri, A., Salama, A. D., Carter, C. R., Landsittel, D., Arumugakani, G., Clark, B., et al. (2017). Reduced human transitional B cell T1/T2 ratio is associated with subsequent deterioration in renal allograft function. *Kidney Int.* 91, 183–195. doi: 10.1016/j.kint.2016.08.028

Cherukuri, A., Salama, A. D., Mehta, R., Mohib, K., Zheng, L., Magee, C., et al. (2021b). Transitional B cell cytokines predict renal allograft outcomes. *Sci. Transl. Med.* 13:eabe4929. doi: 10.1126/scitranslmed.abe4929

Chesneau, M., Pallier, A., Braza, F., Lacombe, G., Le Gallou, S., Baron, D., et al. (2014). Unique B cell differentiation profile in tolerant kidney transplant patients. *Am. J. Transplant.* 14, 144–155. doi: 10.1111/ajt.12508

Chong, A. S., Rothstein, D. M., Safa, K., and Riella, L. V. (2019). Outstanding questions in transplantation: B cells, alloantibodies, and humoral rejection. *Am. J. Transplant.* 19, 2155–2163. doi: 10.1111/ajt.15323

Chung, J. B., Silverman, M., and Monroe, J. G. (2003). Transitional B cells: step by step towards immune competence. *Trends Immunol.* 24, 343–349.

Clement, R. L., Daccache, J., Mohammed, M. T., Diallo, A., Blazar, B. R., Kuchroo, V. K., et al. (2019). Follicular regulatory T cells control humoral and allergic immunity by restraining early B cell responses. *Nat. Immunol.* 20, 1360–1371. doi: 10.1038/s41590-019-0472-4

Crotty, S. (2019). T Follicular Helper Cell Biology: A Decade of Discovery and Diseases. *Immunity* 50, 1132–1148. doi: 10.1016/j.immuni.2019.04.011

Deng, J., Wei, Y., Fonseca, V. R., Graca, L., and Yu, D. (2019). T follicular helper cells and T follicular regulatory cells in rheumatic diseases. *Nat. Rev. Rheumatol.* 15, 475–490. doi: 10.1038/s41584-019-0254-2

Dilillo, D. J., Matsushita, T., and Tedder, T. F. (2010). B10 cells and regulatory B cells balance immune responses during inflammation, autoimmunity, and cancer. *Ann. N Y. Acad. Sci.* 1183, 38–57. doi: 10.1111/j.1749-6632.2009.05137.x

Ding, Q., Yeung, M., Camirand, G., Zeng, Q., Akiba, H., Yagita, H., et al. (2011). Regulatory B cells are identified by expression of TIM-1 and can be induced through TIM-1 ligation to promote tolerance in mice. *J Clin. Invest.* 121, 3645–3656. doi: 10.1172/jci46274

Ding, T., Su, R., Wu, R., Xue, H., Wang, Y., Su, R., et al. (2021). Frontiers of Autoantibodies in Autoimmune Disorders: Crosstalk Between Tfh/Tfr and Regulatory B Cells. *Front. Immunol* 12:641013. doi: 10.3389/fimmu.2021.641013

Fillatreau, S. (2018). Natural regulatory plasma cells. *Curr. Opin. Immunol.* 55, 62–66. doi: 10.1016/j.coi.2018.09.012

Fillatreau, S. (2019). Regulatory functions of B cells and regulatory plasma cells. *Biomed. J.* 42, 233–242. doi: 10.1016/j.bj.2019.05.008

Fonseca, V. R., Ribeiro, F., and Graca, L. (2019). T follicular regulatory (Tfr) cells: Dissecting the complexity of Tfr-cell compartments. *Immunol. Rev.* 288, 112–127. doi: 10.1111/imr.12739

Fonseca, V. R., Romao, V. C., Agua-Doce, A., Santos, M., Lopez-Presa, D., Ferreira, A. C., et al. (2018). Blood T Follicular Regulatory Cells / T Follicular Helper Cells ratio Marks Ectopic Lymphoid Structure Formation and PD-1(+) ICOS(+) T Follicular Helper Cells Indicate Disease Activity in Primary Sjogren's Syndrome. *Arthritis Rheumatol.* 70, 774–784. doi: 10.1002/art.40424

Fu, W., Liu, X., Lin, X., Feng, H., Sun, L., Li, S., et al. (2018). Deficiency in T follicular regulatory cells promotes autoimmunity. *J. Exp. Med.* 215, 815–825. doi: 10.1084/jem.20170901

Giltiay, N. V., Giordano, D., and Clark, E. A. (2019). The Plasticity of Newly Formed B Cells. *J. Immunol.* 203, 3095–3104. doi: 10.4049/jimmunol.1900928

Gonzalez-Figueroa, P., Roco, J. A., Papa, I., Nunez Villacis, L., Stanley, M., Linterman, M. A., et al. (2021). Follicular regulatory T cells produce neuritin to regulate B cells. *Cell* 184, 1775.e–1789.e.

Hasan, M. M., Nair, S. S., O'leary, J. G., Thompson-Snipes, L., Nyarige, V., Wang, J., et al. (2021). Implication of TIGIT(+) human memory B cells in immune regulation. *Nat. Commun.* 12:1534.

Hollbacher, B., Duhen, T., Motley, S., Klicznik, M. M., Gratz, I. K., and Campbell, D. J. (2020). Transcriptomic Profiling of Human Effector and Regulatory T Cell Subsets Identifies Predictive Population Signatures. *Immunohorizons* 4, 585–596. doi: 10.4049/immunohorizons.2000037

Hou, S., Clement, R. L., Diallo, A., Blazar, B. R., Rudensky, A. Y., Sharpe, A. H., et al. (2019). FoxP3 and Ezh2 regulate Tfr cell suppressive function and transcriptional program. *J. Exp. Med.* 216, 605–620. doi: 10.1084/jem.20181134

Huai, G., Markmann, J. F., Deng, S., and Rickert, C. G. (2021). TGF-beta-secreting regulatory B cells: unsung players in immune regulation. *Clin. Transl. Immunol.* 10:e1270.

Kalampokis, I., Yoshizaki, A., and Tedder, T. F. (2013). IL-10-producing regulatory B cells (B10 cells) in autoimmune disease. *Arthritis Res. Ther.* 15(Suppl. 1), S1.

Khiew, S. H., Jain, D., Chen, J., Yang, J., Yin, D., Young, J. S., et al. (2020). Transplantation tolerance modifies donor-specific B cell fate to suppress de novo alloreactive B cells. *J. Clin. Invest.* 130, 3453–3466. doi: 10.1172/jci132814

Kourko, O., Seaver, K., Odoardi, N., Basta, S., and Gee, K. (2019). IL-27, IL-30, and IL-35: A Cytokine Triumvirate in Cancer. *Front. Oncol.* 9:969. doi: 10.3389/fonc.2019.00969

La Muraglia, G. M. II, Wagener, M. E., Ford, M. L., and Badell, I. R. (2019). Circulating T follicular helper cells are a biomarker of humoral alloreactivity and predict donor-specific antibody formation after transplantation. *Am. J. Transplant.* 20, 75–87. doi: 10.1111/ajt.15517

Laidlaw, B. J., Lu, Y., Amezquita, R. A., Weinstein, J. S., Vander Heiden, J. A., Gupta, N. T., et al. (2017). Interleukin-10 from CD4(+) follicular regulatory T cells promotes the germinal center response. *Sci. Immunol.* 2:eaan4767. doi: 10.1126/sciimmunol.aan4767

Lee, K. M., Kim, J. I., Stott, R., Soohoo, J., O'connor, M. R., Yeh, H., et al. (2012). Anti-CD45RB/anti-TIM-1-induced tolerance requires regulatory B cells. *Am. J. Transplant.* 12, 2072–2078. doi: 10.1111/j.1600-6143.2012.04055.x

Lenert, P., Brummel, R., Field, E. H., and Ashman, R. F. (2005). TLR-9 activation of marginal zone B cells in lupus mice regulates immunity through increased IL-10 production. *J. Clin. Immunol.* 25, 29–40. doi: 10.1007/s10875-005-0355-6

Lin, X., Wang, X., Xiao, F., Ma, K., Liu, L., Wang, X., et al. (2019). IL-10-producing regulatory B cells restrain the T follicular helper cell response in primary Sjogren's syndrome. *Cell Mol. Immunol.* 16, 921–931. doi: 10.1038/s41423-019-0227-z

Lindner, S., Dahlke, K., Sontheimer, K., Hagn, M., Kaltenmeier, C., Barth, T. F., et al. (2013). Interleukin 21-induced granzyme B-expressing B cells infiltrate tumors and regulate T cells. *Cancer Res.* 73, 2468–2479. doi: 10.1158/0008-5472.can-12-3450

Lino, A. C., Dang, V. D., Lampropoulou, V., Welle, A., Joedicke, J., Pohar, J., et al. (2018). LAG-3 Inhibitory Receptor Expression Identifies Immunosuppressive Natural Regulatory Plasma Cells. *Immunity* 49, 120–133e129.

Lu, Y., Jiang, R., Freyn, A. W., Wang, J., Strohmeier, S., Lederer, K., et al. (2021). CD4+ follicular regulatory T cells optimize the influenza virus-specific B cell response. *J. Exp. Med.* 218:e20200547.

Lund, F. E. (2008). Cytokine-producing B lymphocytes-key regulators of immunity. *Curr. Opin. Immunol.* 20, 332–338. doi: 10.1016/j.coi.2008.03.003

Maceiras, A. R., Almeida, S. C. P., Mariotti-Ferrandiz, E., Chaara, W., Jebbawi, F., Six, A., et al. (2017). T follicular helper and T follicular regulatory cells have different TCR specificity. *Nat. Commun.* 8:15067.

Matsumoto, M., Baba, A., Yokota, T., Nishikawa, H., Ohkawa, Y., Kayama, H., et al. (2014). Interleukin-10-producing plasmablasts exert regulatory function in autoimmune inflammation. *Immunity* 41, 1040–1051. doi: 10.1016/j.immuni.2014.10.016

Mauri, C., Gray, D., Mushtaq, N., and Londei, M. (2003). Prevention of arthritis by interleukin 10-producing B cells. *J. Exp. Med.* 197, 489–501. doi: 10.1084/jem.20021293

Miller, M. L., Chong, A. S., and Alegre, M. L. (2017). Fifty shades of tolerance. *Curr. Transplant. Rep.* 4, 262–269.

Mirlekar, B., Michaud, D., and Pylayeva-Gupta, Y. (2021). IL-35 Detection in B Cells at the mRNA and Protein Level. *Methods Mol. Biol.* 2270, 125–147. doi: 10.1007/978-1-0716-1237-8_8

Mohammed, M. T., and Sage, P. T. (2020). Follicular T-cell regulation of alloantibody formation. *Curr. Opin. Organ. Transplant.* 25, 22–26. doi: 10.1097/mot.0000000000000715

Mohammed, M. T., Cai, S., Hanson, B. L., Zhang, H., Clement, R. L., Daccache, J., et al. (2021). Follicular T cells Mediate Donor Specific Antibody and Rejection after Solid Organ Transplantation. *Am. J. Transplant.* 21, 1893–1901. doi: 10.1111/ajt.16484

Mohib, K., Cherukuri, A., Zhou, Y., Ding, Q., Watkins, S. C., and Rothstein, D. M. (2020). Antigen-dependent interactions between regulatory B cells and T cells at the T:B border inhibit subsequent T cell interactions with DCs. *Am. J. Transplant.* 20, 52–63. doi: 10.1111/ajt.15546

Morris, H., Dewolf, S., Robins, H., Sprangers, B., Locascio, S. A., Shonts, B. A., et al. (2015). Tracking donor-reactive T cells: Evidence for clonal deletion in tolerant kidney transplant patients. *Sci. Transl. Med.* 7:272ra210. doi: 210.1126/scitranslmed.3010760

Newell, K. A., Asare, A., Kirk, A. D., Gisler, T. D., Bourcier, K., Suthanthiran, M., et al. (2010). Identification of a B cell signature associated with renal transplant tolerance in humans. *J. Clin. Invest.* 120, 1836–1847. doi: 10.1172/jci39933

Niu, Q., Mendoza Rojas, A., Dieterich, M., Roelen, D. L., Clahsen-Van Groningen, M. C., Wang, L., et al. (2020). Immunosuppression Has Long-Lasting Effects on Circulating Follicular Regulatory T Cells in Kidney Transplant Recipients. *Front. Immunol.* 11:1972. doi: 10.3389/fimmu.2020.01972

Nouel, A., Pochard, P., Simon, Q., Segalen, I., Le Meur, Y., Pers, J. O., et al. (2015). B-Cells induce regulatory T cells through TGF-beta/IDO production in A CTLA-4 dependent manner. *J. Autoimmun.* 59, 53–60. doi: 10.1016/j.jaut.2015.02.004

Pallier, A., Hillion, S., Danger, R., Giral, M., Racape, M., Degauque, N., et al. (2010). Patients with drug-free long-term graft function display increased numbers of peripheral B cells with a memory and inhibitory phenotype. *Kidney Int.* 78, 503–513. doi: 10.1038/ki.2010.162

Panduro, M., Benoist, C., and Mathis, D. (2016). Tissue Tregs. *Annu. Rev. Immunol.* 34, 609–633. doi: 10.1146/annurev-immunol-032712-095948

Rebollo-Mesa, I., Nova-Lamperti, E., Mobillo, P., Runglall, M., Christakoudi, S., Norris, S., et al. (2016). Biomarkers of Tolerance in Kidney Transplantation: Are We Predicting Tolerance or Response to Immunosuppressive Treatment? *Am. J. Transplant.* 16, 3443–3457. doi: 10.1111/ajt.13932

Sage, P. T., and Sharpe, A. H. (2016). T follicular regulatory cells. *Immunol. Rev.* 271, 246–259.

Sage, P. T., and Sharpe, A. H. (2020). The multifaceted functions of follicular regulatory T cells. *Curr. Opin. Immunol.* 67, 68–74. doi: 10.1016/j.coi.2020.10.009

Sage, P. T., Francisco, L. M., Carman, C. V., and Sharpe, A. H. (2013). The receptor PD-1 controls follicular regulatory T cells in the lymph nodes and blood. *Nat. Immunol.* 14, 152–161. doi: 10.1038/ni.2496

Sage, P. T., Paterson, A. M., Lovitch, S. B., and Sharpe, A. H. (2014). The coinhibitory receptor ctla-4 controls B cell responses by modulating T follicular helper, T follicular regulatory, and T regulatory cells. *Immunity* 41, 1026–1039. doi: 10.1016/j.immuni.2014.12.005

Sage, P. T., Ron-Harel, N., Juneja, V. R., Sen, D. R., Maleri, S., Sungnak, W., et al. (2016). Suppression by TFR cells leads to durable and selective inhibition of B cell effector function. *Nat. Immunol.* 17, 1436–1446. doi: 10.1038/ni.3578

Sagoo, P., Perucha, E., Sawitzki, B., Tomiuk, S., Stephens, D. A., Miqueu, P., et al. (2010). Development of a cross-platform biomarker signature to detect renal transplant tolerance in humans. *J. Clin. Invest.* 120, 1848–1861. doi: 10.1172/jci39922

Savage, T. M., Shonts, B. A., Obradovic, A., Dewolf, S., Lau, S., Zuber, J., et al. (2018). Early expansion of donor-specific Tregs in tolerant kidney transplant recipients. *JCI Insight* 3:124086. doi: 124010.121172/jci.insight.124086

Saze, Z., Schuler, P. J., Hong, C. S., Cheng, D., Jackson, E. K., and Whiteside, T. L. (2013). Adenosine production by human B cells and B cell-mediated suppression of activated T cells. *Blood* 122, 9–18. doi: 10.1182/blood-2013-02-482406

Shen, P., and Fillatreau, S. (2015). Antibody-independent functions of B cells: a focus on cytokines. *Nat. Rev. Immunol.* 15, 441–451. doi: 10.1038/nri3857

Shen, P., Roch, T., Lampropoulou, V., O'connor, R. A., Stervbo, U., Hilgenberg, E., et al. (2014). IL-35-producing B cells are critical regulators of immunity during autoimmune and infectious diseases. *Nature* 507, 366–370. doi: 10.1038/nature12979

Siewe, B., Stapleton, J. T., Martinson, J., Keshavarzian, A., Kazmi, N., Demarais, P. M., et al. (2013). Regulatory B cell frequency correlates with markers of HIV disease progression and attenuates anti-HIV CD8(+) T cell function in vitro. *J. Leukoc Biol.* 93, 811–818. doi: 10.1189/jlb.0912436

Stolp, J., Turka, L. A., and Wood, K. J. (2014). B cells with immune-regulating function in transplantation. *Nat. Rev. Nephrol.* 10, 389–397. doi: 10.1038/nrneph.2014.80

Sun, J., Wang, J., Pefanis, E., Chao, J., Rothschild, G., Tachibana, I., et al. (2015). Transcriptomics Identify CD9 as a Marker of Murine IL-10-Competent Regulatory B Cells. *Cell Rep.* 13, 1110–1117. doi: 10.1016/j.celrep.2015.09.070

Van De Veen, W., Stanic, B., Yaman, G., Wawrzyniak, M., Sollner, S., Akdis, D. G., et al. (2013). IgG4 production is confined to human IL-10-producing regulatory B cells that suppress antigen-specific immune responses. *J. Allergy Clin. Immunol.* 131, 1204–1212. doi: 10.1016/j.jaci.2013.01.014

Vanderleyden, I., Fra-Bido, S. C., Innocentin, S., Stebegg, M., Okkenhaug, H., Evans-Bailey, N., et al. (2020). Follicular Regulatory T Cells Can Access the Germinal Center Independently of CXCR5. *Cell Rep.* 30, 611–619e614.

Wang, R. X., Yu, C. R., Dambuza, I. M., Mahdi, R. M., Dolinska, M. B., Sergeev, Y. V., et al. (2014). Interleukin-35 induces regulatory B cells that suppress autoimmune disease. *Nat. Med.* 20, 633–641. doi: 10.1038/nm.3554

Wang, Y., Liu, Z., Wu, J., Li, F., Li, G., and Dong, N. (2020). Profiling circulating T follicular helper cells and their effects on B cells in post-cardiac transplant recipients. *Ann. Transl. Med.* 8:1369. doi: 10.21037/atm-20-3027

Wing, J. B., Ise, W., Kurosaki, T., and Sakaguchi, S. (2014). Regulatory T cells control antigen-specific expansion of Tfh cell number and humoral immune responses via the coreceptor CTLA-4. *Immunity* 41, 1013–1025. doi: 10.1016/j.immuni.2014.12.006

Wing, J. B., Lim, E. L., and Sakaguchi, S. (2020). Control of foreign Ag-specific Ab responses by Treg and Tfr. *Immunol. Rev.* 296, 104–119. doi: 10.1111/imr.12888

Wollenberg, I., Agua-Doce, A., Hernandez, A., Almeida, C., Oliveira, V. G., Faro, J., et al. (2011). Regulation of the germinal center reaction by Foxp3+ follicular regulatory T cells. *J. Immunol.* 187, 4553–4560. doi: 10.4049/jimmunol.1101328

Wu, H., Chen, Y., Liu, H., Xu, L. L., Teuscher, P., Wang, S., et al. (2016). Follicular regulatory T cells repress cytokine production by follicular helper T cells and optimize IgG responses in mice. *Eur. J. Immunol.* 46, 1152–1161.

Yan, L., Li, Y., Li, Y., Wu, X., Wang, X., Wang, L., et al. (2019). Increased circulating Tfh to Tfr ratio in chronic renal allograft dysfunction: a pilot study. *BMC Immunol.* 20:26. doi: 10.1186/s12865-019-0308-x

Yang, C., Ge, J., Rosales, I., Yuan, Q., Szuter, E., Acheampong, E., et al. (2020). Kidney-induced systemic tolerance of heart allografts in mice. *JCI Insight* 5:e139331.

Yeung, M. Y., Ding, Q., Brooks, C. R., Xiao, S., Workman, C. J., Vignali, D. A., et al. (2015). TIM-1 signaling is required for maintenance and induction of regulatory B cells. *Am. J. Transplant.* 15, 942–953. doi: 10.1111/ajt.13087

Zhang, J., Zhang, Y., Wang, Q., Li, C., Deng, H., Si, C., et al. (2019). Interleukin-35 in immune-related diseases: protection or destruction. *Immunology* 157, 13–20. doi: 10.1111/imm.13044

Zhang, X. (2013). Regulatory functions of innate-like B cells. *Cell Mol. Immunol.* 10, 113–121. doi: 10.1038/cmi.2012.63

Zhao, G., Moore, D. J., Lee, K. M., Kim, J. I., Duff, P. E., O'connor, M. R., et al. (2010). An unexpected counter-regulatory role of IL-10 in B-lymphocyte-mediated transplantation tolerance. *Am. J. Transplant.* 10, 796–801. doi: 10.1111/j.1600-6143.2010.03027.x

Zhou, Y., Zhang, Y., Han, J., Yang, M., Zhu, J., and Jin, T. (2020). Transitional B cells involved in autoimmunity and their impact on neuroimmunological diseases. *J. Transl. Med.* 18:131.

4

Mast cells as regulators of T cell responses

Silvia Bulfone-Paus and Rajia Bahri*

Manchester Collaborative Centre for Inflammation Research (MCCIR), Institute of Inflammation and Repair, University of Manchester, Manchester, UK

Edited by:
Elisabetta Padovan, University of Basel, Switzerland

Reviewed by:
Carlo Pucillo, University of Udine, Italy
Shahram Salek-Ardakani, University of Florida, USA
Eric Espinosa, University of Toulouse, France

***Correspondence:**
Silvia Bulfone-Paus, Manchester Collaborative Centre for Inflammation Research (MCCIR), Institute of Inflammation and Repair, University of Manchester, Core Technology Facility, Room 2.18a, 46 Grafton Street, Manchester M13 9NT, UK
silvia.bulfone-paus@manchester.ac.uk

Mast cells (MCs) are recognized to participate in the regulation of innate and adaptive immune responses. Owing to their strategic location at the host–environment interface, they control tissue homeostasis and are key cells for starting early host defense against intruders. Upon degranulation induced, e.g., by immunoglobulin E (IgE) and allergen-mediated engagement of the high-affinity IgE receptor, complement or certain neuropeptide receptors, MCs release a wide variety of preformed and newly synthesized products including proteases, lipid mediators, and many cytokines, chemokines, and growth factors. Interestingly, increasing evidence suggests a regulatory role for MCs in inflammatory diseases via the regulation of T cell activities. Furthermore, rather than only serving as effector cells, MCs are now recognized to induce T cell activation, recruitment, proliferation, and cytokine secretion in an antigen-dependent manner and to impact on regulatory T cells. This review synthesizes recent developments in MC–T cell interactions, discusses their biological and clinical relevance, and explores recent controversies in this field of MC research.

Keywords: mast cells, CD4 T cell, CD8 T cell, Treg cells, adaptive immunity

Introduction

Mast cells (MCs) are among the most malleable and rapidly responding cells of the immune system. Within seconds of activation, they release a multitude of preformed biologically active products, followed by marked changes in cytoplasmic composition and volume that enable reconstitution of their morphology and cell content within hours (1, 2). Counterintuitively, this cell-regenerative phase coincides with a striking wave of mediator synthesis and secretion. Therefore, tissue-resident MCs have the potential to strongly shape their tissue microenvironment and direct cell–cell interactions and immune cell responses even while running through a reconstitution phase, during which they are relatively "refractory" to external stimuli.

Derived from either hematopoietic precursors or local, tissue-resident progenitors, mature MCs represent a heterogeneous collective of long lived, granulated cells located in essentially all tissues, which increase in number upon proliferation or increased recruitment, survival, and/or maturation of MC progenitors (1–3). They are particularly abundant at barrier sites, such as the skin, lung, and gut, and play an important role in defense against, and clearance of various pathogens (4, 5).

While the involvement of MCs in allergic/inflammatory reactions triggered by the crosslinking of FcεRI-bound immunoglobulin E (IgE) by antigen has been characterized in detail (6), the extent of MC function in autoimmune diseases is less well understood (7, 8). Upon activation, MCs release a plethora of mediators, including growth factors, cytokines, and chemokines (e.g., IL-1, IL-6, IL-8, IL-10, TNFα, VEGF, TGFβ, CCL2-4) as well as pro-inflammatory lipid mediators, such as prostaglandins and leukotrienes. However, MCs are mostly known for the ability to degranulate and very rapidly release preformed mediators from cytoplasmic granules, such as vasoactive amines (histamine and serotonin), proteoglycans (e.g., heparin), proteases (above all tryptases and chymases), and some pre-stored cytokines (e.g., TNFα) (1, 2, 9).

As players in innate immunity MCs have the capacity to initiate and amplify immune responses. Several lines of evidence have demonstrated that MCs participate in the sensitization phase of acquired immune responses via the secretion of mediators, which sustain dendritic cell (DC) maturation, function, and recruitment to the tissue or their migration to local draining lymph nodes (10). However, MCs also exert important effector function since MCs and T cells of different origin and subsets establish tight cell–cell interactions and modulate their respective effector functions in a bidirectional manner; this has been shown in a variety of models (11–13). Interestingly, MCs can even present antigen to T cells in a MHC class I- or class II-restricted mechanism (11, 13, 14).

This review focuses on MC-mediated regulation of T cell responses (**Figure 1**) since this activity not only shows MCs to be an important element of acquired immunity but also to play a cardinal role in shaping, controlling, sustaining, or arresting inflammatory responses at host–environment interfaces and, thus, of major clinical relevance.

MCs as Regulators of CD4$^+$ T Cell Effector Functions

Historically, MCs have been associated with the regulation of Th2 immune responses, and as such their modulatory activities on CD4$^+$ T cells have been amply documented in many different models (**Figure 1A**).

In 1993, the Mecheri group reported that murine bone marrow-derived mast cells (BMMCs) displayed antigen-presenting cell (APC) functions (15), with these findings later extended to MCs of rat and human origin (16–18). Efficient BMMC antigen presentation to CD4$^+$ T cells was shown to require expression of the costimulatory molecules CD80 and CD86, which are induced by IL-4 and granulocyte/macrophage-colony-stimulating factor (GM-CSF). Interestingly, in their studies, interferon (IFN) γ completely abrogated this phenomenon (19, 20); this IFNγ effect could

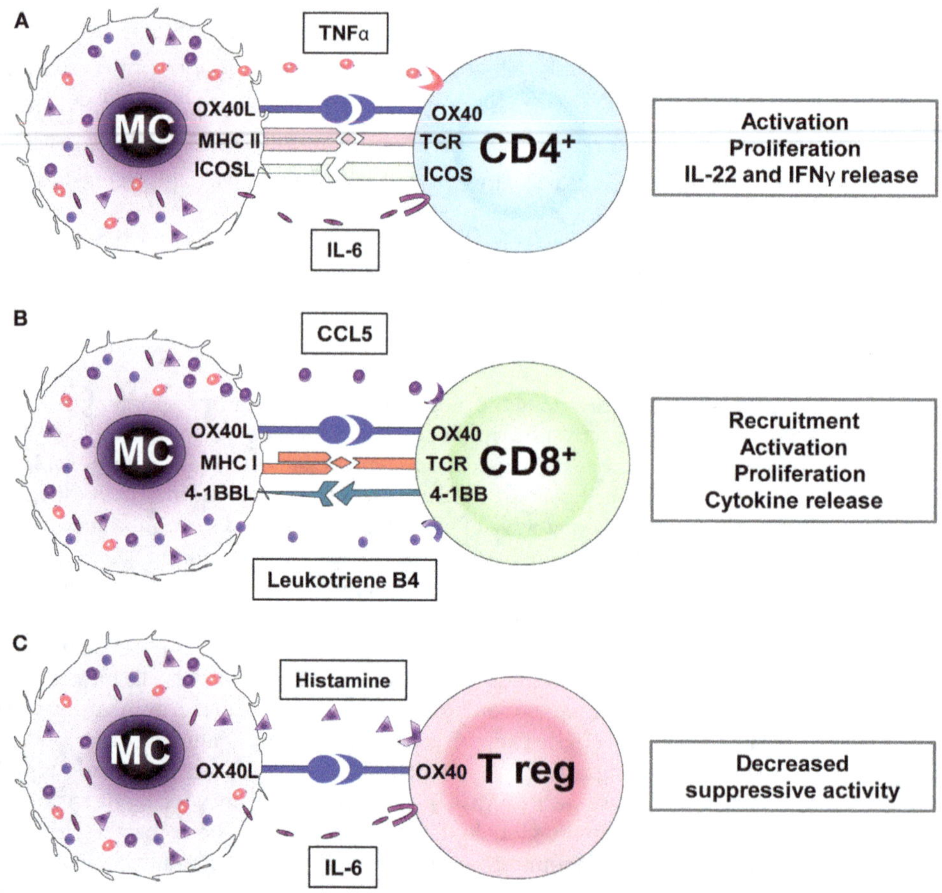

FIGURE 1 | Receptors and mediators involved in the interaction between mast cells (MCs) with CD4$^+$ (A), CD8$^+$ (B), and regulatory T cells (Tregs) (C). **(A)** MCs promote the activation, proliferation, and cytokine secretion (e.g., IL-22, IFNγ) of CD4$^+$ T cells via MHC II and OX40L cell–cell interactions and TNFα secretion. **(B)** MCs induce CD8$^+$ T cell recruitment via the release of chemokines (e.g., CCL5) and leukotriene B4. Furthermore, MC-mediated CD8$^+$ T cell activation requires MHC I/TCR, OX40L/OX40, and 4-1BBL/4-1BB receptors interaction. **(C)** The OX40/OX40L-directed interaction between Treg and MCs and the histamine and IL-6 production by the latter inhibit the suppressive Treg activity.

be counteracted by FcεRI-mediated antigen endocytosis (21). In contrast to the above study, IFNγ-primed mouse MCs in their antigen-mediated interaction with $CD4^+$ T cells were shown to develop a functional immunological synapse (22).

More recently, Gaudenzio and colleagues (23) have defined MCs as "tissue-localized" APCs, which (in inflamed human psoriatic skin) are primed by locally produced IFNγ to present antigen to experienced and recruited $CD4^+$ T cells. IFNγ-primed human MCs establish synaptic contacts with effector/memory $CD4^+$ T cells, thus inducing Th22 and IL-22^+IFNγ^+Th cell subsets via the release of IL-6 and TNFα. Interestingly, in inflammatory conditions in which both MCs and T cells are enriched, as seen in psoriatic skin, the majority of IL-22^+ and IFN$\gamma^+$$CD4^+$ T cells are in close contact with MCs and the latter act as amplifiers of inflammation (23).

Since IL-6 and TNFα are mediators commonly released by activated MCs upon a wide range of stimuli, it remains unclear whether the IFNγ-induced MC search for immune partners is broad or restricted to a specific cell type or T cell subset; and how this encounter is spatially and temporally controlled. Furthermore, whether this cognate interaction leads to bidirectional effector functions, which might shape long-term MC activities is yet to be defined.

The antigen presentation activity of murine MCs and the MC-dependent modulation of effector T cell functions correlates with the induced expression of MHC class II molecules (14, 24) together with the up-regulation of a wide variety of costimulatory molecules, including members of the B7 family (ICOS ligand, PD-L1, and PD-L2) and the TNF/TNFR families (OX40L, CD153, Fas, and 4-1BB) (25).

In conjunction with the secretion of TNFα, the up-regulation of the costimulatory molecule OX40L, in particular, has been demonstrated to be essential for the MC-$CD4^+$ T cell crosstalk and modulation of effector T cell function (25). OX40L expression was reported to be induced by exposure of mouse MCs to stimuli, such as toll-like receptor (TLR) agonists and FcεRI engagement (24). Furthermore, Notch signaling was shown to upregulate MHC class II and OX40L expression on mouse MCs thus promoting the proliferation $CD4^+$ T cells and their differentiation into T helper 2 cells producing IL-4, IL-5, IL-10, and IL-13 (26).

Interestingly, treatment of human MCs with type I IFNs had the opposite effect of down-regulating both TNFα and OX40L expression while inducing IL-10 and TGFβ production with the consequence of restraining $CD4^+$ T cell effector activities (27). This latter report underlies the key role of the inflammatory microenvironment in tightly controlling the outcome of MC–T cell interactions, and also suggests that the antigen presentation ability of MCs is possibly not intrinsic to this cell type but varies in response to time and location.

Gong and colleagues have proposed that the antigen-presenting property is restricted to an $Fc\varepsilon RI^{hi}$, MHC II^+, and c-kit^+ mouse MC subset (28). However, considering the plasticity of MCs, one could interpret the $Fc\varepsilon RI^{hi}$ and MHC II^+ expression on MCs rather as a transitory "activation" state born of environmental (allergen) or inflammatory pressure rather than as a bona fide subset of MCs.

In vitro as well as *in vivo* MCs are a heterogeneous cell population, and their MHC class II expression is variable and inducible. However, MHC class II molecules are not confined to a "professional" MHC class II compartment as it is found in professional APCs, but are stored in mature and immature forms in both lysosomal and secretory granules of MCs [Ref. (29); reviewed in Ref. (11)]. Furthermore, it has been reported that MC-mediated T cell activation is mediated via exosome release (30). It is therefore tempting to speculate that antigen presentation in MCs may be the result of both direct cognate cell–cell interactions between MCs and T cells and MC-secreted MHC class II and costimulatory molecule-loaded exosomes acting upon T cells.

MCs as Modulators of $CD8^+$ T Cell Responses

Recent evidence has suggested a protective role for MCs in antiviral immune responses (31–35). This is based on the observation that MCs are equipped with a full repertoire of pattern recognition receptors, including TLRs (36), which allow MCs to sense and respond to most microbial components, including viruses.

Upon TLR engagement, mouse MCs are activated to secrete chemokines, of which notably CCL5 can recruit effector $CD8^+$ T cells (37). Reovirus-infected human MCs have been shown, through release of chemokines including CCL3, CCL4, and CCL5, to selectively recruit cytotoxic effector cells, thus suggesting their ability to enhance viral immunity (31).

Furthermore, in a model of murine cytomegalovirus (CMV) infection, activated MCs have been described to recruit $CD8^+$ T cells to the lungs via CCL5 release and thus contribute to a reduction in the viral load and the clearance of infection (34). MC activation upon CMV infection is characterized by an immediate TLR3/TRIF signaling-dependent phase and a delayed TLR3/TRIF-independent pathway phase (38). In allergy models, the MC-mediated recruitment of effector, but not central memory, $CD8^+$ T cells to sites of inflammation was shown to be dependent on the production of MC leukotriene B4 (39).

However, the interactions between MCs and $CD8^+$ T cells go far beyond that of chemokine-induced recruitment (**Figure 1B**). MCs have been reported to be capable of antigen presentation via MHC class I molecules to T cells following phagocytosis and processing of bacterial antigens from live bacteria (40). Furthermore, physical MC/$CD8^+$ T-cell contacts have been demonstrated in healthy human skin. In lesional skin from alopecia areata (AA) patients, MCs display an activated phenotype prominently expressing MHC class I and the costimulatory molecules OX40L and 4-1BBL. Furthermore, abnormal MC numbers, effector functions, and increased interactions with $CD8^+$ T cells were observed in the grafted C3H/HeJ mouse model of AA and in a recently developed humanized mouse model for AA (41). Here, in a pathological inflammatory environment, activated MCs may contribute to the collapse of hair follicle immune privilege by initiating/sustaining $CD8^+$ T cell effector functions, thus promoting the disease (41).

Importantly, MC initiated antigen-dependent and MHC class I-mediated cross-presentation to $CD8^+$ T cells has been shown to regulate $CD8^+$ T cell effector functions including proliferation, cytokine secretion, and cytotoxic activity *in vitro*;

this was supported by complementary *in vivo* studies in which antigen-specific CD8$^+$ T cell numbers were reduced in MC-deficient mice, using the experimental autoimmune encephalomyelitis (EAE) model (42). These studies support previously published evidence that MC-deficient mice not only display defective CD4$^+$ but also CD8$^+$ T cell numbers in EAE (43) as well as in *Leishmania major* infection (44).

A specific priming of CD8$^+$ effector T cells in the tissue at the site of inflammation, delivered by resident immune cells, such as MCs, may also be a relevant strategy not only to, initially, promote protective inflammation but also to control and limit excessive and/or chronic cytotoxic activity. However, very little evidence has been published to date on CD8$^+$ T cell/MC interactions. Therefore, closing this important gap in our understanding of MCs functions in health and disease should be a prime future research focus.

MCs as Suppressors of T Cell Effector Functions

Mast cells are also able to suppress T cell effector functions, namely, by their interaction with regulatory T cells (Treg) (**Figure 1C**). Adoptive transfer of Tregs in a mouse model of sepsis correlated with increased MC numbers (45). Furthermore, MCs contribute to the induction of tolerance to alloantigens being recruited to skin allografts in response to IL-9 secreted by Tregs (46, 47).

In line with the previously reported finding that high-FcεRI expression correlates with efficient antigen-presenting abilities in MCs (24, 28), Treg cells down-regulate FcεRI expression in MCs (48). Mouse MCs have been shown to secrete histamine and IL-6 and to use the OX40/OX40L signaling pathway to inhibit Treg functions and to thus promote optimal activation of effector CD4$^+$ and CD8$^+$ T cells (49–52).

However, it remains unclear which conditions promote the suppression of MC functions by Tregs versus the inhibition of Tregs by MCs. Moreover, it is conceivable that, under some conditions, MC activation may overcome Treg-mediated immunosuppression, promote the development of effective antitumor immunity, and boost the immune response in the tissue, while a different signaling environment may contribute to allograft tolerance in transplantation. Only a better definition of the relevant molecular check points will clarify the mechanisms that underlie these opposite functional outcomes and will identify promising targets for therapeutic interventions.

Controversies in the Field

However, it should be acknowledged that the regulatory impact of MCs on T cell functions is still a controversially debated field. Namely, studies utilizing various MC-deficient mouse models have claimed that MCs are non-essential for the regulation of either CD4$^+$ or CD8$^+$ T cell immune responses (53, 54). Yet, this does not necessarily exclude T cell-regulatory MC activities under physiological conditions.

Mast cell function has been classically studied using the MC-deficient C57BL/6-Kit$^{W\text{-}sh/W\text{-}sh}$ or *Kit*$^{W/W\text{-}V}$ mice, whose MC deficiencies arise through loss of function mutations affecting Kit. However, these mice are limited in their usefulness by their perturbed immune cell composition, as such a number of new "Kit-independent" MC-deficient strains have been generated (53, 55, 56). These mice have the great advantage of deleting the MC population without apparently affecting other immune populations, with the exception of basophils (strain dependent), and have called into question findings originally obtained using Kit-dependent MC-deficient mice.

Owing to the use of multiple mouse strains and diseases models, the role of MCs in autoimmune diseases has been very controversial, with some authors tending to conclude that MCs are generally dispensable in autoimmunity (53). However, very recently, Schubert and colleagues investigated in more detail the function of MCs in arthritis using different strains of MC-deficient mice and in models, either based on autoreactive antibody transfer or effector T cells (57). Interestingly, these authors found MCs to be critically relevant in the T cell-dependent mouse model of rheumatoid arthritis [collagen-induced arthritis (CIA)], while being dispensable in the T cell-independent antibody-induced arthritis model. In the CIA model, absence of MCs resulted in dramatic loss of T cell expansion upon immunization and concomitant reduction in T cell cytokine responses (57). These recent findings underscore the critical role of MCs in T cell-dependent autoimmunity.

However, in a T cell-dependent spontaneous diabetes model, using non-obese diabetic (NOD) mice, MCs failed to impact on CD4$^+$ and CD8$^+$ T cell numbers measured at the onset of the disease (54). However, this study left it unclear whether at later time points during disease progression, i.e., when the phenotype divergence between MC deficient and wild-type mice may be greatest, or during spontaneous disease resolution, the absence or presence of MCs would have impacted upon T cell responses and clinical outcome.

Possibly, the most contentious issue has been the role of MCs in multiple sclerosis (MS), particularly in the T cell-dependent surrogate mouse model of EAE, with some studies arguing an important role for MCs (58, 59), while another one claims that they are dispensable (53). This controversial discussion has been very important and productive in the sense that it has brought to light the limitations in the use of each of the presently available MC-deficient mouse strains, and has underscored the urgent need for standardized disease-induction protocols to improve data reproducibility. Furthermore, these discrepancies have served to acutely remind us of the constitutive difficulties one faces in translating murine data to the human condition.

Conclusion and Perspectives

In this review, we have highlighted interactions between MCs and T cells, which regulate adaptive immune responses and have delineated that the antigen-presenting activity of tissue-resident immune cells, such as MCs, is fundamental to the maintenance of productive and protective inflammation. MCs may also actively participate in the fundamental processes, which minimize immune-mediated bystander damage to healthy tissues.

We have also reviewed the evidence that MC can modulate Treg activities. However, the mechanisms and dynamics that interrupt MC-mediated antigen presentation, down-regulate the MC-induced amplification of T cell-dependent immune response, and restore local Treg cell homeostasis, all remain to be dissected by future research.

This review has closed with discussing contradictory results and the ensuing controversial debate on the role of MC in experimental autoimmune disease. It is important to keep in mind that the conflicting findings were generated using different MC-deficient mouse strains. This raises the pertinent question whether models, which rely on the deletion of an entire cell population, such as MCs, which are notoriously heterogeneous, highly plastic and adaptable in nature, and excel in their capacity to rapidly shift the spectrum of mediators released and surface markers expressed in distinct signaling environments (e.g., homeostatic versus inflammatory settings), are not overly simplistic. Can such models possibly reflect the (very transitory) dynamics of MC biology *in vivo*? Therefore, the ultimate research tool for definitively clarifying the contribution of MCs to the regulation of T cell functions under physiological and pathological conditions, which fully takes into account the dynamism and heterogeneity of MCs, may still have to be developed.

Author Contributions

SP and RB drafted and revised the manuscript.

Acknowledgments

We thank Michelle Campbell, Martin Barron, and Ralf Paus for the critical reading of the manuscript. This study was supported by the COST Action BM1007 "Mast cells and Basophils: targets for innovative therapies."

References

1. Galli SJ, Grimbaldeston M, Tsai M. Immunomodulatory mast cells: negative, as well as positive, regulators of immunity. *Nat Rev Immunol* (2008) **8**:478–86. doi:10.1038/nri2327
2. Gurish MF, Austen KF. Developmental origin and functional specialization of mast cell subsets. *Immunity* (2012) **37**:25–33. doi:10.1016/j.immuni.2012.07.003
3. Sugawara K, Bíró T, Tsuruta D, Tóth BI, Kromminga A, Zákány N, et al. Endocannabinoids limit excessive mast cell maturation and activation in human skin. *J Allergy Clin Immunol* (2012) **129**:726–38. doi:10.1016/j.jaci.2011.11.009
4. Janssens AS, Heide R, den Hollander JC, Mulder PG, Tank B, Oranje AP. Mast cell distribution in normal adult skin. *J Clin Pathol* (2005) **58**:285–9. doi:10.1136/jcp.2004.017210
5. Abraham SN, St John AL. Mast cell-orchestrated immunity to pathogens. *Nat Rev Immunol* (2010) **10**:440–52. doi:10.1038/nri2782
6. Galli SJ, Tsai M. IgE and mast cells in allergic disease. *Nat Med* (2012) **18**:693–704. doi:10.1038/nm.2755
7. Walker ME, Hatfield JK, Brown MA. New insights into the role of mast cells in autoimmunity: evidence for a common mechanism of action? *Biochim Biophys Acta* (2012) **1822**:57–65. doi:10.1016/j.bbadis.2011.02.009
8. Rodewald HR, Feyerabend TB. Widespread immunological functions of mast cells: fact or fiction? *Immunity* (2012) **37**:13–24. doi:10.1016/j.immuni.2012.07.007
9. Jobbings CE, Sandig H, Whittingham-Dowd JK, Roberts IS, Bulfone-Paus S. *Listeria monocytogenes* alters mast cell phenotype, mediator and osteopontin secretion in a listeriolysin-dependent manner. *PLoS One* (2013) **8**:e57102. doi:10.1371/journal.pone.0057102
10. McLachlan JB, Shelburne CP, Hart JP, Pizzo SV, Goyal R, Brooking-Dixon R, et al. Mast cell activators: a new class of highly effective vaccine adjuvants. *Nat Med* (2008) **14**:536–41. doi:10.1038/nm1757
11. Valitutti S, Espinosa E. Cognate interactions between mast cells and helper T lymphocytes. *Self Nonself* (2010) **1**:114–22. doi:10.4161/self.1.2.11795
12. Gri G, Frossi B, D'Inca F, Danelli L, Betto E, Mion F, et al. Mast cell: an emerging partner in immune interaction. *Front Immunol* (2012) **3**:120. doi:10.3389/fimmu.2012.00120
13. Mekori YA, Hershko AY, Frossi B, Mion F, Pucillo CE. Integrating innate and adaptive immune cells: mast cells as crossroads between regulatory and effector B and T cells. *Eur J Pharmacol* (2015). doi:10.1016/j.ejphar.2015.03.087
14. Kambayashi T, Laufer TM. Atypical MHC class II-expressing antigen-presenting cells: can anything replace a dendritic cell? *Nat Rev Immunol* (2014) **14**:719–30. doi:10.1038/nri3754
15. Frandji P, Oskéritzian C, Cacaraci F, Lapeyre J, Peronet R, David B, et al. Antigen-dependent stimulation by bone marrow-derived mast cells of MHC class II-restricted T cell hybridoma. *J Immunol* (1993) **151**:6318–28.
16. Fox CC, Jewell SD, Whitacre CC. Rat peritoneal mast cells present antigen to a PPD-specific T cell line. *Cell Immunol* (1994) **158**:253–64. doi:10.1006/cimm.1994.1272
17. Poncet P, Arock M, David B. MHC class II-dependent activation of CD4$^+$ T cell hybridomas by human mast cells through superantigen presentation. *J Leukoc Biol* (1999) **66**:105–12.
18. Suurmond J, van Heemst J, van Heiningen J, Dorjée AL, Schilham MW, van der Beek FB, et al. Communication between human mast cells and CD4$^+$ T cells through antigen-dependent interactions. *Eur J Immunol* (2013) **43**:1758–68. doi:10.1002/eji.201243058
19. Frandji P, Tkaczyk C, Oskéritzian C, Lapeyre J, Peronet R, David B, et al. Presentation of soluble antigens by mast cells: upregulation by interleukin-4 and granulocyte/macrophage colony-stimulating factor and downregulation by interferon-gamma. *Cell Immunol* (1995) **163**:37–46. doi:10.1006/cimm.1995.1096
20. Frandji P, Tkaczyk C, Oskeritzian C, David B, Desaymard C, Mecheri S. Exogenous and endogenous antigens are differentially presented by mast cells to CD4 T lymphocytes. *Eur J Immunol* (1996) **26**:2517–28. doi:10.1002/eji.1830261036
21. Tkaczyk C, Villa I, Peronet R, David B, Mecheri S. FcεRI-mediated antigen endocytosis turns interferon-gamma-treated mouse mast cells from inefficient into potent antigen-presenting cells. *Immunology* (1999) **97**:333–40. doi:10.1046/j.1365-2567.1999.00789.x
22. Gaudenzio N, Espagnolle N, Mars LT, Liblau R, Valitutti S, Espinosa E. Cell-cell cooperation at the T helper cell/mast cell immunological synapse. *Blood* (2009) **114**:4979–88. doi:10.1182/blood-2009-02-202648
23. Gaudenzio N, Laurent C, Valitutti S, Espinosa E. Human mast cells drive memory CD4$^+$ T cells toward an inflammatory IL-22+ phenotype. *J Allergy Clin Immunol* (2013) **131**:1400–7. doi:10.1016/j.jaci.2013.01.029
24. Kambayashi T, Allenspach EJ, Chang JT, Zou T, Shoag JE, Reiner SL, et al. Inducible MHC class II expression by mast cells supports effector and regulatory T cell activation. *J Immunol* (2009) **182**:4686–95. doi:10.4049/jimmunol.0803180
25. Nakae S, Suto H, Iikura M, Kakurai M, Sedgwick JD, Tsai M, et al. Mast cells enhance T cell activation: importance of mast cell costimulatory molecules and secreted TNF. *J Immunol* (2006) **176**:2238–48. doi:10.4049/jimmunol.176.4.2238
26. Nakano N, Nishiyama C, Yagita H, Koyanagi A, Akiba H, Chiba S, et al. Notch signaling confers antigen-presenting cell functions on mast cells. *J Allergy Clin Immunol* (2009) **123**:74–81. doi:10.1016/j.jaci.2008.10.040
27. Fujita T, Kambe N, Uchiyama T, Hori T. Type I interferons attenuate T cell activating functions of human mast cells by decreasing TNF-alpha production and OX40 ligand expression while increasing IL-10 production. *J Clin Immunol* (2006) **26**:512–8. doi:10.1007/s10875-006-9043-1
28. Gong J, Yang NS, Croft M, Weng IC, Sun L, Liu FT, et al. The antigen presentation function of bone marrow-derived mast cells is spatiotemporally restricted to a subset expressing high levels of cell surface FcεRI and MHC II. *BMC Immunol* (2010) **11**:34. doi:10.1186/1471-2172-11-34

29. Raposo G, Tenza D, Mecheri S, Peronet R, Bonnerot C, Desaymard C. Accumulation of major histocompatibility complex class II molecules in mast cell secretory granules and their release upon degranulation. *Mol Biol Cell* (1997) **8**:2631–45. doi:10.1091/mbc.8.12.2631
30. Skokos D, Le Panse S, Villa I, Rousselle JC, Peronet R, David B, et al. Mast cell-dependent B and T lymphocyte activation is mediated by the secretion of immunologically active exosomes. *J Immunol* (2001) **166**:868–76. doi:10.4049/jimmunol.166.2.868
31. McAlpine SM, Issekutz TB, Marshall JS. Virus stimulation of human mast cells results in the recruitment of $CD56_+$ T cells by a mechanism dependent on CCR5 ligands. *FASEB J* (2012) **26**:1280–9. doi:10.1096/fj.11-188979
32. Avirutnan P, Matangkasombut P. Unmasking the role of mast cells in dengue. *Elife* (2013) **30**(2):e00767. doi:10.7554/eLife.00767
33. Liu B, Meng D, Wei T, Zhang S, Hu Y, Wang M. Apoptosis and pro-inflammatory cytokine response of mast cells induced by influenza A viruses. *PLoS One* (2014) **9**(6):e100109. doi:10.1371/journal.pone.0100109
34. Ebert S, Becker M, Lemmermann NA, Büttner JK, Michel A, Taube C, et al. Mast cells expedite control of pulmonary murine cytomegalovirus infection by enhancing the recruitment of protective CD8 T cells to the lungs. *PLoS Pathog* (2014) **10**(4):e1004100. doi:10.1371/journal.ppat.1004100
35. Al-Afif A, Alyazidi R, Oldford SA, Huang YY, King CA, Haidl ID, et al. Respiratory syncytial virus infection of primary human mast cells induces the selective production of type I interferons, CXCL10, and CCL4. *J Allergy Clin Immunol* (2015). doi:10.1016/j.jaci.2015.01.042
36. Sandig H, Bulfone-Paus S. TLR signaling in mast cells: common and unique features. *Front Immunol* (2012) **3**:185. doi:10.3389/fimmu.2012.00185
37. Orinska Z, Bulanova E, Budagian V, Metz M, Maurer M, Bulfone-Paus S. TLR3-induced activation of mast cells modulates $CD8^+$ T-cell recruitment. *Blood* (2005) **106**:978–87. doi:10.1182/blood-2004-07-2656
38. Becker M, Lemmermann NA, Ebert S, Baars P, Renzaho A, Podlech J, et al. Mast cells as rapid innate sensors of cytomegalovirus by TLR3/TRIF signaling-dependent and -independent mechanisms. *Cell Mol Immunol* (2015) **12**:192–201. doi:10.1038/cmi.2014.73
39. Ott VL, Cambier JC, Kappler J, Marrack P, Swanson BJ. Mast cell-dependent migration of effector $CD8^+$ T cells through production of leukotriene B4. *Nat Immunol* (2003) **4**:974–81. doi:10.1038/ni971
40. Malaviya R, Twesten NJ, Ross EA, Abraham SN, Pfeifer JD. Mast cells process bacterial Ags through a phagocytic route for class I MHC presentation to T cells. *J Immunol* (1996) **156**:1490–6.
41. Bertolini M, Zilio F, Rossi A, Kleditzsch P, Emelianov VE, Gilhar A, et al. Abnormal interactions between perifollicular mast cells and CD8+ T-cells may contribute to the pathogenesis of alopecia areata. *PLoS One* (2014) **9**(5):e94260. doi:10.1371/journal.pone.0094260
42. Stelekati E, Bahri R, D'Orlando O, Orinska Z, Mittrücker HW, Langenhaun R, et al. Mast cell-mediated antigen presentation regulates CD8+ T cell effector functions. *Immunity* (2009) **31**:665–76. doi:10.1016/j.immuni.2009.08.022
43. Gregory GD, Robbie-Ryan M, Secor VH, Sabatino JJ Jr, Brown MA. Mast cells are required for optimal autoreactive T cell responses in a murine model of multiple sclerosis. *Eur J Immunol* (2005) **35**:3478–86. doi:10.1002/eji.200535271
44. Maurer M, Lopez Kostka S, Siebenhaar F, Moelle K, Metz M, Knop J, et al. Skin mast cells control T cell-dependent host defense in *Leishmania major* infections. *FASEB J* (2006) **20**:2460–7. doi:10.1096/fj.06-5860com
45. Heuer JG, Zhang T, Zhao J, Ding C, Cramer M, Justen KL, et al. Adoptive transfer of in vitro-stimulated $CD4^+CD25^+$ regulatory T cells increases bacterial clearance and improves survival in polymicrobial sepsis. *J Immunol* (2005) **174**:7141–6. doi:10.4049/jimmunol.174.11.7141
46. Lu LF, Lind EF, Gondek DC, Bennett KA, Gleeson MW, Pino-Lagos K, et al. Mast cells are essential intermediaries in regulatory T-cell tolerance. *Nature* (2006) **442**:997–1002. doi:10.1038/nature05010
47. Eller K, Wolf D, Huber JM, Metz M, Mayer G, McKenzie AN, et al. IL-9 production by regulatory T cells recruits mast cells that are essential for regulatory T cell-induced immune suppression. *J Immunol* (2011) **186**:83–91. doi:10.4049/jimmunol.1001183
48. Kashyap M, Thornton AM, Norton SK, Barnstein B, Macey M, Brenzovich J, et al. Cutting edge: CD4 T cell-mast cell interactions alter IgE receptor expression and signaling. *J Immunol* (2008) **180**:2039–43. doi:10.4049/jimmunol.180.4.2039
49. Piconese S, Gri G, Tripodo C, Musio S, Gorzanelli A, Frossi B, et al. Mast cells counteract regulatory T-cell suppression through interleukin-6 and OX40/OX40L axis toward Th17-cell differentiation. *Blood* (2009) **114**:2639–48. doi:10.1182/blood-2009-05-220004
50. Forward NA, Furlong SJ, Yang Y, Lin TJ, Hoskin DW. Mast cells down-regulate $CD4^+CD25^+$ T regulatory cell suppressor function via histamine H1 receptor interaction. *J Immunol* (2009) **183**:3014–22. doi:10.4049/jimmunol.0802509
51. Frossi B, D'Incà F, Crivellato E, Sibilano R, Gri G, Mongillo M, et al. Single-cell dynamics of mast cell-$CD4^+$ $CD25^+$ regulatory T cell interactions. *Eur J Immunol* (2011) **41**:1872–82. doi:10.1002/eji.201041300
52. Gri G, Piconese S, Frossi B, Manfroi V, Merluzzi S, Tripodo C, et al. $CD4^+CD25^+$ regulatory T cells suppress mast cell degranulation and allergic responses through OX40-OX40L interaction. *Immunity* (2008) **29**:771–81. doi:10.1016/j.immuni.2008.08.018
53. Feyerabend TB, Weiser A, Tietz A, Stassen M, Harris N, Kopf M, et al. Cre-mediated cell ablation contests mast cell contribution in models of antibody- and T cell-mediated autoimmunity. *Immunity* (2011) **35**:832–44. doi:10.1016/j.immuni.2011.09.015
54. Gutierrez DA, Fu W, Schonefeldt S, Feyerabend TB, Ortiz-Lopez A, Lampi Y, et al. Type 1 diabetes in NOD mice unaffected by mast cell deficiency. *Diabetes* (2014) **63**:3827–34. doi:10.2337/db14-0372
55. Lilla JN, Chen CC, Mukai K, BenBarak MJ, Franco CB, Kalesnikoff J, et al. Reduced mast cell and basophil numbers and function in Cpa3-Cre; Mcl-1fl/fl mice. *Blood* (2011) **118**:6930–8. doi:10.1182/blood-2011-03-343962
56. Reber LL, Marichal T, Galli SJ. New models for analyzing mast cell functions in vivo. *Trends Immunol* (2012) **33**:613–25. doi:10.1016/j.it.2012.09.008
57. Schubert N, Dudeck J, Liu P, Karutz A, Speier S, Maurer M, et al. Mast cell promotion of T cell-driven antigen-induced arthritis despite being dispensable for antibody-induced arthritis in which T cells are bypassed. *Arthritis Rheumatol* (2015) **67**:903–13. doi:10.1002/art.38996
58. Brown MA, Hatfield JK, Walker ME, Sayed BA. A game of kit and mouse: the Kit is still in the bag. *Immunity* (2012) **36**:891–2; author reply 893–4. doi:10.1016/j.immuni.2012.05.004
59. Brown MA, Hatfield JK. Mast cells are important modifiers of autoimmune disease: with so much evidence, why is there still controversy? *Front Immunol* (2012) **3**:147. doi:10.3389/fimmu.2012.00147

5

How neutrophils shape adaptive immune responses

*Pieter H. C. Leliefeld[1,2], Leo Koenderman[2,3] and Janesh Pillay[2,4]**

[1] Department of Surgery, University Medical Center Utrecht, Utrecht, Netherlands, [2] Laboratory of Translational Immunology, University Medical Center Utrecht, Utrecht, Netherlands, [3] Department of Respiratory Medicine, University Medical Center Utrecht, Utrecht, Netherlands, [4] Department of Anaesthesiology and Critical Care, University Medical Center Utrecht, Utrecht, Netherlands

Edited by:
Elisabetta Padovan, University of Basel, Switzerland

Reviewed by:
Matteo Iannacone, San Raffaele Scientific Institute, Italy
Marco A. Cassatella, University of Verona, Italy
Dieter Kabelitz, Christian-Albrechts University Kiel, Germany

***Correspondence:**
Janesh Pillay, Department of Anaesthesiology and Critical Care, University Medical Center Utrecht, Heidelberglaan 100, Utrecht GA 3508, Netherlands
j.pillay-2@umcutrecht.nl, jpillay@gmail.com

Neutrophils are classically considered as cells pivotal for the first line of defense against invading pathogens. In recent years, evidence has accumulated that they are also important in the orchestration of adaptive immunity. Neutrophils rapidly migrate in high numbers to sites of inflammation (e.g., infection, tissue damage, and cancer) and are subsequently able to migrate to draining lymph nodes (LNs). Both at the site of inflammation as well as in the LNs, neutrophils can engage with lymphocytes and antigen-presenting cells. This crosstalk occurs either directly via cell–cell contact or via mediators, such as proteases, cytokines, and radical oxygen species. In this review, we will discuss the current knowledge regarding locations and mechanisms of interaction between neutrophils and lymphocytes in the context of homeostasis and various pathological conditions. In addition, we will highlight the complexity of the microenvironment that is involved in the generation of suppressive or stimulatory neutrophil phenotypes.

Keywords: inflammation, immune-regulation, neutrophil, myeloid-derived suppressor cells, immune-paralysis, neutrophil phenotypes, T-cells

Introduction

Neutrophils are particularly known for their potent anti-microbial functions (1). This notion is enforced by various congenital neutrophil deficiencies, which show marked clinical phenotypes characterized by enhanced susceptibility to bacterial and fungal infections (2, 3). Infections, sterile inflammation, and other non-chronic challenges to the immune system are characterized by a rapid influx of neutrophils into the affected tissue (4). These neutrophils respond to chemo-attractants and adhesion molecules expressed on endothelial cells, and their main function is to clear infections and/or debris. In addition, they influence inflammatory responses through interactions with various cells of the immune system, such as antigen-presenting cells (APCs) and lymphocytes (5, 6). This has been observed in both murine models and in *ex vivo* studies with isolated cells from humans. Although neutrophils have long been considered to be composed of a homogenous population, an increasing body of literature supports the presence of multiple neutrophil phenotypes in cancer and inflammation (7–10). This heterogeneity can be induced by specific differentiation programs in the bone marrow or orchestrated by extracellular signals derived from inflammatory tissue (e.g., cytokines, bioactive lipids, or chemokines) (11, 12). The contribution of distinct neutrophil populations to immune suppression has not been resolved. In addition, in murine models and some human studies, clear distinctions were suggested between neutrophils and granulocytic myeloid-derived suppressor cells (G-MDSCs). These issues have been reviewed in detail (13, 14). This review will focus on the location and relevant diseases in which both (suppressive) neutrophils and G-MDSCs modulate adaptive immune responses and the mechanisms behind this process.

Location of the Interaction Between Neutrophils and Lymphocytes

Site of Inflammation – Bystander Response

The early phase of infection is characterized by an influx of neutrophils and monocytes, which precedes the development of an antigen-specific response. Simultaneously, small numbers of T-cells are recruited into the infected tissue. Some of these T-cells can be activated and proliferate "in situ" in response to antigen presentation by myeloid cells (15). In addition, inflammatory cytokines cause proliferation and activation of non-specific T-cells in the profoundly pro-inflammatory microenvironment. This process has been coined the "bystander response" and was first seen in viral infections (16). It has recently been suggested that this bystander response contributes to early pathogen control in mice by enabling bystander memory T-cells to recognize and eliminate micro-organisms, such as *Listeria monocytogenes* infected cells in a NKG2D-dependent manner (17).

It is conceivable that a large and uncontrolled bystander response might predispose for auto-immunity and self-reactivity through the proliferation of self-reactive T-cells (18). It is tempting to speculate that neutrophils are involved to limit and control this bystander T-cell response as the timing of massive neutrophil tissue infiltration and the bystander response coincide.

Lymph Nodes and Primary Lymphatic Tissue

Neutrophils are found both in LNs and spleen particularly under inflammatory conditions (19–24). Dynamic imaging studies have shown that neutrophils are recruited to and form swarms in infected LNs in mice (25, 26). In addition, neutrophil migration to afferent LNs in response to tissue inflammation has been shown in various murine models (19–24).

There are two possible routes for neutrophils to enter LNs, via blood vessels or via afferent lymphatics (**Figure 1**). The first route requires exiting the circulation via high endothelial venules (HEVs). This mechanism is controversial, as human neutrophils seem to lack the expression of CCR7, a receptor for CCL21 and required for lymphocyte exiting through HEVs (27). Nonetheless, it has been shown in a murine model of ovalbumin-induced inflammation that neutrophil homing to LNs via the HEV takes place and requires integrins αMβ2 (MAC-1), αLβ2 (LFA-1), and L- and P-selectin (19). In LN-draining inflammatory tissue, additional chemokines and cytokines could orchestrate the attraction of neutrophils via HEVs. This has also been shown in tumor-draining LNs, when the tumor was subjected to photodynamic therapy. This treatment induces additional sterile inflammation. In this model, neutrophils are recruited to tumor-draining LNs via the HEV in an IL-17-dependent manner (20).

Neutrophil migration to LNs via afferent lymphatics has been observed in various murine models of infections, vaccinations, and cancer and seems to depend on MAC-1 and CXCR4 expression on neutrophils (19, 22) (see **Figure 1**). The area in the LN that is occupied by neutrophils will determine which cells they encounter, and how they can influence subsequent immune responses. Neutrophils have been reported to occupy the medullary region and interfollicular zone (23). Neutrophils migrate to these areas in the LN during infection with *Staphylococcus aureus*. There they exhibit short- and long-term interactions with B-cells, thereby inhibiting production of antibodies, and thus humoral responses (23). Furthermore, neutrophil B-cell interactions have also been observed in primary lymphoid organs in various mouse models. In the marginal zone of the spleen, neutrophils were observed to contribute to antibody production and class switching by activating B-cells by producing BAFF, APRIL, and IL-21 (24). In this study, evidence was provided for the existence of a similar population of neutrophils that modulate B-cell responses in humans. However, this remains controversial as in a subsequent study, no splenic neutrophil–B cell interactions could be observed in humans (28). It seems firmly established, at least in various murine models that neutrophils enter primary and secondary lymphatic sites during the immune response evoked by various inflammatory stimuli. Apart from regulating immunity in inflamed tissue, they may play a role in regulating immune responses at these privileged immune sites (see below).

The Role of Neutrophils in Controlling Immune Responses Evoked by Bacterial and Viral Infections, Sterile Inflammation and Cancer

Viral Infections

Acute viral infections, such as influenza, are ideal models to study cellular kinetics during the immune responses and the putative modulating effects of neutrophils hereon. Influenza and RSV infections are characterized by an early large influx of neutrophils in the lung tissue followed several days later by a virus specific $CD8^+$ T-cell response (29–31). Neutrophils might facilitate the development of this antigen-specific response as they are able to serve as APCs in influenza infection in mice (31, 32). Such antigen presentation by influenza-infected neutrophils has been demonstrated and was found to be mediated by MHC-I and co-stimulatory molecules CD80 and CD86, which leads to induction and activation of anti-viral responses of $CD8^+$ T-cells (32). On the other hand, it is tempting to speculate that neutrophils may also inhibit T-cell responses in viral infections by inhibiting T-cell proliferation and inducing T-cell apoptosis. The mechanisms of this suppression will be discussed below and involve reactive oxygen species (ROS), arginase-I (ARG), and PD-L1. This has also been found in other inflammatory scenarios (33–35). The role of immune suppression by neutrophils *in vivo* in murine models of viral infections has not been adequately experimentally verified, but may be deduced from the fact that pathology in mice is T-cell dependent and that depleting neutrophils often results in an exaggerated response and pathology (31, 36). In chronic viral infections, such as human hepatitis B virus (HBV), it has recently been shown that recruitment of neutrophils to the liver limits immune pathology through inhibiting bystander and HBV specific T-cells in an arginase-dependent way, thus protecting the host from immune-mediated damage (37). These

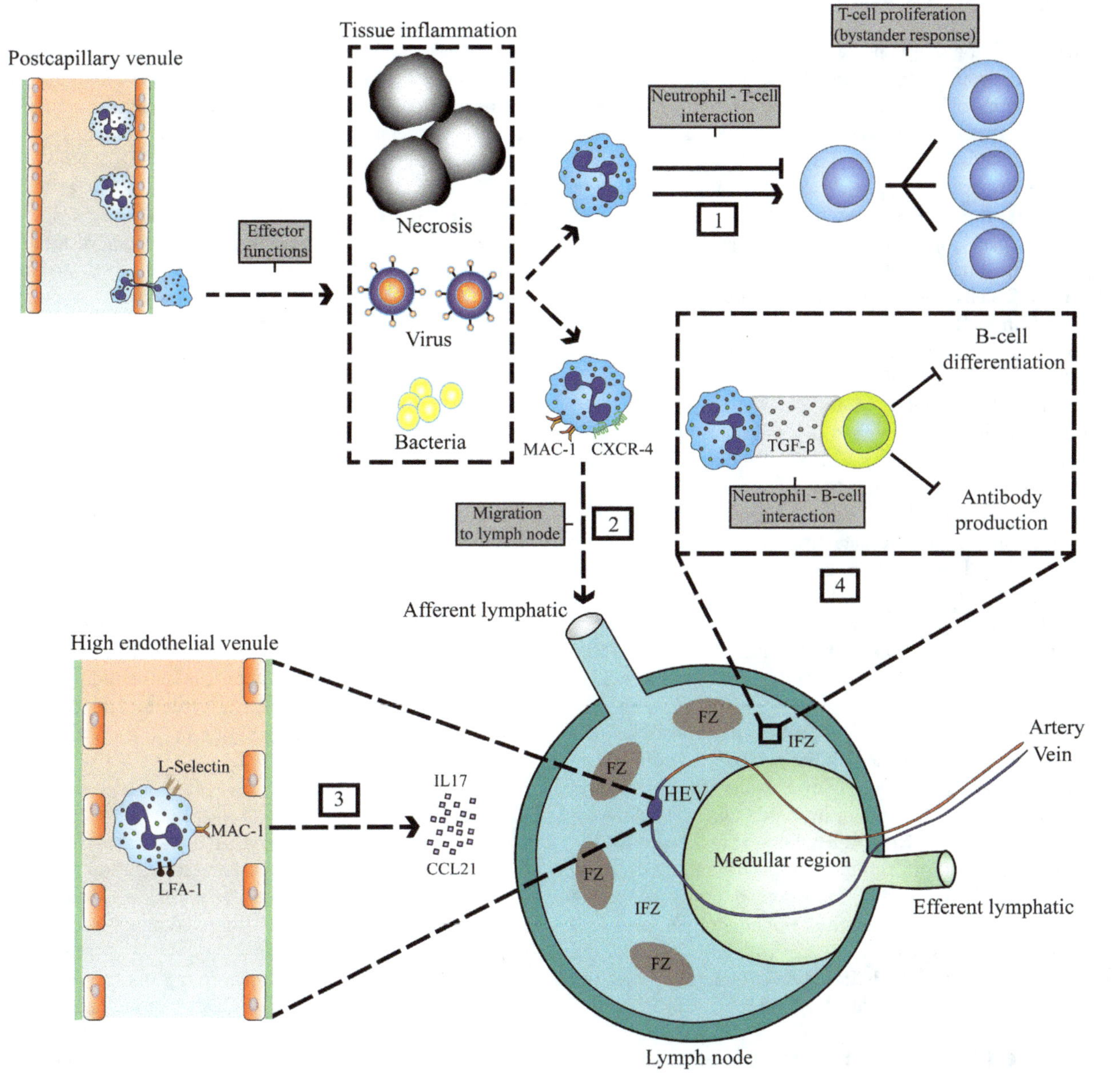

FIGURE 1 | Localization of interaction between neutrophils and lymphocytes at sites of inflammation and in lymphoid tissue. Invasion of pathogens or inflammation due to necrosis and cancer leads to extravasation of neutrophils. (1) Interaction of neutrophils with T-cells in the peripheral tissue. (2) MAC-1 and CXCR4-dependent migration of neutrophils to LNs via afferent lymphatics during inflammation (22). (3) IL17 and CCL21-mediated migration of neutrophils via HEVs to the LN that requires MAC-1, LFA-1, and L-selectin (19, 20). (4) Inhibition of humoral responses by neutrophils in the IFZ and medullar region (23). HEV, high endothelial venule; FZ, follicular zone; IFZ, interfollicular zone.

neutrophils were isolated from the PBMC fraction and were termed G-MDSC (13).

Bacterial Infections

As in viral infections, bacterial infections are associated with a large recruitment of neutrophils. The pivotal difference with viral infections is that phagocytosis and killing of bacterial targets by phagocytes is the principle mechanism of pathogen eradication (1). Ineffective killing of phagocytosed bacteria results in intracellular (phagosomal) survival and can lead to pathogen shuttling to distant sites and LNs (38, 39). Recently, it has been shown that neutrophils from mice infected with *S. aureus* migrated to the draining LNs and limited humoral responses through direct cellular interactions with B-cells. These direct cellular interactions were also found for neutrophil–T-cell interactions in humans (40). Kamenyeva et al. suggested that suppression of antibody production by neutrophils *ex vivo* was dependent on TGF-β (23). However, the contribution of the reduced humoral response to pathogen load was not assessed.

As mentioned above, in the early course of infection, large numbers of neutrophils are recruited to the affected tissue where modulation of T-cell responses most likely occurs with early recruited T-cells. These early lymphocytes mainly belong to the family of γδ-T-cells (41). These γδ-T-cells are thought to play a role in early pathogen clearance through production of cytokines and their crosstalk with innate immune cells (41). Neutrophils play an important role in the initiation of these γδ-T-cell responses. Phagocytosis of bacteria enables neutrophils to activate γδ-T-cells and induce their proliferation (42). This is dependent on (1) the microbial metabolite (E)-4-hydroxy-3-methyl-but-2-enyl pyrophosphate (HMB-PP), which neutrophils release after phagocytosis of bacteria and (2) the presence of monocytes for cellular contact-induced activation (42). However, other human studies have revealed the ability of neutrophils to suppress γδ-T-cells activation, possibly providing a negative-feedback mechanism (43, 44).

The early instruction of γδ-T-cells in humans by neutrophils parallels the role of these innate immune cells in the early instruction of T-cell responses in mice. In a murine model of *Legionella pneumophila*, neutrophils from pulmonary tissue are pivotal for the development of a TH1 response. In this model which resembles human disease, neutrophils were depleted by neutrophil-specific antibody Ly-6G, and this led to more TH2 skewing and more disease (45).

T-cell instruction, activation, and proliferation mostly require antigen-presenting cells, such as dendritic cells, B-cells, and macrophages. Neutrophils have been shown to both negatively and positively affect antigen presentation by these APCs under different conditions. This has extensively been reviewed previously (46, 47). Neutrophils may simply affect the amount of available antigen by phagocytosis, and thus limit antigen presentation by professional APCs (48). Alternatively, neutrophils might function as APCs themselves (49, 50). This possibility is supported by several studies showing the expression of MHCII and co-stimulatory molecules on neutrophils under different clinical conditions (51–53).

Disseminated Bacterial Infections (Sepsis)

Severe bacterial infections can result in systemic dissemination of bacteria that can lead to severe clinical conditions, such as sepsis and septic shock. These conditions are characterized by severe systemic inflammation, which can result in severe inflammatory damage to the host when not properly controlled. Immune inhibitory mechanisms have evolved in order to prevent this exaggerated inflammatory response (54). The specific role of neutrophils in this immune suppression has not been adequately studied. This is a challenging research question as depletion or inhibition of neutrophil functions with the purpose of studying their anti-inflammatory role has profound impact on bacterial clearance. Identification of suppressive mechanisms that do not influence pathogen clearance and neutrophil-specific murine knockout models may aid in answering this question.

In humans, evidence has accumulated that neutrophils might contribute to the immune suppression seen in sepsis. Neutrophils in septic-shock patients express ARG and suppress T-cell functions, probably through depletion of L-arginine as detailed below (55). Immune suppression in sepsis can be at least in part attributed to the PD-1/PD-L1 axis that is involved in control of apoptosis in T-cells (56). Interestingly, expression of PD-L1 on tissue neutrophils has also been shown during chronic inflammation (57). The expression of PD-L1 on human neutrophils was found to be induced by the TH1 cytokine, interferon-γ, *in vitro* (35).

Sterile Inflammation/Vaccination

Neutrophils also play a role in the fine tuning of inflammation under sterile conditions. Many studies have been performed in ovalbumine (OVA)-induced immune responses in murine models. The OVA models are used as vaccination and allergy models and are useful to study the development of adaptive immune responses. The role of neutrophils in the OVA model follows the above-described findings in microbial models. The cells seem to effectively cross-prime $CD8^+$ T-cells in an MHCI-dependent manner (58). They function as APCs or influence the capacity to present antigens by professional APCs (59, 60). For instance, dendritic cells have been shown to take up antigens acquired from phagocytosed apoptotic neutrophils (61).

These examples show that neutrophils can increase antigen presentation as APC or by delivering antigen to APCs. On the other hand, there are reports that neutrophils decrease the level of antigen presentation by APCs through an unknown mechanism during brief cellular interactions (48). These findings show that it is difficult to predict in which circumstances neutrophils stimulate or suppress antigen presentation even when very similar and well-controlled models are used.

Cancer

There is a large body of literature, which shows a heterogeneous population of myeloid cells characterized by their potential to inhibit adaptive immunity, and thus anti-tumor immune responses (14). These myeloid-derived suppressor cells consist of mononuclear cells and neutrophils in different stages of maturation. G-MDSCs facilitate tumor growth in various murine models through suppression of $CD8^+$ responses and production of cytokines (62–64). In addition, in human cancer patients, G-MDSCs and suppressive neutrophils are isolated from the peripheral blood (65, 66). Although the distinction between neutrophils and G-MDSCs is not clear, the modulating role of these cells in the immune responses induced by tumors has become an accepted paradigm, and is extensively reviewed elsewhere (13, 67). Neutrophils are involved in both pro- or anti-tumor immune responses. Importantly, they have recently been shown to promote metastasis (7, 68). Their anti-tumor effects are mediated by their direct antibody-dependent cytotoxicity and their production of pro-inflammatory cytokines near and inside the tumor (69). These properties will not be discussed in this short review.

The pro-tumor effects of neutrophils are mediated by different mechanisms. First, neutrophils play an essential role in angiogenesis through expression of matrix metallo-proteases, such as MMP9 (70, 71). Second, in multiple murine models they inhibit anti-tumor $CD8^+$ T-cell responses through mechanisms described below. The suppression of anti-tumor T-cell responses by neutrophils was recently shown to be pivotal in tumor

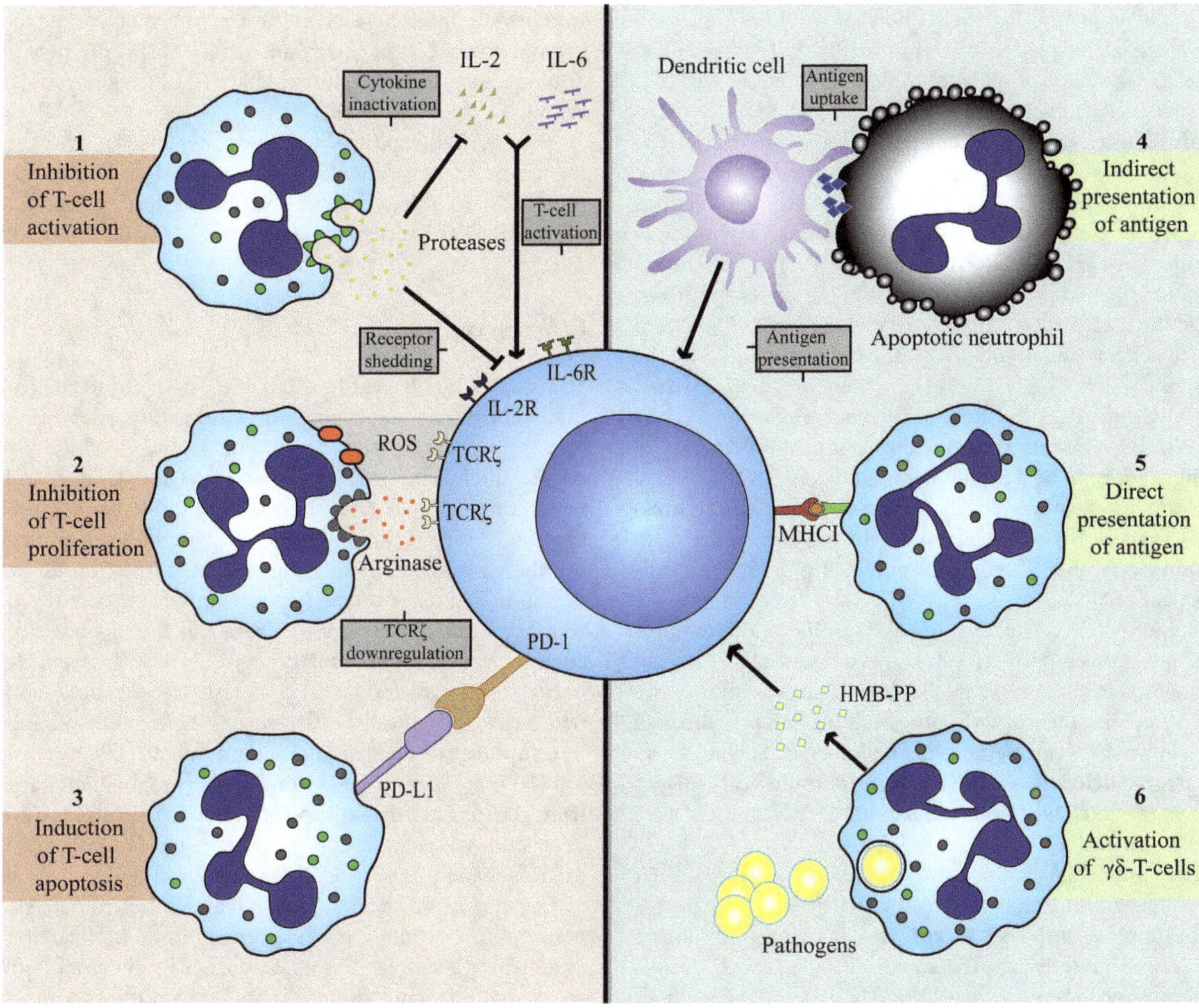

FIGURE 2 | Mechanisms involved in T-cell inhibition (left panel) and activation (right panel) by neutrophils. Neutrophils can establish T-cell inhibition by (1) degranulation of granular constituents. The serine proteases elastase and cathepsin G inactivate T-cell stimulating cytokines, IL-2 and IL-6, and catalyze shedding of cytokine receptors for IL-2 and IL-6 on T-cells (72, 73). (2) Production of ROS and release of arginase. Both agents can result in downregulation of TCRζ on T-cells, thereby arresting the cell in the G0-G1 phase (40, 74–78). (3) Expression of PD-L1. Upregulation of this ligand is associated with interferon-dependent PD1-mediated T-cell apoptosis (35, 56). T-cell activation by neutrophils is attained by (4) indirect antigen presentation. Dendritic cells take up antigens from apoptotic neutrophils and serve as APC for T-cells (61). (5) Direct antigen presentation. Neutrophils posses the capacity to cross-prime CD8$^+$ T-cells directly in a MHCI-dependent manner (32). (6) Release of microbial metabolites (HMB-PP). Neutrophils release bacterial products after ingestion to activate γδ-T-cells (42).

metastasis in a murine model of breast cancer (7). In this study, γδ-T-cells facilitated neutrophil recruitment to the tumor via an IL-17 and G-CSF mediated pathway. The microenvironmental cues for the switch in neutrophil phenotype from pro- to anti-tumor are slowly being unraveled. In a model of lung cancer, TGF-β induces or recruits neutrophils with a pro-tumor phenotype (termed N1), whereas blocking TGF-β induces an anti-tumor neutrophil phenotype (termed N2) (11).

Mechanisms of T-Cell Suppression by Neutrophils and G-MDSCs

Despite the evidence that neutrophils can stimulate T-cell responses, most studies point toward a direct suppressive role of these cells on different T-cell responses in various disease models as described above. The mechanisms of suppression have been reviewed in detail elsewhere and are summarized in **Figure 2** (13). Most of the mechanisms that neutrophils employ to suppress T-cell functions are closely related to their anti-microbial functions, i.e., the same or similar mediators are used. Two of the most frequently reported mechanisms are via ARG and ROS.

ARG is found in the gelatinase containing granules of neutrophils and is thought to contribute to antifungal immunity trough depletion of L-arginine (79, 80). Depletion of L-arginine also results in a cell cycle arrest in activated T-cells in the G0-G1 phase, which limits T-cell proliferation (74). This is thought to occur through downregulation of TCRζ (75, 76). It seems that the expression of TCRζ requires L-arginine for adequate expression and functionality

(81). In addition, L-arginine is required for dephosphorylation of cofilin. Cofilin is pivotal for the stability of the immunological synapse. Therefore, depletion of L-arginine by ARG impairs the formation and stability of an immunological synapse, which is required for T-cell activation and proliferation (82, 83).

ROS are an intricate part of neutrophil anti-microbial defense and the lack of ability to produce ROS as, seen in chronic granulomatous disease, is characterized by severe infections (84–86). One of the products of NADPH oxidase activation is hydrogenperoxide (H_2O_2). H_2O_2 can suppress T-cell proliferation and activation through various mechanisms. It induces apoptosis, decreases Nf-κB activation, and downregulates TCRζ (77, 78). In addition, T-cell suppression by ROS is also accompanied by the oxidation of cofilin (77, 87). Cofilin can, therefore, be influenced by both ARG and ROS: both mechanisms being employed by neutrophils. Therefore, the T-cell suppression by disruption of cofilin might prove to be a useful therapeutic target.

Interestingly, regulatory T-cells are resistant to oxidative stress (88). This suggests that regulatory T-cells are less sensitive to suppression than other T-cells, thus enhancing the overall suppressive effect of H_2O_2.

Suppression of T-cell activation and proliferation requires high concentrations of H_2O_2 (33, 87). This amount of ROS might only be reached in inflammatory tissue with massive neutrophil influx. A more elegant way of suppression via H_2O_2 is through cell-cell contact between neutrophils and T-cells. Such a direct mechanism for delivery of ROS in an immunological synapse has been identified (29). Here, neutrophil-T-cell contacts were mediated by MAC-1.

Another important suppressive pathway requires similar cell-cell contacts: inhibition via T-cell PD-1 by PD-L1, a potent inducer of apoptosis in T-cells 1, expressed on neutrophils during sepsis (25). The underlying mechanism of PD-L1 expression is an interferon dependent process (35). The PD-1/PD-L1 axis is thought to be an important mechanism in the immune suppression found in sepsis patients by inducing lymphocyte apoptosis and monocyte dysfunction (56). Blocking this axis after the induction of sepsis by administering a PD-1 blocking antibody improves survival in mice by increasing pathogen clearance (89). This suppressive mechanism might be protective in tissues with severe inflammatory infiltrates, but may be detrimental as immune suppression aggravates sepsis. At this moment, one can only speculate regarding the role of PD-L1 on neutrophils in this immune suppressed state.

Finally, neutrophils can modulate T-cells by degranulating granular constituents, such as neutrophil elastase. These proteases are able to cleave and inactivate essential cytokines, such as IL-2 and receptors, such as the IL-2 and IL-6 receptor on T-cells (72, 73).

Conclusion

The studies mentioned in this review have led to the consensus that neutrophils are capable of modulating adaptive immune responses through interactions with T- and B-cells and possibly APCs. The mechanistic studies in mice have been corroborated with human *ex vivo* data. These studies show that neutrophils are capable of directly interacting with lymphocytes and modulating their responses at local sites of inflammation as well as in draining LNs. One of the key remaining issues is the question whether human neutrophils show functional plasticity as has been suggested by us and others (13, 90). This plasticity can occur at different levels: (1) the existence of functional subsets, which are intrinsically different or (2) the transdifferentiation into suppressive neutrophils or even into an APC type of hybrid cell (90–92). The microenvironmental cues mediating the switch from classical neutrophils to suppressive neutrophils have barely been studied although TGF-β seems to play an important role in microbial and tumor models (11, 23).

In conclusion, murine and human studies to date show that neutrophils are potent modulators of immunity. The first step of establishing a strategy to target immune modulatory neutrophils without influencing their essential anti-microbial functions is finding relevant human diseases in which this modulation plays a pivotal role (93). The unraveling of microenvironmental cues mediating the recruitment of and/or "switching" into suppressive neutrophils in such diseases is essential in understanding and targeting of this pathway.

References

1. Nauseef WM. How human neutrophils kill and degrade microbes: an integrated view. *Immunol Rev* (2007) **219**:88–102. doi:10.1111/j.1600-065X.2007.00550.x
2. Dinauer MC. Inherited neutrophil disorders: molecular basis and new therapies. *Hematology* (2000) **2000**:303–18. doi:10.1182/asheducation-2000.1.303
3. Keszei M, Westerberg LS. Congenital defects in neutrophil dynamics. *J Immunol Res* (2014) **2014**:303782. doi:10.1155/2014/303782
4. Nathan C. Neutrophils and immunity: challenges and opportunities. *Nat Rev Immunol* (2006) **6**:173–82. doi:10.1038/nri1785
5. Scapini P, Cassatella MA. Social networking of human neutrophils within the immune system. *Blood* (2014) **124**:710–9. doi:10.1182/blood-2014-03-453217
6. Kalyan S, Kabelitz D. When neutrophils meet T cells: beginnings of a tumultuous relationship with underappreciated potential. *Eur J Immunol* (2014) **44**:627–33. doi:10.1002/eji.201344195
7. Coffelt SB, Kersten K, Doornebal CW, Weiden J, Vrijland K, Hau C-S, et al. IL-17-producing γδ T cells and neutrophils conspire to promote breast cancer metastasis. *Nature* (2015) **522**:345–8. doi:10.1038/nature14282
8. Pillay J, Ramakers BP, Kamp VM, Loi ALT, Lam SW, Hietbrink F, et al. Functional heterogeneity and differential priming of circulating neutrophils in human experimental endotoxemia. *J Leukoc Biol* (2010) **88**:211–20. doi:10.1189/jlb.1209793
9. Buckley C, Ross E. Identification of a phenotypically and functionally distinct population of long-lived neutrophils in a model of reverse endothelial migration. *J Leukoc Biol* (2006) **79**:303–11. doi:10.1189/jlb.0905496.Journal
10. Pillay J, Hietbrink F, Koenderman L, Leenen LPH. The systemic inflammatory response induced by trauma is reflected by multiple phenotypes of blood neutrophils. *Injury* (2007) **38**:1365–72. doi:10.1016/j.injury.2007.09.016
11. Fridlender ZG, Sun J, Kim S, Kapoor V, Cheng G, Ling L, et al. Polarization of tumor-associated neutrophil phenotype by TGF-β: "N1" versus "N2" TAN. *Cancer Cell* (2009) **16**:183–94. doi:10.1016/j.ccr.2009.06.017
12. Christoffersson G, Vågesjö E, Vandooren J, Lidén M, Massena S, Reinert RB, et al. VEGF-Arecruits a proangiogenic MMP-9-delivering neutrophil subset that induces angiogenesis in transplanted hypoxic tissue. *Blood* (2012) **120**:4653–62. doi:10.1182/blood-2012-04-421040
13. Pillay J, Tak T, Kamp VM, Koenderman L. Immune suppression by neutrophils and granulocytic myeloid-derived suppressor cells: similarities and differences. *Cell Mol Life Sci* (2013) **70**:3813–27. doi:10.1007/s00018-013-1286-4
14. Gabrilovich DI, Nagaraj S. Myeloid-derived suppressor cells as regulators of the immune system. *Nat Rev Immunol* (2009) **9**:162–74. doi:10.1038/nri2506

15. McGill J, Legge KL. Cutting edge: contribution of lung-resident T cell proliferation to the overall magnitude of the antigen-specific CD8 T cell response in the lungs following murine influenza virus infection. *J Immunol* (2009) **183**:4177–81. doi:10.4049/jimmunol.0901109
16. Tough DF, Borrow P, Sprent J. Induction of bystander T cell proliferation by viruses and type I interferon in vivo. *Science* (1996) **272**:1947–50. doi:10.1126/science.272.5270.1947
17. Chu T, Tyznik AJ, Roepke S, Berkley AM, Woodward-Davis A, Pattacini L, et al. Bystander-activated memory CD8 T cells control early pathogen load in an innate-like, NKG2D-dependent manner. *Cell Rep* (2013) **3**:701–8. doi:10.1016/j.celrep.2013.02.020
18. Burroughs NJ, Ferreira M, Oliveira BMPM, Pinto AA. Autoimmunity arising from bystander proliferation of T cells in an immune response model. *Math Comput Model* (2011) **53**:1389–93. doi:10.1016/j.mcm.2010.01.020
19. Gorlino CV, Ranocchia RP, Harman MF, García IA, Crespo MI, Morón G, et al. Neutrophils exhibit differential requirements for homing molecules in their lymphatic and blood trafficking into draining lymph nodes. *J Immunol* (2014) **193**:1966–74. doi:10.4049/jimmunol.1301791
20. Brackett CM, Muhitch JB, Evans SS, Gollnick SO. IL-17 promotes neutrophil entry into tumor-draining lymph nodes following induction of sterile inflammation. *J Immunol* (2013) **191**:4348–57. doi:10.4049/jimmunol.1103621
21. De Veer M, Neeland M, Burke M, Pleasance J, Nathanielsz J, Elhay M, et al. Cell recruitment and antigen trafficking in afferent lymph after injection of antigen and poly(I: C) containing liposomes, in aqueous or oil-based formulations. *Vaccine* (2013) **31**:1012–8. doi:10.1016/j.vaccine.2012.12.049
22. Hampton HR, Bailey J, Tomura M, Brink R, Chtanova T. Microbe-dependent lymphatic migration of neutrophils modulates lymphocyte proliferation in lymph nodes. *Nat Commun* (2015) **6**:7139. doi:10.1038/ncomms8139
23. Kamenyeva O, Boularan C, Kabat J, Cheung GYC, Cicala C, Yeh AJ, et al. Neutrophil recruitment to lymph nodes limits local humoral response to *Staphylococcus aureus*. *PLoS Pathog* (2015) **11**:e1004827. doi:10.1371/journal.ppat.1004827
24. Puga I, Cols M, Barra CM, He B, Cassis L, Gentile M, et al. B cell–helper neutrophils stimulate the diversification and production of immunoglobulin in the marginal zone of the spleen. *Nat Immunol* (2011) **13**:170–80. doi:10.1038/ni.2194
25. Chtanova T, Schaeffer M, Han SJ, van Dooren GG, Nollmann M, Herzmark P, et al. Dynamics of neutrophil migration in lymph nodes during infection. *Immunity* (2008) **29**:487–96. doi:10.1016/j.immuni.2008.07.012
26. Lämmermann T, Afonso PV, Angermann BR, Wang JM, Kastenmüller W, Parent CA, et al. Neutrophil swarms require LTB4 and integrins at sites of cell death in vivo. *Nature* (2013) **498**:371–5. doi:10.1038/nature12175
27. Förster R, Davalos-Misslitz AC, Rot A. CCR7 and its ligands: balancing immunity and tolerance. *Nat Rev Immunol* (2008) **8**:362–71. doi:10.1038/nri2297
28. Nagelkerke SQ, Aan De Kerk DJ, Jansen MH, Van Den Berg TK, Kuijpers TW. Failure to detect functional neutrophil B helper cells in the human spleen. *PLoS One* (2014) **9**:1–6. doi:10.1371/journal.pone.0088377
29. Narasaraju T, Yang E, Samy RP, Ng HH, Poh WP, Liew AA, et al. Excessive neutrophils and neutrophil extracellular traps contribute to acute lung injury of influenza pneumonitis. *Am J Pathol* (2011) **179**:199–210. doi:10.1016/j.ajpath.2011.03.013
30. Lukens MV, van de Pol AC, Coenjaerts FEJ, Jansen NJG, Kamp VM, Kimpen JLL, et al. A systemic neutrophil response precedes robust CD8(+) T-cell activation during natural respiratory syncytial virus infection in infants. *J Virol* (2010) **84**:2374–83. doi:10.1128/JVI.01807-09
31. Tate MD, Brooks AG, Reading PC, Mintern JD. Neutrophils sustain effective CD8+ T-cell responses in the respiratory tract following influenza infection. *Immunol Cell Biol* (2012) **90**:197–205. doi:10.1038/icb.2011.26
32. Hufford MM, Richardson G, Zhou H, Manicassamy B, García-Sastre A, Enelow RI, et al. Influenza-infected neutrophils within the infected lungs act as antigen presenting cells for anti-viral CD8+ T cells. *PLoS One* (2012) **7** e46581. doi:10.1371/journal.pone.0046581
33. Schmielau J, Finn OJ. Activated granulocytes and granulocyte-derived hydrogen peroxide are the underlying mechanism of suppression of t-cell function in advanced cancer patients. *Cancer Res* (2001) **61**:4756–60.
34. Highfill SL, Rodriguez PC, Zhou Q, Goetz CA, Koehn BH, Veenstra R, et al. Bone marrow myeloid-derived suppressor cells (MDSC) inhibit graft-versus-host (GVHD) disease via an arginase-1 dependent mechanism that is upregulated by IL-13. *Blood* (2010) **116**:612–26. doi:10.1182/blood-2010-06-287839
35. De Kleijn S, Langereis JD, Leentjens J, Kox M, Netea MG, Koenderman L, et al. IFN-γ-stimulated neutrophils suppress lymphocyte proliferation through expression of PD-L1. *PLoS One* (2013) **8** e72249. doi:10.1371/journal.pone.0072249
36. Rygiel TP, Rijkers ESK, de Ruiter T, Stolte EH, van der Valk M, Rimmelzwaan GF, et al. Lack of CD200 enhances pathological T cell responses during influenza infection. *J Immunol* (2009) **183**:1990–6. doi:10.4049/jimmunol.0900252
37. Pallett LJ, Gill US, Quaglia A, Sinclair LV, Jover-Cobos M, Schurich A, et al. Metabolic regulation of hepatitis B immunopathology by myeloid-derived suppressor cells. *Nat Med* (2015) **21**:591–600. doi:10.1038/nm.3856
38. Thwaites GE, Gant V. Are bloodstream leukocytes Trojan horses for the metastasis of *Staphylococcus aureus*? *Nat Rev Microbiol* (2011) **9**:215–22. doi:10.1038/nrmicro2508
39. Bland DM, Anderson DM. Imaging early pathogenesis of bubonic plague: are neutrophils commandeered for lymphatic transport of bacteria? *MBio* (2013) **4**:e837–813. doi:10.1128/mBio.00837-13
40. Pillay J, Kamp VM, Van Hoffen E, Visser T, Tak T, Lammers J, et al. A subset of neutrophils in human systemic inflammation inhibits T cell responses through Mac-1. *J Clin Invest* (2012) **122**:327–36. doi:10.1172/JCI57990DS1
41. Bonneville M, O'Brien RL, Born WK. Gammadelta T cell effector functions: a blend of innate programming and acquired plasticity. *Nat Rev Immunol* (2010) **10**:467–78. doi:10.1038/nri2781
42. Davey MS, Lin C-Y, Roberts GW, Heuston S, Brown AC, Chess JA, et al. Human neutrophil clearance of bacterial pathogens triggers anti-microbial γδ T cell responses in early infection. *PLoS Pathog* (2011) **7**:e1002040. doi:10.1371/journal.ppat.1002040
43. Sabbione F, Gabelloni ML, Ernst G, Gori MS, Salamone G, Oleastro M, et al. Neutrophils suppress γδ T-cell function. *Eur J Immunol* (2014) **44**:819–30. doi:10.1002/eji.201343664
44. Kalyan S, Chandrasekaran V, Quabius ES, Lindhorst TK, Kabelitz D. Neutrophil uptake of nitrogen-bisphosphonates leads to the suppression of human peripheral blood γδ T cells. *Cell Mol Life Sci* (2014) **71**:2335–46. doi:10.1007/s00018-013-1495-x
45. Tateda K, Moore TA, Deng JC, Newstead MW, Zeng X, Matsukawa A, et al. Early recruitment of neutrophils determines subsequent T1/T2 host responses in a murine model of *Legionella pneumophila* pneumonia. *J Immunol* (2001) **166**:3355–61. doi:10.4049/jimmunol.166.5.3355
46. Soehnlein O, Weber C, Lindbom L. Neutrophil granule proteins tune monocytic cell function. *Trends Immunol* (2009) **30**:538–46. doi:10.1016/j.it.2009.06.006
47. Appelberg R. Neutrophils and intracellular pathogens: beyond phagocytosis and killing. *Trends Microbiol* (2007) **15**:87–92. doi:10.1016/j.tim.2006.11.009
48. Yang C-W, Strong BSI, Miller MJ, Unanue ER. Neutrophils influence the level of antigen presentation during the immune response to protein antigens in adjuvants. *J Immunol* (2010) **185**:2927–34. doi:10.4049/jimmunol.1001289
49. Müller I, Munder M, Kropf P, Hänsch GM. Polymorphonuclear neutrophils and T lymphocytes: strange bedfellows or brothers in arms? *Trends Immunol* (2009) **30**:522–30. doi:10.1016/j.it.2009.07.007
50. Potter NS, Harding CV. Neutrophils process exogenous bacteria via an alternate class I MHC processing pathway for presentation of peptides to T lymphocytes. *J Immunol* (2001) **167**:2538–46. doi:10.4049/jimmunol.167.5.2538
51. Wagner C, Iking-Konert C, Hug F, Stegmaier S, Heppert V, Wentzensen A, et al. Cellular inflammatory response to persistent localized *Staphylococcus aureus* infection: phenotypical and functional characterization of polymorphonuclear neutrophils (PMN). *Clin Exp Immunol* (2006) **143**:70–7. doi:10.1111/j.1365-2249.2005.02963.x
52. Gosselin EJ, Wardwell K, Rigby WF, Guyre PM. Induction of MHC class II on human polymorphonuclear neutrophils by granulocyte/macrophage colony-stimulating factor, IFN-gamma, and IL-3. *J Immunol* (1993) **151**:1482–90.
53. Radsak M, Iking-Konert C, Stegmaier S, Andrassy K, Hänsch GM. Polymorphonuclear neutrophils as accessory cells for T-cell activation: major histocompatibility complex class II restricted antigen-dependent induction of T-cell proliferation. *Immunology* (2000) **101**:521–30. doi:10.1046/j.1365-2567.2000.00140.x
54. Boomer JS. Immunosuppression in patients who die of sepsis and multiple organ failure. *JAMA* (2011) **306**:2594. doi:10.1001/jama.2011.1829
55. Darcy CJ, Minigo G, Piera KA, Davis JS, McNeil YR, Chen Y, et al. Neutrophils with myeloid derived suppressor function deplete arginine and constrain T

cell function in septic shock patients. *Crit Care* (2014) **18**:R163. doi:10.1186/cc14003

56. Hotchkiss RS, Monneret G, Payen D. Sepsis-induced immunosuppression: from cellular dysfunctions to immunotherapy. *Nat Rev Immunol* (2013) **13**:862–74. doi:10.1038/nri3552
57. Tak T, Hilvering B, Tesselaar K, Koenderman L. Similar activation state of neutrophils in sputum of asthma patients irrespective of sputum eosinophilia. *Clin Exp Immunol* (2015). doi:10.1111/cei.12676
58. Beauvillain C, Delneste Y, Scotet M, Peres A, Gascan H, Guermonprez P, et al. Neutrophils efficiently cross-prime naive T cells in vivo. *Blood* (2007) **110**:2965–73. doi:10.1182/blood-2006-12-063826
59. Maletto BA, Ropolo AS, Alignani DO, Liscovsky MV, Ranocchia RP, Moron VG, et al. Presence of neutrophil-bearing antigen in lymphoid organs of immune mice. *Blood* (2006) **108**:3094–102. doi:10.1182/blood-2006-04-016659
60. Abdallah DSA, Egan CE, Butcher BA, Denkers EY. Mouse neutrophils are professional antigen-presenting cells programmed to instruct Th1 and Th17 T-cell differentiation. *Int Immunol* (2011) **23**:317–26. doi:10.1093/intimm/dxr007
61. Schuster S, Hurrell B, Tacchini-Cottier F. Crosstalk between neutrophils and dendritic cells: a context-dependent process. *J Leukoc Biol* (2013) **94**:671–5. doi:10.1189/jlb.1012540
62. Tecchio C, Scapini P, Pizzolo G, Cassatella MA. On the cytokines produced by human neutrophils in tumors. *Semin Cancer Biol* (2013) **23**:159–70. doi:10.1016/j.semcancer.2013.02.004
63. Youn J-I, Nagaraj S, Collazo M, Gabrilovich DI. Subsets of myeloid-derived suppressor cells in tumor-bearing mice. *J Immunol* (2008) **181**:5791–802. doi:10.4049/jimmunol.181.8.5791
64. Youn J-I, Collazo M, Shalova IN, Biswas SK, Gabrilovich DI. Characterization of the nature of granulocytic myeloid-derived suppressor cells in tumor-bearing mice. *J Leukoc Biol* (2012) **91**:167–81. doi:10.1189/jlb.0311177
65. Rodriguez PC, Ernstoff MS, Hernandez C, Atkins M, Zabaleta J, Sierra R, et al. Arginase I-producing myeloid-derived suppressor cells in renal cell carcinoma are a subpopulation of activated granulocytes. *Cancer Res* (2009) **69**:1553–60. doi:10.1158/0008-5472.CAN-08-1921
66. Khaled YS, Ammori BJ, Elkord E. Increased levels of granulocytic myeloid-derived suppressor cells in peripheral blood and tumour tissue of pancreatic cancer patients. *J Immunol Res* (2014) **2014**:879897. doi:10.1155/2014/879897
67. Dumitru CA, Moses K, Trellakis S, Lang S, Brandau S. Neutrophils and granulocytic myeloid-derived suppressor cells: immunophenotyping, cell biology and clinical relevance in human oncology. *Cancer Immunol Immunother* (2012) **61**:1155–67. doi:10.1007/s00262-012-1294-5
68. Fridlender ZG, Albelda SM, Granot Z. Promoting metastasis: neutrophils and T cells join forces. *Cell Res* (2015) **25**:765–6. doi:10.1038/cr.2015.62
69. Brandau S, Dumitru CA, Lang S. Protumor and antitumor functions of neutrophil granulocytes. *Semin Immunopathol* (2013) **35**:163–76. doi:10.1007/s00281-012-0344-6
70. Kuang DM, Zhao Q, Wu Y, Peng C, Wang J, Xu Z, et al. Peritumoral neutrophils link inflammatory response to disease progression by fostering angiogenesis in hepatocellular carcinoma. *J Hepatol* (2011) **54**:948–55. doi:10.1016/j.jhep.2010.08.041
71. Jablonska J, Leschner S, Westphal K, Lienenklaus S, Weiss S. Neutrophils responsive to endogenous IFN-beta regulate tumor angiogenesis and growth in a mouse tumor model. *J Clin Invest* (2010) **120**:1151–64. doi:10.1172/JCI37223
72. Bank U, Reinhold D, Schneemilch C, Kunz D, Synowitz HJ, Ansorge S. Selective proteolytic cleavage of IL-2 receptor and IL-6 receptor ligand binding chains by neutrophil-derived serine proteases at foci of inflammation. *J Interferon Cytokine Res* (1999) **19**:1277–87. doi:10.1089/107999099312957
73. Bank U, Ansorge S. More than destructive: neutrophil-derived serine proteases in cytokine bioactivity control. *J Leukoc Biol* (2001) **69**:197–206.
74. Rodriguez PC, Quiceno DG, Ochoa AC. L-arginine availability regulates T-lymphocyte cell-cycle progression. *Blood* (2007) **109**:1568–73. doi:10.1182/blood-2006-06-031856
75. Makarenkova VP, Bansal V, Matta BM, Perez LA, Ochoa JB. CD11b+/Gr-1+ myeloid suppressor cells cause T cell dysfunction after traumatic stress. *J Immunol* (2006) **176**:2085–94. doi:10.4049/jimmunol.176.4.2085
76. Yachimovich-Cohen N, Even-Ram S, Shufaro Y, Rachmilewitz J, Reubinoff B. Human embryonic stem cells suppress T cell responses via arginase I-dependent mechanism. *J Immunol* (2010) **184**:1300–8. doi:10.4049/jimmunol.0804261
77. Gelderman KA, Hultqvist M, Holmberg J, Olofsson P, Holmdahl R. T cell surface redox levels determine T cell reactivity and arthritis susceptibility. *Proc Natl Acad Sci U S A* (2006) **103**:12831–6. doi:10.1073/pnas.0604571103
78. Malmberg KJ, Arulampalam V, Ichihara F, Petersson M, Seki K, Andersson T, et al. Inhibition of activated/memory (CD45RO(+)) T cells by oxidative stress associated with block of NF-kappaB activation. *J Immunol* (2001) **167**:2595–601. doi:10.4049/jimmunol.167.5.2595
79. Jacobsen LC, Theilgaard-Mönch K, Christensen EI, Borregaard N. Arginase 1 is expressed in myelocytes/metamyelocytes and localized in gelatinase granules of human neutrophils. *Blood* (2007) **109**:3084–7. doi:10.1182/blood-2006-06-032599
80. Munder M, Mollinedo F, Calafat J, Canchado J, Gil-lamaignere C, Fuentes M, et al. Arginase I is constitutively expressed in human granulocytes and participates in fungicidal activity. *Immunobiology* (2005) **105**:2549–56. doi:10.1182/blood-2004-07-2521.Supported
81. Rodriguez PC, Zea AH, Culotta KS, Zabaleta J, Ochoa JB, Ochoa AC. Regulation of T cell receptor CD3zeta chain expression by L-arginine. *J Biol Chem* (2002) **277**:21123–9. doi:10.1074/jbc.M110675200
82. Feldmeyer N, Wabnitz G, Leicht S, Luckner-minden C, Schiller M, Franz T, et al. Arginine deficiency leads to impaired cofilin dephosphorylation in activated human T lymphocytes. *Int Immunol* (2012) **24**:303–13. doi:10.1093/intimm/dxs004
83. Burkhardt JK, Carrizosa E, Shaffer MH. The actin cytoskeleton in T cell activation. *Annu Rev Immunol* (2008) **26**:233–59. doi:10.1146/annurev.immunol.26.021607.090347
84. Klebanoff SJ, White LR. Iodination defect in the leukocytes of a patient with chronic granulomatous disease of childhood. *N Engl J Med* (1969) **280**:460–6. doi:10.1056/NEJM196902272800902
85. Seger RA. Chronic granulomatous disease: recent advances in pathophysiology and treatment. *Neth J Med* (2010) **68**:334–40.
86. Nathan C, Ding A. Snapshot: reactive oxygen intermediates (ROI). *Cell* (2010) **140**:8–10. doi:10.1016/j.cell.2010.03.008
87. Klemke M, Wabnitz GH, Funke F, Funk B, Kirchgessner H, Samstag Y. Oxidation of cofilin mediates T cell hyporesponsiveness under oxidative stress conditions. *Immunity* (2008) **29**:404–13. doi:10.1016/j.immuni.2008.06.016
88. Mougiakakos D, Johansson CC, Kiessling R. Naturally occurring regulatory T cells show reduced sensitivity toward oxidative stress-induced cell death. *Blood* (2009) **113**:3542–5. doi:10.1182/blood-2008-09-181040
89. Brahmamdam P, Inoue S, Unsinger J, Chang KC, McDunn JE, Hotchkiss RS. Delayed administration of anti-PD-1 antibody reverses immune dysfunction and improves survival during sepsis. *J Leukoc Biol* (2010) **88**:233–40. doi:10.1189/jlb.0110037
90. Matsushima H, Geng S, Lu R, Okamoto T, Yao Y, Mayuzumi N, et al. Neutrophil differentiation into a unique hybrid population exhibiting dual phenotype and functionality of neutrophils and dendritic cells. *Blood* (2013) **121**:1677–89. doi:10.1182/blood-2012-07-445189
91. Oehler L, Majdic O, Pickl WF, Stöckl J, Riedl E, Drach J, et al. Neutrophil granulocyte-committed cells can be driven to acquire dendritic cell characteristics. *J Exp Med* (1998) **187**:1019–28. doi:10.1084/jem.187.7.1019
92. Mantovani A, Cassatella MA, Costantini C, Jaillon S. Neutrophils in the activation and regulation of innate and adaptive immunity. *Nat Rev Immunol* (2011) **11**:519–31. doi:10.1038/nri3024
93. Bruijnzeel PLB, Uddin M, Koenderman L. Targeting neutrophilic inflammation in severe neutrophilic asthma: can we target the disease-relevant neutrophil phenotype? *J Leukoc Biol* (2015) **98**. doi:10.1189/jlb.3VMR1214-600RR

6

Contribution of basophils to cutaneous immune reactions and Th2-mediated allergic responses

Atsushi Otsuka[1]* *and Kenji Kabashima*[1,2]*

[1] Department of Dermatology, Kyoto University Graduate School of Medicine, Kyoto, Japan, [2] PRESTO, Japan Science and Technology Agency, Kawaguchi, Saitama, Japan

Edited by:
Elisabetta Padovan,
University of Basel, Switzerland

Reviewed by:
F. Ronchese,
Malaghan Institute of Medical Research, New Zealand
Daniel Yerly,
University Hospital of Bern, Switzerland

***Correspondence:**
Atsushi Otsuka and Kenji Kabashima,
Department of Dermatology, Kyoto University Graduate School of Medicine, 54 Shogoin Kawara, Sakyo-ku, Kyoto 606-8507, Japan
otsukamn@kuhp.kyoto-u.ac.jp;
kaba@kuhp.kyoto-u.ac.jp

Basophils are potent effector cells of innate immunity and also play a role in T helper 2 (Th2)-mediated allergic responses. But, although their *in vitro* functions are well studied, their *in vivo* functions remain largely unknown. However, several mouse models of basophil depletion have recently been developed and used to investigate basophil functions. For example, in a croton oil-induced model of irritant contact dermatitis in conditionally basophil-depleted transgenic mice, we found that basophils rapidly infiltrate inflamed skin and subsequently induce infiltration of eosinophils. We also showed that basophils induce Th2 skewing upon epicutaneous sensitization with various haptens and peptide antigens. Intriguingly, basophils also promoted Th2 polarization upon protein antigen exposure in the presence of dendritic cells (DCs). The dermal DC subset associated with Th2 skewing was recently identified as $CD301b^{+}$ DC. Such studies with basophil-deficient mouse models have significantly improved our understanding of the mechanisms involved in human immune-related diseases. In this review, we will focus on the relative contribution of basophils and DCs to Th2-mediated allergic responses.

Keywords: basophil, dendritic cell, Th2, contact dermatitis, IgE-CAI

Introduction

T helper 2 (Th2) immune responses, which develop in response to allergens and parasites, are characterized by high levels of immunoglobulin E (IgE) and the presence of Th2 cells (1). Basophils are intimately involved in Th2 immune responses, and upon activation of the high-affinity receptor for IgE (FcεRI) or other surface receptors, they release multiple effector molecules, including proteases, vasodilating substances, such as histamine, cytokines, pro-inflammatory chemokines, and lipid mediators (2, 3). However, the mechanisms that initiate Th2 responses are not fully understood. Previous reports have shown that dendritic cells (DCs), the most efficient antigen-presenting cells (APCs) in the immune system, play a crucial role (4). However, recent experiments in newly developed basophil-deficient mouse models have highlighted the importance of basophils as well. For example, Th2 skewing is considered to be mainly induced by DCs, but recent studies in basophil-depletion mouse models indicate that basophils also play a pivotal role in this process (5–7). Here, we review the roles of basophils in cutaneous immune reactions and Th2-mediated allergic responses associated with cutaneous allergic diseases, focusing on the possibility that basophils and DCs function cooperatively in inducing Th2-mediated allergic responses.

Cutaneous Allergic Diseases Associated with Basophil Infiltration

Basophils have been detected in the vicinity of eosinophils in several human cutaneous allergic diseases, and infiltration of basophils has been reported in several skin diseases, including atopic dermatitis (AD), prurigo, and urticaria (8). It is noteworthy that skin lesions of bullous pemphigoid, classical eosinophilic pustular folliculitis (Ofuji's disease), and Henoch–Schönlein purpura also frequently exhibit tissue basophilia (8–11) (**Table 1**). We recently demonstrated the presence of both basophils and eosinophils in inflamed skin of patients with irritant contact dermatitis (ICD) (12). Further, we showed that basophils rapidly infiltrate into the inflamed skin, and subsequently induce infiltration of eosinophils with a croton oil-induced model of ICD. But it is still unclear exactly how basophils infiltrate into the lesional skin. There are several candidate basophil attractants, such as α(1,3)-fucosyltransferases IV and VII, for the initial recruitment of basophils in chronic allergic inflammation (CAI) (13). Subsequently, basophils attract eosinophils directly or indirectly via eotaxin-mediated interaction with mesenchymal fibroblasts (12).

IgE-Mediated Chronic Allergic Inflammation and Chronic Idiopathic Urticaria

Immunoglobulin E-mediated chronic allergic inflammation (IgE-CAI) is a novel type of chronic inflammation of the skin that follows the immediate-type and late-phase responses in mice (14). It has been reported that IgE-CAI is independent of mast cells and T cells, but is dependent on basophils expressing FceRIa and CD49b phenotypic markers (14). Interestingly, although the number of basophils infiltrating the lesional skin is very low, their depletion led to a marked reduction in inflammation, concomitantly with decreased numbers of eosinophils and neutrophils and attenuation of the increased ear thickness (14). Recent studies have shown that inflammatory monocytes recruited to IgE-CAI lesions acquire an anti-inflammatory phenotype via basophil-derived IL-4 (15). Collectively, these results suggest a specific and non-redundant role for basophils in the initiation and maintenance of chronic IgE-mediated inflammatory responses in mice (16).

It is important to note that there are some functional differences between human basophils and mouse basophils. In mice, activated basophils produce platelet-activating factors and contribute to the development of anaphylaxis in response to penicillin-IgG antibody complexes. On the other hand, human basophils do not respond to IgG immune complexes (17, 18). Nevertheless, some findings in mouse basophils appear to shed light on the pathogenesis of human cutaneous diseases. Antibodies to FcεRIα were found in 40% of patients with chronic idiopathic urticaria (CIU). Some CIU patients exhibited urticaria in response to anti-FcεRIα IgG and/or IgE antibodies, which may stimulate mast cells or basophils (19). In addition, an activation marker on basophils, CD203c, was upregulated upon incubation of donor basophils with sera from patients with CIU (20). Furthermore, infiltration of basophils is increased in urticarial lesions of CIU (8, 21). Consistently with this finding, basopenia in CIU appears to be due to the migration of basophils from the peripheral blood to urticarial lesions (1, 8, 21). Therefore, the phenomena seen in the mouse IgE-CAI model might explain the pathogenesis of human CIU.

TABLE 1 | Dermatological diseases accompanied with basophil infiltration.

Atopic dermatitis (8)
Irritant contact dermatitis (12)
Prurigo (8)
Urticaria (8)
Pemphigus vulgaris (8)
Bullous vulgaris (8)
Drug eruption (8)
Henoch–Schönlein purpura (8)
Insect bite (tick bite) (11)
Scabies (8)
Dermatomyositis (8)
Eosinophilic pustular folliculitis (10)
Leprosy (LL type) (9)

Dendritic Cell-Specific and Basophil-Specific Depletion Models

Although the CD11c-based system is the most common depletion model of DCs, it has the disadvantage of imperfectly separating conventional DCs (cDCs) and macrophages (22, 23). On the other hand, since there are no natural mouse mutants with basophil deficiencies, antibodies that recognize either FcεRI (clone MAR-1) or the orphan-activating receptor CD200 receptor 3 (CD200R3) (clone Ba103) have been used to investigate the role of basophils. However, these antibody clones not only deplete basophils but also stimulate mast cells (24, 25). In addition, Ba103 activates myeloid cells and NK cells (26), and MAR-1 depletes a subset of FcεRI-positive DCs (27). **Table 2** summarizes currently available mouse strains with constitutive or inducible depletion of basophils. Three groups have developed basophil-depletion models through regulation of *Mcpt8*, a basophil-specific gene in the conserved chymase locus (24, 28–30). In these mice, basophils were depleted in peripheral blood without side effects. A different basophil-depletion model utilizing the P1-Runx gene was reported by Mukai et al. (31) These mice show depletion of basophils, but not eosinophils, neutrophils, or mast cells. Sawaguchi et al. developed Bas-TRECK Tg mice, using a diphtheria-toxin receptor (DTR) transgene under the control of the DNase I-hypersensitive site 4 (HS4) region of IL-4 (32).

Basophils are Associated with Th2 Skewing in Response to Haptens

Mature DCs are generally considered to be required for naïve T cells to proliferate and acquire Th2 effector functions in response to antigen encounters (33). Recently, however, the function of DCs in Th2 induction has been questioned because basophils also appear to play a pivotal role in this process (5–7). Basophils migrate into draining lymph nodes (LNs) from the site of papain injection or helminth infection and act as APCs by taking up and processing antigens (5–7). In addition, basophils are capable of expressing MHC class II and costimulatory molecules, such

TABLE 2 | Mouse models of basophil depletion.

Model system	Experimental strategy	Method of depletion	Depletion efficiency	Reference
Basoph8	Knock-in of IRES–YFP–Cre cassette before the Mcpt8 start codon	Cross to R-DTA mice	>90%	(28)
Mcpt8-Cre	BAC transgene (Cre inserted after the Mcpt8 start codon)	Constitutive depletion	>90%	(24)
Mcpt8^{DTR}	Knock-in of IRES–DTR–EGFP cassette in 3′-UTR of Mcpt8	DT injection	>90%	(29)
P1-Runx1	Knockout	P1-Runx1 seems to be essential for the basophil lineage	>90%	(31)
Bas-TRECK	DTR transgene (under control of HS4 region of IL-4)	DT injection	>90%	(32)

BAC, bacterial artificial chromosome; DTR, diphtheria toxin receptor; IL-4, interleukin-4; IRES, internal ribosome entry site; Mcpt, mast cell protease; NA, not applicable; NR, not reported; R-DTA, ROSA-diphtheria toxin-α; UTR, untranslated region; YFP, yellow fluorescent protein.

as CD40, CD80, and CD86. They also secrete several cytokines critical for Th2 development, including IL-4 and thymic stromal lymphopoietin (TSLP). Thus, under certain conditions, basophils alone, without DCs, can cause Th2 induction from naïve T cells. However, the role of basophils in Th2 skewing has again been questioned since several of the above experiments used bone marrow-derived basophils (BMBaso) containing FcεRI-expressing inflammatory DC (27).

Recently, we demonstrated that basophils play a role in Th2 skewing in response to haptens and peptide antigens, but not protein antigens, in a basophil-deficient mouse model, Bas TRECK Tg (34). In addition, we showed that basophils were capable of Th2 skewing by using CD11c-depleted BMBaso in order to avoid contamination with inflammatory DCs. Basophils express MHC class II, CD40, CD80, CD86, and IL-4 in the hapten-induced cutaneous Th2 model. However, using the DQ-OVA system, we confirmed that basophils did not efficiently take up or process protein antigens (34). A different experimental system using OVA coupled to fluorescein isothiocyanate showed that basophils could take up protein antigens (6), but our results showed that hapten antigens and peptides might bind directly to MHC class II on basophils, and they could be acquired and presented by basophils. On the other hand, basophils hardly digest protein and so cannot efficiently present protein antigens (**Figures 1** and **2**). Although the OVA-peptide system is totally artificial, complex inflammatory environments, such as post-*Schistosoma mansoni* or *Trichuris muris* infection, probably contain small soluble antigens as well as larger proteins. In addition, cutaneous immunization with papain protease allergen promotes MHC class II expression on basophils in LNs, probably after the generation of peptide antigens from the protein *in vivo* (6). A recent report showed that basophils are capable of inducing Th2 upon exposure to OVA proteins complexed with specific IgE (7). They pulsed basophils with various doses of DNP-OVA in the presence of monoclonal antibody to DNP (IgE anti-DNP) and showed that Th2 skewing by basophils was enhanced with the effect of IgE anti-DNP, especially when basophils were pulsed with low concentrations of DNP-OVA (7). House dust mites, which possess cysteine protease activity, are incapable of inducing Th2 when presented by basophils, even though cysteine protease may play a role in processing protein antigen into peptides *in vivo* (27), because the expressions of HLA-DM and of the invariant chain on basophils, those were sorted from the LNs 3 days after house dust mites administration, were very low (27).

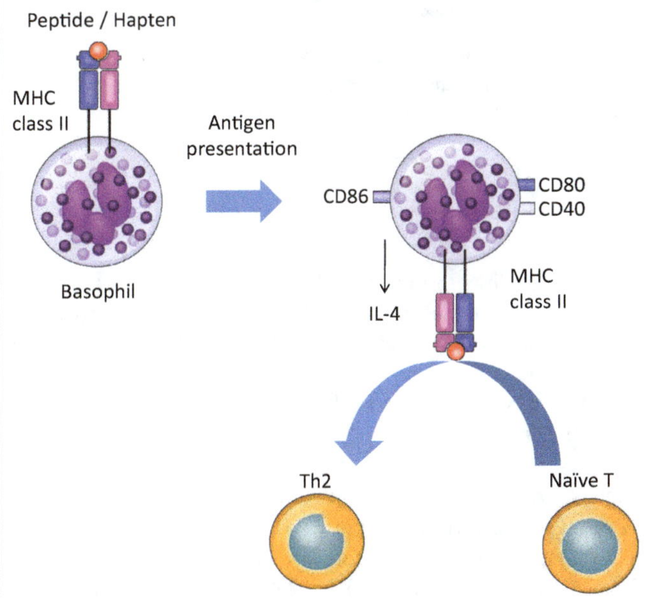

FIGURE 1 | Basophils promote Th2 skewing in response to haptens and peptide antigens. Basophils promote Th2 skewing upon peptide and hapten exposure by expressing MHC class II, CD40, CD80, CD86, and IL-4.

Although several studies show that murine basophils can serve as APCs, the situation is less clear for human basophils. Human basophils express MHC class II (35, 36), but it was not able to induce antigen-specific T cell activation or proliferation in response to house dust mite allergen exposure (36). Another group reported that HLA-DR in human basophils is upregulated by IL-3 and IFN-γ, but the basophils cannot work as APCs for pollen allergen (37). It has been confirmed that human basophils lack some features of APCs (38, 39). Additional studies are needed to determine whether human basophils can act as APCs under various pathophysiological conditions.

Interaction between DCs and Basophils for Th2 Skewing

It has been reported that basophils contribute to the strength of the Th2 response in the lungs, but they cannot present antigens or express chaperones involved in antigen presentation (27). Therefore, it was suggested that DCs are necessary and sufficient

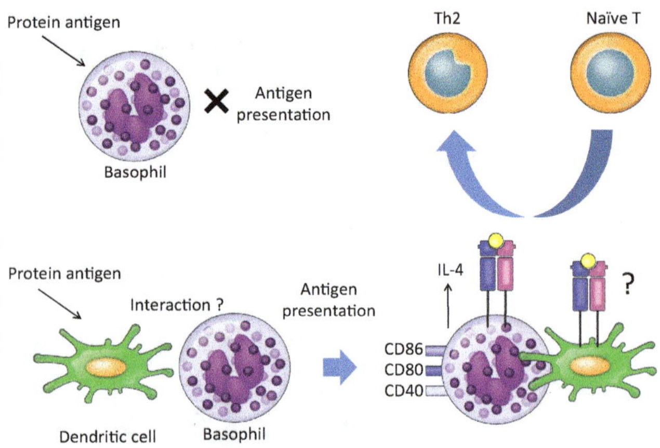

FIGURE 2 | Basophils promote Th2 skewing in response to protein antigens in the presence of dendritic cells. Upon exposure to OVA protein, basophils do not work as APCs, since basophils cannot take up or process OVA protein. In the presence of dendritic cells, however, basophils promote Th2 skewing. The precise mechanisms of interaction between basophils and dendritic cells remain unclear.

for inducing Th2 immunity to house dust mites in the lungs, and basophils are not required. In accordance with this idea, Th2 responses were severely impaired after *Schistosoma mansoni* egg injection and during active *Schistosoma mansoni* infection by depletion of CD11c$^+$ cells, but not by depletion of basophils with anti-FcεRIα antibody (4). These findings suggest that some DC subsets induce Th2 skewing upon exposure to protein antigens.

Recently, two different groups have shown that Th2 skewing in response to *Nippostrongylus brasiliensis* infection depends on dermal CD301b$^+$ DCs (40, 41). Depletion of CD301b$^+$ DCs prior to infection reduces the number of IL-4-producing CD4$^+$ T cells (40, 41). CD301b$^+$ DCs also express programed death ligand-2 (PDL2), and a subset of PDL2$^+$CD301b$^+$ DCs that express the transcription factor interferon regulatory factor 4 (IRF4) was shown to be required for Th2 induction *in vivo* (41). In accordance with these findings, CD11c$^+$MHC class II$^+$ dermal DCs expressing PDL2, and CD301b were identified as a Th2-inducing DC subset in *Nippostrongylus brasiliensis* infection (42). However, CD301b$^+$ DCs alone are incapable of inducing a Th2 response *in vitro* (41) or *in vivo* (40).

We have shown that basophils are capable of inducing Th2 skewing upon exposure to protein antigens in the presence of DCs (34). Because basophils are not able to take up or process protein antigens efficiently, DCs may prepare peptides from protein antigens for antigen presentation by basophils or may promote IL-4 production from basophils to skew Th2. In line with this, we had previously demonstrated that Langerhans cells, an epidermal DC subset, mediate epicutaneous sensitization with OVA protein antigen to induce Th2-type immune responses (43). Further studies are needed to show direct evidence whether DCs prepare peptides from protein antigens for the Th2 induction by basophils. In addition, Th2 reaction in response to schistosome infection or protein antigens was reduced in a CD11c-depletion model (4, 27). Therefore, DCs seem to be necessary for inducing Th2 reaction upon exposure to protein antigen both *in vivo* and *in vitro*.

Furthermore, basophils were found in the vicinity of T-cells in the T-cell zone of draining LNs by epicutaneous sensitization with haptens (34). Optimal localization of DCs within LNs may play a crucial role in Th2 skewing in each condition. CXCR5-expressing CD11c$^+$ DCs migrate to the LNs and localize adjacent to B cell follicles in *Heligmosomoides polygyrus* infection, whereas depletion of CXCR5 or B cell-derived lymphotoxin alters the localization of DCs and impairs the development of Th2 cells (44). Therefore, although the location of DCs on draining LNs for Th2 induction is still controversial, it is possible that basophils, T cells, and DCs promote Th2 induction in a coordinated way. Similarly, reactive oxygen species (ROS) were generated in dermal DCs and in LN DCs upon subcutaneous exposure to papain plus antigen. ROS promoted Th2 response via formation of oxidized lipids that triggered TSLP production by epithelial cells. In addition, ROS enhanced Th2 induction by inducing release of CCL7 from DCs, leading to the recruitment of basophils to the draining LNs (45). Another group showed that IL-3 plays a role in basophil recruitment to draining LNs using helminth infection model with mice deficient in IL-3 or IL-3Rβ (46). However, they found that helminth-induced Th2 response was not diminished in an MAR-1 antibody-induced basophil-depletion model. Further studies are needed to determine whether DCs present peptides to basophils directly or whether plasma membrane fragments are transferred from APCs to lymphocytes by trogocytosis.

Conclusion

Studies in basophil-deficient mouse models over the last decade have greatly improved our understanding of the mechanisms of development of Th2 immune reactions. Nevertheless, some key questions remain unanswered, including how DCs cooperate with basophils during Th2 skewing, especially in response to protein antigen exposure. In addition, the precise role of basophils in Th2 skewing, especially their function as APCs, remains controversial (27, 46). One possibility is that basophils may work as early IL-4-producing cells for the induction of Th2. An issue in some previous studies has been the imperfect separation of cDC in CD11c-based systems, and one possible approach to overcome this would be to use *CD11c*-DTR and *Zbtb46*-DTR, a marker specifically expressed by cDCs in lymphoid and non-lymphoid tissues but not by other myeloid or lymphoid cell types (47). Newly developed DC-deficient and basophil-deficient models are expected to provide further information on the mechanisms involved in Th2 skewing. Such studies may provide a basis for novel therapeutic approaches to controlling allergic diseases.

Acknowledgments

This work was supported in part by Grants-in-Aid (6-Itaku(men)-ippan-007 and Kiban S 15H05890) for Scientific Research from the Ministry of Education, Culture, Sports, Science and Technology, and for Precursory Research on Embryonic Science and Technology from the Ministry of Health, Labour and Welfare, Japan.

References

1. Otsuka A, Kabashima K. Mast cells and basophils in cutaneous immune responses. *Allergy* (2015) **70**:131–40. doi:10.1111/all.12526
2. Migalovich-Sheikhet H, Friedman S, Mankuta D, Levi-Schaffer F. Novel identified receptors on mast cells. *Front Immunol* (2012) **3**:238. doi:10.3389/fimmu.2012.00238
3. Schneider E, Thieblemont N, De Moraes ML, Dy M. Basophils: new players in the cytokine network. *Eur Cytokine Netw* (2010) **21**:142–53. doi:10.1684/ecn.2010.0197
4. Phythian-Adams AT, Cook PC, Lundie RJ, Jones LH, Smith KA, Barr TA, et al. CD11c depletion severely disrupts Th2 induction and development in vivo. *J Exp Med* (2010) **207**:2089–96. doi:10.1084/jem.20100734
5. Perrigoue JG, Saenz SA, Siracusa MC, Allenspach EJ, Taylor BC, Giacomin PR, et al. MHC class II-dependent basophil-CD4+ T cell interactions promote T(H)2 cytokine-dependent immunity. *Nat Immunol* (2009) **10**:697–705. doi:10.1038/ni.1740
6. Sokol CL, Chu NQ, Yu S, Nish SA, Laufer TM, Medzhitov R. Basophils function as antigen-presenting cells for an allergen-induced T helper type 2 response. *Nat Immunol* (2009) **10**:713–20. doi:10.1038/ni.1738
7. Yoshimoto T, Yasuda K, Tanaka H, Nakahira M, Imai Y, Fujimori Y, et al. Basophils contribute to T(H)2-IgE responses in vivo via IL-4 production and presentation of peptide-MHC class II complexes to CD4+ T cells. *Nat Immunol* (2009) **10**:706–12. doi:10.1038/ni.1737
8. Ito Y, Satoh T, Takayama K, Miyagishi C, Walls AF, Yokozeki H. Basophil recruitment and activation in inflammatory skin diseases. *Allergy* (2011) **66**:1107–13. doi:10.1111/j.1398-9995.2011.02570.x
9. Otsuka A, Ozaki M, Horiguchi Y, Murata Y, Kumano K, Nogami R, et al. Basophils infiltrate the skin lesions in lepromatous leprosy. *Acta Derm Venereol* (2013) **93**:88–9. doi:10.2340/00015555-1329
10. Otsuka A, Miyagawa-Hayashino A, Walls AF, Miyachi Y, Kabashima K. Comparison of basophil infiltration into the skin between eosinophilic pustular folliculitis and neutrophilic folliculitis. *J Eur Acad Dermatol Venereol* (2012) **26**:527–9. doi:10.1111/j.1468-3083.2011.04091.x
11. Nakahigashi K, Otsuka A, Tomari K, Miyachi Y, Kabashima K. Evaluation of basophil infiltration into the skin lesions of tick bites. *Case Rep Dermatol* (2013) **5**:48–51. doi:10.1159/000348650
12. Nakashima C, Otsuka A, Kitoh A, Honda T, Egawa G, Nakajima S, et al. Basophils regulate the recruitment of eosinophils in a murine model of irritant contact dermatitis. *J Allergy Clin Immunol* (2014) **134**:100–7. doi:10.1016/j.jaci.2014.02.026
13. Saeki K, Satoh T, Yokozeki H. α(1, 3) fucosyltransferases IV and VII are essential for the initial recruitment of basophils in chronic allergic inflammation. *J Invest Dermatol* (2013) **133**:2161–9. doi:10.1038/jid.2013.160
14. Mukai K, Matsuoka K, Taya C, Suzuki H, Yokozeki H, Nishioka K, et al. Basophils play a critical role in the development of IgE-mediated chronic allergic inflammation independently of T cells and mast cells. *Immunity* (2005) **23**:191–202. doi:10.1016/j.immuni.2005.06.011
15. Egawa M, Mukai K, Yoshikawa S, Iki M, Mukaida N, Kawano Y, et al. Inflammatory monocytes recruited to allergic skin acquire an anti-inflammatory M2 phenotype via basophil-derived interleukin-4. *Immunity* (2013) **38**:570–80. doi:10.1016/j.immuni.2012.11.014
16. Siracusa MC, Perrigoue JG, Comeau MR, Artis D. New paradigms in basophil development, regulation and function. *Immunol Cell Biol* (2010) **88**:275–84. doi:10.1038/icb.2010.1
17. Tsujimura Y, Obata K, Mukai K, Shindou H, Yoshida M, Nishikado H, et al. Basophils play a pivotal role in immunoglobulin-G-mediated but not immunoglobulin-E-mediated systemic anaphylaxis. *Immunity* (2008) **28**:581–9. doi:10.1016/j.immuni.2008.02.008
18. Siracusa MC, Kim BS, Spergel JM, Artis D. Basophils and allergic inflammation. *J Allergy Clin Immunol* (2013) **132**:789–801. doi:10.1016/j.jaci.2013.07.046
19. Eckman JA, Hamilton RG, Gober LM, Sterba PM, Saini SS. Basophil phenotypes in chronic idiopathic urticaria in relation to disease activity and autoantibodies. *J Invest Dermatol* (2008) **128**:1956–63. doi:10.1038/jid.2008.55
20. Yasnowsky KM, Dreskin SC, Efaw B, Schoen D, Vedanthan PK, Alam R, et al. Chronic urticaria sera increase basophil CD203c expression. *J Allergy Clin Immunol* (2006) **117**:1430–4. doi:10.1016/j.jaci.2006.02.016
21. Ying S, Kikuchi Y, Meng Q, Kay AB, Kaplan AP. TH1/TH2 cytokines and inflammatory cells in skin biopsy specimens from patients with chronic idiopathic urticaria: comparison with the allergen-induced late-phase cutaneous reaction. *J Allergy Clin Immunol* (2002) **109**:694–700. doi:10.1016/S0091-6749(02)81367-7
22. Murphy KM. Comment on "activation of beta-catenin in dendritic cells regulates immunity versus tolerance in the intestine". *Science* (2011) **333**:405. doi:10.1126/science.1198277
23. Manicassamy S, Reizis B, Ravindran R, Nakaya H, Salazar-Gonzalez RM, Wang YC, et al. Activation of beta-catenin in dendritic cells regulates immunity versus tolerance in the intestine. *Science* (2010) **329**:849–53. doi:10.1126/science.1188510
24. Ohnmacht C, Schwartz C, Panzer M, Schiedewitz I, Naumann R, Voehringer D. Basophils orchestrate chronic allergic dermatitis and protective immunity against helminths. *Immunity* (2010) **33**:364–74. doi:10.1016/j.immuni.2010.08.011
25. Kojima T, Obata K, Mukai K, Sato S, Takai T, Minegishi Y, et al. Mast cells and basophils are selectively activated in vitro and in vivo through CD200R3 in an IgE-independent manner. *J Immunol* (2007) **179**:7093–100. doi:10.4049/jimmunol.179.10.7093
26. Obata K, Mukai K, Tsujimura Y, Ishiwata K, Kawano Y, Minegishi Y, et al. Basophils are essential initiators of a novel type of chronic allergic inflammation. *Blood* (2007) **110**:913–20. doi:10.1182/blood-2007-01-068718
27. Hammad H, Plantinga M, Deswarte K, Pouliot P, Willart MA, Kool M, et al. Inflammatory dendritic cells – not basophils – are necessary and sufficient for induction of Th2 immunity to inhaled house dust mite allergen. *J Exp Med* (2010) **207**:2097–111. doi:10.1084/jem.20101563
28. Sullivan BM, Liang HE, Bando JK, Wu D, Cheng LE, McKerrow JK, et al. Genetic analysis of basophil function in vivo. *Nat Immunol* (2011) **12**:527–35. doi:10.1038/ni.2036
29. Wada T, Ishiwata K, Koseki H, Ishikura T, Ugajin T, Ohnuma N, et al. Selective ablation of basophils in mice reveals their nonredundant role in acquired immunity against ticks. *J Clin Invest* (2010) **120**:2867–75. doi:10.1172/JCI42680
30. Poorafshar M, Helmby H, Troye-Blomberg M, Hellman L. MMCP-8, the first lineage-specific differentiation marker for mouse basophils. Elevated numbers of potent IL-4-producing and MMCP-8-positive cells in spleens of malaria-infected mice. *Eur J Immunol* (2000) **30**:2660–8. doi:10.1002/1521-4141(200009)30:9<2660::AID-IMMU2660>3.0.CO;2-I
31. Mukai K, BenBarak MJ, Tachibana M, Nishida K, Karasuyama H, Taniuchi I, et al. Critical role of P1-Runx1 in mouse basophil development. *Blood* (2012) **120**:76–85. doi:10.1182/blood-2011-12-399113
32. Sawaguchi M, Tanaka S, Nakatani Y, Harada Y, Mukai K, Matsunaga Y, et al. Role of mast cells and basophils in IgE responses and in allergic airway hyperresponsiveness. *J Immunol* (2012) **188**:1809–18. doi:10.4049/jimmunol.1101746
33. Lambrecht BN. Dendritic cells and the regulation of the allergic immune response. *Allergy* (2005) **60**:271–82. doi:10.1111/j.1398-9995.2005.00708.x
34. Otsuka A, Nakajima S, Kubo M, Egawa G, Honda T, Kitoh A, et al. Basophils are required for the induction of Th2 immunity to haptens and peptide antigens. *Nat Commun* (2013) **4**:1739. doi:10.1038/ncomms2740
35. Poulsen BC, Poulsen LK, Jensen BM. Detection of MHC class II expression on human basophils is dependent on antibody specificity but independent of atopic disposition. *J Immunol Methods* (2012) **381**:66–9. doi:10.1016/j.jim.2012.04.009
36. Voskamp AL, Prickett SR, Mackay F, Rolland JM, O'Hehir RE. MHC class II expression in human basophils: induction and lack of functional significance. *PLoS One* (2013) **8**:e81777. doi:10.1371/journal.pone.0081777
37. Kitzmüller C, Nagl B, Deifl S, Walterskirchen C, Jahn-Schmid B, Zlabinger GJ, et al. Human blood basophils do not act as antigen-presenting cells for the major birch pollen allergen Bet v 1. *Allergy* (2012) **67**:593–600. doi:10.1111/j.1398-9995.2011.02764.x
38. Eckl-Dorna J, Ellinger A, Blatt K, Ghanim V, Steiner I, Pavelka M, et al. Basophils are not the key antigen-presenting cells in allergic patients. *Allergy* (2012) **67**:601–8. doi:10.1111/j.1398-9995.2012.02792.x
39. Sharma M, Hegde P, Aimanianda V, Beau R, Maddur MS, Sénéchal H, et al. Circulating human basophils lack the features of professional antigen presenting cells. *Sci Rep* (2013) **3**:1188. doi:10.1038/srep01188
40. Kumamoto Y, Linehan M, Weinstein JS, Laidlaw BJ, Craft JE, Iwasaki A. CD301b(+) dermal dendritic cells drive T helper 2 cell-mediated immunity. *Immunity* (2013) **39**:733–43. doi:10.1016/j.immuni.2013.08.029

41. Gao Y, Nish SA, Jiang R, Hou L, Licona-Limón P, Weinstein JS, et al. Control of T helper 2 responses by transcription factor IRF4-dependent dendritic cells. *Immunity* (2013) **39**:722–32. doi:10.1016/j.immuni.2013.08.028
42. Connor LM, Tang SC, Camberis M, Le Gros G, Ronchese F. Helminth-conditioned dendritic cells prime CD4+ T cells to IL-4 production in vivo. *J Immunol* (2014) **193**:2709–17. doi:10.4049/jimmunol.1400374
43. Nakajima S, Igyártó BZ, Honda T, Egawa G, Otsuka A, Hara-Chikuma M, et al. Langerhans cells are critical in epicutaneous sensitization with protein antigen via thymic stromal lymphopoietin receptor signaling. *J Allergy Clin Immunol* (2012) **129**:1048–55.e1046. doi:10.1016/j.jaci.2012.01.063
44. León B, Ballesteros-Tato A, Browning JL, Dunn R, Randall TD, Lund FE. Regulation of T(H)2 development by CXCR5+ dendritic cells and lymphotoxin-expressing B cells. *Nat Immunol* (2012) **13**:681–90. doi:10.1038/ni.2309
45. Tang H, Cao W, Kasturi SP, Ravindran R, Nakaya HI, Kundu K, et al. The T helper type 2 response to cysteine proteases requires dendritic cell-basophil cooperation via ROS-mediated signaling. *Nat Immunol* (2010) **11**:608–17. doi:10.1038/ni.1883
46. Kim S, Prout M, Ramshaw H, Lopez AF, LeGros G, Min B. Cutting edge: basophils are transiently recruited into the draining lymph nodes during helminth infection via IL-3, but infection-induced Th2 immunity can develop without basophil lymph node recruitment or IL-3. *J Immunol* (2010) **184**:1143–7. doi:10.4049/jimmunol.0902447
47. Meredith MM, Liu K, Darrasse-Jeze G, Kamphorst AO, Schreiber HA, Guermonprez P, et al. Expression of the zinc finger transcription factor zDC (Zbtb46, Btbd4) defines the classical dendritic cell lineage. *J Exp Med* (2012) **209**:1153–65. doi:10.1084/jem.20112675

7

Maintenance of immune homeostasis through ILC/T cell interactions

Nicole von Burg*[1,2], *Gleb Turchinovich*[1,2] and *Daniela Finke*[1,2]

[1] *Department of Biomedicine, University of Basel, Basel, Switzerland,* [2] *University of Basel Children's Hospital, Basel, Switzerland*

Edited by:
Stefan F. Martin, University of Freiburg, Germany

Reviewed by:
Peter John Lane, Birmingham University, UK
Shahram Salek-ardakani, University of Florida, USA

***Correspondence:**
Daniela Finke, Department of Biomedicine, University of Basel Children's Hospital, Mattenstrasse 28, Basel 4058, Switzerland daniela.finke@unibas.ch

Innate lymphoid cells (ILCs) have emerged as a new family of immune cells with crucial functions in innate and adaptive immunity. ILC subsets mirror the cytokine and transcriptional profile of CD4$^+$ T helper (T_H) cell subsets. Hence, group 1 (ILC1), group 2 (ILC2), and group 3 (ILC3) ILCs can be distinguished by the production of T_H1, T_H2, and T_H17-type cytokines, respectively. Cytokine release by ILCs not only shapes early innate immunity but can also orchestrate T_H immune responses to microbial or allergen exposure. Recent studies have identified an unexpected effector function of ILCs as antigen presenting cells. Both ILC2s and ILC3s are able to process and present foreign antigens (Ags) via major histocompatibility complex class II, and to induce cognate CD4$^+$ T cell responses. In addition, Ag-stimulated T cells promote ILC activation and effector functions indicating a reciprocal interaction between the adaptive and innate immune system. A fundamental puzzle in ILC function is how ILC/T cell interactions promote host protection and prevent autoimmune diseases. Furthermore, the way in which microenvironmental and inflammatory signals determine the outcome of ILC/T cell immune responses in various tissues is not yet understood. This review focuses on recent advances in understanding the mechanisms that coordinate the collaboration between ILCs and T cells under homeostatic and inflammatory conditions. We also discuss the potential roles of T cells and other immune cells to regulate ILC functions and to maintain homeostasis in mucosal tissues.

Keywords: innate lymphoid cell, cytokine, T helper cell, immune response, antigen presentation

Introduction

Adaptive immune responses are tightly controlled by the selection of the T and B cell receptor repertoire and by transcriptional networks regulating commitment, expansion, and contraction of the responses. Upon cognate antigen (Ag)–peptide–major histocompatibility complex (MHC) recognition Ag-specific T helper (T_H) cells proliferate and differentiate into effector T_H cell subsets with distinguishable cytokine profiles. Almost 30 years ago, interferon (IFN)-γ-secreting T_H1 cells were discriminated from T_H2 cells, whose cytokine profile includes interleukin (IL)-4, IL-5, and IL-13 (1). Additional subsets of T_H cells, such as T_H17 (2), regulatory T (T_{reg}) cells (3), T_H9 (4), T follicular helper cells (5), and more recently granulocyte-macrophage colony-stimulating factor (GM-CSF) producing T_H cells (6–8), were described.

In the past 5 years, new subsets of innate immune cells have emerged as a first line of defense at mucosal barriers. Like conventional natural killer (cNK) cells, they belong to the lymphoid lineage and develop from common lymphoid progenitor (CLP) cells but unlike T and B cells, they lack rearranged Ag-receptors. Hence, they were termed innate lymphoid cells (ILCs). ILCs are found in various tissues including mucosa, lymphoid tissue, liver, skin, and fat. They depend on the expression of the common cytokine receptor γ chain (γ_c chain) and the transcriptional repressor inhibitor of DNA binding 2 (ID2) for their development (9–11). The factors involved in regulating different stages of ILC commitment from CLPs have been recently reviewed in Ref. (12). ILCs resemble T_H cells in their developmental requirements, transcriptional regulation, and in their cytokine secretion pattern. Thus, they were classified into three groups, which are able to immediately react to microbial and inflammatory challenge with cytokine production thereby limiting pathogen spread and tissue injury (9). Group 1 ILCs consist of cNK cells and so-called helper ILC1s; both secrete the T_H1-type cytokine IFN-γ. Group 2 ILCs are characterized by the production of T_H2-type cytokines IL-4, IL-5, and/or IL-13. Group 3 ILCs include fetal lymphoid tissue-inducer (LTi) cells, as well as adult ILC3s either expressing the natural cytotoxicity receptor (NCR) NKp46 (NCR^+ILC3s) or lacking this molecule (NCR^-ILC3s). Cells within this group produce the T_H17-type cytokines, IL-17 and/or IL-22 (9). The classification into ILC1, 2, and 3 is sometimes unhelpfully restrictive because ILCs have the potential to modulate their phenotypic and transcriptional signature upon activation and inflammation. When exposed to inflammatory conditions, NCR^-ILC3s can produce IFNγ (13, 14), and NCR^+ILC3s are able to convert into IFNγ-producing ILC1-like cells (15, 16). Moreover, in multiple sclerosis patients, blockade of CD25 (IL-2Rα) induces phenotypic changes of ILC3s toward cNK cells (17). Additional evidence for heterogeneity among ILC subsets comes from clonal analysis in humans demonstrating that the spectrum of cytokines produced by ILC3s is diverse (18) and in some cases, both ILC2 and ILC3 cytokines are produced (19). Finally, environmental factors, such as retinoic acid, short chain fatty acids, vitamins, aryl hydrocarbon receptor (AHR) ligands, stearyl sulfate, and probably bacterial metabolites, can shape ILC phenotypes and functions (20–24). Together, these data now provide convincing evidence that, similar to T_H cells, ILCs have a degree of plasticity in their cytokine profile. As for T_H cell commitment, cytokine-mediated conditioning, as well as epigenetic (25, 26) and transcriptional regulation (27) may account for changes of ILC subset-determining transcription factors and cytokines.

The biological relevance of ILCs is based on their capacity to sense environmental and inflammatory signals, and to respond with the secretion of cytokines important for immune defense, allergic reactions, and tissue repair. Recent data provide additional evidence that ILCs can condition T cell responses, either through cytokines, direct cell–cell contact, or through effects on accessory cells. This review will focus on the effects of ILC–T cell interactions for maintaining immune homeostasis. We will highlight major questions on how ILCs may cooperate with T cells thereby regulating T cell responses.

Induction and Skewing of T Cell Responses

Dendritic cells (DCs) are professional Ag-presenting cells (APCs) known for their robust capacity to activate naïve T cells and to modulate innate and adaptive immune responses (28). Distinct DC subsets have decisive roles in engaging pathways responsible for skewing the type of effector T_H cell response (29, 30). Moreover, DCs can suppress immune responses in order to maintain peripheral immune homeostasis and tolerance to self-Ags (31). As a key step in shaping the type of T_H cell response, cytokines secreted by innate immune cells including APCs can account for the expression of T_H subset-specific transcription factors (32). For example, IL-12 activates signal transducer and activator of transcription (STAT)-4 and induces the expression of the T-box transcription factor T-bet, which is critical for T_H1 cell commitment (33, 34). T-bet expression and T_H1 cell differentiation are further promoted by IL-2 (35). IL-4 induces STAT6 activation, which enhances Gata3 expression thereby initiating differentiation into T_H2 cell lineage (36). Additionally, IL-2 signaling followed by STAT5 activation plays a crucial role in T_H2 cell commitment by the induction of IL-4 transcription (37, 38). IL-6 signaling through STAT3, together with transforming growth factor (TGF)-β, induces retinoic acid-related orphan receptor (ROR)-γt expression and consequently the differentiation of pathogenic T_H17 cells from naïve T_H cells (39). A key issue in establishing immune homeostasis is the induction of T_{reg} cells that prevent immunopathology by maintaining tolerance. In addition, active suppression of inappropriate T cell responses is mediated by the induction of immune-regulatory cytokines, such as IL-10 (40), the expression of inhibitory receptors including cytotoxic T-lymphocyte-associated protein (CTLA)-4 or programed cell death (PD)-1 or the lack of co-stimulation and bystander signals. Altogether, cytokines and activating or inhibiting receptors of innate immune cells are pivotal for generating and conditioning T_H cell responses.

Group 1 ILCs

The group 1 ILCs comprised cNK cells and helper ILC1s. Both subsets secrete IFNγ and express the transcription factor T-bet (15, 16, 41–43). The expression of Eomesodermin (Eomes) is considered as a key factor for distinguishing cNK cells ($Eomes^+$) from ILC1s ($Eomes^-$) (43). However, splenic $NK1.1^+$ CD127 $(IL\text{-}7R\alpha)^+$ cells, which are in some studies referred to as ILC1s, express considerable levels of Eomes (44). Nfil3, another transcription factor, has been attributed a role in specifying cNK cells versus ILC1s. Although important for the development of all ILC lineages, studies of Nfil3-deficient mice (42, 45, 46) revealed that cNK cells have greater dependency on Nfil3 than ILC1s (47, 48). This is probably due to direct transcriptional control of Eomes expression by Nfil3 (49). Thus, NK cells resident in the salivary gland appear to be a prototype of ILC1s, as they also do not require Nfil3 for their development (48). Cells defined as ILC1s in the intestinal epithelium in humans and mice express the epithelial homing marker CD103 and readily produce IFNγ upon stimulation (41). $CD103^+$ intraepithelial ILC1s, similar to cNK cells, express Eomes and T-bet, and are Nfil3-dependent, but in contrast to cNK cells do not require IL-15 for their development. Phenotypically, cNK cells express DX5 and, unlike most ILC1s, lack Trail or CD127 expression (43, 47, 48). Some ILC1-like cells derive from $ROR\gamma t^+$ ILC3s by a process that is accompanied by the loss of RORγt expression and the upregulation of T-bet in both mice and humans (15, 16, 50). Future research on $T\text{-}bet^+$

IFNγ-secreting subsets will help to clarify the developmental and functional relationship of group 1 ILCs.

Group 1 ILC–T Cell Interactions

Unlike group 2 and group 3 ILCs, murine cNK cells and ILC1s do not express MHC class II (MHC II) molecules, thus being incapable of direct Ag-dependent interaction with $CD4^+$ T_H cells (**Table 1**). Nevertheless, in recent years, a number of reports described new aspects of a direct crosstalk between T and cNK/ILC1 cells. Several studies defined a regulatory role for cNK cells in controlling T cell-dependent immune responses by direct cytotoxic activity toward $CD4^+$ and $CD8^+$ T cells (51–53), as well as toward APCs required for T cell priming. Two recent publications demonstrated that type 1 IFN confer the resistance to cNK cell-mediated lysis of activated $CD8^+$ T cells (54, 55). $CD8^+$ T cells isolated from IFN-α-receptor-1-deficient (*Ifnar1*$^{-/-}$) mice were preferentially targeted by cNK cells resulting in the elimination of cytotoxic $CD8^+$ T cells in response to viral infection through a perforin-dependent pathway. Another study proposed a role for NKp46 in limiting graft versus host disease (GVHD) (56), although it has remained obscure whether NKp46 is required for the direct killing of host-reactive T cells, or if it operates via targeting of accessory APCs. More recently, Schuster et al. reported that cNK cells specifically limit the number of virus-reactive $CD4^+$ T cells in a model of chronic murine cytomegalovirus (MCMV) infection in the salivary gland (57). Intriguingly, this process is dependent on the TNF-superfamily ligand Trail, which is, in addition to NKp46 also expressed by ILC1s. This suggests a possible contribution of ILC1s to the processes described above. Additionally, in humans, activated cNK cells could be shown to positively regulate $CD4^+$ T_H cell activity (58). cNK cells stimulated by cytokines or through activating receptors were shown to upregulate the co-stimulatory molecules, OX40L and members of B7 family (CD80/CD86). Interaction with such cNK cells led to augmented IFNγ production and enhanced T cell receptor-dependent proliferation of autologous $CD4^+$ T_H cells.

Conventional natural killer/ILC1 and T cell crosstalk operates in a reverse direction as well. Two studies showed that T_{reg} cells play an important role in keeping cNK cell activity in check (59, 60). Gasteiger et al. demonstrated that upon depletion of T_{reg}

TABLE 1 | Phenotype of mouse and human ILCs.

	Mouse				Human			
	cNK	ILC1	ILC2	ILC3	cNK	ILC1	ILC2	ILC3
SURFACE MOLECULES								
CD90	+	+	+	+	ND	ND	ND	ND
CD127	–[a]	+	+	+	lo	–[a]	+	+
CD117	lo	+	+[c]	+	lo	sub[l]	±	+
NK1.1	+	+	–	lo	+	+	+	+[o]
NKp46/NKp44	+	+	+	sub	sub	+[a]	–	sub[o]
CD25	–	–[b]	+	+	+	–	+	+[o]
ST-2	–	–	+[d]	–	–	–	+	–
Sca-1	–	–	+[e]	lo	ND	ND	ND	ND
TRANSCRIPTION FACTORS								
ID2	+	+	+	+	ND	ND	ND	+[o]
Gata3	–	lo	+	lo	lo	lo	+	lo
RORγt	–	–	lo	+	–	lo	lo	+
T-bet	+	+	–	sub	+	+	–	–
Eomes	+	–	–	–	+	–	–	–
NFIL3	+	+	+	+	ND	ND	ND	ND
MOLECULES INVOLVED IN ILC–T CELL INTERACTION/ILC ACTIVATION								
CD69	lo	lo	–[f]	ind, +[h]	+	sub[m]	sub[m]	sub[m, p]
MHC class II	–	–	+	+[i]	ind, +[k]	ND	+[n]	+
CD80	–	–	ind[g]	ind[j]	ind, +[k]	ND	+[n]	ND
CD86	–	–	ind[g]	ind[j]	ind, +[k]	ND	+[n]	ND
CD40	–	–	–	ind[j]	–	ND	ND	ND
CD30L	–	lo	–	+	ind, +[k]	ND	ND	ND
OX40L	–	–	–	+	ind, +[k]	ND	ND	+
ICOS	–	–	+	ND	ind, +[k]	ND	+	+
ICOSL	–	lo	+	ND	ND	ND	+	lo
RANKL	–	–	ND	+	–	ND	ND	+
TRAIL	–	+	ND	lo	ind, +[k]	ND	ND	ND

+ indicates expression; – indicates no expression; lo indicates low expression; sub indicates expression on a subset; ind indicates activation-induced expression; ND indicates expression is not determined.

[a]Expressed in certain tissues; [b]Intestinal ILC1s are $CD25^+$ (44); [c]Skin ILC2s are $CD117^-$ (62); [d]Small intestinal ILC2s are ST-2^- (73); [e]Liver ILC2s are Sca-1^- (71); [f]Fat-associated lymphoid cluster-derived and intestinal ILC2s are $CD69^+$ (69); [g]Expressed on mediastinal LN-derived ILC2s from IL-33 treated mice (93); [h]Expressed on splenic ILC3s under inflammatory conditions (130); constitutively expressed on intestinal ILC3s (44); [i]Expression increased on splenic ILC3s under inflammatory conditions (130); [j]Expressed on splenic, but not intestinal ILC3s under inflammatory conditions (130, 133); [k]Expressed after activation (159, 160); expressed at steady state (161); [l]Molecule expressed on certain subsets (16); [m]Human peripheral blood ILCs heterogeneously express CD69 (162); [n]Human ILC2s express CD80/CD86 and HLA-DR (93); [o]Human ILC population resembling ILC3s (122); [p]Human splenic ILCs are $CD69^+$ (122).

cells, cNK cells become hyper-responsive toward MHC I-deficient target cells that are recognized via missing-self mechanism. This was attributed to the increased availability of IL-2 produced by activated $CD4^+$ T cells (59). Another report demonstrated in a genetic model of type 1 diabetes that the acute removal of T_{reg} cells leads to the accumulation of activated cNK cells in pancreatic islets (60). On the contrary, in this experimental setting, depletion of T_{reg} cells did not result in an increase of IL-2 secretion by $CD4^+$ T_H cells, but more likely increased the availability of IL-2 to cNK cells by decreasing IL-2 consumption by T_{reg} cells. Interestingly, the accumulating cNK cells express CD127 (61) and might therefore constitute an "ILC1-like" subset. These studies provide the first example of T_{reg} cell-dependent control of cNK cell and possibly ILC1 activity. Given the importance of IL-2 for the expansion of other ILC subsets (45, 62), T_{reg} cells might also be involved in controlling their activity. Taken together, these findings illustrate the reciprocal immuno-regulatory relationship between group 1 ILCs and T cells.

Group 2 ILCs

ILC2s are the most homogenous ILC subset albeit with a specific phenotypic signature in the lung and intestine (44, 63). They express CD127, CD90.2 (Thy1), various levels of CD25, and the IL-33-receptor subunit ST2 (**Table 1**). The development of ILC2s depends on the transcription factors, ROR-α, Gata3, and T cell factor (TCF)-1 (64–67). ILC2s in both humans and mice secrete T_H2-type cytokines IL-4, IL-5, and/or IL-13 in response to IL-9, IL-25, IL-33, and thymic stromal lymphopoietin (TSLP), as well as during pulmonary inflammation or infection with *Nippostrongylus brasiliensis*, a helminth controlled by T_H2-type cytokine responses (63, 68–78). In addition to ILC2s, another cell type, the multipotent progenitor type 2 (MPP^{type2}) is described. MPP^{type2} cells exhibit similar phenotypic and functional characteristics with ILC2s (79), but do not produce T_H2-type cytokines in response to IL-33 (80). The release of T_H2-type cytokines by ILC2s is not only involved in *N. brasiliensis* expulsion (81) but can also trigger airway inflammation and allergic responses in humans (82–84). Together, ILC2s share developmental and inducible cytokine signatures with T_H2 cells suggesting a role in type 2 immune responses.

Group 2 ILC–T Cell Interactions

Type 2 immune responses are severely impaired in IL-4-receptor-α-deficient ($Il4R\alpha^{-/-}$) and IL-4-deficient ($Il4^{-/-}$) mice indicating that IL-4 has a role in T_H2 cell differentiation (85, 86). Further, the accumulation of T_H2 cells after *N. brasiliensis*/ovalbumin challenge is dramatically reduced in IL-4 and IL-13-double-deficient ($Il4^{-/-}Il13^{-/-}$) mice as compared to wild type (*WT*) mice (87). T_H2 cell differentiation is most likely initiated by innate immune cells, which become activated in the early phase of immune responses. Beside basophils and mast cells (88–90), it is now well established that ILC2s can secrete IL-4 suggesting a role for these cells in the induction of T_H2 cell differentiation and type 2 immune responses. Indeed, several reports provide evidence that ILC2s and $CD4^+$ T cells cooperate at multiple levels (91–97). In mice, which either have dramatically reduced numbers or a complete lack of ILC2s, the generation of type 2 immune responses upon *N. brasiliensis* infection, challenge with house dust mite Ag or with protease-allergen papain is impaired indicating a contribution of ILC2s to T_H2 cell responses (91, 93, 95). The addition of ILC2s to cultures of naïve $CD4^+$ T cells promotes the differentiation into T_H2 cells, while inhibiting the differentiation into T_H1 cells even in the presence of IL-12, a cytokine that drives T_H1 differentiation (33, 34, 92). In line with this finding, type 2 cytokines are not detectable when T_H cells are co-cultured with ILC2s unable to secrete IL-4 (94). On the other hand, *in vivo* differentiation of T_H1/T_H17 cells occurs independently of ILC2s, since mice, which lack ILC2s, show normal responses when exposed to *Saccharopolyspora rectivirgula*, a bacterium inducing T_H1/T_H17 inflammatory responses (95). Together, there is evidence that ILC2-derived IL-4 contributes to type 2 cytokine production of T_H cells, although an IL-4-independent pathway for ILC2-driven type 2 immune responses may also occur (91). Beside the direct effect of ILC2s on T_H2 differentiation, T_H2-type cytokines secreted by ILC2s can also affect $CD4^+$ T cells indirectly via DCs. Evidence for this comes from the finding that ILC2-derived IL-13 promotes migration of DCs into lung-draining lymph nodes (LNs), where activated DCs induce the differentiation of $CD4^+$ T cells into T_H2 cells (91).

Interleukin-33, a pro-inflammatory cytokine expressed by a variety of cell types can trigger the generation of inducible regulatory T (iT_{reg}) cells (98) and the activation of ILC2s to produce type 2 cytokines and amphiregulin (AREG). AREG is an epithelial growth factor that promotes restoration of airway epithelial integrity following influenza virus-induced damage (63). Importantly, analysis of ILC2-depleted, influenza virus-infected mice revealed a strong reduction in AREG mRNA suggesting that ILC2s are the main source of AREG under such inflammatory conditions. In other inflammatory models, mast cells were thought to be the major source of AREG and importantly, in these models, AREG was found to be critical for efficient T_{reg} cell function (99). In view of their abundance in the skin, lung, and colon, their strong responsiveness to IL-33, and early inflammatory signals, AREG-secreting ILC2s may have a function in tissue repair and likely also in triggering T_{reg} cell responses.

Another mechanism through which ILC2s have an influence on $CD4^+$ T_H cells is by their ability to serve as APCs. Co-stimulatory signals via OX40 are crucial for effector/memory T cell responses and for initiating T_H2 differentiation (100, 101). OX40-ligand (OX40L) is detectable on ILC2s, and the production of T_H2-type cytokines in ILC2-T cell co-cultures is significantly inhibited when anti-OX40L antibodies (Abs) are added, suggesting that ILC2s promote T_H2-responses via OX40/OX40L interactions (94). Further evidence for cell–cell interactions between ILC2s and $CD4^+$ T cells is provided by the finding that human and mouse ILC2s express both inducible T cell co-stimulator (ICOS) and ICOS-ligand (ICOSL) (70, 102), a co-stimulatory receptor/ligand pair known for its function for survival, proliferation, and cytokine secretion of T_H cell subsets (103). Moreover, ILC2s can process Ags and present peptides on MHC II. They express the co-stimulatory molecules, CD80 and CD86, and induce proliferation of T_H2 cells, albeit to a lesser extent than professional APCs (92, 93). Interestingly, the expression of MHC II is higher on LN-, spleen-, and Peyer's Patch (PP)-derived ILC2s than on peritoneal lavage-, bronchoalveolar lavage-, and lung-derived ILC2s. Therefore, lymphoid tissue-specific factors might be responsible for sustained MHC II expression.

Together with the finding that ILC2s can express MHC II and co-stimulatory molecules, the direct ILC2–T cell interaction not only promotes T_H responses but also extends to cytokine-mediated help from activated T_H cells for ILC2 effector functions. During the acute phase of *N. brasiliensis* infection, Rag2-deficient (*Rag2*$^{-/-}$) mice show a similar expansion of ILC2s as *WT* mice. However, adaptive immune cells are required for prolonged ILC2 expansion and complete clearance of the infection (70). In a papain-induced inflammation model, IL-9 production by ILC2s is severely reduced in *Rag2*$^{-/-}$ mice suggesting that cytokine secretion by ILC2s is also dependent on the adaptive immune system (68). *In vitro* co-culture of CD4$^+$ T cells and ILC2s results in the upregulation of IL-4 mRNA in ILC2s, suggesting that T_H cells induce type 2 cytokine production by ILC2s (94). Additionally, activated CD4$^+$ T cells in co-culture with ILC2s can directly induce ILC2 proliferation and IL-5/IL-13 secretion (92). This effect is partially impaired by adding anti-IL-2-neutralizing Abs but not by separating CD4$^+$ T cells from ILC2s in transwell assays, suggesting an IL-2-driven feedback mechanism from activated CD4$^+$ T cells to ILC2s (92). In line with this, treatment of mice with IL-2/anti-IL-2 complexes results in increased *in vivo* proliferation of ILC2s (62) and expansion of ILC2 progenitors in the bone marrow (BM) (45). IL-2 can also promote IL-9 release by ILC2s, whereas IL-33 induces the upregulation of the IL-2-receptor subunit CD25 on ILC2s (104). The induction of CD25 expression may help ILC2s to become more sensitive to T cell-derived IL-2. It is currently unclear to what extent ILC2s and T_{reg} cells, which express high levels of CD25, or other T_H subsets, compete for IL-2. Hence, the expression of CD25 by ILC2s may also reduce the availability of IL-2 for T cells. Based on these observations, we propose the following model (**Figure 1**): ILC2s can be rapidly activated by various alarm signals leading to the release of T_H2-type cytokines, which help to induce T_H2 cell responses and DC migration into LNs toward T cell zones. Further, activated ILC2s secrete AREG, and it remains to be investigated whether this can trigger T_{reg} cell responses. The cognate interaction between ILC2s and CD4$^+$ T cells via MHC II–Ag presentation, co-stimulatory signals, and cytokines helps to amplify both ILC2 and CD4$^+$ T cell responses.

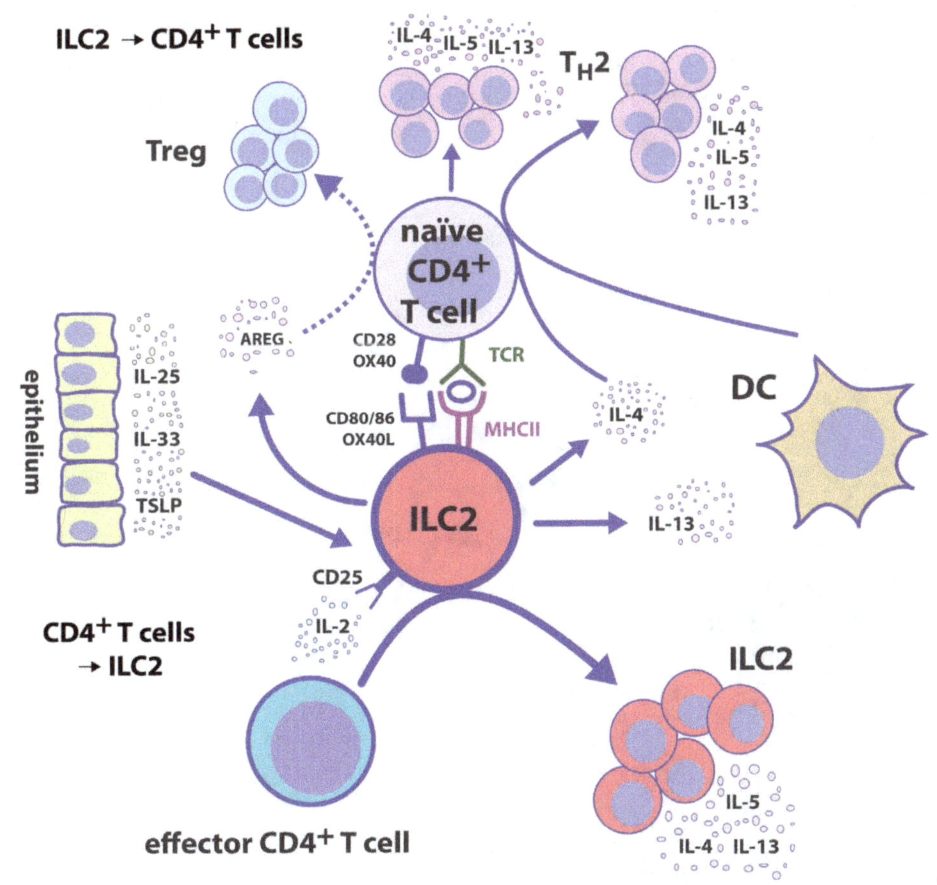

FIGURE 1 | Group 2 ILC–CD4$^+$ T cell interactions. ILC2s polarize CD4$^+$ T cell responses toward T_H2 immunity directly by presenting cognate Ag and by secreting T_H2-inducing cytokines. Reciprocally, activated CD4$^+$ T cells produce IL-2, which serves as a growth factor leading to the expansion of ILC2s.

Group 3 ILCs

All ILC3 subsets depend on the transcription factor RORγt for their development (105–107), and produce the T_H17-type cytokine IL-22 (107–111). IL-22 has a major role in protecting intestinal epithelial cells from bacterial infections and in promoting tissue repair through induction of epithelial cell proliferation and production of antimicrobial peptides (112). Group 3 ILCs can be phenotypically classified into a subset of fetal $ROR\gamma t^+$ $CD127^+$ $CD117^+$ LTi cells (106, 113–116), and adult NCR^+ or $NCR^-ROR\gamma t^+$ ILC3s (107, 108, 111, 117).

Group 3 ILC–T Cell Interactions

ILC3s can modulate T_H cell immune responses in several ways. One pathway involves the development of lymphoid tissue and T cell zone stroma. Already before birth, the cellular crosstalk of fetal lymphotoxin (LT)$\alpha_1\beta_2$-expressing LTi cells with mesenchymal stromal cells (MSCs) plays a pivotal role in the formation of LNs and PPs, in which immune responses are generated. Adult ILC3s retain the capacity to induce lymphoid tissue formation (118, 119). Following lymphocytic choriomeningitis virus (LCMV) infection in mice, the crosstalk between $LT\alpha_1\beta_2$-expressing ILC3s and T cell zone fibroblastic reticular cells helps to restore the disrupted T-zone compartment and hence the structure to generate proper immune responses (120). Similarly, $LT\alpha_1\beta_2^+$ ILC3s can restore lymphoid follicle organization in the colon of mice infected with *Citrobacter rodentium* (121). The interaction of ILC3s with MSCs is also reciprocal. In humans, the crosstalk between $LT\alpha_1\beta_2^+$ ILC3s and marginal reticular cells (MRCs), a subset of marginal zone stromal cells, induces the production of MRC-derived survival factors for ILC3s, such as IL-7 (122). A second pathway, by which ILC3s can modulate T_H cell immune responses, is through altering the recruitment of $CD4^+$ T_H cells. ILC3s are able to release soluble $LT\alpha_3$, which promotes the homing of $CD4^+$ T_H cells to the gut lamina propria where they differentiate into functional T_H cell subsets (**Figure 2**) (123). In a model of airway inflammation, ILC3-derived IL-22 reduces CCL17 production by epithelial cells thereby limiting T_H2 cell recruitment and immune responses to allergens in the lung (124). These data show that ILC3s have an impact on generating functional T cell compartments and recruitment of $CD4^+$ T_H cells to mucosal sites.

In the adult spleen, ILC3s are localized in the marginal zone and around the central arterioles, and in LNs in proximity to

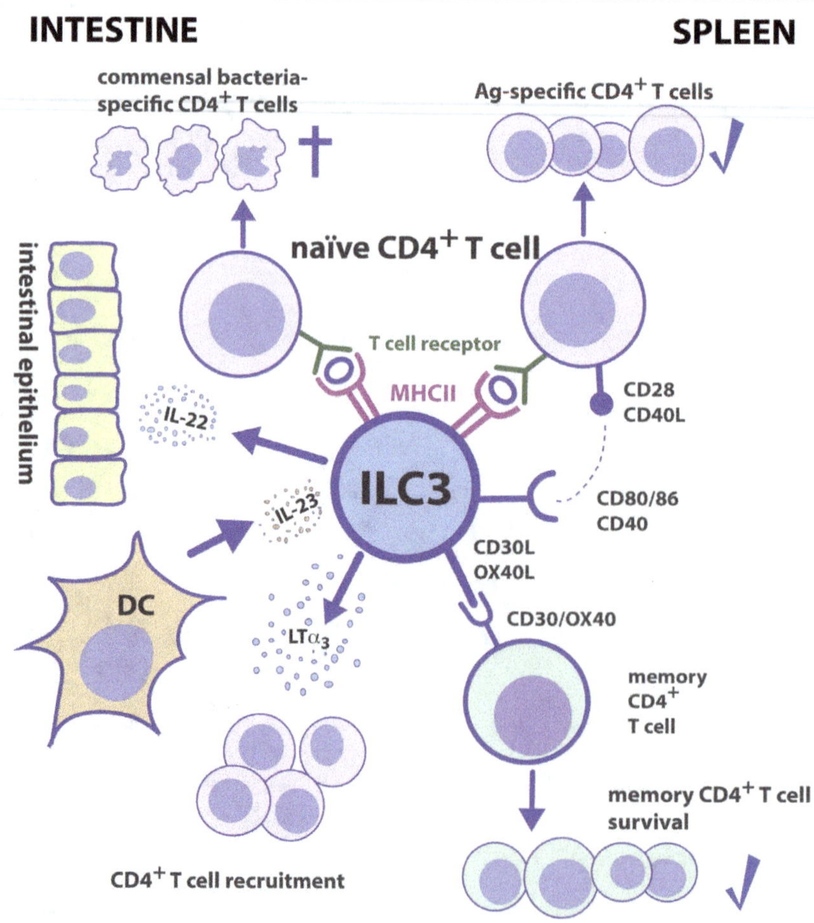

FIGURE 2 | Group 3 ILC–CD4+ T cell interactions. Tissue localization greatly affects the outcome of Ag-dependent T cell–ILC3 interaction. Intestinal ILC3s maintain tolerance toward commensal microbiota, while splenic ILC3s are efficient in the induction of Ag-specific $CD4^+$ T cell responses and memory $CD4^+$ T cell survival.

high endothelial venules and interfollicular areas (122, 125–127). Because of the close association of splenic ILC3s to Ag-entry sites and T cells as well as their expression of the co-stimulatory molecules, CD30-ligand (CD30L) and OX40L, it has been assumed that they may directly interact with T cells during adaptive immune responses (125). Mice with a deficiency in CD30 and OX40 (*CD30*$^{-/-}$*OX40*$^{-/-}$ mice) lack proper memory Ab responses due to a failure in survival of primed CD4^{+} T$_{H}$ cells (128). *In vitro*, ILC3s can promote survival of memory CD4^{+} T$_{H}$ cells from *WT* but not from *CD30*$^{-/-}$*OX40*$^{-/-}$ mice suggesting that both CD30L and OX40L molecules expressed by ILC3s are essential for CD4^{+} T$_{H}$ memory responses (128). This possibility was supported by an *in vivo* study, which identified ILC3s as the key players in the maintenance of CD4^{+} memory T$_{H}$ cells (**Figure 2**) (129).

A third mechanism by which ILC3s interact with CD4^{+} T$_{H}$ cells is through receptors required for immune recognition. ILC3s isolated from various tissues of fetal, neonatal, and adult mice express MHC II and MHC II-associated gene transcripts (44, 113, 130–132). NCR^{-}ILC3s are able to internalize, process, and present foreign Ags to CD4^{+} T$_{H}$ cells (130, 131). Under non-inflammatory conditions, ILC3s express neither CD40 and CD80 nor CD86 (130, 131). However, following stimulation with IL-1β splenic but not intestinal, NCR^{-}ILC3s can upregulate co-stimulatory molecules (130). A recent study confirmed that even after toll-like receptor ligand (TLRL) or pro-inflammatory cytokine exposure, intestinal ILC3s do not upregulate co-stimulatory molecules (133). The finding that mLN-derived ILC3s are as well unable to express co-stimulatory molecules upon stimulation is likely due to the fact that ILC3s found in the mLNs are originally intestinal ILC3s, which were trafficking from the intestine to the mLNs (127). It is noteworthy that genome-wide transcriptional profiling of splenic ILC3s reveals an enrichment for genes involved in cell activation and immune responses (63). In contrast to splenic ILC3s, intestinal ILC3s express the activation marker, CD69 (44), a glycoprotein involved in establishing oral tolerance (134) and limiting dextran sodium sulfate (DSS)-induced inflammation (135). Moreover, ILC3s present in the small intestine express neuropilin-1 (Nrp1) (44), which promotes T$_{reg}$ cell survival and functional activity (136–138). It is therefore conceivable that ILC3s exert tissue-specific immune functions with immunogenic versus tolerogenic activity in the spleen and intestine, respectively. This hypothesis is further supported by the notion that splenic NCR^{-}ILC3s promote CD4^{+} T$_{H}$ cell responses *in vitro* and *in vivo*, whereas intestinal ILC3s fail to efficiently stimulate CD4^{+} T$_{H}$ cells (**Figure 2**) (130). In mice, intestinal ILC3s express lower levels of MHC II as compared to ILC3s identified in other tissues (130, 131, 133). Together with the observation that intestinal ILC3s lack co-stimulatory molecules, this may contribute to maintaining intestinal T cell tolerance, similar to immature DCs expressing low surface levels of MHC II and co-stimulatory molecules (139).

Hepworth et al. reported the development of spontaneous intestinal inflammation in mice lacking MHC II exclusively on ILC3s (ILC3Δ^{MHCII} mice) and found a role for intestinal ILC3s in limiting commensal bacteria-specific pro-inflammatory colonic CD4^{+} T$_{H}$ cell responses through induction of PD (131, 133). Since other laboratories failed to detect spontaneous signs of inflammation in ILC3Δ^{MHCII} mice (130, 132), it is possible that the development of immunopathology is triggered by microbial co-factors. In the intestine, ILC3s can inhibit T$_{H}$17 cell-mediated inflammation through AHR signaling, release of IL-22, and by preventing the expansion of aberrant segmented filamentous bacteria (SFB) (140). In pediatric Crohn's disease (CD) patients, MHC II levels on intestinal ILC3s are significantly reduced, and such low expression correlates with increased frequencies of colonic T$_{H}$17 cells and circulating commensal bacteria-specific IgG (133). This study is the first to describe an association of ILC3-mediated Ag presentation and control of commensal bacteria-specific adaptive immunity in humans. It remains unclear which are the mechanisms that underlie loss of MHC II in CD patients and whether this is sufficient to trigger inflammatory bowel disease. Together, these findings suggest that intestinal ILC3s can inhibit expansion of T$_{H}$17 cells and immunopathology after exposure to pro-inflammatory stimuli.

Analogously to ILC2–T cell interactions, the crosstalk between ILC3s and CD4^{+} T$_{H}$ cells might be bidirectional and depends on cytokines. This is further supported by the findings that the presence of the adaptive immune system has an effect on the number and IL-22 production of intestinal ILC3s, most likely through competition for growth factors (141, 142). Human and activated mouse ILC3s produce IL-2 (19, 130), and conversely, TLR2-driven proliferation of human ILC3s is partially dependent on IL-2 (19). Availability of IL-2 alone or in combination with Pam3Cys promotes increased CD25 expression in human ILC3s suggesting that CD25 expression might help ILC3s to win the competition for IL-2 against T cells (19). Moreover, there is some evidence that mouse ILC3s have a higher capacity to bind IL-2 than activated CD4^{+} T$_{H}$ cells (133). Therefore, the availability of IL-2 can restrict ILC3 and T$_{H}$ responses as a result of receptor density, efficiency of binding, and kinetics of IL-2 consumption.

Immune Homeostasis in the Gut: Tolerance Versus Inflammation

The critical question regarding maintenance of immune homeostasis is where, when, and how immune responses prevent tissue injury. The intestine is a prime example that has been extensively studied with respect to cellular networks and pathways patrolling tissue integrity and regulating inflammation. T$_{reg}$ and T$_{H}$17 cells are the most abundant CD4^{+} T$_{H}$ cells in the intestinal mucosa under steady state (143–145). The balance between the two subsets is crucial for the outcome of mucosal immune responses (146). Commensal bacteria have a specific impact on the number of both T$_{H}$ subsets (147) and on the capacity of ILC3s to regulate T$_{H}$ subset responses (148). On the other hand, ILC3s contribute to maintenance of intestinal epithelial barrier function thereby limiting microbes entry and inflammatory T$_{H}$ cell responses (108, 109, 117, 141, 148). Whereas under steady-state conditions, intestinal ILC3s produce high levels of IL-22, the production of IL-17 is rather low (44). Importantly, T$_{H}$17 cells are induced by SFB (149, 150) by a mechanism that requires SFB presentation by DCs (132, 151). In contrast, ILC3 presentation of Ag prevents amplification of SFB-independent T$_{H}$17 cells (132). In line with this, the expansion of SFB and pathogenic T_H17 cells inversely correlates with the number of intestinal ILC3s (140). In an IL-17-dependent autoimmune mouse model, it was recently shown that SFB colonization was associated with enhanced auto-Ab titers (152). The increase in IL-17-producing cells, as observed in CD patients (153), is probably not sufficient *per se* to induce immunopathology. Specificity of inflammatory T_H cells, intestinal infections, pro-inflammatory bystander cells, and loss of functional T_{reg} cells might be required to trigger intestinal inflammation.

All these studies published in recent years raised the question of whether and how ILC–T cell interactions regulate pro- or anti-inflammatory responses in the gut. Since ILC3s can prevent dissemination of commensal bacteria in the gut and commensal bacteria-specific T_H cell responses (123, 131, 132, 148), they probably promote an immunological tolerogenic state in the gut. In addition, the production of GM-CSF by ILC3s has the potential to enhance iT_{reg} cell numbers and function thereby promoting intestinal homeostasis (154). In some colitis models, however, ILC3s were reported to enhance intestinal inflammation (13, 15), and pathogenic ILC1 numbers were increased in patients with CD (16, 41). The functional polarization toward IFNγ-producing ILC1s or IL-22-producing ILC3s appears to depend on tissue-specific and pro-inflammatory conditions. Environmental changes may immediately affect the ratio and/or polarization of ILC and T cell subsets. For example, induction of pro-inflammatory cytokines, such as IL-23, was shown to counteract the responsiveness toward IL-33, and the generation of iTregs in the intestine (98). As for T_H cell differentiation, it is likely that the amount of cytokines determines ILC cytokine polarization. Under homeostatic conditions, the intestine provides a microenvironment enriched of cytokines with inhibitory effects, such as TGF-β. At high dose, TGF-β inhibits T_H17 responses, whereas low-dose TGF-β promotes T_H17-differentiation (155–157). A similar impact of cytokine concentrations for immune homeostasis has also been discussed for IL-22 (158). Therefore, excessive release of cytokines by ILCs may contribute to immunopathology, whereas under steady-state conditions, ILCs rather promote epithelial tissue integrity and tolerogenic T cell responses. During inflammation, ILC3s can switch off RORγt expression, which may eventually be regained at later time points. The modulation of cytokine receptors during a critical time window of ILC activation and ILC-T cell interaction might also contribute to prevent excessive immunopathology. This has been shown for a number of receptors controlling growth and survival of both ILCs and T cells. Finally, the polarization toward protective versus inflammatory response in the gut likely requires a tight balance between temporal regulation, amount, and combination of cytokines co-expressed by individual ILCs.

Conclusion

Our understanding of immune homeostasis has been challenged by the notion that environmental factors, including commensal bacteria and nutritional components, as well as cholinergic and metabolic signals can regulate immune functions and pro-inflammatory processes. ILCs are important "early sentinel" cells, which connect innate and adaptive immunity by sensing environmental changes, such as infections and inflammation and by the release of immuno-regulatory cytokines. They not only contribute to T cell immune homeostasis by promoting T_H cell differentiation and effector functions but can also directly interact with $CD4^+$ T_H cells. Both ILC2s and ILC3s internalize and present Ag to T_H cells. Considering the fact that the number of ILCs in most tissues is rather low as compared to other immune cells, they appear to have a surprising *in vivo* impact on immune homeostasis. The localization of ILCs in relatively high density at Ag-entry sites and T cell areas as well as bystander effects on classical DCs might explain this effect. In addition, advances in two-photon microscopy have shown that several $CD4^+$ T_H cells are often clustering with the same APC, a fact that may increase local cytokine concentrations for optimal cell–cell interactions. The capacity to elicit cognate T_H cell proliferation or rather prevent T_H cell responses strongly depends on environmental factors and the nature of Ag, and it will be important to further investigate the mechanisms by which ILCs prevent or promote T cell responses in various tissues. For example, it will be interesting to unravel whether ILCs can express inhibitory receptors and/or collaborate with T_{reg} cells. Finally, there are clearly cytokine-driven reciprocal effects between ILCs and T cells, which might help to coordinate and/or limit immune responses. Taken together, a better understanding of the regulation of cytokine expression by ILCs and their interaction with T cells will help to develop new strategies to treat inflammatory diseases in humans.

Acknowledgments

The authors sincerely apologize to all colleagues whose work has been omitted due to space limitations. We would like to thank A. Baerenwaldt, T. Rolink, E. Palmer, G. de Libero, and all members of the lab for comments on the manuscript. DF is supported by the Swiss National Science Foundation (SNF) grant 310030-153247/1. NB is supported by the Horton foundation. GT is supported by the Basel University Research Fund Junior Researcher.

References

1. Mosmann TR, Cherwinski H, Bond MW, Giedlin MA, Coffman RL. Two types of murine helper T cell clone. I. Definition according to profiles of lymphokine activities and secreted proteins. *J Immunol* (1986) **136**(7):2348–57.
2. Yao Z, Painter SL, Fanslow WC, Ulrich D, Macduff BM, Spriggs MK, et al. Human IL-17: a novel cytokine derived from T cells. *J Immunol* (1995) **155**(12):5483–6.
3. Sakaguchi S, Sakaguchi N, Asano M, Itoh M, Toda M. Immunologic self-tolerance maintained by activated T cells expressing IL-2 receptor alpha-chains (CD25). Breakdown of a single mechanism of self-tolerance causes various autoimmune diseases. *J Immunol* (1995) **155**(3):1151–64.
4. Veldhoen M, Uyttenhove C, van Snick J, Helmby H, Westendorf A, Buer J, et al. Transforming growth factor-beta 'reprograms' the differentiation of T helper 2 cells and promotes an interleukin 9-producing subset. *Nat Immunol* (2008) **9**(12):1341–6. doi:10.1038/ni.1659

5. Breitfeld D, Ohl L, Kremmer E, Ellwart J, Sallusto F, Lipp M, et al. Follicular B helper T cells express CXC chemokine receptor 5, localize to B cell follicles, and support immunoglobulin production. *J Exp Med* (2000) **192**(11):1545–52. doi:10.1084/jem.192.11.1545
6. El-Behi M, Ciric B, Dai H, Yan Y, Cullimore M, Safavi F, et al. The encephalitogenicity of T(H)17 cells is dependent on IL-1- and IL-23-induced production of the cytokine GM-CSF. *Nat Immunol* (2011) **12**(6):568–75. doi:10.1038/ni.2031
7. Codarri L, Gyülvészi G, Tosevski V, Hesske L, Fontana A, Magnenat L, et al. RORgammat drives production of the cytokine GM-CSF in helper T cells, which is essential for the effector phase of autoimmune neuroinflammation. *Nat Immunol* (2011) **12**(6):560–7. doi:10.1038/ni.2027
8. Sheng W, Yang F, Zhou Y, Yang H, Low PY, Kemeny DM, et al. STAT5 programs a distinct subset of GM-CSF-producing T helper cells that is essential for autoimmune neuroinflammation. *Cell Res* (2014) **24**(12):1387–402. doi:10.1038/cr.2014.154
9. Spits H, Artis D, Colonna M, Diefenbach A, Di Santo JP, Eberl G, et al. Innate lymphoid cells – a proposal for uniform nomenclature. *Nat Rev Immunol* (2013) **13**(2):145–9. doi:10.1038/nri3365
10. Yokota Y, Mansouri A, Mori S, Sugawara S, Adachi S, Nishikawa S, et al. Development of peripheral lymphoid organs and natural killer cells depends on the helix-loop-helix inhibitor Id2. *Nature* (1999) **397**(6721):702–6. doi:10.1038/17812
11. Boos MD, Yokota Y, Eberl G, Kee BL. Mature natural killer cell and lymphoid tissue-inducing cell development requires Id2-mediated suppression of E protein activity. *J Exp Med* (2007) **204**(5):1119–30. doi:10.1084/jem.20061959
12. Lim AW, McKenzie AN. Deciphering the transcriptional switches of innate lymphoid cell programming: the right factors at the right time. *Genes Immun* (2015) **16**(3):177–86. doi:10.1038/gene.2014.83
13. Buonocore S, Ahern PP, Uhlig HH, Ivanov II, Littman DR, Maloy KJ, et al. Innate lymphoid cells drive interleukin-23-dependent innate intestinal pathology. *Nature* (2010) **464**(7293):1371–5. doi:10.1038/nature08949
14. Klose CS, Kiss EA, Schwierzeck V, Ebert K, Hoyler T, d'Hargues Y, et al. A T-bet gradient controls the fate and function of CCR6-RORgammat+ innate lymphoid cells. *Nature* (2013) **494**(7436):261–5. doi:10.1038/nature11813
15. Vonarbourg C, Mortha A, Bui VL, Hernandez PP, Kiss EA, Hoyler T, et al. Regulated expression of nuclear receptor RORgammat confers distinct functional fates to NK cell receptor-expressing RORgammat(+) innate lymphocytes. *Immunity* (2010) **33**(5):736–51. doi:10.1016/j.immuni.2010.10.017
16. Bernink JH, Peters CP, Munneke M, te Velde AA, Meijer SL, Weijer K, et al. Human type 1 innate lymphoid cells accumulate in inflamed mucosal tissues. *Nat Immunol* (2013) **14**(3):221–9. doi:10.1038/ni.2534
17. Perry JS, Han S, Xu Q, Herman ML, Kennedy LB, Csako G, et al. Inhibition of LTi cell development by CD25 blockade is associated with decreased intrathecal inflammation in multiple sclerosis. *Sci Transl Med* (2012) **4**(145):145ra106. doi:10.1126/scitranslmed.3004140
18. Crellin NK, Trifari S, Kaplan CD, Cupedo T, Spits H. Human NKp44+IL-22+ cells and LTi-like cells constitute a stable RORC+ lineage distinct from conventional natural killer cells. *J Exp Med* (2010) **207**(2):281–90. doi:10.1084/jem.20091509
19. Crellin NK, Trifari S, Kaplan CD, Satoh-Takayama N, Di Santo JP, Spits H. Regulation of cytokine secretion in human CD127(+) LTi-like innate lymphoid cells by toll-like receptor 2. *Immunity* (2010) **33**(5):752–64. doi:10.1016/j.immuni.2010.10.012
20. Spencer SP, Wilhelm C, Yang Q, Hall JA, Bouladoux N, Boyd A, et al. Adaptation of innate lymphoid cells to a micronutrient deficiency promotes type 2 barrier immunity. *Science* (2014) **343**(6169):432–7. doi:10.1126/science.1247606
21. van de Pavert SA, Ferreira M, Domingues RG, Ribeiro H, Molenaar R, Moreira-Santos L, et al. Maternal retinoids control type 3 innate lymphoid cells and set the offspring immunity. *Nature* (2014) **508**(7494):123–7. doi:10.1038/nature13158
22. Kiss EA, Vonarbourg C, Kopfmann S, Hobeika E, Finke D, Esser C, et al. Natural aryl hydrocarbon receptor ligands control organogenesis of intestinal lymphoid follicles. *Science* (2011) **334**(6062):1561–5. doi:10.1126/science.1214914
23. Hu X, Wang Y, Hao LY, Liu X, Lesch CA, Sanchez BM, et al. Sterol metabolism controls T(H)17 differentiation by generating endogenous RORgamma agonists. *Nat Chem Biol* (2015) **11**(2):141–7. doi:10.1038/nchembio.1714
24. Qiu J, Heller JJ, Guo X, Chen ZM, Fish K, Fu YX, et al. The aryl hydrocarbon receptor regulates gut immunity through modulation of innate lymphoid cells. *Immunity* (2012) **36**(1):92–104. doi:10.1016/j.immuni.2011.11.011
25. Zhou L, Chong MM, Littman DR. Plasticity of CD4+ T cell lineage differentiation. *Immunity* (2009) **30**(5):646–55. doi:10.1016/j.immuni.2009.05.001
26. Shih HY, Sciumè G, Poholek AC, Vahedi G, Hirahara K, Villarino AV, et al. Transcriptional and epigenetic networks of helper T and innate lymphoid cells. *Immunol Rev* (2014) **261**(1):23–49. doi:10.1111/imr.12208
27. Murphy KM, Stockinger B. Effector T cell plasticity: flexibility in the face of changing circumstances. *Nat Immunol* (2010) **11**(8):674–80. doi:10.1038/ni.1899
28. Steinman RM, Cohn ZA. Identification of a novel cell type in peripheral lymphoid organs of mice. I. Morphology, quantitation, tissue distribution. *J Exp Med* (1973) **137**(5):1142–62. doi:10.1084/jem.137.5.1142
29. Maldonado-López R, De Smedt T, Michel P, Godfroid J, Pajak B, Heirman C, et al. CD8alpha+ and CD8alpha- subclasses of dendritic cells direct the development of distinct T helper cells in vivo. *J Exp Med* (1999) **189**(3):587–92. doi:10.1084/jem.189.3.587
30. Feili-Hariri M, Falkner DH, Morel PA. Polarization of naive T cells into Th1 or Th2 by distinct cytokine-driven murine dendritic cell populations: implications for immunotherapy. *J Leukoc Biol* (2005) **78**(3):656–64. doi:10.1189/jlb.1104631
31. Pulendran B, Tang H, Manicassamy S. Programming dendritic cells to induce T(H)2 and tolerogenic responses. *Nat Immunol* (2010) **11**(8):647–55. doi:10.1038/ni.1894
32. Zhu J, Yamane H, Paul WE. Differentiation of effector CD4 T cell populations (*). *Annu Rev Immunol* (2010) **28**:445–89. doi:10.1146/annurev-immunol-030409-101212
33. Szabo SJ, Kim ST, Costa GL, Zhang X, Fathman CG, Glimcher LH. A novel transcription factor, T-bet, directs Th1 lineage commitment. *Cell* (2000) **100**(6):655–69. doi:10.1016/S0092-8674(00)80702-3
34. Thierfelder WE, van Deursen JM, Yamamoto K, Tripp RA, Sarawar SR, Carson RT, et al. Requirement for Stat4 in interleukin-12-mediated responses of natural killer and T cells. *Nature* (1996) **382**(6587):171–4. doi:10.1038/382171a0
35. Liao W, Lin JX, Wang L, Li P, Leonard WJ. Modulation of cytokine receptors by IL-2 broadly regulates differentiation into helper T cell lineages. *Nat Immunol* (2011) **12**(6):551–9. doi:10.1038/ni.2030
36. Kaplan MH, Schindler U, Smiley ST, Grusby MJ. Stat6 is required for mediating responses to IL-4 and for development of Th2 cells. *Immunity* (1996) **4**(3):313–9. doi:10.1016/S1074-7613(00)80439-2
37. Cote-Sierra J, Foucras G, Guo L, Chiodetti L, Young HA, Hu-Li J, et al. Interleukin 2 plays a central role in Th2 differentiation. *Proc Natl Acad Sci U S A* (2004) **101**(11):3880–5. doi:10.1073/pnas.0400339101
38. Zhu J, Cote-Sierra J, Guo L, Paul WE. Stat5 activation plays a critical role in Th2 differentiation. *Immunity* (2003) **19**(5):739–48. doi:10.1016/S1074-7613(03)00292-9
39. Bettelli E, Carrier Y, Gao W, Korn T, Strom TB, Oukka M, et al. Reciprocal developmental pathways for the generation of pathogenic effector TH17 and regulatory T cells. *Nature* (2006) **441**(7090):235–8. doi:10.1038/nature04753
40. Moore KW, de Waal Malefyt R, Coffman RL, O'Garra A. Interleukin-10 and the interleukin-10 receptor. *Annu Rev Immunol* (2001) **19**:683–765. doi:10.1146/annurev.immunol.19.1.683
41. Fuchs A, Vermi W, Lee JS, Lonardi S, Gilfillan S, Newberry RD, et al. Intraepithelial type 1 innate lymphoid cells are a unique subset of IL-12- and IL-15-responsive IFN-gamma-producing cells. *Immunity* (2013) **38**(4):769–81. doi:10.1016/j.immuni.2013.02.010
42. Klose CS, Flach M, Möhle L, Rogell L, Hoyler T, Ebert K, et al. Differentiation of type 1 ILCs from a common progenitor to all helper-like innate lymphoid cell lineages. *Cell* (2014) **157**(2):340–56. doi:10.1016/j.cell.2014.03.030
43. Daussy C, Faure F, Mayol K, Viel S, Gasteiger G, Charrier E, et al. T-bet and Eomes instruct the development of two distinct natural killer cell lineages in the liver and in the bone marrow. *J Exp Med* (2014) **211**(3):563–77. doi:10.1084/jem.20131560
44. Robinette ML, Fuchs A, Cortez VS, Lee JS, Wang Y, Durum SK, et al. Transcriptional programs define molecular characteristics of innate lymphoid cell classes and subsets. *Nat Immunol* (2015) **16**(3):306–17. doi:10.1038/ni.3094
45. Seillet C, Rankin LC, Groom JR, Mielke LA, Tellier J, Chopin M, et al. Nfil3 is required for the development of all innate lymphoid cell subsets. *J Exp Med* (2014) **211**(9):1733–40. doi:10.1084/jem.20140145

46. Geiger TL, Abt MC, Gasteiger G, Firth MA, O'Connor MH, Geary CD, et al. Nfil3 is crucial for development of innate lymphoid cells and host protection against intestinal pathogens. *J Exp Med* (2014) **211**(9):1723–31. doi:10.1084/jem.20140212
47. Seillet C, Huntington ND, Gangatirkar P, Axelsson E, Minnich M, Brady HJ, et al. Differential requirement for Nfil3 during NK cell development. *J Immunol* (2014) **192**(6):2667–76. doi:10.4049/jimmunol.1302605
48. Cortez VS, Fuchs A, Cella M, Gilfillan S, Colonna M. Cutting edge: salivary gland NK cells develop independently of Nfil3 in steady-state. *J Immunol* (2014) **192**(10):4487–91. doi:10.4049/jimmunol.1303469
49. Male V, Nisoli I, Kostrzewski T, Allan DS, Carlyle JR, Lord GM, et al. The transcription factor E4bp4/Nfil3 controls commitment to the NK lineage and directly regulates Eomes and Id2 expression. *J Exp Med* (2014) **211**(4):635–42. doi:10.1084/jem.20132398
50. Rankin LC, Groom JR, Chopin M, Herold MJ, Walker JA, Mielke LA, et al. The transcription factor T-bet is essential for the development of NKp46+ innate lymphocytes via the Notch pathway. *Nat Immunol* (2013) **14**(4):389–95. doi:10.1038/ni.2545
51. Lu L, Ikizawa K, Hu D, Werneck MB, Wucherpfennig KW, Cantor H. Regulation of activated CD4+ T cells by NK cells via the Qa-1-NKG2A inhibitory pathway. *Immunity* (2007) **26**(5):593–604. doi:10.1016/j.immuni.2007.03.017
52. Soderquest K, Walzer T, Zafirova B, Klavinskis LS, Polić B, Vivier E, et al. Cutting edge: CD8+ T cell priming in the absence of NK cells leads to enhanced memory responses. *J Immunol* (2011) **186**(6):3304–8. doi:10.4049/jimmunol.1004122
53. Waggoner SN, Cornberg M, Selin LK, Welsh RM. Natural killer cells act as rheostats modulating antiviral T cells. *Nature* (2012) **481**(7381):394–8. doi:10.1038/nature10624
54. Crouse J, Bedenikovic G, Wiesel M, Ibberson M, Xenarios I, Von Laer D, et al. Type I interferons protect T cells against NK cell attack mediated by the activating receptor NCR1. *Immunity* (2014) **40**(6):961–73. doi:10.1016/j.immuni.2014.05.003
55. Xu HC, Grusdat M, Pandyra AA, Polz R, Huang J, Sharma P, et al. Type I interferon protects antiviral CD8+ T cells from NK cell cytotoxicity. *Immunity* (2014) **40**(6):949–60. doi:10.1016/j.immuni.2014.05.004
56. Ghadially H, Ohana M, Elboim M, Gazit R, Gur C, Nagler A, et al. NK cell receptor NKp46 regulates graft-versus-host disease. *Cell Rep* (2014) **7**(6):1809–14. doi:10.1016/j.celrep.2014.05.011
57. Schuster IS, Wikstrom ME, Brizard G, Coudert JD, Estcourt MJ, Manzur M, et al. TRAIL+ NK cells control CD4+ T cell responses during chronic viral infection to limit autoimmunity. *Immunity* (2014) **41**(4):646–56. doi:10.1016/j.immuni.2014.09.013
58. Zingoni A, Sornasse T, Cocks BG, Tanaka Y, Santoni A, Lanier LL. Cross-talk between activated human NK cells and CD4+ T cells via OX40-OX40 ligand interactions. *J Immunol* (2004) **173**(6):3716–24. doi:10.4049/jimmunol.173.6.3716
59. Gasteiger G, Hemmers S, Firth MA, Le Floc'h A, Huse M, Sun JC, et al. IL-2-dependent tuning of NK cell sensitivity for target cells is controlled by regulatory T cells. *J Exp Med* (2013) **210**(6):1167–78. doi:10.1084/jem.20122462
60. Sitrin J, Ring A, Garcia KC, Benoist C, Mathis D. Regulatory T cells control NK cells in an insulitic lesion by depriving them of IL-2. *J Exp Med* (2013) **210**(6):1153–65. doi:10.1084/jem.20122248
61. Gasteiger G, Hemmers S, Bos PD, Sun JC, Rudensky AY. IL-2-dependent adaptive control of NK cell homeostasis. *J Exp Med* (2013) **210**(6):1179–87. doi:10.1084/jem.20122571
62. Roediger B, Kyle R, Yip KH, Sumaria N, Guy TV, Kim BS, et al. Cutaneous immunosurveillance and regulation of inflammation by group 2 innate lymphoid cells. *Nat Immunol* (2013) **14**(6):564–73. doi:10.1038/ni.2584
63. Monticelli LA, Sonnenberg GF, Abt MC, Alenghat T, Ziegler CG, Doering TA, et al. Innate lymphoid cells promote lung-tissue homeostasis after infection with influenza virus. *Nat Immunol* (2011) **12**(11):1045–54. doi:10.1031/ni.2131
64. Wong SH, Walker JA, Jolin HE, Drynan LF, Hams E, Camelo A, et al. Transcription factor RORalpha is critical for nuocyte development. *Nat Immunol* (2012) **13**(3):229–36. doi:10.1038/ni.2208
65. Hoyler T, Klose CS, Souabni A, Turqueti-Neves A, Pfeifer D, Rawlins EL, et al. The transcription factor GATA-3 controls cell fate and maintenance of type 2 innate lymphoid cells. *Immunity* (2012) **37**(4):634–48. doi:10.1016/j.immuni.2012.06.020
66. Halim TY, MacLaren A, Romanish MT, Gold MJ, McNagny KM, Takei F. Retinoic-acid-receptor-related orphan nuclear receptor alpha is required for natural helper cell development and allergic inflammation. *Immunity* (2012) **37**(3):463–74. doi:10.1016/j.immuni.2012.06.012
67. Yang Q, Monticelli LA, Saenz SA, Chi AW, Sonnenberg GF, Tang J, et al. T cell factor 1 is required for group 2 innate lymphoid cell generation. *Immunity* (2013) **38**(4):694–704. doi:10.1016/j.immuni.2012.12.003
68. Wilhelm C, Hirota K, Stieglitz B, Van Snick J, Tolaini M, Lahl K, et al. An IL-9 fate reporter demonstrates the induction of an innate IL-9 response in lung inflammation. *Nat Immunol* (2011) **12**(11):1071–7. doi:10.1038/ni.2133
69. Moro K, Yamada T, Tanabe M, Takeuchi T, Ikawa T, Kawamoto H, et al. Innate production of T(H)2 cytokines by adipose tissue-associated c-Kit(+)Sca-1(+) lymphoid cells. *Nature* (2010) **463**(7280):540–4. doi:10.1038/nature08636
70. Neill DR, Wong SH, Bellosi A, Flynn RJ, Daly M, Langford TK, et al. Nuocytes represent a new innate effector leukocyte that mediates type-2 immunity. *Nature* (2010) **464**(7293):1367–70. doi:10.1038/nature08900
71. Price AE, Liang HE, Sullivan BM, Reinhardt RL, Eisley CJ, Erle DJ, et al. Systemically dispersed innate IL-13-expressing cells in type 2 immunity. *Proc Natl Acad Sci U S A* (2010) **107**(25):11489–94. doi:10.1073/pnas.1003988107
72. Nussbaum JC, Van Dyken SJ, von Moltke J, Cheng LE, Mohapatra A, Molofsky AB, et al. Type 2 innate lymphoid cells control eosinophil homeostasis. *Nature* (2013) **502**(7470):245–8. doi:10.1038/nature12526
73. Halim TY, Krauss RH, Sun AC, Takei F. Lung natural helper cells are a critical source of Th2 cell-type cytokines in protease allergen-induced airway inflammation. *Immunity* (2012) **36**(3):451–63. doi:10.1016/j.immuni.2011.12.020
74. Mjösberg JM, Trifari S, Crellin NK, Peters CP, van Drunen CM, Piet B, et al. Human IL-25- and IL-33-responsive type 2 innate lymphoid cells are defined by expression of CRTH2 and CD161. *Nat Immunol* (2011) **12**(11):1055–62. doi:10.1038/ni.2104
75. Hurst SD, Muchamuel T, Gorman DM, Gilbert JM, Clifford T, Kwan S, et al. New IL-17 family members promote Th1 or Th2 responses in the lung: in vivo function of the novel cytokine IL-25. *J Immunol* (2002) **169**(1):443–53. doi:10.4049/jimmunol.169.1.443
76. Chang YJ, Kim HY, Albacker LA, Baumgarth N, McKenzie AN, Smith DE, et al. Innate lymphoid cells mediate influenza-induced airway hyper-reactivity independently of adaptive immunity. *Nat Immunol* (2011) **12**(7):631–8. doi:10.1038/ni.2045
77. Kim BS, Siracusa MC, Saenz SA, Noti M, Monticelli LA, Sonnenberg GF, et al. TSLP elicits IL-33-independent innate lymphoid cell responses to promote skin inflammation. *Sci Transl Med* (2013) **5**(170):170ra116. doi:10.1126/scitranslmed.3005374
78. Yasuda K, Muto T, Kawagoe T, Matsumoto M, Sasaki Y, Matsushita K, et al. Contribution of IL-33-activated type II innate lymphoid cells to pulmonary eosinophilia in intestinal nematode-infected mice. *Proc Natl Acad Sci U S A* (2012) **109**(9):3451–6. doi:10.1073/pnas.1201042109
79. Saenz SA, Siracusa MC, Perrigoue JG, Spencer SP, Urban JF Jr, Tocker JE, et al. IL25 elicits a multipotent progenitor cell population that promotes T(H)2 cytokine responses. *Nature* (2010) **464**(7293):1362–6. doi:10.1038/nature08901
80. Saenz SA, Siracusa MC, Monticelli LA, Ziegler CG, Kim BS, Brestoff JR, et al. IL-25 simultaneously elicits distinct populations of innate lymphoid cells and multipotent progenitor type 2 (MPPtype2) cells. *J Exp Med* (2013) **210**(9):1823–37. doi:10.1084/jem.20122332
81. Fallon PG, Ballantyne SJ, Mangan NE, Barlow JL, Dasvarma A, Hewett DR, et al. Identification of an interleukin (IL)-25-dependent cell population that provides IL-4, IL-5, and IL-13 at the onset of helminth expulsion. *J Exp Med* (2006) **203**(4):1105–16. doi:10.1084/jem.20051615
82. Barlow JL, Bellosi A, Hardman CS, Drynan LF, Wong SH, Cruickshank JP, et al. Innate IL-13-producing nuocytes arise during allergic lung inflammation and contribute to airways hyperreactivity. *J Allergy Clin Immunol* (2012) **129**(1):.e1–4. doi:10.1016/j.jaci.2011.09.041
83. Bartemes KR, Iijima K, Kobayashi T, Kephart GM, McKenzie AN, Kita H. IL-33-responsive lineage- CD25+ CD44(hi) lymphoid cells mediate innate type 2 immunity and allergic inflammation in the lungs. *J Immunol* (2012) **188**(3):1503–13. doi:10.4049/jimmunol.1102832
84. Kim HY, Chang YJ, Subramanian S, Lee HH, Albacker LA, Matangkasombut P, et al. Innate lymphoid cells responding to IL-33 mediate airway hyperreactivity independently of adaptive immunity. *J Allergy Clin Immunol* (2012) **129**(1):.e1–6. doi:10.1016/j.jaci.2011.10.036

85. Kopf M, Le Gros G, Bachmann M, Lamers MC, Bluethmann H, Köhler G. Disruption of the murine IL-4 gene blocks Th2 cytokine responses. *Nature* (1993) **362**(6417):245–8. doi:10.1038/362245a0
86. Noben-Trauth N, Shultz LD, Brombacher F, Urban JF Jr, Gu H, Paul WE. An interleukin 4 (IL-4)-independent pathway for CD4+ T cell IL-4 production is revealed in IL-4 receptor-deficient mice. *Proc Natl Acad Sci U S A* (1997) **94**(20):10838–43. doi:10.1073/pnas.94.20.10838
87. Voehringer D, Reese TA, Huang X, Shinkai K, Locksley RM. Type 2 immunity is controlled by IL-4/IL-13 expression in hematopoietic non-eosinophil cells of the innate immune system. *J Exp Med* (2006) **203**(6):1435–46. doi:10.1084/jem.20052448
88. Perrigoue JG, Saenz SA, Siracusa MC, Allenspach EJ, Taylor BC, Giacomin PR, et al. MHC class II-dependent basophil-CD4+ T cell interactions promote T(H)2 cytokine-dependent immunity. *Nat Immunol* (2009) **10**(7):697–705. doi:10.1038/ni.1740
89. Sokol CL, Chu NQ, Yu S, Nish SA, Laufer TM, Medzhitov R. Basophils function as antigen-presenting cells for an allergen-induced T helper type 2 response. *Nat Immunol* (2009) **10**(7):713–20. doi:10.1038/ni.1738
90. Yoshimoto T, Yasuda K, Tanaka H, Nakahira M, Imai Y, Fujimori Y, et al. Basophils contribute to T(H)2-IgE responses in vivo via IL-4 production and presentation of peptide-MHC class II complexes to CD4+ T cells. *Nat Immunol* (2009) **10**(7):706–12. doi:10.1038/ni.1737
91. Halim TY, Steer CA, Mathä L, Gold MJ, Martinez-Gonzalez I, McNagny KM, et al. Group 2 innate lymphoid cells are critical for the initiation of adaptive T helper 2 cell-mediated allergic lung inflammation. *Immunity* (2014) **40**(3):425–35. doi:10.1016/j.immuni.2014.01.011
92. Mirchandani AS, Besnard AG, Yip E, Scott C, Bain CC, Cerovic V, et al. Type 2 innate lymphoid cells drive CD4+ Th2 cell responses. *J Immunol* (2014) **192**(5):2442–8. doi:10.4049/jimmunol.1300974
93. Oliphant CJ, Hwang YY, Walker JA, Salimi M, Wong SH, Brewer JM, et al. MHCII-mediated dialog between group 2 innate lymphoid cells and CD4(+) T cells potentiates type 2 immunity and promotes parasitic helminth expulsion. *Immunity* (2014) **41**(2):283–95. doi:10.1016/j.immuni.2014.06.016
94. Drake LY, Iijima K, Kita H. Group 2 innate lymphoid cells and CD4+ T cells cooperate to mediate type 2 immune response in mice. *Allergy* (2014) **69**(10):1300–7. doi:10.1111/all.12446
95. Gold MJ, Antignano F, Halim TY, Hirota JA, Blanchet MR, Zaph C, et al. Group 2 innate lymphoid cells facilitate sensitization to local, but not systemic, TH2-inducing allergen exposures. *J Allergy Clin Immunol* (2014) **133**(4):1142–8. doi:10.1016/j.jaci.2014.02.033
96. Liu B, Lee JB, Chen CY, Hershey GK, Wang YH. Collaborative interactions between type 2 innate lymphoid cells and antigen-specific CD4+ Th2 cells exacerbate murine allergic airway diseases with prominent eosinophilia. *J Immunol* (2015) **194**(8):3583–93. doi:10.4049/jimmunol.1400951
97. Bouchery T, Kyle R, Camberis M, Shepherd A, Filbey K, Smith A, et al. ILC2s and T cells cooperate to ensure maintenance of M2 macrophages for lung immunity against hookworms. *Nat Commun* (2015) **6**:6970. doi:10.1038/ncomms7970
98. Schiering C, Krausgruber T, Chomka A, Fröhlich A, Adelmann K, Wohlfert EA, et al. The alarmin IL-33 promotes regulatory T-cell function in the intestine. *Nature* (2014) **513**(7519):564–8. doi:10.1038/nature13577
99. Zaiss DM, van Loosdregt J, Gorlani A, Bekker CP, Gröne A, Sibilia M, et al. Amphiregulin enhances regulatory T cell-suppressive function via the epidermal growth factor receptor. *Immunity* (2013) **38**(2):275–84. doi:10.1016/j.immuni.2012.09.023
100. Croft M, So T, Duan W, Soroosh P. The significance of OX40 and OX40L to T-cell biology and immune disease. *Immunol Rev* (2009) **229**(1):173–91. doi:10.1111/j.1600-065X.2009.00766.x
101. So T, Song J, Sugie K, Altman A, Croft M. Signals from OX40 regulate nuclear factor of activated T cells c1 and T cell helper 2 lineage commitment. *Proc Natl Acad Sci U S A* (2006) **103**(10):3740–5. doi:10.1073/pnas.0600205103
102. Maazi H, Patel N, Sankaranarayanan I, Suzuki Y, Rigas D, Soroosh P, et al. ICOS:ICOS-ligand interaction is required for type 2 innate lymphoid cell function, homeostasis, and induction of airway hyperreactivity. *Immunity* (2015) **42**(3):538–51. doi:10.1016/j.immuni.2015.02.007
103. Hutloff A, Dittrich AM, Beier KC, Eljaschewitsch B, Kraft R, Anagnostopoulos I, et al. ICOS is an inducible T-cell co-stimulator structurally and functionally related to CD28. *Nature* (1999) **397**(6716):263–6. doi:10.1038/16717
104. Wilhelm C, Stockinger B. Innate lymphoid cells and type 2 (th2) mediated immune responses – pathogenic or beneficial? *Front Immunol* (2011) **2**:68. doi:10.3389/fimmu.2011.00068
105. Sun Z, Unutmaz D, Zou YR, Sunshine MJ, Pierani A, Brenner-Morton S, et al. Requirement for RORgamma in thymocyte survival and lymphoid organ development. *Science* (2000) **288**(5475):2369–73. doi:10.1126/science.288.5475.2369
106. Eberl G, Marmon S, Sunshine MJ, Rennert PD, Choi Y, Littman DR. An essential function for the nuclear receptor RORgamma(t) in the generation of fetal lymphoid tissue inducer cells. *Nat Immunol* (2004) **5**(1):64–73. doi:10.1038/ni1022
107. Sanos SL, Bui VL, Mortha A, Oberle K, Heners C, Johner C, et al. RORgammat and commensal microflora are required for the differentiation of mucosal interleukin 22-producing NKp46+ cells. *Nat Immunol* (2009) **10**(1):83–91. doi:10.1038/ni.1684
108. Satoh-Takayama N, Vosshenrich CA, Lesjean-Pottier S, Sawa S, Lochner M, Rattis F, et al. Microbial flora drives interleukin 22 production in intestinal NKp46+ cells that provide innate mucosal immune defense. *Immunity* (2008) **29**(6):958–70. doi:10.1016/j.immuni.2008.11.001
109. Sonnenberg GF, Monticelli LA, Elloso MM, Fouser LA, Artis D. CD4(+) lymphoid tissue-inducer cells promote innate immunity in the gut. *Immunity* (2011) **34**(1):122–34. doi:10.1016/j.immuni.2010.12.009
110. Takatori H, Kanno Y, Watford WT, Tato CM, Weiss G, Ivanov II, et al. Lymphoid tissue inducer-like cells are an innate source of IL-17 and IL-22. *J Exp Med* (2009) **206**(1):35–41. doi:10.1084/jem.20072713
111. Luci C, Reynders A, Ivanov II, Cognet C, Chiche L, Chasson L, et al. Influence of the transcription factor RORgammat on the development of NKp46+ cell populations in gut and skin. *Nat Immunol* (2009) **10**(1):75–82. doi:10.1038/ni.1681
112. Ouyang W, Rutz S, Crellin NK, Valdez PA, Hymowitz SG. Regulation and functions of the IL-10 family of cytokines in inflammation and disease. *Annu Rev Immunol* (2011) **29**:71–109. doi:10.1146/annurev-immunol-031210-101312
113. Mebius RE, Rennert P, Weissman IL. Developing lymph nodes collect CD4+CD3- LTbeta+ cells that can differentiate to APC, NK cells, and follicular cells but not T or B cells. *Immunity* (1997) **7**(4):493–504. doi:10.1016/S1074-7613(00)80371-4
114. Adachi S, Yoshida H, Kataoka H, Nishikawa S. Three distinctive steps in Peyer's patch formation of murine embryo. *Int Immunol* (1997) **9**(4):507–14. doi:10.1093/intimm/9.4.507
115. Finke D, Acha-Orbea H, Mattis A, Lipp M, Kraehenbuhl J. CD4+CD3- cells induce Peyer's patch development: role of alpha4beta1 integrin activation by CXCR5. *Immunity* (2002) **17**(3):363–73. doi:10.1016/S1074-7613(02)00395-3
116. Yoshida H, Honda K, Shinkura R, Adachi S, Nishikawa S, Maki K, et al. IL-7 receptor alpha+ CD3(-) cells in the embryonic intestine induces the organizing center of Peyer's patches. *Int Immunol* (1999) **11**(5):643–55. doi:10.1093/intimm/11.5.643
117. Cella M, Fuchs A, Vermi W, Facchetti F, Otero K, Lennerz JK, et al. A human natural killer cell subset provides an innate source of IL-22 for mucosal immunity. *Nature* (2009) **457**(7230):722–5. doi:10.1038/nature07537
118. Schmutz S, Bosco N, Chappaz S, Boyman O, Acha-Orbea H, Ceredig R, et al. Cutting edge: IL-7 regulates the peripheral pool of adult ROR gamma+ lymphoid tissue inducer cells. *J Immunol* (2009) **183**(4):2217–21. doi:10.4049/jimmunol.0802911
119. Tsuji M, Suzuki K, Kitamura H, Maruya M, Kinoshita K, Ivanov II, et al. Requirement for lymphoid tissue-inducer cells in isolated follicle formation and T cell-independent immunoglobulin A generation in the gut. *Immunity* (2008) **29**(2):261–71. doi:10.1016/j.immuni.2008.05.014
120. Scandella E, Bolinger B, Lattmann E, Miller S, Favre S, Littman DR, et al. Restoration of lymphoid organ integrity through the interaction of lymphoid tissue-inducer cells with stroma of the T cell zone. *Nat Immunol* (2008) **9**(6):667–75. doi:10.1038/ni.1605
121. Ota N, Wong K, Valdez PA, Zheng Y, Crellin NK, Diehl L, et al. IL-22 bridges the lymphotoxin pathway with the maintenance of colonic lymphoid structures during infection with *Citrobacter rodentium*. *Nat Immunol* (2011) **12**(10):941–8. doi:10.1038/ni.2089
122. Magri G, Miyajima M, Bascones S, Mortha A, Puga I, Cassis L, et al. Innate lymphoid cells integrate stromal and immunological signals to enhance

antibody production by splenic marginal zone B cells. *Nat Immunol* (2014) **15**(4):354–64. doi:10.1038/ni.2830
123. Kruglov AA, Grivennikov SI, Kuprash DV, Winsauer C, Prepens S, Seleznik GM, et al. Nonredundant function of soluble LTalpha3 produced by innate lymphoid cells in intestinal homeostasis. *Science* (2013) **342**(6163):1243–6. doi:10.1126/science.1243364
124. Taube C, Tertilt C, Gyülveszi G, Dehzad N, Kreymborg K, Schneeweiss K, et al. IL-22 is produced by innate lymphoid cells and limits inflammation in allergic airway disease. *PLoS One* (2011) **6**(7):e21799. doi:10.1371/journal.pone.0021799
125. Kim MY, Gaspal FM, Wiggett HE, McConnell FM, Gulbranson-Judge A, Raykundalia C, et al. CD4(+)CD3(-) accessory cells costimulate primed CD4 T cells through OX40 and CD30 at sites where T cells collaborate with B cells. *Immunity* (2003) **18**(5):643–54. doi:10.1016/S1074-7613(03)00110-9
126. Kim MY, McConnell FM, Gaspal FM, White A, Glanville SH, Bekiaris V, et al. Function of CD4+CD3- cells in relation to B- and T-zone stroma in spleen. *Blood* (2007) **109**(4):1602–10. doi:10.1182/blood-2006-04-018465
127. Mackley EC, Houston S, Marriott CL, Halford EE, Lucas B, Cerovic V, et al. CCR7-dependent trafficking of RORgamma(+) ILCs creates a unique microenvironment within mucosal draining lymph nodes. *Nat Commun* (2015) **6**:5862. doi:10.1038/ncomms6862
128. Gaspal FM, Kim MY, McConnell FM, Raykundalia C, Bekiaris V, Lane PJ. Mice deficient in OX40 and CD30 signals lack memory antibody responses because of deficient CD4 T cell memory. *J Immunol* (2005) **174**(7):3891–6. doi:10.4049/jimmunol.174.7.3891
129. Withers DR, Gaspal FM, Mackley EC, Marriott CL, Ross EA, Desanti GE, et al. Cutting edge: lymphoid tissue inducer cells maintain memory CD4 T cells within secondary lymphoid tissue. *J Immunol* (2012) **189**(5):2094–8. doi:10.4049/jimmunol.1201639
130. von Burg N, Chappaz S, Baerenwaldt A, Horvath E, Bose Dasgupta S, Ashok D, et al. Activated group 3 innate lymphoid cells promote T-cell-mediated immune responses. *Proc Natl Acad Sci U S A* (2014) **111**(35):12835–40. doi:10.1073/pnas.1406908111
131. Hepworth MR, Monticelli LA, Fung TC, Ziegler CG, Grunberg S, Sinha R, et al. Innate lymphoid cells regulate CD4+ T-cell responses to intestinal commensal bacteria. *Nature* (2013) **498**(7452):113–7. doi:10.1038/nature12240
132. Goto Y, Panea C, Nakato G, Cebula A, Lee C, Diez MG, et al. Segmented filamentous bacteria antigens presented by intestinal dendritic cells drive mucosal Th17 cell differentiation. *Immunity* (2014) **40**(4):594–607. doi:10.1016/j.immuni.2014.03.005
133. Hepworth MR, Fung TC, Masur SH, Kelsen JR, McConnell FM, Dubrot J, et al. Group 3 innate lymphoid cells mediate intestinal selection of commensal bacteria-specific CD4+ T cells. *Science* (2015) **348**(6238):1031–5. doi:10.1126/science.aaa4812
134. Radulovic K, Manta C, Rossini V, Holzmann K, Kestler HA, Wegenka UM, et al. CD69 regulates type I IFN-induced tolerogenic signals to mucosal CD4 T cells that attenuate their colitogenic potential. *J Immunol* (2012) **188**(4):2001–13. doi:10.4049/jimmunol.1100765
135. Radulovic K, Rossini V, Manta C, Holzmann K, Kestler HA, Niess JH. The early activation marker CD69 regulates the expression of chemokines and CD4 T cell accumulation in intestine. *PLoS One* (2013) **8**(6):e65413. doi:10.1371/journal.pone.0065413
136. Yadav M, Louvet C, Davini D, Gardner JM, Martinez-Llordella M, Bailey-Bucktrout S, et al. Neuropilin-1 distinguishes natural and inducible regulatory T cells among regulatory T cell subsets in vivo. *J Exp Med* (2012) **209**(10):S1–19. doi:10.1084/jem.20120822
137. Weiss JM, Bilate AM, Gobert M, Ding Y, Curotto de Lafaille MA, Parkhurst CN, et al. Neuropilin 1 is expressed on thymus-derived natural regulatory T cells, but not mucosa-generated induced Foxp3+ T reg cells. *J Exp Med* (2012) **209**(10):1723–42,S1721. doi:10.1084/jem.20120914
138. Delgoffe GM, Woo SR, Turnis ME, Gravano DM, Guy C, Overacre AE, et al. Stability and function of regulatory T cells is maintained by a neuropilin-1-semaphorin-4a axis. *Nature* (2013) **501**(7466):252–6. doi:10.1038/nature12428
139. Steinman RM, Nussenzweig MC. Avoiding horror autotoxicus: the importance of dendritic cells in peripheral T cell tolerance. *Proc Natl Acad Sci U S A* (2002) **99**(1):351–8. doi:10.1073/pnas.231606698
140. Qiu J, Guo X, Chen ZM, He L, Sonnenberg GF, Artis D, et al. Group 3 innate lymphoid cells inhibit T-cell-mediated intestinal inflammation through aryl hydrocarbon receptor signaling and regulation of microflora. *Immunity* (2013) **39**(2):386–99. doi:10.1016/j.immuni.2013.08.002
141. Sawa S, Lochner M, Satoh-Takayama N, Dulauroy S, Bérard M, Kleinschek M, et al. RORgammat+ innate lymphoid cells regulate intestinal homeostasis by integrating negative signals from the symbiotic microbiota. *Nat Immunol* (2011) **12**(4):320–6. doi:10.1038/ni.2002
142. Korn LL, Thomas HL, Hubbeling HG, Spencer SP, Sinha R, Simkins HM, et al. Conventional CD4+ T cells regulate IL-22-producing intestinal innate lymphoid cells. *Mucosal Immunol* (2014) **7**(5):1045–57. doi:10.1038/mi.2013.121
143. Ivanov II, de Frutos RL, Manel N, Yoshinaga K, Rifkin DB, Sartor RB, et al. Specific microbiota direct the differentiation of IL-17-producing T-helper cells in the mucosa of the small intestine. *Cell Host Microbe* (2008) **4**(4):337–49. doi:10.1016/j.chom.2008.09.009
144. Ivanov II, McKenzie BS, Zhou L, Tadokoro CE, Lepelley A, Lafaille JJ, et al. The orphan nuclear receptor RORgammat directs the differentiation program of proinflammatory IL-17+ T helper cells. *Cell* (2006) **126**(6):1121–33. doi:10.1016/j.cell.2006.07.035
145. Denning TL, Norris BA, Medina-Contreras O, Manicassamy S, Geem D, Madan R, et al. Functional specializations of intestinal dendritic cell and macrophage subsets that control Th17 and regulatory T cell responses are dependent on the T cell/APC ratio, source of mouse strain, and regional localization. *J Immunol* (2011) **187**(2):733–47. doi:10.4049/jimmunol.1002701
146. Honda K, Littman DR. The microbiome in infectious disease and inflammation. *Annu Rev Immunol* (2012) **30**:759–95. doi:10.1146/annurev-immunol-020711-074937
147. Ivanov II, Honda K. Intestinal commensal microbes as immune modulators. *Cell Host Microbe* (2012) **12**(4):496–508. doi:10.1016/j.chom.2012.09.009
148. Sonnenberg GF, Monticelli LA, Alenghat T, Fung TC, Hutnick NA, Kunisawa J, et al. Innate lymphoid cells promote anatomical containment of lymphoid-resident commensal bacteria. *Science* (2012) **336**(6086):1321–5. doi:10.1126/science.1222551
149. Gaboriau-Routhiau V, Rakotobe S, Lécuyer E, Mulder I, Lan A, Bridonneau C, et al. The key role of segmented filamentous bacteria in the coordinated maturation of gut helper T cell responses. *Immunity* (2009) **31**(4):677–89. doi:10.1016/j.immuni.2009.08.020
150. Ivanov II, Atarashi K, Manel N, Brodie EL, Shima T, Karaoz U, et al. Induction of intestinal Th17 cells by segmented filamentous bacteria. *Cell* (2009) **139**(3):485–98. doi:10.1016/j.cell.2009.09.033
151. Lécuyer E, Rakotobe S, Lengliné-Garnier H, Lebreton C, Picard M, Juste C, et al. Segmented filamentous bacterium uses secondary and tertiary lymphoid tissues to induce gut IgA and specific T helper 17 cell responses. *Immunity* (2014) **40**(4):608–20. doi:10.1016/j.immuni.2014.03.009
152. Van Praet JT, Donovan E, Vanassche I, Drennan MB, Windels F, Dendooven A, et al. Commensal microbiota influence systemic autoimmune responses. *EMBO J* (2015) **34**(4):466–74. doi:10.15252/embj.201489966
153. Geremia A, Arancibia-Cárcamo CV, Fleming MP, Rust N, Singh B, Mortensen NJ, et al. IL-23-responsive innate lymphoid cells are increased in inflammatory bowel disease. *J Exp Med* (2011) **208**(6):1127–33. doi:10.1084/jem.20101712
154. Mortha A, Chudnovskiy A, Hashimoto D, Bogunovic M, Spencer SP, Belkaid Y, et al. Microbiota-dependent crosstalk between macrophages and ILC3 promotes intestinal homeostasis. *Science* (2014) **343**(6178):1249288. doi:10.1126/science.1249288
155. Yang L, Anderson DE, Baecher-Allan C, Hastings WD, Bettelli E, Oukka M, et al. IL-21 and TGF-beta are required for differentiation of human T(H)17 cells. *Nature* (2008) **454**(7202):350–2. doi:10.1038/nature07021
156. Volpe E, Servant N, Zollinger R, Bogiatzi SI, Hupé P, Barillot E, et al. A critical function for transforming growth factor-beta, interleukin 23 and proinflammatory cytokines in driving and modulating human T(H)-17 responses. *Nat Immunol* (2008) **9**(6):650–7. doi:10.1038/ni.1613
157. Manel N, Unutmaz D, Littman DR. The differentiation of human T(H)-17 cells requires transforming growth factor-beta and induction of the nuclear receptor RORgammat. *Nat Immunol* (2008) **9**(6):641–9. doi:10.1038/ni.1610
158. Colonna M. Interleukin-22-producing natural killer cells and lymphoid tissue inducer-like cells in mucosal immunity. *Immunity* (2009) **31**(1):15–23. doi:10.1016/j.immuni.2009.06.008
159. Zamai L, Ahmad M, Bennett IM, Azzoni L, Alnemri ES, Perussia B. Natural killer (NK) cell-mediated cytotoxicity: differential use of TRAIL and Fas

ligand by immature and mature primary human NK cells. *J Exp Med* (1998) **188**(12):2375–80. doi:10.1084/jem.188.12.2375

160. Spits H, Lanier LL. Natural killer or dendritic: what's in a name? *Immunity* (2007) **26**(1):11–6. doi:10.1016/j.immuni.2007.01.004
161. Kashii Y, Giorda R, Herberman RB, Whiteside TL, Vujanovic NL. Constitutive expression and role of the TNF family ligands in apoptotic killing of tumor cells by human NK cells. *J Immunol* (1999) **163**(10):5358–66.
162. Munneke JM, Björklund AT, Mjösberg JM, Garming-Legert K, Bernink JH, Blom B, et al. Activated innate lymphoid cells are associated with a reduced susceptibility to graft-versus-host disease. *Blood* (2014) **124**(5):812–21. doi:10.1182/blood-2013-11-536888

8

Regulation of T cell immunity in atopic dermatitis by microbes: the Yin and Yang of cutaneous inflammation

Tilo Biedermann[1], Yuliya Skabytska[2], Susanne Kaesler[2] and Thomas Volz[1]*

[1] Department of Dermatology and Allergy, Technische Universität München, Munich, Germany, [2] Department of Dermatology, University Hospital, Tübingen, Germany

Edited by:
Stefan F. Martin,
University of Freiburg, Germany

Reviewed by:
Gabrielle Belz,
Walter and Eliza Hall Institute of Medical Research, Australia
Shahram Salek-Ardakani,
University of Florida, USA

***Correspondence:**
Tilo Biedermann,
Department of Dermatology and Allergy, Technische Universität München, Biedersteinerstrasse 29, Munich 80802, Germany
tilo.biedermann@tum.de

Atopic dermatitis (AD) is a chronic inflammatory skin disease predominantly mediated by T helper cells. While numerous adaptive immune mechanisms in AD pathophysiology have been elucidated in detail, deciphering the impact of innate immunity in AD pathogenesis has made substantial progress in recent years and is currently a fast evolving field. As innate and adaptive immunity are intimately linked, cross-talks between these two branches of the immune system are critically influencing the resulting immune response and disease. Innate immune recognition of the cutaneous microbiota was identified to substantially contribute to immune homeostasis and shaping of protective adaptive immunity in the absence of inflammation. Disturbances in the composition of the skin microbiome with reduced microbial diversity and overabundance of *Staphylococcus spp*. have been shown to be associated with AD inflammation. Distinct *Staphylococcus aureus* associated microbial associated molecular patterns (MAMPs) binding to TLR2 heterodimers could be identified to initiate long-lasting cutaneous inflammation driven by T helper cells and consecutively local immune suppression by induction of myeloid-derived suppressor cells further favoring secondary skin infections as often seen in AD patients. Moreover dissecting cellular and molecular mechanisms in cutaneous innate immune sensing in AD pathogenesis paved the way for exploiting regulatory and anti-inflammatory pathways to attenuate skin inflammation. Activation of the innate immune system by MAMPs of non-pathogenic bacteria on AD skin alleviated cutaneous inflammation. The induction of tolerogenic dendritic cells, interleukin-10 expression and regulatory Tr1 cells were shown to mediate this beneficial effect. Thus, activation of innate immunity by MAMPs of non-pathogenic bacteria for induction of regulatory T cell phenotypes seems to be a promising strategy for treatment of inflammatory skin disorders such as AD. These new findings demonstrate how detailed analyses identify partly opposing consequences of microbe sensing by the innate immune system and how these mechanisms translate into AD pathogenesis as well as new therapeutic strategies.

Keywords: atopic dermatitis, bacteria, dendritic cells, microbiota, non-pathogenic, T cell, tolerance, skin

Introduction

The skin is the body's outer interface organ forming a multi-layered barrier between the environment and the individual. To maintain integrity of the host and protect from potentially detrimental influences by pathogens or toxic substances, effective defense mechanisms have evolved. In addition, the skin is colonized by a multitude of bacteria forming the cutaneous microbiome that provides essential functions for skin homeostasis. Thus anti-bacterial immune responses must be tightly controlled to allow pathogen defense but also to preserve the composition of the microbiota in the absence of inflammation. Innate and adaptive immunity interact and orchestrate different qualities of immune responses. A breakdown in the symbiotic relationship between the cutaneous microbiota and its host has been identified and is associated with skin inflammation in atopic dermatitis (AD) (1). Deciphering mechanisms of the innate immune system which promote skin inflammation in AD patients and identifying counter regulatory pathways that limit inflammation by shaping T helper cell responses have not only broadened our understanding of disease pathology but also opened up new therapeutic perspectives.

Atopic Dermatitis Pathogenesis: In the Beginning, It is All About T Cells

Atopic dermatitis is a frequent inflammatory skin disease affecting up to 10–20% of the children and approximately 3% of adults in western countries (2). Innate (mast cells, eosinophils, basophils, different types of dendritic cells (DC), innate lymphocytes, and myeloid-derived suppressor cells) and adaptive immune cells (B cells and T cells) are believed to contribute to the complex immune network underlying cutaneous inflammation in AD. Few of the experimental setups and studies trying to disclose a role for these different cell types for AD allow defining one of these cell types as causal for cutaneous inflammation with the exception of $CD4^+$ T helper cells which have been shown in several studies, clinical trials, and mechanistic analyses to drive AD (3–5). Consequently, a closer look at the state of the art in regard to T cells in AD is essential to create a modern concept of AD pathogenesis and to develop new therapeutic strategies.

In AD, a dense infiltrate of activated CD4+ T cells can be detected in the dermis especially in acute lesions (**Figure 1**) (6). To better understand the initiation of AD, analyses of atopy patch test lesions has contributed substantially. Analyses of cytokine expression revealed that T helper cells of early lesions produce IL-4, IL-5, and IL-13, hallmark cytokines of Th2 cells (7). Thus, the concept that was developed within the last 20 years was based on the interpretation that Th2 cytokines in the skin promote cutaneous inflammation in AD. As examples of Th2-associated pathology, the Th2-induced isotype switch in B cells leading to the production of IgE is frequently cited and IL-5 promoting maturation and survival of eosinophils are highlighted to play a role in some types of AD and other atopic diseases (8, 9). Mechanistic analyses have helped to understand how these Th2 cells are recruited to the skin also disclosing possible targets of new therapeutic strategies: cutaneous leukocyte antigen (CLA) as adhesion molecule allowing Th2 cells to roll on the luminal side of the high endothelial venules proved to be a good marker for T cells prone to migrate to the skin (10, 11). CCR4 and CCR10 were shown to be prominent chemokine receptors allowing T cells to migrate through endothelia in the skin upon binding with the respective chemokines such as CCL17, CCL22, and CCL27 (11–13), and the chemokines binding CCR4 are among the best biomarkers for AD inflammation (14). Once

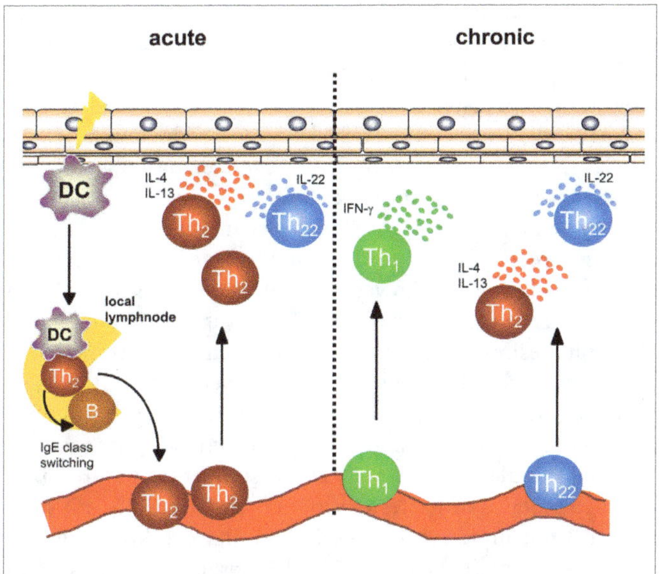

FIGURE 1 | Overview of T helper cell populations in acute and chronic dermatitis. In acute atopic dermatitis activated skin-resident DC migrate to local lymphnodes to prime naïve T helper cells and polarize them into a Th2 phenotype. Th2 cells induce IgE class switching in B cells accounting for enhanced IgE levels regularly found in atopic dermatitis patients. Th2 cells are recruited back to the skin and induce cutaneous inflammation by effector cytokines accompanied by Th22 cells. In chronic atopic dermatitis, Th1 cells are increasingly part of the skin infiltrate consisting of Th1, Th2, and Th22 cells.

Th2 cells are recruited to AD skin, Th2 cell activation leads to the accumulation of high levels of Th2 cytokines. Interestingly, IL-4 orchestrates monocytes and DC to produce high amounts of CCR4-binding chemokines further amplifying Th2 cell recruitment to the skin (15–17). Besides the effect on these immune cells, Th2 cytokines also fundamentally influence keratinocytes and how the epidermis responds to different stimuli. Th2 cytokines suppress the expression of terminal differentiation proteins of keratinocytes (filaggrin, loricrin and involucrin) therefore destabilizing cutaneous barrier function. In addition, Th2 cytokines have been shown to suppress the upregulation of antimicrobial peptides (AMP) in the skin upon stimulation such as beta defensin (HBD)-2, HBD-3, and LL-37 in keratinocytes. This failure to secrete AMPs to reach levels found in psoriasis has been argued to be the underlying mechanism of the susceptibility to bacterial and viral infections found in AD (18–20). Bacterial colonization on AD skin may be further supported by IL-4-mediated enhanced expression of fibronectin and fibrinogen acting as adhesion molecules for *Staphylococcus aureus* (21, 22). The Th1 cell and Th17 cell subsets are known for their potent anti-infectious properties controlling for intracellular and extracellular bacterial and fungal infections (23). Thus, demonstrating that IL-4 potently suppresses Th1 and Th17 cell immunity (24–28) further emphasized that AD skin is fundamentally more susceptible to cutaneous colonization and infection than normal or psoriasis skin. Most recent analyses even demonstrated that IL-4 reduces the Th17 inducing and maintaining cytokine IL-23 in antigen presenting cells both *in vitro* and *in vivo* in humans (28). These findings highlight that analyzing the recruitment, persistence, and function of different Th cell subtypes into AD skin is of pivotal importance for better understanding AD and for disclosing the impact of bacteria for AD inflammation, its prevention, and resolution.

Th17 cells were characterized by the production of IL-17 and IL-22 (29, 30). Following Th17 characterization, screening analyses were carried out for different diseases and tissues to better understand the Th17 cell function. Immunohistochemical studies revealed IL-17 production in acute AD lesions and confirmatory studies showed correlation of AD severity with the number of IL-17-producing T cells in peripheral blood and acute lesions (31, 32). Further characterization of IL-17-producing T cells in acute AD lesions revealed that IL-17 was produced by newly described subsets of Th2/IL-17$^+$ and Th0/IL-17$^+$ cells (33). Interestingly, IL-17 production by these subsets required stimulation by staphylococcal superantigens indicating interdependence of bacterial products and IL-17 in AD skin. It is still not understood why despite Th2 cytokines such as IL-4 suppressing IL-17 and IL-23, IL-17-producing cells are still detected in AD and whether IL-17 contributes to AD initiation or represents an epiphenomenon of cutaneous colonization and infection with bacteria in AD (27, 28, 33). Thus, the role of IL-17 in AD needs further clarification and new drugs being available targeting IL-17 and IL-17R for the treatment of psoriasis such as secukinumab will soon shed light into the hitherto unknown role of IL-17 for AD. As microbiota also induce or condition for IL-17 production, defining the role of IL-17 for skin homeostasis, defense, and inflammation requires functional analyses, disclosure of the cellular network, and spatiotemporal differentiation.

More recently, another unique subset of T helper cells enriched in inflamed human skin producing IL-22 in the absence of IL-17 was identified and characterized (34). These Th22 cells express the skin homing chemokine receptors CCR4 and CCR10 like Th2 cells and are distinct from Th17 cells as shown by transcriptome analyses (34, 35). Accumulation of Th22 cells was demonstrated in acute and chronic lesions of AD (36, 37) as were IL-22-producing CD8+ T cells (33, 36). IL-22 binds to a complex of IL-22R1 and IL-10R2 for induction of downstream signaling (38). IL-22R1 is not expressed on hematopoietic cells but rather can be detected on tissue-resident cells including keratinocytes (39). Functional consequences of IL-22 production are dependent on the target organ and the presence or absence of other cytokines, such as IL-17 or TNFα leading to either protective immune responses or inflammation (38, 40). IL-22 acting on keratinocytes has been reported to downregulate filaggrin expression and to affect expression of profilaggrin processing enzymes leading to further impairment of the epithelial barrier (41). Furthermore, IL-22 was reported to inhibit terminal differentiation of keratinocytes and to induce epidermal hyperplasia which is prominently seen in chronic AD (34). Thus IL-22-producing T cells may well play a crucial role in the pathogenesis of AD (42), however, the exact role cannot be defined based on the data available. Functions enhancing processes of both inflammation and regeneration describe Th22 cells as a Janus-like player for AD.

Atopic Dermatitis Pathogenesis: Chronic and Self-Perpetuating Inflammation Through Bacterial Exposure

While acute flares of AD are characterized by an infiltrate consisting of Th2 and Th22 cells, Th1 cells can be detected in chronic lesions of AD (**Figure 1**) in addition to Th2 and Th22 cells as early as 48 hours following elicitation of dermatitis (7, 37, 43). Th1 cells are characterized by the transcription factor T-bet and the secretion of the inflammatory cytokine IFN-γ (44). In regard to the pathogenesis of chronic AD, IFN-γ was postulated to contribute to skin hypertrophy in chronic AD (45). IFN-γ strongly induces IL-22R1 on keratinocytes allowing IFN-γ and IL-22 to act together for induction of epidermal hyperplasia (39).

Th1 cells can be polarized from naïve T helper cells by DC secreting large amounts of IL-12p70 (46, 47). As DC are at the interface of innate and adaptive immunity and build a dense network of immune sentinels in the skin, innate immune signals activating skin-resident DC were postulated to contribute to enhanced priming of Th1 cells in AD leading to chronic skin inflammation (48, 49). *S. aureus* colonization found in the majority of AD skin lesions and very early during lesion development has been shown to contribute to the release of pharmacological relevant amounts of Toll-like receptor (TLR2) agonists such as lipoteichoic acid (50). Binding of *S. aureus*-derived lipoteichoic acid to TLR2 on DC *in vitro* leads to DC maturation and production of the pro-inflammatory cytokines IL-12p70 and IL-23 resulting in enhanced Th1 and Th17 priming (51). Amplification of Th1 polarization is further achieved by the presence of the Th2 cytokine IL-4 acting on DC resulting in enhanced IL-12p70 production during T cell priming (52–54). As IL-4 is abundantly present in the skin of acute flares of AD as is *S. aureus*, combinatorial activation of DC by IL-4 and TLR2-ligands is a constant feature in AD skin. Based on this combined stimulation of cutaneous DC, a profound shaping of consecutive immune response can be anticipated (55). Indeed, TLR2 activation together with IL-4R signaling transfers acute Th2-driven dermatitis (48 h before dermatitis resolution) into long-lasting skin inflammation (14 days) with enhanced expression of the Th1 cytokine IFN-γ (56). A key role could be ascribed to the Th2 cytokine IL-4 mediating suppression of the anti-inflammatory cytokine IL-10 while enhancing IL-12 (**Figure 2**). Administration of exogenous IL-10 reverted chronic skin inflammation induced by TLR2 ligands and IL-4 indicating a crucial role for sustained production of IL-10 in response to cutaneous exposure to microbes. In conclusion, innate immune signals derived from *S. aureus* colonization or infection play a pivotal role in the transition of acute dermatitis into chronic skin inflammation and disease exacerbation highlighting a crucial role for microbes in the pathogenesis of AD (56). Furthermore, these mechanistic studies in AD models also revealed that IL-4 is responsible for the transition of early self-limiting AD into chronic self-perpetuating AD as found in most of AD patients. These findings demonstrate that Th2 cytokines such as IL-4 and IL-13 are not only responsible for early AD lesions but also for the development and maintenance of chronic AD. This also explains why targeting AD by the recently described antibody dupilumab blocking both IL-4 and IL-13 is highly effective in AD patients.

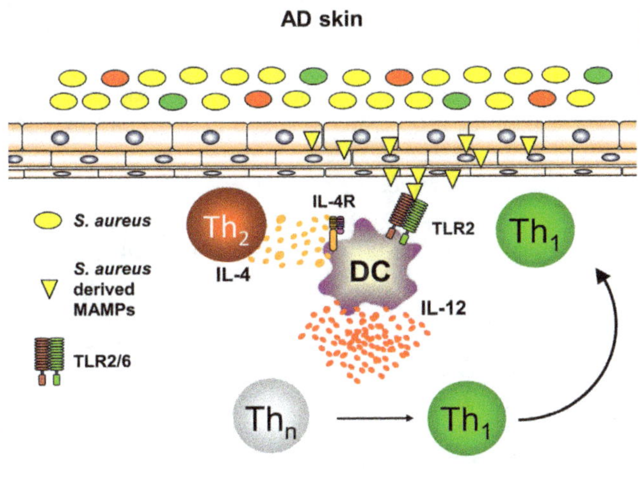

FIGURE 2 | Dual activation of skin-resident DC by IL-4 and TLR2 ligands promotes IL-12 expression and Th1 polarization. In atopic dermatitis skin, Th2 cells secreting IL-4 are abundantly present. Skin-resident DC are activated by *S. aureus* derived TLR2 ligands (lipoproteins, lipoteichoic acid) in an IL-4 rich environment leading to DC maturation and enforced IL-12 secretion by combinatorial activation of TLR2- and IL-4R-signaling while IL-10 production is markedly attenuated. As a consequence in the local lymph nodes, naïve T helper cells are preferentially polarized into a Th1 phenotype promoting long-lasting cutaneous inflammation after homing to atopic dermatitis skin.

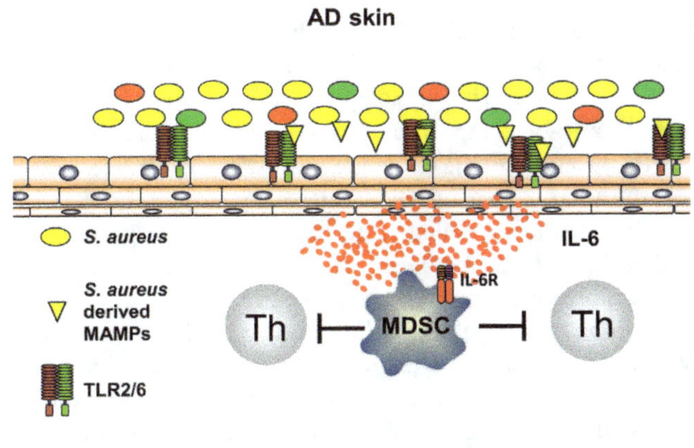

FIGURE 3 | *S. aureus*-derived lipoproteins induce MDSC. TLR2/6 heterodimers are expressed on skin-resident cells. Binding of diacylated bacterial lipoproteins induces IL-6 secretion leading to accumulation and activation of MDSC in the skin. T cell activation is vigorously suppressed by a NO-dependent mechanism.

Dupilumab is expected to be the first biologic being launched for AD treatment after having shown efficacy in several clinical trials (57). However, these analyses clearly highlight an intrinsic failure to terminate IL-4- and TLR2-driven chronic self-perpetuating AD as prominent feature of AD pathogenesis.

It can be anticipated that all types of inflammation, including those of anti-infectious immune responses, induce immune pathways that are capable to terminate inflammation and to prevent exaggerated and self-perpetuating potentially harmful courses of inflammation. Recently, it could be shown that innate immune recognition of *S. aureus* induces, following TLR2-induced inflammation, immune suppression by induction of myeloid-derived suppressor cells (MDSC) in a mouse model of AD (58). *S. aureus*-derived lipoproteins binding exclusively to the TLR2/6 heterodimer on skin-resident cells trigger IL-6 secretion that leads to activation and recruitment of $CD11b^+$ $Gr1^+$ MDSC into the skin (**Figure 3**). These $CD11b^+$ $Gr1^+$ MDSC efficiently suppressed T cell recall responses in the skin by an iNOS-dependent pathway. These MDSC, however, fail to suppress AD inflammation, but rather inhibit anti-infectious immune responses allowing *S. aureus* to further spread and drive AD and possibly also herpes viruses to mount a dangerous AD complication, eczema herpeticum (58). These investigations show that innate immune recognition of pathogenic bacteria on the skin induces an anti-inflammatory pathway presumably to limit damage induced by inflammatory responses. Distinct temporal and spatial distributions may coordinate these different and counter regulatory immune responses and understanding underlying mechanisms of attempts to prevent or resolve inflammation are important areas of research to identify new targets of treatments. Some of these mechanisms may be identified by the analyses that focus on the skin microbiome and immune consequences derived of the communication between the microbiome, the skin, and the cutaneous immune system.

Skin Microbiome

The skin is constantly colonized by myriads of bacteria with approximately 10^6 bacteria homing per square centimeter resulting in a total of 10^{10} bacteria covering the whole skin (59). The composition and distribution of the cutaneous microbiota have been deciphered in yet unknown details using deep sequencing techniques (60, 61). These techniques revealed a much more diverse microbiota as previously anticipated and detected using culture-based methods (61). The majority of bacteria identified by 16S ribosomal RNA sequencing can be assigned to four major phyla: Actinobacteria, Firmicutes, Bacteroidetes, and Proteobacteria (62). Importantly, 16S rRNA sequencing also detected Gram-negative species at dry skin areas, which were previously seen as contaminants but not residents using culture-based techniques (63).

Examining different skin sites, it was found that the skin microbiota differs between topographical locations (60). The colonization of bacteria on the different areas of human skin is largely dependent on the physiology of the respective skin site. Whether the area is predominantly "moist," "dry" or "sebaceous" impacts the respective microbiota to a large extent. At moist areas, *Staphylococcus spp.* and *Corynebacterium spp.* are the most abundant bacterial communities detected (59, 60). The highest diversity of phylotypes can be observed at dry skin areas like forearms, buttocks, and part of the hands with multiple species from the phyla Actinobacteria, Firmicutes, Bacteroidetes, and Proteobacteria being detected.

In contrast, sebaceous sites have the lowest diversity of phylotypes with a predominance of *Propionibacterium spp.* confirming culture-based approaches showing that *Propionibacterium spp.* are commensals in areas rich in the "pilosebaceous units" consisting of hair, hair follicle, and sebaceous gland (60).

Comparing interpersonal and intrapersonal variations of the skin microbiota at distinct topographical sites, it was shown that interpersonal variations are less than anticipated indicating that the colonized niche and its physiological features are a much stronger determinant for composition of the bacterial colonization than genetic variations of the individuals investigated (59, 62). In addition, the microbiota of one individual of, e.g., some sebaceous sites that share the same ecological features display a large similarity, further supporting the concept of cutaneous habitats determining the compositions of microbes by the cutaneous milieu.

Microbial colonization of the skin is established early in life. With birth, transition of the newborn's surfaces derived from a sterile uterine milieu then exposed to a microbial-rich environment occurs. Thus, immediately after birth the skin of the newborn is being colonized (64). The mode of delivery has been shown to play a major impact on the composition of the skin microbiota of the newborn. Following vaginal delivery, the skin microbiota resembles the mother's vaginal microbiota. In contrast, following cesarean delivery, the skin microbiota of the mother and the skin microbiota of the newborn show striking differences (64). The impact of these observations on the composition of the individual microbiota and the infant's health is largely unknown, but consequences for immune responses have been postulated. Interestingly, the composition of the skin microbiota of 1 to 3-month-old children did not differ in regard to mode of delivery (65), whereas other studies demonstrated a striking stability of individual microbiota over time. Indeed, the microbiome of adults is maintained over time whereas the microbiome of children shows less stability and even an increase in microbial diversity over time (65). The consequences of individual microbiota developing at different time points for immune responses, immune tolerance development, and the "readiness" for defense are still a matter of debate. Whether disturbances and dysbiosis during the process of microbiota development influence susceptibility to skin diseases associated with dyscolonization of the skin remains to be established.

Functional Consequences of the Skin Microbiome

The studies of the intestinal and the cutaneous microbiome are for the most part descriptive in nature and associations of certain microbiota or of compositions within detected microbiota with diseases are increasingly being detected. However, functional consequences still need to be proven, underlying mechanisms of diseases need firm linkage to microbial exposure, and pathways of translating surface exposure to microbes into immune responses and memory still need to be established. Only few mechanisms of how the skin microbiome or specific microorganisms contribute to cutaneous immune homeostasis have been identified so far. Importantly, functional studies need to also involve pre-clinical analyses in disease models. However, animals with fur may not follow the same rules and algorithms as human skin in the absence of fur.

Much attention has been given to consequences of cutaneous exposure to *staphylococci* with the assumption of *Staphylococcus epidermidis* being the "good" part of the microbiome and *S. aureus* being the "bad" causing infections and disease. Indeed, cutaneous colonization of severe barrier-disrupted murine skin with *S. aureus* leads to expression of IL-1β, IL-6, and TNFα lasting for up to 6 days demonstrating a pivotal role for *S. aureus* in promoting skin inflammation in susceptible hosts (66). After skin wounding and subsequently initiated inflammation due to TLR3-mediated detection of damaged cells, the skin commensal *Staphylococcus epidermidis* was identified to mediate resolution of cutaneous inflammation. Binding of *Staphylococcus epidermidis* derived lipoteichoic acid to TLR2 on keratinocytes was crucial in mediating this anti-inflammatory function via a TRAF1 dependent pathway (67). Recently, it was shown that recognition of *S. epidermidis* by the innate immune system profoundly shapes adaptive immune responses (68). Colonization of the skin with *S. epidermidis* activates antigen-specific T cells secreting IL-17 and IFN-γ in an IL-1R- and MyD88-dependent manner at steady-state conditions (68). Lack of commensals lead to a failure of induction of dermal IL-17- and IFN-γ-producing αβ T cells but raised the numbers of $FoxP3^+$ regulatory T cells in the skin. To identify functional consequences of cutaneous *S. epidermidis* exposure, a model of Leishmania infection was applied showing that in the absence of sufficient immune sensing of *S. epidermidis*, Leishmania infection could not be controlled sufficiently (68). Further analysis of the cellular pathways involved in this process showed that IL-17-producing T cells induced by *S. epidermidis* belong to the CD8+ subset displaying a unique and previously unknown role for these T cells in providing immune defense mechanisms in the skin (69). Thus, colonization of the skin with the commensal *S. epidermidis* provides innate immune signals to set up a functional threshold for adaptive immunity to establish pathogen control. Adaptive immune responses induced by the microbiota are required not only to fight pathogens but also to control colonization of the skin with commensals as in the absence of adaptive immunity commensal bacteria were detected in the local lymph nodes indicating microbial invasion (70). Skin microbiota therefore seems to induce a feedback loop to control microbial colonization with commensals to maintain epithelial integrity and immune homeostasis.

Changes of the skin microbiota composition might therefore contribute to cutaneous inflammation seen in various skin diseases (71). Detailed analysis of the cutaneous microbiota of AD patients demonstrated dramatically reduced diversity of the microbiome analyzed from acute flares presenting at the antecubital and popliteal crease (1). Instead of microbiota diversity overabundance of *S. aureus* and *S. epidermidis* was detected and correlated with disease severity confirming previous observations demonstrating *S. aureus* colonization and worsening of AD (1, 72). Of note, the "hen and egg problem" is not solved. Loss of microbiome diversity leading to skin flares or skin flares orchestrating dramatically reduced diversity of the microbiome are both possible scenarios. While for humans, the latter was thought to be the more likely cascade of events, new insights were brought forward by a mouse model.

A new model to study these changes from humans in detail including possibly causal relations was established most recently: mice lacking epidermal ADAM17 ($Adam17^{\Delta Sox9}$, $A17^{\Delta KC}$) exhibit skin barrier disruption with enhanced transepidermal water loss (TEWL) and subsequently develop eczematous lesions with a lymphocytic infiltrate resembling human AD (73, 74). The skin microbiome of mice with disrupted barrier function due to epidermal deficiency of ADAM17 (*Adam17*$^{\Delta Sox9}$) was indistinguishable from wildtype littermates in the first 2 weeks after birth but showed decreased bacterial diversity and an abundance of *Staphylococcus spp.* and *Corynebacterium spp.* compared to wildtype controls starting 4 weeks after birth (74). Administration of antibiotics in *Adam17*$^{\Delta Sox9}$ mice targeting *S. aureus* prevented the development of eczematous lesions and TEWL as well as cytokine production by CD4+ T cells and an increased number of skin-infiltrating T cells. Moreover, the microbiome showed a higher diversity – despite the use of antibiotics – and was comparable to the one of wildtype controls. In crossover experiments, antibiotic depletion of *S. aureus* in *Adam17*$^{\Delta Sox9}$ mice resulted in reduction of eczematous lesions, reduced TEWL, attenuation of skin-infiltrating T cells, and reversal of dysbiosis. By contrast, withdrawal of antibiotics in previously administered *Adam17*$^{\Delta Sox9}$ mice resulted in development of eczema, enhanced TEWL, increased skin-infiltrating T cells, and severe dysbiosis with excessive *S. aureus* colonization (74). These data clearly demonstrate that a shift of the microbiome resulting in dysbiosis with reduced microbial diversity and overrepresentation of *S. aureus* strikingly contributes to development of cutaneous inflammation and acute atopic flares in both mice with disrupted barrier and susceptible humans (1, 74). Thus enhancing the diversity of the microbiome to support colonization with putative non-pathogenic beneficial bacteria and/or targeting *S. aureus* colonization may be a therapeutic strategy in treatment of AD.

Resolution and Prevention of Atopic Skin Inflammation

While functional analysis of the skin microbiome is currently in its beginnings, much more details on the functional properties of the gut microbiota were gathered (75, 76). At steady-state conditions, IL-17A- and IFN-γ-producing T cells can be found in the gut-associated lymphoid tissue (GALT) and are required for prevention of inflammation by intestinal pathogens (77). Induction of these T cell populations has been shown to be dependent on the presence of the gut microbiota because in germ-free mice their numbers are significantly reduced (77, 78). This situation closely resembles what was found in the skin, namely turning off the local immune response by commensals to avoid inflammation by pathogens (71, 79). In contrast to the skin, FoxP3^{+} regulatory T cells (Tregs) are abundantly present in the GALT especially lining the lamina propria and Treg induction is dependent on the intestinal microbiota (79, 80). Several distinct mechanisms for induction of these regulatory T cells by the microbiota have been elucidated. Polysaccharide A (PsA) from Gram-negative *Bacteroides fragilis* has been shown to bind to TLR2 and to exert immune modulatory capacities in murine models of intestinal inflammation (81). The regulatory effects of PsA are due to induction of FoxP3^{+} iTregs and IL-10 secretion. Furthermore PsA is critical for maintaining immune homeostasis in the gut epithelium (81). A mixture of non-pathogenic *Clostridium spp* lacking toxins and virulence factors was identified to induce FoxP3^{+} Tregs in a TGF-β dependent manner preventing experimentally induced intestinal inflammation (82, 83). Whether analogous approaches performed in animal models for the gut are also feasible to attenuate skin inflammation was not yet investigated.

Recently, it was shown by investigating humans that the diversity of the environmental microbiota and the prevalence of atopic diseases are interrelated and in atopic individuals a significant reduced diversity of Gammaproteobacteria at their surroundings and on their skin could be found (84). Relative abundance of Gammaproteobacteria was correlated with IL-10 secretion by PBMCs of human healthy individuals while this IL-10 secretion was lacking in atopic patients. Investigations on the level of genus revealed that the reduced frequency of Gram-negative *Acinetobacter* best correlated with diminished IL-10 production in atopic individuals (84). Moreover, it was shown that heat-inactivated *Acinetobacter Iwoffi* induces IL-10 production in DC and primary human keratinocytes *in vitro* and when applied intradermally (85). This work extends investigations that showed that *Acinetobacter Iwoffi* exposure of pregnant mice avoids allergic asthma development in their off springs (86). These findings highlighting a possibly beneficial role for Gram-negative bacteria both for prevention of atopic diseases and for maintaining skin microbiota propose to investigate new therapeutic strategies extending the regulation of the skin microbiome beyond the focus on Gram-positive bacteria such as *S. epidermidis*. We performed the first proof-of-concept RCT in humans to investigate whether signals derived from non-pathogenic Gram-negative bacteria may mediate beneficial effects for the skin with mild AD. Therefore, we initiated a randomized double-blind placebo-controlled clinical trial on AD patients using a lysate from Gram-negative *Vitreoscilla filiformis*. Groups of patients with AD received either vehicle cream or this vehicle cream supplemented with a lysate of *V. filiformis* for 29 days. A first analysis following 15 days of treatment already detected a significant change in the group treated with the *V. filiformis* supplemented cream. Following 29 days of treatment with *V. filiformis*-derived substances, a significant reduction of disease activity in patients receiving topical therapy with a cream containing *V. filiformis* was observed, moreover, intergroup comparison revealed a significant difference between groups demonstrating clinical efficacy of immune signals derived from Gram-negative *V. filiformis* (87). Consecutive work focused on underlying mechanisms mediating immune modulation induced by immune signals derived from Gram-negative *V. filiformis*. To be able to analyze this mechanism of action possibly inducing tolerogenic immune responses effective on the skin, a mouse model for AD was utilized. Topical application of a lysate of *V. filiformis*, the Gram-negative, non-pathogenic bacterium, was shown to suppress skin inflammation in Th2-dominated hypersensitivity in the AD-prone NC/Nga mice (88). To unravel the underlying mechanisms, a series of *in vitro* and *in vivo* experiments was performed. It could be shown that *V. filiformis* lysate predominantly induces IL-10-producing DC in a TLR2-and MyD88-dependent manner. Priming of naïve T cells with DC activated by *V. filiformis* lead to the induction of Tr1 cells, which are characterized by their cytokine profile with high IL-10 and low IFN-γ levels (88, 89). The induction of IL-10^{high} IFN-γ^{low} Tr1 cells by innate immune signals from *V. filiformis* was dependent on DC-derived IL-10 and TLR2-signaling in DC. *V. filiformis* induced Tr1 cells had the capacity to suppress effector T cell proliferation and function demonstrating their regulatory function (**Figure 4**). Enhanced IL-10 production, reduced IFN-γ levels and diminished T cell proliferation in skin draining lymph

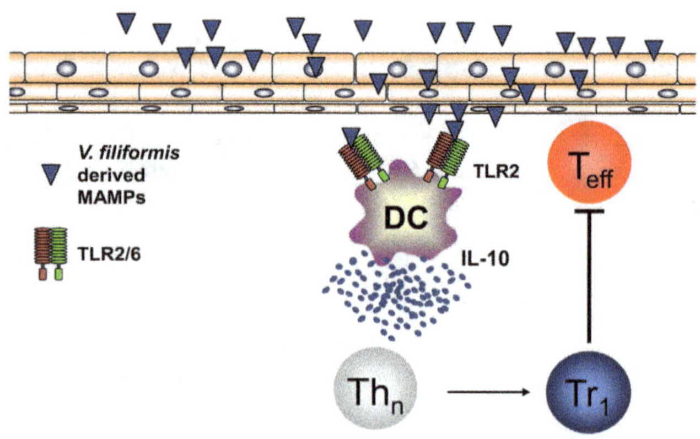

FIGURE 4 | Non-pathogenic bacterium *V. filiformis*-derived MAMPs induce tolerogenic DC and Tr1 cells. *V. filiformis*-derived MAMPs activate DC to produce IL-10 via a TLR2-dependent mechanism. DC-derived IL-10 is required to subsequently polarize naïve T helper cells into a Tr1 phenotype characterized by low IFN-γ and high IL-10 secretion. Vf-induced Tr1 cells efficiently block effector T cells (T_{eff}) demonstrating regulatory function for attenuating skin inflammation.

nodes of mice topically treated with *V. filiformis* lysate compared to controls was observed demonstrating *in vivo* functionality of this approach (88). These data demonstrate that cutaneous exposure to innate immune signals derived of non-pathogenic Gram-negative bacteria is sufficient to induce long-lasting immune tolerance by induction of IL-10, that limited cutaneous exposure is capable to induce also systemic immune modulation, and that indirect supplementation of IL-10 lacking in atopic individuals by innate immune signals from non-pathogenic Gram-negative bacteria may be a feasible therapeutic approach to stabilize both the cutaneous barrier and immune homeostasis.

Summary

T helper cells play a key role in eliciting and maintaining AD inflammation. Therefore, modulating T cell-elicited immune responses is a promising therapeutic approach. Th1- and Th1/Th17-mediated skin inflammation leading to psoriasis or cutaneous delayed-type hypersensitivity reactions could be treated successfully by immune deviation approaches targeting T helper cell polarization and inducing immune deviation (25, 26, 28). The contribution of various T helper cell subsets (Th2, Th1 Th22, maybe Th17) to AD pathophysiology precludes application of this successful principle as it could be detrimental and result in worsening of disease severity. Thus, induction of tolerogenic immune responses promises to be a feasible strategy. Innate immune recognition of specific components or bacteria derived from the gut microbiota has been shown to induce tolerance based on induction of tolerogenic DC, regulatory T cells, and anti-inflammatory cytokines. This approach could by successfully applied to dampen AD inflammation by activating DC with innate immune signals of non-pathogenic bacteria resulting in induction of tolerogenic DC, priming of regulatory Tr1 cells, and attenuation of cutaneous inflammation. After identification of diminished bacterial diversity in the skin microbiome of atopic individuals with consecutive loss of anti-inflammatory and tolerogenic IL-10, substitution of these tolerance promoting innate immune signals using microbes or microbial components is a new and promising therapeutic strategy.

References

1. Kong HH, Oh J, Deming C, Conlan S, Grice EA, Beatson MA, et al. Temporal shifts in the skin microbiome associated with disease flares and treatment in children with atopic dermatitis. *Genome Res* (2012) **22**:850–9. doi:10.1101/gr.131029.111
2. Bieber T. Atopic dermatitis. *N Engl J Med* (2008) **358**:1483–94. doi:10.1056/NEJMra074081
3. Woodward AL, Spergel JM, Alenius H, Mizoguchi E, Bhan AK, Castigli E, et al. An obligate role for T-cell receptor alphabeta+ T cells but not T-cell receptor gammadelta+ T cells, B cells, or CD40/CD40L interactions in a mouse model of atopic dermatitis. *J Allergy Clin Immunol* (2001) **107**:359–66. doi:10.1067/mai.2001.112695
4. Schmitt J, Schmitt N, Meurer M. Cyclosporin in the treatment of patients with atopic eczema – a systematic review and meta-analysis. *J Eur Acad Dermatol Venereol* (2007) **21**:606–19. doi:10.1111/j.1468-3083.2006.02023.x
5. Staumont-Salle D, Fleury S, Lazzari A, Molendi-Coste O, Hornez N, Lavogiez C, et al. CX(3)CL1 (fractalkine) and its receptor CX(3)CR1 regulate atopic dermatitis by controlling effector T cell retention in inflamed skin. *J Exp Med* (2014) **211**:1185–96. doi:10.1084/jem.20121350
6. Leung DY, Bieber T. Atopic dermatitis. *Lancet* (2003) **361**:151–60. doi:10.1016/S0140-6736(03)12193-9
7. Grewe M, Walther S, Gyufko K, Czech W, Schöpf E, Krutmann J. Analysis of the cytokine pattern expressed in situ in inhalant allergen patch test reactions of atopic dermatitis patients. *J Invest Dermatol* (1995) **105**:407–10. doi:10.1111/1523-1747.ep12321078
8. Phipps S, Flood-Page P, Menzies-Gow A, Ong YE, Kay AB. Intravenous anti-IL-5 monoclonal antibody reduces eosinophils and tenascin deposition in allergen-challenged human atopic skin. *J Invest Dermatol* (2004) **122**:1406–12. doi:10.1111/j.0022-202X.2004.22619.x
9. Ortega HG, Liu MC, Pavord ID, Brusselle GG, Fitzgerald JM, Chetta A, et al. Mepolizumab treatment in patients with severe eosinophilic asthma. *N Engl J Med* (2014) **371**:1198–207. doi:10.1056/NEJMoa1403290
10. Berg EL, Yoshino T, Rott LS, Robinson MK, Warnock RA, Kishimoto TK, et al. The cutaneous lymphocyte antigen is a skin lymphocyte homing receptor for the vascular lectin endothelial cell-leukocyte adhesion molecule 1. *J Exp Med* (1991) **174**:1461–6. doi:10.1084/jem.174.6.1461
11. Biedermann T, Schwärzler C, Lametschwandtner G, Thoma G, Carballido-Perrig N, Kund J, et al. Targeting CLA/E-selectin interactions prevents CCR4-mediated recruitment of human Th2 memory cells to human skin in vivo. *Eur J Immunol* (2002) **32**:3171–80. doi:10.1002/1521-4141(200211)32:11<3171:AID-IMMU3171>3.0.CO;2-4
12. Campbell JJ, Haraldsen G, Pan J, Rottman J, Qin S, Ponath P, et al. The chemokine receptor CCR4 in vascular recognition by cutaneous but not intestinal memory T cells. *Nature* (1999) **400**:776–80. doi:10.1038/23495
13. Homey B, Alenius H, Muller A, Soto H, Bowman EP, Yuan W, et al. CCL27-CCR10 interactions regulate T cell-mediated skin inflammation. *Nat Med* (2002) **8**:157–65. doi:10.1038/nm0202-157
14. Jahnz-Rozyk K, Targowski T, Paluchowska E, Owczarek W, Kucharczyk A. Serum thymus and activation-regulated chemokine, macrophage-derived chemokine and eotaxin as markers of severity of atopic dermatitis. *Allergy* (2005) **60**:685–8. doi:10.1111/j.1398-9995.2005.00774.x
15. Andrew DP, Chang MS, Mcninch J, Wathen ST, Rihanek M, Tseng J, et al. STCP-1 (MDC) CC chemokine acts specifically on chronically activated Th2 lymphocytes and is produced by monocytes on stimulation with Th2 cytokines IL-4 and IL-13. *J Immunol* (1998) **161**:5027–38.

16. Vulcano M, Albanesi C, Stoppacciaro A, Bagnati R, D'Amico G, Struyf S, et al. Dendritic cells as a major source of macrophage-derived chemokine/CCL22 in vitro and in vivo. *Eur J Immunol* (2001) **31**:812–22. doi:10.1002/1521-4141(200103)31:3<812::AID-IMMU812>3.0.CO;2-L
17. Xiao T, Fujita H, Saeki H, Mitsui H, Sugaya M, Tada Y, et al. Thymus and activation-regulated chemokine (TARC/CCL17) produced by mouse epidermal Langerhans cells is upregulated by TNF-alpha and IL-4 and downregulated by IFN-gamma. *Cytokine* (2003) **23**:126–32. doi:10.1016/S1043-4666(03)00221-7
18. Ong PY, Ohtake T, Brandt C, Strickland I, Boguniewicz M, Ganz T, et al. Endogenous antimicrobial peptides and skin infections in atopic dermatitis. *N Engl J Med* (2002) **347**:1151–60. doi:10.1056/NEJMoa021481
19. Nomura I, Goleva E, Howell MD, Hamid QA, Ong PY, Hall CF, et al. Cytokine milieu of atopic dermatitis, as compared to psoriasis, skin prevents induction of innate immune response genes. *J Immunol* (2003) **171**:3262–9. doi:10.4049/jimmunol.171.6.3262
20. Howell MD, Wollenberg A, Gallo RL, Flaig M, Streib JE, Wong C, et al. Cathelicidin deficiency predisposes to eczema herpeticum. *J Allergy Clin Immunol* (2006) **117**:836–41. doi:10.1016/j.jaci.2005.12.1345
21. Cho SH, Strickland I, Boguniewicz M, Leung DY. Fibronectin and fibrinogen contribute to the enhanced binding of *Staphylococcus aureus* to atopic skin. *J Allergy Clin Immunol* (2001) **108**:269–74. doi:10.1067/mai.2001.117455
22. Cho SH, Strickland I, Tomkinson A, Fehringer AP, Gelfand EW, Leung DY. Preferential binding of *Staphylococcus aureus* to skin sites of Th2-mediated inflammation in a murine model. *J Invest Dermatol* (2001) **116**:658–63. doi:10.1046/j.0022-202x.2001.01331.x
23. O'Connor W Jr, Zenewicz LA, Flavell RA. The dual nature of T(H)17 cells: shifting the focus to function. *Nat Immunol* (2010) **11**:471–6. doi:10.1038/ni.1882
24. Racke MK, Bonomo A, Scott DE, Cannella B, Levine A, Raine CS, et al. Cytokine-induced immune deviation as a therapy for inflammatory autoimmune disease. *J Exp Med* (1994) **180**:1961–6. doi:10.1084/jem.180.5.1961
25. Biedermann T, Mailhammer R, Mai A, Sander C, Ogilvie A, Brombacher F, et al. Reversal of established delayed type hypersensitivity reactions following therapy with IL-4 or antigen-specific Th2 cells. *Eur J Immunol* (2001) **31**:1582–91. doi:10.1002/1521-4141(200105)31:5<1582:AID-IMMU1582>3.0.CO;2-M
26. Ghoreschi K, Thomas P, Breit S, Dugas M, Mailhammer R, Van Eden W, et al. Interleukin-4 therapy of psoriasis induces Th2 responses and improves human autoimmune disease. *Nat Med* (2003) **9**:40–6. doi:10.1038/nm804
27. Park H, Li Z, Yang XO, Chang SH, Nurieva R, Wang YH, et al. A distinct lineage of CD4 T cells regulates tissue inflammation by producing interleukin 17. *Nat Immunol* (2005) **6**:1133–41. doi:10.1038/ni1261
28. Guenova E, Skabytska Y, Hoetzenecker W, Weindl G, Sauer K, Tham M, et al. IL-4 abrogates TH17 cell-mediated inflammation by selective silencing of IL-23 in antigen-presenting cells. *Proc Natl Acad Sci U S A* (2015) **112**:2163–8. doi:10.1073/pnas.1416922112
29. Harrington LE, Hatton RD, Mangan PR, Turner H, Murphy TL, Murphy KM, et al. Interleukin 17-producing CD4+ effector T cells develop via a lineage distinct from the T helper type 1 and 2 lineages. *Nat Immunol* (2005) **6**:1123–32. doi:10.1038/ni1254
30. Ghoreschi K, Laurence A, Yang XP, Hirahara K, O'Shea JJ. T helper 17 cell heterogeneity and pathogenicity in autoimmune disease. *Trends Immunol* (2011) **32**:395–401. doi:10.1016/j.it.2011.06.007
31. Toda M, Leung DYM, Molet S, Boguniewicz M, Taha R, Christodoulopoulos P, et al. Polarized in vivo expression of IL-11 and IL-17 between acute and chronic skin lesions. *J Allergy Clin Immunol* (2003) **111**:875–81. doi:10.1067/mai.2003.1414
32. Koga C, Kabashima K, Shiraishi N, Kobayashi M, Tokura Y. Possible pathogenic role of Th17 cells for atopic dermatitis. *J Invest Dermatol* (2008) **128**:2625–30. doi:10.1038/jid.2008.111
33. Eyerich K, Pennino D, Scarponi C, Foerster S, Nasorri F, Behrendt H, et al. IL-17 in atopic eczema: linking allergen-specific adaptive and microbial-triggered innate immune response. *J Allergy Clin Immunol* (2009) **123**(59–66):e54. doi:10.1016/j.jaci.2008.10.031
34. Eyerich S, Eyerich K, Pennino D, Carbone T, Nasorri F, Pallotta S, et al. Th22 cells represent a distinct human T cell subset involved in epidermal immunity and remodeling. *J Clin Invest* (2009) **119**:3573–85. doi:10.1172/JCI40202
35. Duhen T, Geiger R, Jarrossay D, Lanzavecchia A, Sallusto F. Production of interleukin 22 but not interleukin 17 by a subset of human skin-homing memory T cells. *Nat Immunol* (2009) **10**:857–63. doi:10.1038/ni.1767
36. Nograles KE, Zaba LC, Shemer A, Fuentes-Duculan J, Cardinale I, Kikuchi T, et al. IL-22-producing "T22" T cells account for upregulated IL-22 in atopic dermatitis despite reduced IL-17-producing TH17 T cells. *J Allergy Clin Immunol* (2009) **123**(1244–1252):e1242. doi:10.1016/j.jaci.2009.03.041
37. Gittler JK, Shemer A, Suarez-Farinas M, Fuentes-Duculan J, Gulewicz KJ, Wang CQ, et al. Progressive activation of T(H)2/T(H)22 cytokines and selective epidermal proteins characterizes acute and chronic atopic dermatitis. *J Allergy Clin Immunol* (2012) **130**:1344–54. doi:10.1016/j.jaci.2012.07.012
38. Eyerich S, Eyerich K, Cavani A, Schmidt-Weber C. IL-17 and IL-22: siblings, not twins. *Trends Immunol* (2010) **31**:354–61. doi:10.1016/j.it.2010.06.004
39. Wolk K, Kunz S, Witte E, Friedrich M, Asadullah K, Sabat R. IL-22 increases the innate immunity of tissues. *Immunity* (2004) **21**:241–54. doi:10.1016/j.immuni.2004.07.007
40. Sonnenberg GF, Fouser LA, Artis D. Border patrol: regulation of immunity, inflammation and tissue homeostasis at barrier surfaces by IL-22. *Nat Immunol* (2011) **12**:383–90. doi:10.1038/ni.2025
41. Gutowska-Owsiak D, Schaupp AL, Salimi M, Taylor S, Ogg GS. Interleukin-22 downregulates filaggrin expression and affects expression of profilaggrin processing enzymes. *Br J Dermatol* (2011) **165**:492–8. doi:10.1111/j.1365-2133.2011.10400.x
42. Guttman-Yassky E, Nograles KE, Krueger JG. Contrasting pathogenesis of atopic dermatitis and psoriasis – part II: immune cell subsets and therapeutic concepts. *J Allergy Clin Immunol* (2011) **127**:1420–32. doi:10.1016/j.jaci.2011.01.054
43. Biedermann T, Röcken M, Carballido JM. TH1 and TH2 lymphocyte development and regulation of TH cell-mediated immune responses of the skin. *J Investig Dermatol Symp Proc* (2004) **9**:5–14. doi:10.1111/j.1087-0024.2004.00829.x
44. Zhu J, Yamane H, Paul WE. Differentiation of effector CD4 T cell populations. *Annu Rev Immunol* (2010) **28**:445–89. doi:10.1146/annurev-immunol-030409-101212
45. Spergel JM, Mizoguchi E, Oettgen H, Bhan AK, Geha RS. Roles of TH1 and TH2 cytokines in a murine model of allergic dermatitis. *J Clin Invest* (1999) **103**:1103–11. doi:10.1172/JCI5669
46. Hsieh CS, Macatonia SE, Tripp CS, Wolf SF, O'Garra A, Murphy KM. Development of TH1 CD4+ T cells through IL-12 produced by *Listeria*-induced macrophages. *Science* (1993) **260**:547–9. doi:10.1126/science.8097338
47. Walsh KP, Mills KH. Dendritic cells and other innate determinants of T helper cell polarisation. *Trends Immunol* (2013) **34**:521–30. doi:10.1016/j.it.2013.07.006
48. Baker BS. The role of microorganisms in atopic dermatitis. *Clin Exp Immunol* (2006) **144**:1–9. doi:10.1111/j.1365-2249.2005.02980.x
49. Biedermann T. Dissecting the role of infections in atopic dermatitis. *Acta Derm Venereol* (2006) **86**:99–109. doi:10.2340/00015555-0047
50. Travers JB, Kozman A, Mousdicas N, Saha C, Landis M, Al-Hassani M, et al. Infected atopic dermatitis lesions contain pharmacologic amounts of lipoteichoic acid. *J Allergy Clin Immunol* (2010) **125**(146–152):e141–2. doi:10.1016/j.jaci.2009.09.052
51. Volz T, Nega M, Buschmann J, Kaesler S, Guenova E, Peschel A, et al. Natural *Staphylococcus aureus*-derived peptidoglycan fragments activate NOD2 and act as potent costimulators of the innate immune system exclusively in the presence of TLR signals. *FASEB J* (2010) **24**:4089–102. doi:10.1096/fj.09-151001
52. Biedermann T, Zimmermann S, Himmelrich H, Gumy A, Egeter O, Sakrauski AK, et al. IL-4 instructs TH1 responses and resistance to *Leishmania* major in susceptible BALB/c mice. *Nat Immunol* (2001) **2**:1054–60. doi:10.1038/ni725
53. Yao Y, Li W, Kaplan MH, Chang CH. Interleukin (IL)-4 inhibits IL-10 to promote IL-12 production by dendritic cells. *J Exp Med* (2005) **201**:1899–903. doi:10.1084/jem.20050324
54. Guenova E, Volz T, Sauer K, Kaesler S, Müller MR, Wölbing F, et al. IL-4-mediated fine tuning of IL-12p70 production by human DC. *Eur J Immunol* (2008) **38**:3138–49. doi:10.1002/eji.200838463
55. Volz T, Kaesler S, Biedermann T. Innate immune sensing 2.0 – from linear activation pathways to fine tuned and regulated innate immune networks. *Exp Dermatol* (2012) **21**:61–9. doi:10.1111/j.1600-0625.2011.01393.x
56. Kaesler S, Volz T, Skabytska Y, Köberle M, Hein U, Chen KM, et al. Toll-like receptor 2 ligands promote chronic atopic dermatitis through IL-4-mediated suppression of IL-10. *J Allergy Clin Immunol* (2014) **134**:92–9. doi:10.1016/j.jaci.2014.02.017
57. Beck LA, Thaci D, Hamilton JD, Graham NM, Bieber T, Rocklin R, et al. Dupilumab treatment in adults with moderate-to-severe atopic dermatitis. *N Engl J Med* (2014) **371**:130–9. doi:10.1056/NEJMoa1314768
58. Skabytska Y, Wölbing F, Günther C, Koberle M, Kaesler S, Chen KM, et al. Cutaneous innate immune sensing of toll-like receptor 2-6 ligands suppresses

T cell immunity by inducing myeloid-derived suppressor cells. *Immunity* (2014) **41**:762–75. doi:10.1016/j.immuni.2014.10.009
59. Grice EA, Kong HH, Renaud G, Young AC, Bouffard GG, Blakesley RW, et al. A diversity profile of the human skin microbiota. *Genome Res* (2008) **18**:1043–50. doi:10.1101/gr.075549.107
60. Grice EA, Kong HH, Conlan S, Deming CB, Davis J, Young AC, et al. Topographical and temporal diversity of the human skin microbiome. *Science* (2009) **324**:1190–2. doi:10.1126/science.1171700
61. Kong HH, Segre JA. Skin microbiome: looking back to move forward. *J Invest Dermatol* (2012) **132**:933–9. doi:10.1038/jid.2011.417
62. Grice EA, Segre JA. The skin microbiome. *Nat Rev Microbiol* (2011) **9**:244–53. doi:10.1038/nrmicro2537
63. Roth RR, James WD. Microbial ecology of the skin. *Annu Rev Microbiol* (1988) **42**:441–64. doi:10.1146/annurev.mi.42.100188.002301
64. Dominguez-Bello MG, Costello EK, Contreras M, Magris M, Hidalgo G, Fierer N, et al. Delivery mode shapes the acquisition and structure of the initial microbiota across multiple body habitats in newborns. *Proc Natl Acad Sci U S A* (2010) **107**:11971–5. doi:10.1073/pnas.1002601107
65. Capone KA, Dowd SE, Stamatas GN, Nikolovski J. Diversity of the human skin microbiome early in life. *J Invest Dermatol* (2011) **131**:2026–32. doi:10.1038/jid.2011.168
66. Wanke I, Skabytska Y, Kraft B, Peschel A, Biedermann T, Schittek B. *Staphylococcus aureus* skin colonization is promoted by barrier disruption and leads to local inflammation. *Exp Dermatol* (2013) **22**:153–5. doi:10.1111/exd.12083
67. Lai Y, Di Nardo A, Nakatsuji T, Leichtle A, Yang Y, Cogen AL, et al. Commensal bacteria regulate Toll-like receptor 3-dependent inflammation after skin injury. *Nat Med* (2009) **15**:1377–82. doi:10.1038/nm.2062
68. Naik S, Bouladoux N, Wilhelm C, Molloy MJ, Salcedo R, Kastenmuller W, et al. Compartmentalized control of skin immunity by resident commensals. *Science* (2012) **337**:1115–9. doi:10.1126/science.1225152
69. Naik S, Bouladoux N, Linehan JL, Han SJ, Harrison OJ, Wilhelm C, et al. Commensal-dendritic-cell interaction specifies a unique protective skin immune signature. *Nature* (2015) **520**:104–8. doi:10.1038/nature14052
70. Shen W, Li W, Hixon JA, Bouladoux N, Belkaid Y, Dzutzev A, et al. Adaptive immunity to murine skin commensals. *Proc Natl Acad Sci U S A* (2014) **111**:E2977–86. doi:10.1073/pnas.1401820111
71. Belkaid Y, Segre JA. Dialogue between skin microbiota and immunity. *Science* (2014) **346**:954–9. doi:10.1126/science.1260144
72. Breuer K, Kapp A, Werfel T. *Staphylococcus aureus*: colonizing features and influence of an antibacterial treatment in adults with atopic dermatitis. *Br J Dermatol* (2002) **147**:55–61. doi:10.1046/j.1365-2133.2002.04872.x
73. Franzke CW, Cobzaru C, Triantafyllopoulou A, Loffek S, Horiuchi K, Threadgill DW, et al. Epidermal ADAM17 maintains the skin barrier by regulating EGFR ligand-dependent terminal keratinocyte differentiation. *J Exp Med* (2012) **209**:1105–19. doi:10.1084/jem.20112258
74. Kobayashi T, Glatz M, Horiuchi K, Kawasaki H, Akiyama H, Kaplan DH, et al. Dysbiosis and *Staphylococcus aureus* colonization drives inflammation in atopic dermatitis. *Immunity* (2015) **42**:756–66. doi:10.1016/j.immuni.2015.03.014
75. Kamada N, Seo SU, Chen GY, Nunez G. Role of the gut microbiota in immunity and inflammatory disease. *Nat Rev Immunol* (2013) **13**:321–35. doi:10.1038/nri3430
76. Sommer F, Bäckhed F. The gut microbiota – masters of host development and physiology. *Nat Rev Microbiol* (2013) **11**:227–38. doi:10.1038/nrmicro2974
77. Ivanov II, Atarashi K, Manel N, Brodie EL, Shima T, Karaoz U, et al. Induction of intestinal Th17 cells by segmented filamentous bacteria. *Cell* (2009) **139**:485–98. doi:10.1016/j.cell.2009.09.033
78. Maynard CL, Elson CO, Hatton RD, Weaver CT. Reciprocal interactions of the intestinal microbiota and immune system. *Nature* (2012) **489**:231–41. doi:10.1038/nature11551
79. Belkaid Y, Bouladoux N, Hand TW. Effector and memory T cell responses to commensal bacteria. *Trends Immunol* (2013) **34**:299–306. doi:10.1016/j.it.2013.03.003
80. Geuking MB, Cahenzli J, Lawson MA, Ng DC, Slack E, Hapfelmeier S, et al. Intestinal bacterial colonization induces mutualistic regulatory T cell responses. *Immunity* (2011) **34**:794–806. doi:10.1016/j.immuni.2011.03.021
81. Round JL, Mazmanian SK. The gut microbiota shapes intestinal immune responses during health and disease. *Nat Rev Immunol* (2009) **9**:313–23. doi:10.1038/nri2515
82. Atarashi K, Tanoue T, Shima T, Imaoka A, Kuwahara T, Momose Y, et al. Induction of colonic regulatory T cells by indigenous *Clostridium* species. *Science* (2011) **331**:337–41. doi:10.1126/science.1198469
83. Atarashi K, Tanoue T, Oshima K, Suda W, Nagano Y, Nishikawa H, et al. Treg induction by a rationally selected mixture of Clostridia strains from the human microbiota. *Nature* (2013) **500**:232–6. doi:10.1038/nature12331
84. Hanski I, Von Hertzen L, Fyhrquist N, Koskinen K, Torppa K, Laatikainen T, et al. Environmental biodiversity, human microbiota, and allergy are interrelated. *Proc Natl Acad Sci U S A* (2012) **109**:8334–9. doi:10.1073/pnas.1205624109
85. Fyhrquist N, Ruokolainen L, Suomalainen A, Lehtimaki S, Veckman V, Vendelin J, et al. *Acinetobacter* species in the skin microbiota protect against allergic sensitization and inflammation. *J Allergy Clin Immunol* (2014) **134**(1301–1309):e1311. doi:10.1016/j.jaci.2014.07.059
86. Conrad ML, Ferstl R, Teich R, Brand S, Blumer N, Yildirim AO, et al. Maternal TLR signaling is required for prenatal asthma protection by the nonpathogenic microbe *Acinetobacter lwoffii* F78. *J Exp Med* (2009) **206**:2869–77. doi:10.1084/jem.20090845
87. Gueniche A, Knaudt B, Schuck E, Volz T, Bastien P, Martin R, et al. Effects of nonpathogenic Gram-negative bacterium *Vitreoscilla filiformis* lysate on atopic dermatitis: a prospective, randomized, double-blind, placebo-controlled clinical study. *Br J Dermatol* (2008) **159**:1357–63. doi:10.1111/j.1365-2133.2008.08836.x
88. Volz T, Skabytska Y, Guenova E, Chen KM, Frick JS, Kirschning CJ, et al. Nonpathogenic bacteria alleviating atopic dermatitis inflammation induce IL-10-producing dendritic cells and regulatory Tr1 cells. *J Invest Dermatol* (2014) **134**:96–104. doi:10.1038/jid.2013.291
89. Cottrez F, Hurst SD, Coffman RL, Groux H. T regulatory cells 1 inhibit a Th2-specific response in vivo. *J Immunol* (2000) **165**:4848–53. doi:10.4049/jimmunol.165.9.4848

9

Emerging functions of regulatory T Cells in tissue homeostasis

*Amit Sharma[1,2] and Dipayan Rudra[1,2]**

[1] *Academy of Immunology and Microbiology, Institute for Basic Science (IBS), Pohang, South Korea,* [2] *Division of Integrative Biosciences and Biotechnology, Pohang University of Science and Technology (POSTECH), Pohang, South Korea*

Edited by:
Amit Awasthi,
Translational Health Science and Technology Institute, India

Reviewed by:
Koji Yasutomo,
Tokushima University, Japan
Zhaocai Zhou,
Institute of Biochemistry and Cell Biology, Shanghai Institutes for Biological Sciences (CAS), China

***Correspondence:**
Dipayan Rudra
rudrad@ibs.re.kr

CD4⁺Foxp3⁺ regulatory T-cells (Tregs) are a unique subset of helper T-cells, which regulate immune response and establish peripheral tolerance. Tregs not only maintain the tone and tenor of an immune response by dominant tolerance but, in recent years, have also been identified as key players in resolving tissue inflammation and as mediators of tissue healing. Apart from being diverse in their origin (thymic and peripheral) and location (lymphoid and tissue resident), Tregs are also phenotypically heterogeneous as per the orientation of ongoing immune response. In this review, we discuss the recent advances in the field of Treg biology in general, and non-lymphoid and tissue-resident Tregs in particular. We elaborate upon well-known visceral adipose tissue, colon, skin, and tumor-infiltrating Tregs and newly identified tissue Treg populations as in lungs, skeletal muscle, placenta, and other tissues. Our attempt is to differentiate Tregs based on distinctive properties of their location, origin, ligand specificity, chemotaxis, and specific suppressive mechanisms. Despite ever expanding roles in maintaining systemic homeostasis, Tregs are employed by large varieties of tumors to dampen antitumor immunity. Thus, a comprehensive understanding of Treg biology in the context of inflammation can be instrumental in effectively managing tissue transplantation, autoimmunity, and antitumor immune responses.

Keywords: immune tolerance, autoimmunity, regulatory T cells, regulatory T-cells, Foxp3, tissue Treg, tumor Treg, regeneration

INTRODUCTION

Vertebrate immune and nervous system are two systems which are cognitive and under continuous interaction with the environment. This probably explains why both share common paradigms like recognition, learning or modulation, and memory. For long, immunology has been defined as a science of "self/non-self" discrimination (1). However, overtime, the immunological concept of "self" has evolved, where the very definition of an individual with defined anatomic borders, compatible balance between its parts, physiological autonomy, and ability to replicate as a unit is rapidly challenged by symbionts. Immune identity is now considered more fluid than restricted in strict borders (2). Hence, apart from generating a protective and offensive backdrop, the immune system must work to maintain an organismal identity by mediating dynamic exchange processes with the environment. This not only entails to generate robust defense against pathogens and toxins but also makes it rather paramount to suppress an overzealous immune response, curb autoimmune reactions, and maintain equilibrium toward commensals and food. Several mechanisms like clonal deletion, editing, anergy, ignorance, and immune deviation have evolved to safeguard against self-directed immunity (3). Specialized cells with immunosuppressive capabilities like tolerogenic dendritic cells (DCs) (4–6), regulatory B cells (7, 8), regulatory innate lymphoid cells (9), type 1 regulatory (Tr1) T-cells (10), and Foxp3$^+$ regulatory T-cells (Tregs) (11–13) have also evolved.

Regulatory T-cells are arguably the most versatile immunosuppressive cells and work like immunological sentinels across various tissues. Both in mice and men, loss of these cells essentially results in breakdown of tolerance and multi-organ autoimmunity. Since their discovery, biology of Tregs has been a most dynamic field of immunological research and as a result, Tregs, which were once considered as a homogenous immunosuppressive population, have been found to be highly adaptable and diversified cell type. Their heterogeneity is now appreciated in the context of origin, localization, differentiation, and mechanisms of immunosuppression. In the first part of this review, we will briefly discuss the events which put Tregs to the center stage of immune research, following which we will attempt to elaborate on the various layers of Treg heterogeneity especially pertaining to non-lymphoid and tissue-resident Tregs.

CONCEPT OF "DOMINANT" TOLERANCE AND THE EMERGENCE OF REGULATORY T-CELL RESEARCH

T-cell tolerance is pivotal for regulating adaptive immune responses as T-cell help is essential for mounting an antibody response *via* B cells (14). T-cell tolerance for long, was studied in light of "recessive tolerance," wherein T-cells with high affinity TCRs toward self-antigens are clonally deleted (15), or undergo "receptor editing" in thymus (16, 17). The runaway cells which escape these central processes encounter anergy or activation induced cell death in the periphery (15, 18). However, studies on tolerance ushered into an "active" or "dominant" era with the seminal discovery of suppressive CD4$^+$ T-cells expressing high levels of high efficiency α-chain receptor of IL2 (CD25) (19).

The Outset of Treg Research

Preliminary evidences of suppressive cells maintained in thymus started emerging when several investigators reported that neonatal thymectomy (3 day postnatal, 3dTx) could induce various autoimmune diseases in suitable mouse strains (20–25). Even more astonishing was the fact that similarly induced disease processes in rats could be reversed by reconstitution with normal lymphoid cells (26). Several groups tried to identify specific markers to distinguish suppressive cells from pathogenic T-cells in the thymus. It was reported that T-cells depleted of CD4$^+$CD5^{hi} cells induced autoimmune phenotype akin to 3dTx in BALB/c and C3H mice (27). Two other groups demonstrated the capability of CD4$^+$CD45RB^{hi} T-cells in inducing inflammatory bowel disease in BALB/c SCID mice (28, 29) and its resolution upon reconstitution with total T-cells. While these studies demonstrated that phenotypically distinct subsets of T-cells are capable of mounting discrete immune responses, specific identity of tolerance inducing counterparts remained elusive. Sakaguchi et al. in 1995 (19) discovered high surface expression of CD25 on about 8–10% of CD4$^+$ T-cells, which were both CD5^{hi} and CD45RB^{lo} in concordance with previous studies. Asano et al. (30) demonstrated that CD4$^+$CD25$^+$ T-cells appear around day 3 postnatal and increase up to the adult levels by day 10. These authors were the first to propose the term "regulatory" for this subtype.

Discovery of Foxp3

While subsequent studies involving numerous experimental models of autoimmunity established its functional existence (31), the usage of CD25 as a marker for Tregs remained controversial for a number of years due to its upregulation in all activated T-cells. Furthermore, it seemed possible that a subset of the activated T-cells, by virtue of marked upregulation of the IL2 receptor α on their surface, restrained immune response simply by competing for IL2.

A mouse line dubbed "scurfy," with spontaneous autoimmunity (originally appeared as a spontaneous mutation at the Oak ridge national laboratory, USA under the Manhattan project), was immunologically characterized in 1991. Scurfy mice have an X-linked recessive mutation which leads to scaly skin, lymphoproliferation, hypergammaglobulinemia, lymphadenomegaly, anemia, runting, and early death (32). Thymectomy reduced the severity of the disease but did not totally ameliorate it. However, crossing the strain with *nu/nu* mice totally prevented the disease, suggesting thymic origin of disease causing cells. Several other studies revealed scurfy to be mainly a T-cell dependent disorder (33–35) much similar to Cytotoxic T-Lymphocyte Associated Protein 4 (CTLA4) (36) and Transforming growth factor β1 (TGFβ1) deficient animals (37). These similarities instigated investigations to identify the gene responsible for scurfy phenotype. In 2001, Brunkow et al. (38) identified 20 putative genes in a 500-kb region of X-chromosome by sequencing four overlapping bacterial artificial chromosomes. Out of these, one possessed an ORF highly homologous with DNA-binding domain of the forkhead/HNF3/winged helix family of proteins. This gene in scurfy mouse was found to harbor a 2-bp insertion mutation, resulting in a truncated gene product, deleting the C-terminal forkhead domain (38). Investigators designated this gene as *Foxp3*. Functional complementation experiments by mating scurfy carrier females with *Foxp3* transgenic lines resulted in complete rescue of the scurfy phenotype, corroborating *Foxp3* mutation as the cause (38).

At around same time, mutations in *FOXP3* gene and its 3′ untranslated region were confirmed in human patients of IPEX syndrome (39, 40). IPEX syndrome is immunodysregulation polyendocrinopathy enteropathy X-linked, originally described in 1982 by Powell et al. (41). The striking similarity in autoimmune phenotype of IPEX patients, scurfy and 3dTx mice led several groups to examine the function of *Foxp3* in Tregs. Subsequently, in 2003, three studies reported that indeed *Foxp3* is uniquely expressed by CD4$^+$CD8$^-$CD25$^+$ thymocytes and CD4$^+$CD25$^+$ peripheral regulatory T-cells (42–44) in mice. Retroviral transduction of *Foxp3* induced CD25 expression in CD4$^+$CD25$^-$ T-cells which were functionally suppressive and expressed Treg associated molecules CTLA4 and GITR. Deletion of *Foxp3* in mice resulted in lymphoproliferative disorder identical to scurfy mice (43, 44). Mixed bone marrow chimera experiments demonstrated that indeed only *Foxp3*-sufficient bone marrows were capable of generating $CD4^+CD25^+$ Tregs (44). Conclusive evidence for Foxp3 as lineage specific marker for mice Tregs came from $Foxp3^{eGFP}$ reporter mice (45) in which GFP expression was found only in $TCR\beta^+$ T-cells among all hematopoietic cellular compartments. Conditional deletion of *Foxp3* in $CD4^+$ T-cells led to a lymphoproliferative disorder mirroring scurfy phenotype. These series of experiments established Foxp3 as the molecular identity responsible for implementing Treg transcriptional signature. Further investigations revealed that the *Foxp3* gene itself is regulated by three conserved non-coding sequences (CNS) 1–3. Detailed epigenetic analyses have identified CNS1 as the TGFβ responsive element which is required for peripheral generation of Tregs, CNS2 is involved with heritable maintenance of Foxp3 expression while CNS3 acts as a pioneering element for thymic induction of *Foxp3* (46). Proteomic analyses demonstrated Foxp3 to be interacting with more than 350 proteins in multiprotein complexes, many of which are transcription-related factors (47). A detailed review on regulation of *Foxp3* and Foxp3 mediated regulation of the Treg transcriptome can be found in Lu et al. (12).

DEVELOPMENTAL AND PHENOTYPIC DIVERSITY IN Tregs

Neonatal thymectomy experiments in mice confirmed beyond doubt that early development of Tregs happens in thymus. A detailed discussion on thymic development of Tregs can be found in Ref. (13, 48, 49). Briefly, cell surface markers indicative of strength of TCR interaction (CD25, CD5, etc.) suggested the involvement of TCR signaling. TCR repertoires of Tregs have limited overlap with that of non-Tregs and are largely self-reactive (50). Nur77-GFP reporter mice which express GFP under *Nur77* gene locus, an early gene expressed upon TCR stimulation have higher GFP expression in thymic Tregs (tTregs) (51). With regard to cytokines, it was reported earlier that mice lacking either IL2 or CD25 (45) are able to generate Tregs, albeit at a reduced level. However, if common γ chain is deleted, Tregs are not formed (45). This suggests cooperation among γ chain cytokines in *Foxp3* expression and maintenance. Thus, the current model of Treg generation in thymus gravitates toward an instructive one wherein TCR signaling substantially above the strength required for positive selection and relatively near the strength that induces negative selection initiates specification toward pre-Treg state. In the second step, cytokines induce *Foxp3* expression. More recently, Satb1, a genome organizer and transcription factor was shown to at least partially mediate the genomic arrangement of super-enhancers responsible for Treg development (52). The Treg specific super-enhancer patterns were found "poised" for activation even in conventional peripheral T-cells.

Though thymic regulatory T-cells are adept at suppressing autoimmune responses against self-antigens, a reasonably tolerant immune environment cannot be developed if repeated immune responses are mounted against beneficial and innocuous microbes as well as food antigens. In part, this is achieved by generation of Tregs in the periphery. Indeed, initial evidences suggested that Tregs can be generated by oral antigen feeding (53, 54) as well as by antigen-specific APCs (55) in the absence of functioning thymus. Also, conventional $CD4^+CD25^-$ naïve T-cells could be converted to $CD4^+CD25^+CD45RB^{-/low}$ suppressor cells by costimulation with TCR and TGFβ. TGFβ activates Smad2 and 3 transcription factors (56) which redundantly, help in peripheral Treg generation by initiating a cascade of interactions with specific enhancer regions within the *Foxp3* locus (56–58).

Contrary to initial interpretations of Tregs being a universal immunosuppressive population, diligent interrogations led to identification of a rather diverse and distinct pool of heterogenous subsets. Other than the site of induction, Tregs were classified into two separate populations: central Tregs (cTregs) and effector Tregs (eTregs) (59, 60). cTregs are comparatively quiescent Tregs in the lymphoid tissues. They express the lymphoid homing molecules CD62L and CCR7 and are dependent on IL2 secreted by Tconv in T-cell zones of lymphoid tissues (60). On the other hand, eTregs are primarily non-lymphoid Tregs which downregulate lymphoid homing molecules and upregulate CD44, ICOS, GITR, and other activation-induced markers. For maintenance, they are dependent on sustained ICOS signaling (60). Most of these cells express transcription factor BLIMP1 and produce high IL10, akin to a population of $ICOS^+IL10^+$ Tregs in humans (61).

Investigations into Treg mediated suppression of distinct helper T-cell immune responses imply a contextual T helper–Treg coupled viewpoint of Treg heterogeneity. It was reported that Tregs express high amount of the interferon (IFN) regulatory factor IRF4, Treg specific ablation of which resulted in selective Th2 related pathologies (62). These findings initiated similar investigations in other helper T-cell contexts and indeed, now a well-established paradigm exists wherein, in a Th1 inflammatory context Tregs express transcription factor Tbet, responsible for Th1 speciation, and express CXCR3 to accumulate at such sites (63). Transcription factor STAT3 is expressed in Tregs in a Th17 context (64) which helps in upregulation of CCR6 to migrate to intestine and production of IL10 (65). Similarly, Bcl6 expression in Tregs was shown to be important for regulating Tfh cells and expression of CXCR5 (66, 67).

Moving a step further and increasing complexity and diversity among Tregs, several Treg subpopulations are discovered in non-lymphoid tissues. These Tregs are not only found to be instrumental in suppression of inflammatory responses but also integrate into a larger biological paradigm for the benefit of organ and organismal homeostasis. In the following sections, we will review the characteristics of non-lymphoid Tregs, how they originate and function in maintaining homeostasis of tissues. We will attempt to elucidate if, apart from location, these cell types can be further identified by virtue of tissue-specific phenotypic and functional characteristics. We will elaborately discuss the well-characterized Treg populations in adipose tissues (AT), intestines, and skin, as well as attempt to highlight upon some of the recently identified ones in other tissues like muscles, lungs, and placenta. While overzealous Tregs in malignancies not necessarily can be clubbed with normal tissue Tregs, but at certain level, as Tregs perceive the context of the environment they reside in and are hijacked by tumors for their benefit, we will also discuss tumor infiltrated Tregs in order to elucidate on the general principles that might integrate such heterogeneity.

FAT Tregs: IMMUNOSUPPRESSION FOR METABOLIC HOMEOSTASIS

Adipose tissue is natural calorie reservoir of the body. Overall, the tissue is classified as two somewhat functionally antagonistic tissue types: white adipose tissue (WAT) and brown adipose tissue (BAT). WAT stores the excessive nutrients in the form of fat droplets during over-nutrition and releases it under energy deficit conditions. BAT, by virtue of higher expression of the uncoupling protein 1 (UCP1) protein, enhances energy utilization by non-shivering thermogenesis (68). WAT is abundantly available and found mainly in subcutaneous tissue, omenta, mesenteries, perirenal tissues, and bone marrow, while BAT has a restricted distribution occurring mainly in interscapular and inguinal regions.

AT Architecture

Structurally, AT is a loose connective tissue comprising mainly of fat cells (adipocytes), each surrounded by its own basal lamina and separated by a thin layer of extracellular matrix composed of reticular and collagen fibers and supplied with numerous capillaries. Several other resident as well as transient cells are strewn around in AT namely fibroblasts, myofibroblasts, and immune cells like macrophages, mast cells, eosinophils, neutrophils, and T-cells. WAT are the professional fat depots (69) which store excess energy as triglycerides without the common lipotoxicity experienced by other cell types (70). WAT adipocytes are usually spherical with a single fat droplet occupying 90% cell volume and a thin elongated mitochondrion on one side. On the other hand, BAT integrates environmental conditions *via* brain adrenergic responses toward cold temperatures. Adipocytes in BAT are typically polygonal, containing triglycerides in multiple small vacuoles, and are characterized by numerous large, spherical mitochondria.

Fat Treg Origin and Accumulating Factors

The plethora of adipokines and cross-talk with nervous as well as immune system has underscored the importance of AT as an endocrine organ with profound effects on body's metabolic homeostasis. However, as adipocyte increase in size due to excess calories, hypoxia sets in leading to accumulation of inflammatory macrophages (**Figure 1**) in obese adipose (71). Subsequent upregulation of several inflammatory adipokines (72) can activate CD4^{+} T-cells independent of macrophages. Any immune response shall be regulated so that it does not outlive its utility; a task largely achieved by several anti-inflammatory immune cell types already resident in the adipose (73–77).

In a seminal study, Feuerer et al. (76) identified unique fat-residing Tregs in mouse and human ATs. Surprisingly, unlike peripheral lymphoid compartment where normally 10–15% of CD4^{+} T-cells are Foxp3^{+} Tregs, almost half of the fat CD4^{+} T-cells are Foxp3^{+} Tregs, which were found to accumulate primarily in visceral fat over a period of time since birth, peaking at around

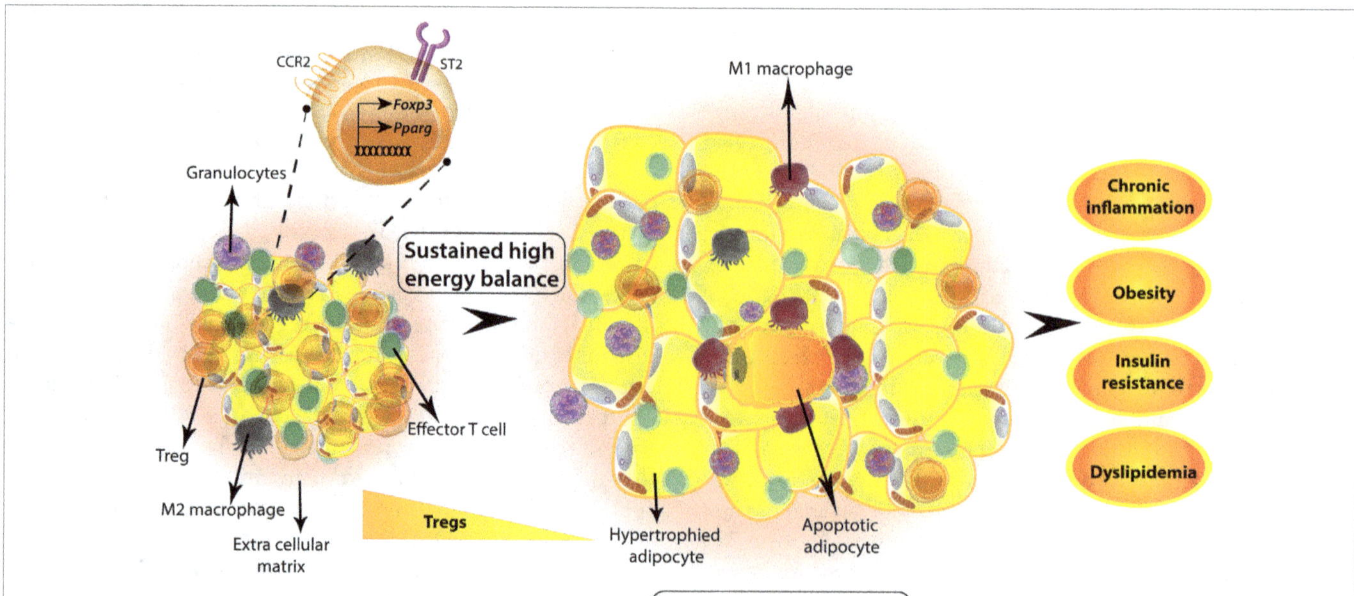

FIGURE 1 | Visceral white adipose tissue (WAT) regulatory T-cells (Tregs) are involved in metabolic homeostasis. WAT Tregs adapt to adipose environment by expression of PPARγ that regulates genes involved in lipid metabolism. These Tregs also express alarmin IL33 receptor ST2 and adipose chemokine receptor CCR2. Tregs are abundant in lean adipose tissue of adult mouse; however, if there is a sustained positive energy balance as in high-fat diet-induced obesity animal model, then the Treg numbers decrease drastically. This is concomitant to a change in macrophage phenotype from anti-inflammatory M2 to inflammatory M1 macrophages and unhealthy hypertrophy of adipocytes. Sustained hypertrophy leads to adipocyte apoptosis and exacerbated inflammation. Overall, decrease in adipose Tregs is accompanied by obesity, insulin resistance, dyslipidemia, and chronic low-grade inflammation.

25 weeks of age. In one study, this characteristic accumulation of Tregs was found to be accompanied by a sudden drop to fifth week levels (78) in mice aged further, suggesting a negative correlation between the frequency of visceral WAT resident Tregs and age-related metabolic inflammation (**Figure 2**). In contrast to this finding, a recent study, reported even greater accumulation of Tregs in older mice, implicating an alternative viewpoint instead (79) (**Figure 2**). The cause of this discrepancy might be different colonies, husbandry practices, as well as microbial and dietary composition. Nonetheless, the aged visceral WAT Tregs were found to be functional (79).

As far as origin of AT Tregs are concerned, visceral WAT Tregs appear to be largely of thymic origin. A thymectomy beyond 3 weeks of life does not affect visceral WAT Tregs population in mice (80). TCRα sequencing experiments from "Limited" mice [mice with limited focused diversity restricted to CDR3α (81)] showed that TCR repertoire of fat Tregs are different from conventional fat T-cells. Furthermore, visceral fat Treg repertoire was only a restricted subset of lymph node (LN) Tregs TCR repertoire (76), suggestive of an abdominal WAT specific distinct TCR repertoire of Tregs. This indicates either a continuous supply of Tregs from peripheral LNs or an initial seeding of tTregs followed by selected clonal expansion in AT. Adoptive transfer of congenically marked Tregs confirmed that visceral WAT Tregs are not significantly derived from circulating Tregs (80). Also, very high expression of both Helios and Neuropilin1 (Nrp1) as well as transcriptomic analysis of visceral WAT Tregs suggest their thymic origin and little to no conversion of naïve T-cells into visceral WAT Tregs (80).

Origin of subcutaneous WAT Tregs and BAT Tregs have not been studied in much detail. Naïve T-cells isolated from both these tissues, however, produce significantly high number of induced Tregs than visceral WAT in *in vitro* conversion assays (82).

Tissue Adaptation and Phenotype

That extralymphoid Tregs adapt to the context and microenvironment is best explained by higher expression of transcription factor PPARγ in fat Tregs (83, 84). Co-immunoprecipitation studies confirmed PPARγ interaction with Foxp3, suggesting a visceral WAT-specific Foxp3-PPARγ-mediated gene expression axis (83). Using a Blimp1-GFP reporter mouse, Vasanthkumar et al. (84) showed that most of the visceral WAT Tregs fall in the category of eTregs. For identifying the survival factors for eTregs, they reported that visceral WAT Tregs specifically express *Il1rl1*, which encodes alarmin IL33 receptor ST2. Both IL33 deficiency in general, as well as T-cell intrinsic ST2 deficiency resulted in specific reduction in number and percentage of visceral WAT Treg compartment (84). In *in vitro* settings, both IL2 and IL33

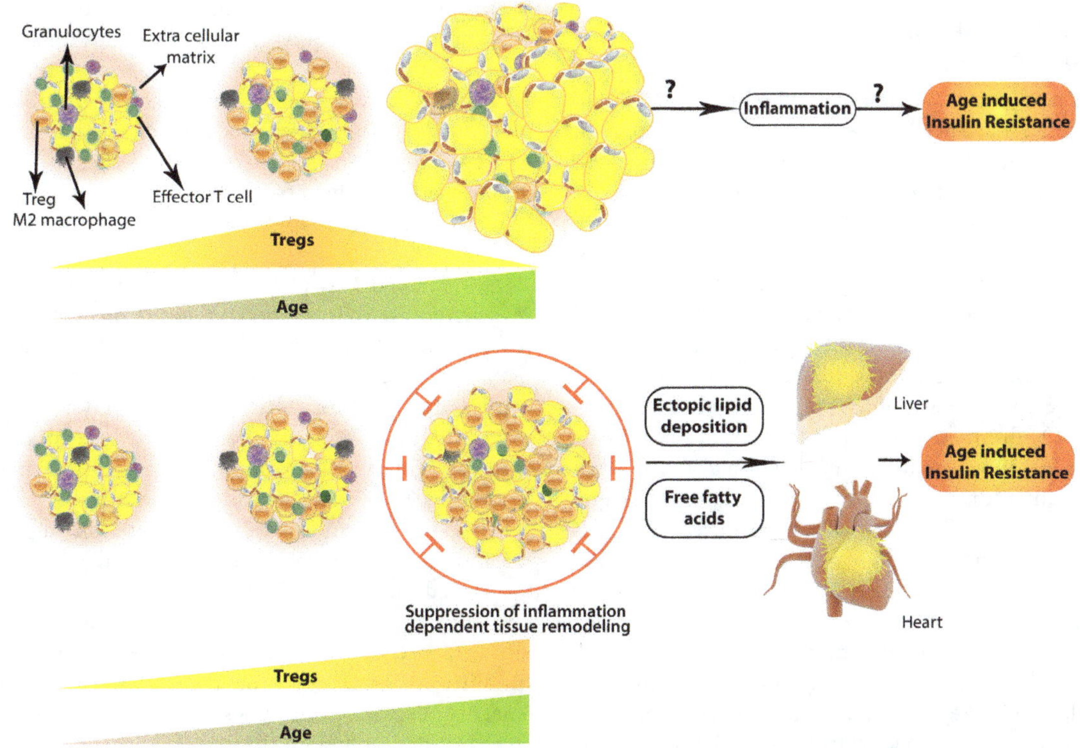

FIGURE 2 | Two contrasting scenarios of regulatory T-cells (Treg) numbers and their outcome in aged white adipose tissue (WAT). WAT Tregs increase with age reaching a plateau and then decrease abruptly in aged (~45 weeks) mouse (top). Whether this results in inflammation leading to age-associated insulin resistance is not explored; however, (bottom part) contrasting evidence suggest that white adipose Tregs keep on increasing even in the aged adipose tissue, which in concordance with "adipose tissue expandability hypothesis" (see text) results in suppression of healthy inflammation required for remodeling of adipose. This results in a storage space problem leading to ectopic deposition of fat in visceral organs, like liver and pericardium. This is accompanied by free fatty acid induced lipotoxicity and age-associated insulin resistance.

were able to induce proliferation and ST2 upregulation in a fraction of T-cells upon TCR stimulation which was dependent on MyD88 (84). Development and proliferation of visceral WAT Tregs appears to be dependent on two signals: (1) TCR crosslinking which induces PPARγ and ST2 expression *via* BATF and IRF4, both of which bind to the intronic regions of *Pparg* and *Il1rl1* genes (84) and (2) IL33 which *via* MyD88 feeds forward the expression of ST2 (84). In accordance to the concept of local adaptation, PPARγ in visceral WAT Tregs upregulates the expression of lipid metabolism genes like *Dgat1* (diacylglycerol *O*-acyltransferase 1), coding for an enzyme which catalyzes the terminal step in triacylglycerol synthesis by using diacylglycerol and fatty acyl CoA as substrates; and *Pcyt1a* (choline-phosphate cytidylyl transferase A), an enzyme involved in regulation of phosphatidylcholine biosynthesis (83). It is possible that these gene products enable visceral WAT Tregs to survive in a lipotoxic environment and/or enable the utilization of fatty acids as metabolic fuel. Other than these essential factors, visceral WAT Tregs also express high levels of GATA3, Klrg1, early activation marker CD69, and adipose signature chemokine receptor CCR2. BAT Tregs are found to be very similar to WAT Tregs at transcriptional level with higher expressions of PPARγ, IL10 and chemokine X ligands 1 and 2 (85). The under-expressed transcripts were those encoding for TCR signaling specific T Cell Factor 7 and cytokine IFNγ (85).

WAT Tregs Are Important Players in Metabolic Syndrome

Adipose originated pro-inflammatory cytokines, like TNFα, IL6, and type1 IFNs, have been suggested as causative of insulin resistance and metabolic syndrome (86–88). Also, human obese subjects were found to be deficient in circulating Tregs, whose levels were inversely correlated with body weight and BMI (89). Considering the primarily immunosuppressive phenotype of Tregs, it is expected that fat Tregs play a major role in controlling adipose inflammation, and in turn, affect the overall metabolic homeostasis of the body. Indeed, in Foxp3^{DTR} mice, in which the gene encoding diphtheria toxin receptor (DTR) is knocked into the *Foxp3* locus (90), Treg depletion upon diphtheria toxin (DT) administration, leads to visceral WAT tissue inflammation (76). However, total Treg deletion also initiates a strong systemic inflammatory response (90). Hence, a visceral WAT specific model for Treg deletion was required. This was achieved by Treg specific deletion of PPARγ, which resulted in more than 80% reduction in visceral WAT Tregs, without any effect on splenic Treg population (83). This decrease in Treg population was accompanied with marked inflammatory cell infiltration in visceral WAT (83). In a high-fat diet-induced obesity model, WAT Treg numbers are reduced drastically (**Figure 1**), which can be rescued by treatment with a synthetic PPAR ligand pioglitazone, which improves insulin sensitivity by working on PPARγ1 and 2 and affecting lipid metabolism (91). Its administration was able to improve the metabolic parameters in wild-type mice but not in mice harboring PPARγ-deficient Tregs, suggesting a direct role of PPARγ expression in visceral WAT Tregs.

Interestingly, the role of visceral WAT Tregs in aging animals has been reported to be opposite to what was observed in comparatively young animals. Contrary to obese animals, depletion of visceral WAT Tregs in aged animals improved the metabolic parameters and rescued aging induced insulin resistance (79) (**Figure 2**). Treg specific deletion of PPARγ led to less increase in fat and more in lean weight with age (more than 45 weeks). The adipocyte size was less and hepatic triglyceridosis was decreased. An increase in total Tregs by IL2–IL2 antibody immune complex resulted in reduced glucose uptake by aged adipocytes, suggesting compromised storage function (79). Similar results were obtained upon external IL33 administration. Overall this study reveals an unexpected cooperative role of visceral WAT Tregs in age-associated insulin resistance and metabolic inflammation. One explanation of this seemingly counter-intuitive finding might be extended by the so called "adipose tissue expandability" hypothesis. This hypothesis posits that in a state of "positive energy balance" metabolic complications arise because WAT is not able to expand further and accommodate excess calories, essentially propounding that metabolic syndrome coming out of excessive nutrition and obesity is actually a storage space problem (92). Indeed, animal models where AT inflammation is controlled result in decreased AT hyperplasia in a high-fat diet-induced mouse model of obesity (93), which causes ectopic lipid depositions (hepatic steatosis, dyslipidemia, etc.) and worsened metabolic parameters (93). Also, obese ob/ob mice which were made transgenic for full-length adiponectin and thus had adiponectin levels equivalent to treatment with a PPARγ agonist, showed uninhibited WAT expansion leading to morbid obesity but improved insulin sensitivity and other metabolic parameters (94) owing to reduced ectopic lipid deposition in liver and muscles (94). Given these observations, whether and how age-related accumulation of the visceral WAT Tregs results in compromised AT hyperplasia, remains to be seen.

BAT Tregs Help in Thermogenesis

A generalized Treg ablation alters the metabolic profile of mice with regard to BAT as well. DT mediated deletion of Tregs in Foxp3^{DTR} mice resulted in reduced whole-body oxygen consumption in a short-term cold temperature exposure model (85). That the Tregs are at forefront of metabolic homeostasis and their interventions are highly context dependent is further strengthened by a recent study analyzing BAT Tregs in detail. While a short-term (2 weeks) high-fat high-sugar (HFHS) diet, promoting thermogenesis (95), increased BAT Tregs, it actually decreased visceral WAT Tregs in young adult mice (82). On the contrary, a long-term HFHS diet (16 weeks) significantly reduced visceral WAT Tregs but made no impact on percent of BAT Tregs. This suggests that the tenor of caloric intake can have specific effect on tissue Tregs. In accordance to the role of BAT Tregs in non-shivering thermogenesis, treatment with ADRB3 (β-3 adrenergic receptor) agonist increased Tregs in BAT. However, "betaless" mice which are deficient in all three (β-1, 2, and 3 adrenergic receptors) did not have a reduced percentage of BAT Tregs, suggesting a redundant role of adrenergic signaling in BAT Treg accumulation *per se*. Treg depletion, followed by β-3 stimulation on the other hand did result in reduced levels of BAT thermogenic and lipolytic genes (*Ucp1*, *Ppargc1a*, *Pparg*, *Prdm16*, *Lpl*, etc.) confirming Treg functionality in BAT thermogenesis (82). It will be interesting to know if this results in reduced metabolic adaptation in cold exposure. Also, whether these effects are intrinsic to Tregs can only be ascertained with Treg specific *Adrb3* deletion. Thus, these studies confirm a role of Tregs in BAT which goes beyond immunosuppression and actively associates Tregs with cold adaptations of the body by regulating lipolysis and thermogenesis.

INTESTINAL Tregs: PRESERVING THE HOLOBIONT

The mammalian digestive system performs two very vital functions—digestion and absorption of food and shaping a gut microbial ecosystem. According to recent estimates, human colon harbors about 4×10^{13} bacteria (96, 97), a density (10^{11}/mL) highest among any microbial habitat (98). It has a perplexing task to efficiently implement a "goldilocks" balance between two seemingly opposite events; permit absorption of nutrients but check exposure to harmful substances, guard against invasive pathogens but facilitate colonization of commensals and help them thrive.

Architecture

Incessant provision of food and microbial antigens has resulted in typical structural adaptations in gut (99, 100) and evolution of specialized gut immune cells for immunosurveillance and maintenance of tolerance (101). The small intestine (duodenum, jejunum, and ileum) with maximum absorptive surface created by large circular folds (plicae) and finger like projections (villi and microvilli), has evolved as the primary organ for food absorption. The folding results in formation of deep invaginations, crypts of Lieberkühn, which house Paneth cells that secrete antimicrobial molecules upon exposure to bacterial antigens. Several enteroendocrine cells and mucus producing Goblet cells are also interspersed among small intestinal epithelial cells. The large intestine (cecum, colon, and rectum) harbor majority of commensals and perform the vital functions of absorbing water and vitamins while converting the undigested food into feces. The large intestinal walls are protected from luminal contents by two layers of mucus, the outer (luminal) thin mucus layer which hosts most of the bacteria, and the inner thick mucus layer which is largely sterile (102, 103).

Histologically, intestinal tract contains four layers—mucosa, submucosa, muscularis propria, and adventitia or serosa. The mucosa is the layer where most of the immune processes take place. It consists of an epithelial layer, which has scattered intraepithelial lymphocytes (IELs), underlying lamina propria (LP) and a thin muscle layer muscularis mucosa. The LP consist of non-cellular connective tissue, like collagen and elastin, blood and lymphatics, myofibroblasts, and nerve endings, and is densely packed with immune cells including mononuclear cells, plasma cells, B and T lymphocytes including Tregs, eosinophils, macrophages, and mast cells (104).

Different parts of intestine drain into separate LNs, like duodenum drains into a LN embedded in pancreatic tissue; mesenteric LNs drain jejunum, ileum, cecum, and ascending colon; two small LNs in pancreatic tissue drain transverse colon and descending colon and rectum primarily drains to caudal LNs (101). Anatomic variations largely define the antigenic variations of intestine as well. While small intestine grapples for equilibrium against food antigens, large intestines have an overwhelming load of microbial antigens. As much as these are foreign to the body, they are equally essential. Thus, for the economy of immune response it is highly desirable to assimilate those in the immunological self. The intestinal population of Tregs is arguably the most important cell type to contain the immune response against both food and innocuous microbial antigens and maintenance of intestinal homeostasis (105, 106).

Origin of Intestinal Tregs

Like other non-lymphoid tissues, Tregs are also enriched in intestinal LP with colon harboring 25–35% (107–109) and small intestine harboring 10–15% (109, 110) Tregs among total $CD4^+$ T-cells. Apropos to the prevalent inflammatory milieu and antigenic environment, the colonic Tregs are largely developed against microbial antigens. GF mice, devoid of any microbiota, have several folds less number of colonic Tregs compared to specific pathogen-free (SPF) mice (111, 112). A long-term broad-spectrum antibiotic treatment also reduces colonic Tregs in SPF mice (111). As small intestine is seat for nutrient absorption, most of the small intestine LP (siLP) Tregs do not develop against bacterial antigens as evident by comparable number of Tregs in SPF and GF mice (109). However, once the GF mice are brought up as antigen-free (AF) mice by provision of only elemental diet post-weaning, there is a marked decrease in siLP Tregs (109). A subset of Tregs, however, remains in colon as well as small intestine of GF and AF mice, presumably specific to gastrointestinal self-antigens.

Sequencing of colonic Treg TCRs of genetically engineered mice with limited polyclonal repertoires found that TCR usage of colonic Tregs was different from that of other tissues (113). Also, there was very little similarity of TCR usage between Tregs and naïve or effector $Foxp3^-$ T-cells (113). Stable chimeras made from retroviral transduction of colonic Treg TCRs to bone marrow progenitors resulted in induction of respective TCR expressing Tregs preferentially in colon while no specific TCR bearing cells were found in thymus (113). Adoptive transfer of naïve T-cells from the transgenic lines made from colonic TCRs resulted in very efficient conversion to peripherally induced Tregs (pTregs) in mesenteric LNs and colon (114). Other than the specific TCR repertoire, high surface expression of Helios, an Ikaros family transcription factor (115), and Nrp1, a membrane-bound co-receptor for vascular endothelial growth factor and semaphorin (116, 117), has been found to be associated with tTregs. Although the precise origin of Tregs based on these markers is debatable since their expression can be upregulated in inflammatory settings (118, 119), nevertheless, most of the studies have reported enrichment of $Helios^-$ and/or $Nrp1^-$ pTregs in colonic Treg compartment (107, 114). Also, the frequency of colonic $Foxp3^+Helios^-Nrp1^-$ Tregs is significantly reduced in GF mice compared to SPF mice (116). Furthermore, treatment of SPF mice with broad-spectrum antibiotics decreased the Helios⁻ colonic Tregs (111). Molecular studies on *Foxp3* gene locus have identified an enhancer, CNS1, to have a prominent role in pTreg generation in gut-associated lymphoid tissues (46). CNS1 contains a TGFβ-NFAT response element (46) and binding sites for retinoic acid receptor (RAR) and retinoid X receptor heterodimer, receptor for retinoic acid (RA) (120). It has been shown that TGFβ and RA can induce *de novo* generation of pTregs upon antigen activation *via* $CD103^+$ DCs (121, 122) (**Figure 3**). Indeed, CNS1-deficient mice have fewer LP Tregs at weaning (46). However, it was recently reported that CNS1 deficiency in colonic TCR transgenic T-cells only delays the pTreg generation and ultimately T-cells do convert to $Foxp3^+$ Tregs (114).

While pTregs are largely accepted to be the primary source of intestinal Treg population, at least under an experimental setting where generation of extra-thymic Tregs are compromised, thymically generated Tregs can migrate to intestinal LP and proliferate to fill up the niche (**Figure 3**). It has been reported that in a limited TCR model, the TCR repertoire of tTregs and colonic Tregs overlap considerably (123). Another study utilizing K14-Aβb (Keratin 14 transgenic, K14) mice, which have restricted MHCII expression in thymic cortical epithelium and thus, cannot provide peripheral MHCII signals for extra-thymic Treg

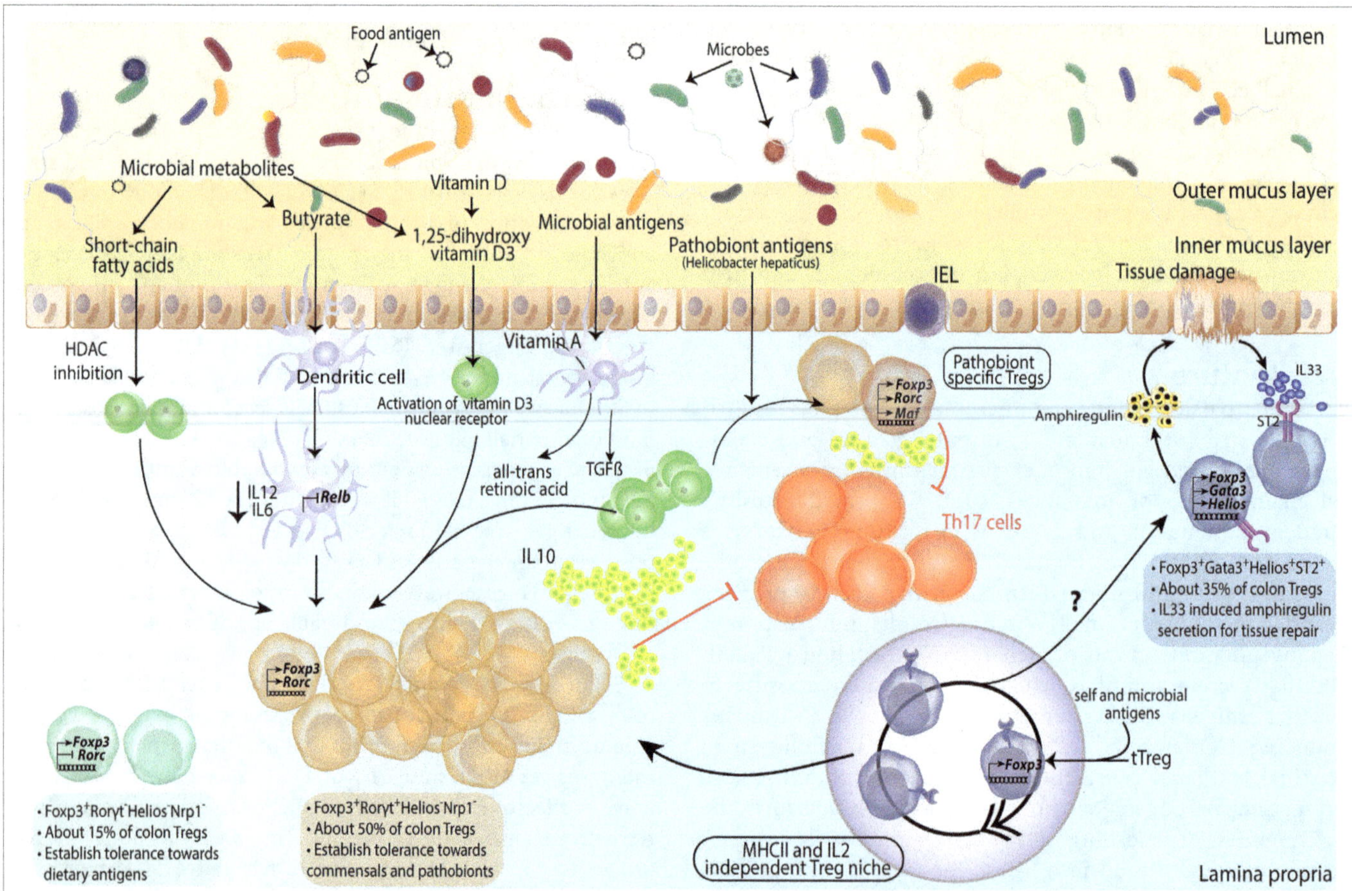

FIGURE 3 | Subtype differentiation of regulatory T-cells (Tregs) in large intestine. Colonic Tregs differentiate into three different subtypes based on RORγt (Rorc) and GATA3 expression along with Foxp3. $Foxp3^+ROR\gamma t^-$ cells comprise ~ 15% of colonic Tregs, their function in colon is not much elucidated but presumably these are responsible for establishing tolerance to dietary antigens. Second and major subset of colonic Tregs is $Foxp3^+ROR\gamma t^+$ Tregs, constituting about 50% of total colonic Tregs. These cells are primarily involved in microbial tolerance and several mechanisms contributing to their generation has been described. From left, short chain fatty acids generated by microbial fermentation can differentiate naive T cells into $Foxp3^+ROR\gamma t^+$ Tregs in lamina propria (LP). Butyrate, specifically, can contribute to Foxp3 expression and function by virtue of its histone deacetylase (HDAC) inhibitory function, as well as can turn dendritic cells (DCs) into Treg generating tolerogenic cells by suppressing their IL12 and IL6 levels and expression of NFκB subunit Relb. Vitamin D metabolite 1,25-dihydroxy vitamin D3 differentiates naive T cells into Tregs by activating its nuclear receptor. TGFβ along with DC generated vitamin A metabolite all-trans retinoic acid differentiates naive T cells into Tregs in presence of microbial antigens. $Foxp3^+ROR\gamma t^+$ Tregs deploy various mechanisms toward establishing dominant tolerance with IL10 production and direct suppression of Th17 cells as prominent ones. A special subset of $Foxp3^+ROR\gamma t^+$ Tregs express cMAF and is instrumental in establishing tolerance to pathobionts in homeostasis. $Foxp3^+ROR\gamma t^+cMaf^+$ Tregs are identified against specific epitopes of *Helicobacter hepaticus* and suppress epitope specific Th17 cells. It has been shown that in absence of pTregs, early seeding of thymic Tregs (tTregs) happens in colonic LP. These tTregs expand into a niche which is independent of MHCII and IL2 signaling but depends on microbial antigens. These Tregs subsequently fill up the LP Treg compartment. However, whether these can differentiate into all Treg subtypes is not known. A third subtype of Tregs express GATA3 (not RORγt) and constitutes about a third of total Tregs. These $Foxp3^+GATA3^+$ Tregs express ST2 receptor which bind to tissue damage-induced alarmin IL33. $Foxp3^+GATA3^+$ Tregs are instrumental in suppressing inflammation and facilitating tissue repair by secretion of amphiregulin upon tissue damage.

generation, showed that while Treg population was significantly decreased in mLNs and spleen, the intestinal Treg compartment was rather intact (124). The LP Treg niche of these mice was found to be inhabited by Tregs of thymic origin at young age. This niche filling phenomenon was not IL2 dependent but was induced by microbial presence, as broad-spectrum antibiotic treatment decreased both large and siLP-Tregs (siTregs) (**Figure 3**). At an older age however; newly generated tTregs were excluded from the LP, presumably due to already occupied Treg niche (124). Taken together, therefore, the available data suggest a peripheral origin of majority of intestinal Tregs and thymic origin of a small subset. However, these mechanisms of origin and development cannot be mutually exclusive and contributions from different pathways are likely to fine tune the ultimate composition of the intestinal Treg compartment.

Tregs Specialize into Multiple Subsets in Intestines

Transcriptomic and functional analyses of intestinal Tregs have largely identified three specialized subsets. Based on transcription factor and surface molecular expression these subsets are GATA3$^+$Helios$^+$(Nrp1$^+$), retinoic acid receptor related orphan receptor γt (RORγt) expressing RORγt$^+$Helios$^-$ and RORγt$^-$ Nrp1$^-$(Helios$^-$) subsets (**Figures 3** and **4A**).

GATA3 is expressed by about a third of intestinal Tregs and can be induced in CD4$^+$Foxp3$^+$ Tregs upon TCR engagement (110). That most of these Tregs are Helios$^+$ and are unaffected by microbial presence suggests their thymic origin (107). However, upon TCR engagement, GATA3 can be induced in CD4$^+$Foxp3$^-$ naïve T-cells as well, in both *in vivo* and Treg polarizing *in vitro* settings (110). While expression of GATA3 is not required under homeostatic conditions, under inflammatory conditions lack of GATA3 in Tregs hampers their accumulation at inflammatory sites (110). GATA3 and Foxp3 interact both at protein and gene levels in Tregs (47). GATA3 binds to *Foxp3* locus and its deletion in Tregs reduces Foxp3 expression (47, 125). It occupies significant number of genes, which are direct targets of Foxp3 and thus, collaborates with Foxp3 to establish Treg gene expression program. Indeed, Treg-specific GATA3 deletion results in intestinal pathology with heightened Th2 cytokine production from large intestinal effector T-cells (47). Most of the GATA3$^+$ Tregs in colon express ST2, which is regulated by GATA3 expression in a feed-forward manner (108). Alarmins like IL33 are produced upon local tissue damage (126, 127) and thus limit self-injury in part by activating GATA3$^+$ST2$^+$ Tregs (108). ST2$^+$ Tregs show enhanced production and activation of IL10 and TGFβ (128). IL23 on the other hand appears to regulate the effect of IL33 in thymus-derived Tregs *via* STAT3 signaling (108).

CD4$^+$Foxp3$^+$RORγt$^+$ Tregs in the intestine are another subset of Tregs specialized toward microbial immunity. These comprise about 50% of total Tregs in colon, which are readily lost in GF mice or upon antibiotic treatment (107, 129) (**Figure 3**). A small population consisting of about 10–15% of Tregs is also found in small intestine (107) (**Figure 4**). Most of the RORγt$^+$ Tregs do not express Helios (107, 129) or Nrp1 (130), suggestive of their

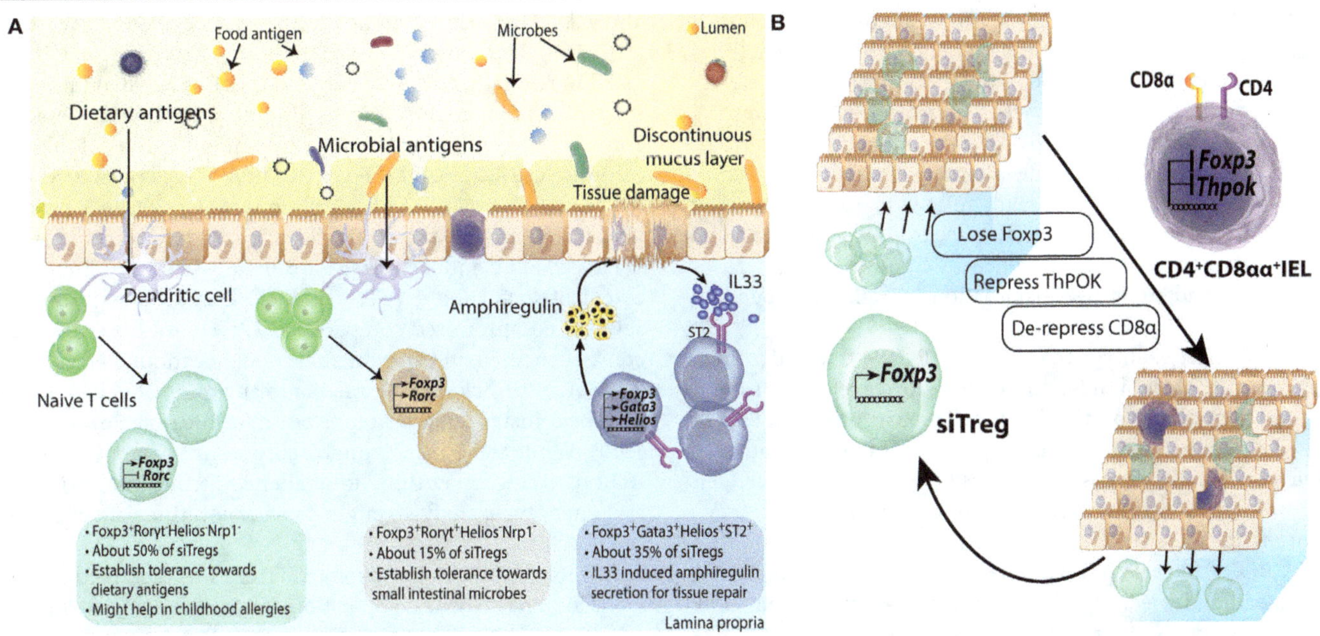

FIGURE 4 | Subtype differentiation of regulatory T-cells (Tregs) in small intestine. **(A)** Small intestine lamina propria (LP) Tregs are differentiated into all three subtypes mentioned in **Figure 3**; however, Foxp3$^+$RORγt$^-$ Tregs are primary population forming about 50% of siTreg compartment. They are primarily generated in response to dietary macromolecules and are proposed to be helpful in containing childhood allergies. Foxp3$^+$RORγt$^+$ and Foxp3$^+$GATA3$^+$ Tregs are about 15% and 35% of total siTregs, respectively. **(B)** Some siTregs continuously traverse in and out of small intestinal epithelial compartment. While most of these Tregs return back to LP, a fraction of these lose their Foxp3 expression and repress ThPOK expression inside epithelial layer. They subsequently, de-repress *CD8a* locus to convert into CD4$^+$CD8αα$^+$ double positive intra epithelial lymphocytes.

extra-thymic origin. However, these cells have substantially reduced CpG methylation within the CNS2 enhancer region of *Foxp3* locus, which is known to be well correlated with stable Foxp3 expression (130, 131). Not all bacteria can elicit similar population of RORγt⁺ Tregs, as it was found that a gradation of Treg inducing capacity exists (107). Mechanistic insights on why certain bacteria have superior capacity of inducing intestinal Tregs than others have started to emerge only recently. It has been reported that short chain fatty acids produced upon fermentation of starch and other dietary fibers by clostridia strains, mainly butyrate and propionate but not acetate, can contribute to colonic Treg generation. Mechanistically, this is attributed to their histone deacetylase inhibitory properties (132) resulting in increased acetylation of *Foxp3* locus (133, 134) (**Figure 3**). Apart from directly acting on T-cells, butyrate also affects DC ability to induce Treg differentiation. Knockdown of *Relb*, which encodes NFκB subunit, has been shown to generate tolerogenic DCs by inhibiting their maturation (135, 136). Indeed, *in vitro* treatment with butyrate represses lipopolysachharide response genes, including *Il12*, *Il6*, and *Relb* in DCs (133) (**Figure 3**). On a translational note, in human IBD patients, colonic butyrate producing bacteria are decreased (137) and mucosal butyrate transporter, monocarboxylate transporter 1, is downregulated (138). It is also possible that colonic Tregs are generated in an antigen-specific manner. Indeed, colonic Treg TCRs have been reported to interact with colonic bacteria *in vitro* (113). Very recently, colonic T cells with TCRs cognate to epitopes of a pathobiont *Helicobacter hepaticus* are shown to induce pTregs under homeostatic conditions (139). This study establishes the role of colonic pTregs in induction and maintenance of tolerance to pathobionts as well. Surprisingly, it was found that although such Tregs are RORγt⁺, their major functional suppressive capabilities are implemented by expression of the transcription factor cMAF (139) (**Figure 3**). cMAF offsets Th17 polarization by producing IL10 downstream to TGFβ1-STAT3 signaling (140). *H. hepaticus* colonized mice with Treg specific *Rorc* deletion had no significant increase in colonic Th17 cells while mice with Treg specific *Maf* deletion had significantly high Th17 cells (139). Thus, RORγt⁺ pTregs in colon establish tolerance to commensals as well as pathobionts and suppress inflammation in a cMAF-dependent manner.

The third Treg subtype (CD4⁺Foxp3⁺RORγt⁻) was identified very recently. Most of these cells express low levels of Nrp1 and thus are, supposedly, pTregs. These cells constitute about 50% of siLP Tregs and 15% of colonic Tregs (109) (**Figures 3** and **4A**). Their localization suggests that these are primarily generated against dietary antigens. Indeed, long-term antibiotic treatment of SPF mice could not reduce their numbers in intestine while RORγt⁺Nrp1^{lo} pTregs were reduced several folds. On the other hand, weaning SPF mice onto AF diet dramatically reduced RORγt⁻Nrp1⁻ pTregs (109). Adoptive transfer of naïve OTII CD4⁺ T-cells in mice on AF diet primarily elicits Th1 cell immune response while Th17 and Th2 responses were comparable to SPF animals. However, pTregs generated in this model were primarily RORγt⁺Nrp1⁻ pTregs, suggesting that dietary antigens can also generate RORγt⁺ pTregs in the absence of microbiota (109).

While TGFβ is by far the most important factor as far as generation and intestinal accumulation of pTregs is concerned (141–143), a generalized modulation of intestinal pTregs can be achieved by several other factors like dietary vitamin A, vitamin D, Niacin (Vitamin B3), Folic acid (Vitamin B9), and tryptophan [reviewed in Ref. (144)]. All-trans retinoic acid, a metabolite of Vitamin A, produced by DCs facilitates *de novo* generation of Foxp3⁺ Tregs from naive CD4⁺CD25⁻ T-cell populations in mice (121, 145) (**Figure 3**). It also plays an important role in upregulating gut-homing markers CCR9 and CD103 (integrin αE) on pTregs (146). Feeding mice with Vitamin A-deficient diet or treatment with RAR inhibitors reduces the RORγt⁺ pTregs in colon while GATA3⁺ Tregs are not affected (129). Similarly, RORγt⁻ pTregs in small intestine are also not affected by vitamin A or RA (109). Vitamin D metabolite 1, 25-dihyroxyvitamin D3 binds to Vitamin D3 nuclear receptor in CD4⁺ T-cells and promotes *Foxp3* expression (147) (**Figure 3**). Recently, it was shown that in human patients of ulcerative colitis a Vitamin D3 agonist can convert CD4⁺ T-cells to pTregs (148).

Functions of Intestinal Tregs

Foxp3⁺GATA3⁺ intestinal Tregs express high level of ST2 (108). These Tregs express high levels of tissue repair factor, an EGF like growth factor Amphiregulin (108, 149) (**Figures 3** and **4A**). It appears that Amphiregulin mediated tissue repair might be a generalized mechanism employed by tissue-resident Tregs as exemplified by its evolving role in lung resident as well as intratumoral Tregs (150, 151). Foxp3⁺RORγt⁺ Tregs express increased levels of ICOS, CTLA4, and the nucleotidases CD39 and CD73 altogether, indicating robust regulatory functions (107, 129). Interestingly, Foxp3⁺RORγt⁺ Tregs have been implicated in regulating both Th2 and Th1/Th17 mediated immunity in two independent studies, implicating animal housing conditions as an important determinant of the type of immune response (107, 129). siLP Foxp3⁺RORγt⁻ Tregs primarily work toward containment of Th1 immunity. When OTII T-cells are transferred in AF mice, T-cells primarily convert to IFNγ⁺ OTII cells and induced Tregs are mainly Tbet⁺, although the extent of such RORγt⁻ pTreg induction in AF conditions was severely compromised compared to SPF conditions (109). As a consequence, in an experimental model of food allergy, where SPF BALB/c mice were weaned onto an amino acid diet, higher diarrheal instances were reported than mice on normal chow (109). While these results underscore an important function of RORγt⁻ pTregs in curbing food allergy, further transcriptomic and phenotypic analyses might provide additional clues to their functions.

Of note, one more function of siTregs was identified recently while looking at the IEL population. It was observed that LP Tregs migrate to epithelial compartment as well, where a fraction of them lose Foxp3 expression (152). Further, these Tregs then give up ThPOK expression leading to de-repression of *Cd8* locus and thus, get converted into a CD4⁺CD8αα⁺ IELs (152) (**Figure 4B**). IELs have cytotoxic as well as immunoregulatory machinery suggesting a role in both mucosal barrier maintenance and elimination of stressed intestinal epithelial cells (153).

SKIN Tregs: KEEPS YOUR HAIR ON

Skin is the largest organ amounting to almost 15% of adult human body weight. Being our exterior, it is always exposed to environmental, microbial, physical, and chemical insults. Skin also harbors more than 10^{12} bacteria/m^2 (154) in the surface intercorneocytic spaces.

Skin Architecture

Anatomically, skin is composed of three layers, the outer epidermis, middle dermis, and inner subcutaneous tissue layer (155). The terminally differentiated keratinocytes in epidermis synthesize long, thread-like protective protein keratin and form a physical barrier. Products of various sweat and sebaceous glands interspersed at epidermal–dermal junction along with antimicrobial peptides develop an acidic hydrophilic skin which acts as a biochemical barrier (154). The epidermal–dermal junction also hosts hair follicles. Cellular component of epidermis comprises of Langerhans cells (specialized skin DCs) and T lymphocytes. The dermis is composed of layers of thick and thin collagen fibers which provide mechanical framework to host blood vessels and various immune cells like dermal DCs, αβ and γδ T-cells, NK cells, B cells, macrophages, and mast cells (154). Understandably, given the exposed nature of skin, it is highly vulnerable to overzealous immune responses against skin commensals and self-antigens. Tregs are an important component of establishing tolerance and homeostasis in the skin. Indeed, both scurfy mouse and human IPEX patients present fulminating immune responses in skin. A study, examining children with IPEX syndrome reported that more than 70% children presented Atopic Dermatitis and eczema with 1.5 months as median age of onset of symptoms (156).

Skin Treg Origin and Accumulation

Normally, 30–50% and 20–30% of total CD4$^+$ T-cells are Tregs in mouse and human skin, respectively (157, 158). It is difficult to establish the origin of cutaneous Tregs, given the paucity of specific information. However, a wave of Tregs has been shown to populate the skin in early neonatal period in a skin bacterial colonization model in mice (159). Furthermore, restricting lymphoid emigration of T-cells by treating with sphingosine-1-phosphate receptor antagonist FTY720 resulted in preferential accumulation of Tregs in thymus instead of skin draining LNs, suggesting their migration directly from thymus (159). In humans, the cutaneous Tregs and Tconv cells share very few TCRβ sequences and these Tregs present a fully demethylated *FOXP3* CNS2 region, suggestive of their stability and thymic origin (157, 160, 161). This is little surprising as skin Tregs establish tolerance to not only self-antigens but also to commensals. How are then commensal antigen-specific Tregs generated in thymus? One possibility appears to be plasmacytoid DCs (pDCs) that have been shown to be able to take up innocuous peripheral antigens to thymus (162) and LNs (163) to induce tolerance. Generally, pDCs are not present in skin but can accumulate in the presence of inflammatory conditions (164, 165). Another probability is that some tTregs have TCRs with sufficient cross-reactivity to microbial antigens and thus can specifically expand and accumulate at sites where antigen is present. However, if indeed skin Tregs are thymic by origin, the concerning mechanisms remain to be elucidated.

Modeling of inducible expression of a self-antigen, by fusing transferrin receptor transmembrane domain, GFP and amino acids 230–359 of chicken ovalbumin in mouse epidermis, revealed that circulating Tregs are not able to suppress primary immune response against OVA, though it initiated activation of Tregs (166). The inflammation resolved spontaneously and any subsequent antigen expression led to an attenuated and short immune response. Further analysis revealed that a fraction of Tregs persisted in the skin which expressed low level of CD25 but higher KLRG1, CTLA4, and CD127, akin to the memory T-cells (166). It is to be noted here that a recent study examining the transcriptional, epigenomic, and functional changes in inflammation experienced Tregs employing the Foxp3^{DTR} system, presented that Tregs revert most of the activation induced changes and lose the accentuated suppressive ability over time (167). An earlier report revealed that cutaneous Tregs express CCR4 and adhesion molecule Integrin αE, CD103 (168). In a mixed bone marrow chimera study, CCR4-deficient Tregs could not reconstitute the skin Treg compartment (168). CCL17 and CCL22 are known chemokine ligands for CCR4 (169, 170), which are differentially expressed in inflamed skin mainly by endothelial cells and dermal DCs, respectively (171). These molecules sequentially manage T-cell homing to skin, where CCL17 promotes vascular recognition and extravasation and CCL22 guides subsequent migration in skin (172). More than 70% skin Tregs express GATA3, although its deletion in Tregs does not alter Treg profile or cause overt skin related phenotype under homeostatic conditions (110).

Since skin is heavily exposed to commensals as well as pathogens, it is imperative to speculate that a fine tuning of effector and suppressive immune responses has evolved. The commensal microbiota residing within skin has been shown to calibrate barrier immunity (173, 174). To identify mechanisms behind development of tolerance to skin commensals, Scharschmidt et al. performed some elegant experiments with model peptide antigen expressing *Staphylococcous epidermidis*, a human skin commensal which efficiently colonizes mouse skin (159). Surprisingly, skin colonization in adult mice did not evoke any tolerance to bacteria, as seen by inflammatory response upon re-challenge. However, when neonatal mice were colonized for a week during postnatal week 2, there was an appreciable attenuation of inflammatory response upon re-challenge after 3–4 weeks. Subdued response was associated with marked enrichment of antigen-specific Tregs in skin and draining LNs and the tolerance could be reversed upon FTY720 treatment (159). Another study has also shown that Tregs, generated very early in life in a defined perinatal window, play a very distinct role in maintaining self-tolerance (175). Thus, in mice, an abrupt wave of Treg infiltration occurs in a defined early postnatal period to establish dominant tolerance toward skin commensals (159) (**Figure 5**).

Both Tregs and skin commensals are localized to hair follicles and in mouse, the time of Treg infiltration (week 2 postnatal) is coincident with hair follicle development (176, 177). Thus, it was speculated that hair follicles might have a role in ingress of

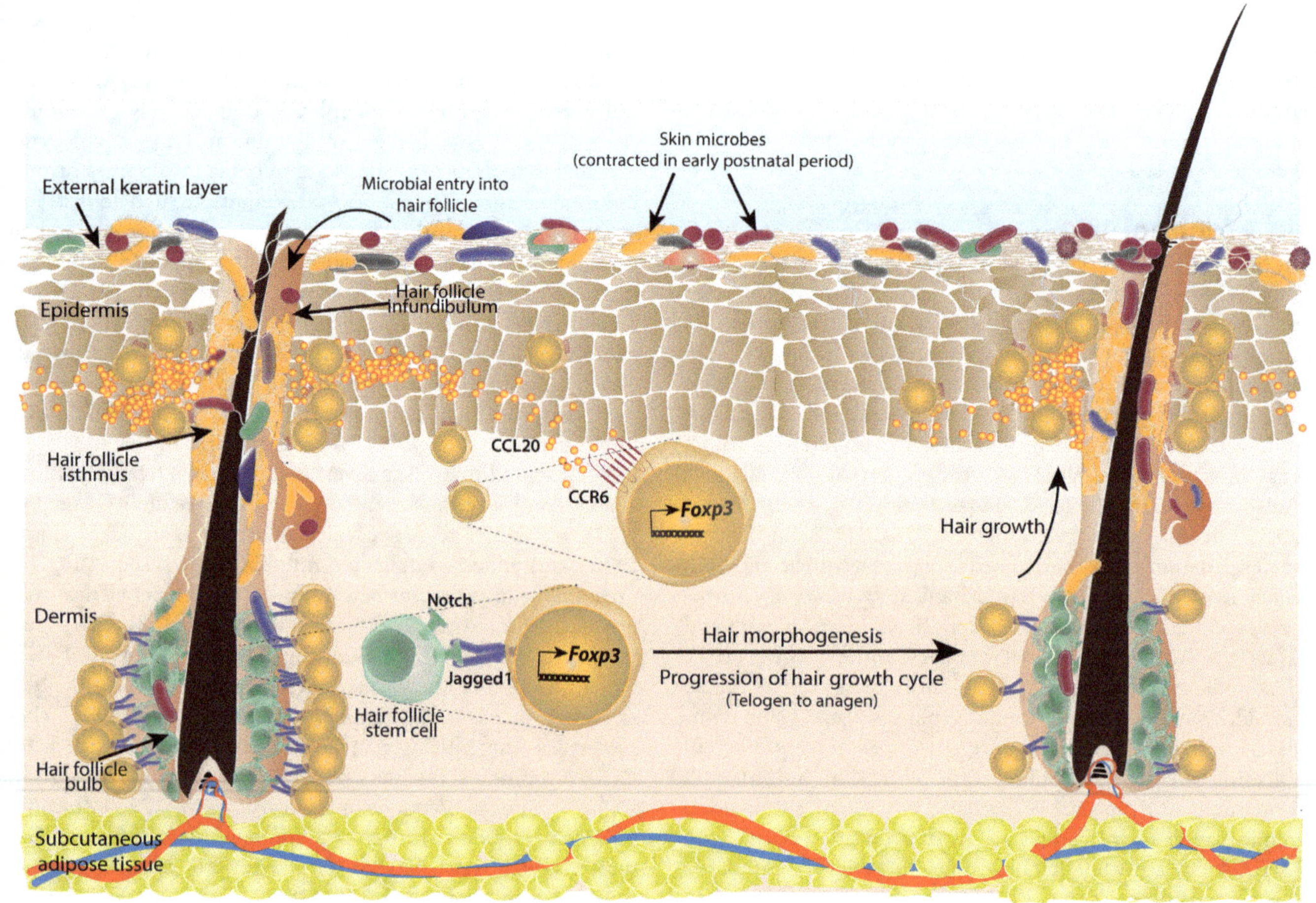

FIGURE 5 | Cutaneous regulatory T-cells (Tregs) facilitate hair morphogenesis and establish tolerance to skin commensals. Skin Tregs colonize mouse skin in early postnatal period coinciding with initial microbial colonization and hair follicle development. Skin microbes enter the hair follicle which induces production of chemokine CCL20 from infundibular cells that attracts large number of Tregs expressing corresponding receptor CCR6. The accumulated Tregs subsequently establish tolerance to these commensals. Also, during the resting phase of hair growth (telogen) which initially coincides with commensal entry in hair follicle, large number of Tregs are seen in contact with hair follicle stem cells (HFSCs) in the bulb of follicle. These Tregs provide notch ligand Jagged1 to the stem cells. Notch signaling triggers the active phase of hair growth cycle (anagen). Tregs are reduced in anagen phase around HFSCs.

Tregs in skin. It has been shown that chemokines from different parts of hair follicles like CCL2 from isthmus, CCL20 from infundibulum, and CCL8 from bulge keratinocytes generate specific type of Langerhans cells (178). Similarly, in a mouse model of skin specific hair follicle morphogenesis arrest, skin Treg population was reduced without affecting Treg population in intestine or draining LNs in neonatal mice (179). Further investigations revealed that neonatal SPF mouse skin produces high amount of chemokine CCL20 whose receptor CCR6 was found to be enriched on cutaneous Tregs (**Figure 5**). It was confirmed by adoptive transfer experiments that CCR6-deficient Tregs were at a competitive disadvantage to reconstitute skin T-cell compartment (179). Tregs in neonates also express high CCR8 and its ligand CCL22 is, in turn, expressed in skin. However, their contribution in establishing and/or maintenance of skin Tregs is yet to be examined. CCL20 mRNA expression also increases in human fetal skin explants upon exposure to cutaneous commensals and bacterial components (179). Thus, tissue morphogenesis (hair follicle generation and subsequent chemokine production by the cells of hair follicle) and commensals are shown to cooperate in developing a tissue-specific immune tolerance. It would be interesting to extrapolate this model to other microbe inhabited organ systems. Whether, these mechanisms sustain throughout the life span particularly in adult life is not known. Earlier, 8- to 12-week-old GF mice were reported to have about twofold more cutaneous Tregs than SPF animals (180). It is possible that yet unknown factors other than commensals increase Treg population in adult GF skin or a lack of tuned immune response against commensals diverts immune resources toward self-antigens and in turn, progressively enrich self-antigen-specific Tregs in skin.

Short wavelength Ultraviolet (UVB) exposure also enriches and accumulates Tregs in mouse skin (181). UVB exposure damages self-RNA in keratinocytes which is sensed by TLR3 to generate an inflammatory response (182). Indeed, the Tregs accumulating post-UVB exposure were Nrp1^{+} with highly demethylated *Foxp3* CNS2 (181). These Tregs highly expressed homing molecules like CD103, CCR4, and P-lig and thus, were able to migrate to the non-UVB exposed parts of the skin as well (181) (**Figure 6**). Interestingly, UVB phototherapy is an effective treatment in autoimmune skin conditions, like psoriasis (183) and atopic dermatitis (184).

Tissue Adaptations and Homeostatic Functions

True to the nature of tissue-resident Tregs where they have been shown to not only develop immune tolerance but also get accustomed to and help local physiology, cutaneous Tregs in hair follicles have been found to modulate hair follicle stem cells (HFSCs) in addition to establishing tolerance to commensals. In mouse skin, an abundance of Tregs was found during telogen phase of hair follicle growth which is characterized by quiescence only to be followed by an active proliferation phase called anagen. Treg population decreases during anagen phase. And as these phases alternate in mouse skin so are the numbers of hair follicle associated Tregs (158) (**Figure 5**). Animals with transient depletion of Tregs during telogen, failed to progress to anagen phase and could not re-grow hairs (158). It was not inflammation related, as transient depletion of Tregs did not elicit any major inflammatory event in skin and co-depletion of either effector CD4⁺, CD8⁺, Gr-1 expressing neutrophils or CD11C⁺ myeloid cells did not rescue HFSC proliferation (158). This suggested a non-immune role of Tregs in HFSC proliferation. Akin to Tregs in hematopoietic system which form an immune-privileged site to provide a protective niche to hematopoietic stem cells (185), hair follicle Tregs were found to co-localize with HFSCs. These Tregs highly express *"jagged1"* which encodes a ligand for notch signaling pathway responsible for HFSC proliferation (158) (**Figure 5**).

Regulatory T-cells play an important role in cutaneous wound healing as well. They accumulate in large numbers at the site soon after a wound injury in skin (186). These Tregs are of activated

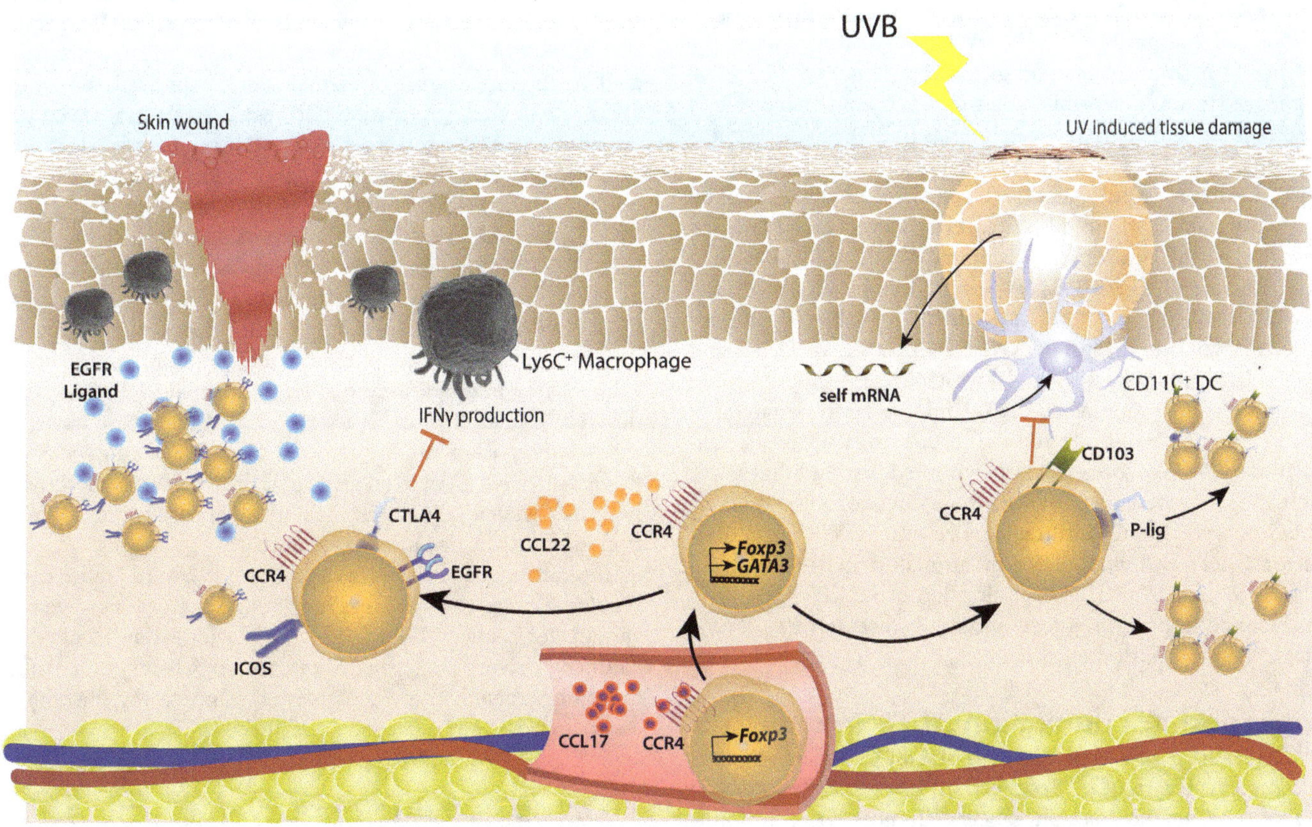

FIGURE 6 | Cutaneous regulatory T-cells (Tregs) actively repair skin tissue damage. Tregs migrate to skin by virtue of sequential interactions of chemokines CCL17 and CCL22 with their receptor CCR4. CCL17 is secreted by endothelial cells in inflamed skin and helps in extravasation of Tregs, CCL22 manages subsequent migration of Tregs. In case of skin wound-induced inflammation, Tregs acquire a highly activated phenotype with higher surface expression of CTLA4 and ICOS. These Tregs actively suppress IFNγ production from inflammatory Ly6C⁺ macrophages. Also, Tregs express high amount of EGFR, helping in their tissue repair ability. In case of short wave UVB light induced skin damage, self mRNA from keratinocytes are taken up by CD103⁺ dendritic cells (DCs) which induce the cutaneous inflammation. These DCs are suppressed by Tregs which have high surface expression of CD103 and P-lig and thus can migrate into non-inflamed skin as well, subsequent to UV exposure.

phenotype with high CD25, CTLA4, and ICOS expression and limit the IFNγ producing T-cells and inflammatory macrophages in wounds (186). The Tregs involved in cutaneous wound healing were shown to be dependent on EGFR pathway (186) as in lung and muscle-healing Tregs (150, 187, 188) (**Figure 6**).

TUMOR-INFILTRATING REGULATORY T-CELLS (TI-Tregs): A BATTLE WON, WAR LOST

Tumors are wounds that do not heal (189–191). Solid tumors, in particular, heterogeneously indulge in various stages of wound healing, which provide essential growth factors for the tumor growth. This hijack of natural processes results in heightened inflammation and its subsequent resolution in the tumor microenvironment, presumably setting up a vicious cycle. Inflammation on one hand provides growth and metastasis opportunities; resolution of inflammation helps the tumor to escape antitumor immunity. Therefore, it is not surprising that many solid tumors including hepatocellular (192), gastric (193), lung (194), breast (195), ovarian (196), cervical (197), and melanomas (198) summon comparatively large numbers of Tregs which sometimes account for even more than 50% of CD4$^+$ T-cell compartment (199). For most of the tumors, the presence of high number of Tregs indicates a guarded to grave prognosis. However, several studies reported a favorable role of FOXP3$^+$ T-cells in colorectal carcinomas (CRC) (200–202). It is to be noted that FOXP3 expression is not exclusive to *bona fide* Tregs in humans, often, effector T-cells express FOXP3, albeit transiently (203, 204). Based on expression levels of FOXP3 and Protein tyrosine phosphatase isoform A (CD45RA), human peripheral blood FOXP3$^+$CD4$^+$ T-cells can be classified into FOXP3^{hi}CD45RA$^-$ *bona fide* Tregs which are highly suppressive and phenotypically eTregs; FOXP3^{lo}CD45RA$^+$ naïve T-cells and FOXP3^{lo}CD45RA$^-$ effector T-cells which are not suppressive in an *in vitro* suppression assay (203). Indeed, careful analysis of TILs in human CRC by Saito et al. (205) revealed the heterogeneity of FOXP3 expression. The authors identified that CRC, where higher expression of FOXP3 was associated with favorable outcomes, were actually infiltrated more with FOXP3^{lo}CD45RA$^+$ effector T-cells and upregulated inflammatory genes like *Il12a*, *Il12b*, *Tgfb1*, and *Tnf*. Higher infiltration of FOXP3^{hi}CD45RA$^-$ cells resulted in poor prognosis and lower disease-free survival (205) as reported for other tumors.

Origin and Accumulation of TI-Tregs

As tTregs and pTregs differ in their stability, conclusive information about origin of TI-Tregs can be very valuable to design TI-Treg specific therapies in cancers. Tumors drive immune responses against tumor-associated self-antigens as well as tumor-specific neo-self antigens. Thus, in theory, Tregs against self-antigens (tTregs) and pTregs against neo-self antigens are possible. Presence of high levels of TGFβ in most solid tumors reinforces the idea of generation of pTregs in tumor microenvironments (206, 207). However, TI-Tregs in several murine tumors have been shown to express high levels of Nrp1 and Helios proteins, suggestive of a thymic origin (208). Attempts for *in situ* conversion of conventional CD4$^+$ T-cells to Tregs against tumors expressing model antigens did result in intratumoral pTregs generation (209, 210), but monoclonal populations of antigen-specific T-cells do not recapitulate physiological conditions where antigen-specific T-cells represent less than 5% of TILs (211–213). TCR repertoire analyses have revealed almost no overlap in Foxp3$^+$ and Foxp3$^-$ T-cells in autochthonous prostate tumors (214), carcinogen-induced tumors (215), and in heterotopic transplanted tumors in mice (216). Further, these studies confirmed that there is enrichment and expansion of selective TCR bearing Tregs inside tumor microenvironment (214, 216). In human breast cancers (217) and hepatitis B virus positive hepatocellular carcinomas (HCC) (192), very low TCR repertoire overlap between TI-Tregs and conventional T-cells suggests little to no conversion of conventional CD4$^+$ T-cells into Tregs (**Figure 7A**). Malchow et al. (214) developed a transgenic mouse expressing the model oncogene SV40 T antigen in prostate and a fixed TCRβ chain (TRAMP-Foxp3^{eGFP}TCRβ^{Tg}). They found that Tregs expressing a single TCR (MJ23), reactive to a normally expressed prostate antigen, consistently populated the tumors (214). This TCR was able to drive a tTreg clone development. However, a deficiency of the transcription factor autoimmune regulator abolished development of these clones (214), suggesting that at least in these experimental settings, TI-Tregs are generated in thymus against a normal tissue expressed self-antigen (**Figure 7A**). Recently, two MHCII restricted natural self-antigen ligands of MJ23 Tregs were discovered. Both of these ligands are non-overlapping peptides originating from same prostatic protein (Tcaf3) and while one is expressed in mouse prostate tumors (MJ23), the other is associated with prostatic autoimmune lesions (SP33) (218). Another study focusing on epigenetic hallmarks of tTregs found that TI-Tregs had consistently hypomethylated *Foxp3* CNS2 in various orthotopic and heterotopic transplanted tumor models, even at different time points of tumor growth (219). These findings were further confirmed in TI-Tregs from different human tumors. It is to be noted that there have been equivocal reports about the demethylated CNS2 being specific for tTregs, since *Foxp3* CNS2 region in pTregs has also been shown to be demethylated (220, 221), most likely upon eventual stabilization following its *de novo* induction.

Overall, available evidences largely point toward higher enrichment and expansion of tTregs inside solid tumors. However, why should not higher TGFβ levels and an activating tumor environment drive pTreg generation and expansion is a baffling question. Probably more conclusive lineage tracing experiments across tumors can be proven more insightful.

TI-Tregs Add Another Layer of Diversification

Recent studies analyzing transcriptome of TI-Tregs from human cancers have identified that though TI-Tregs are largely similar to normal tissue-resident Tregs, these have some specific characteristics and molecular patterns which can be utilized for selective therapy (192, 217, 222). Plitas et al. (217) found that breast cancers, with rather aggressive phenotype, were enriched

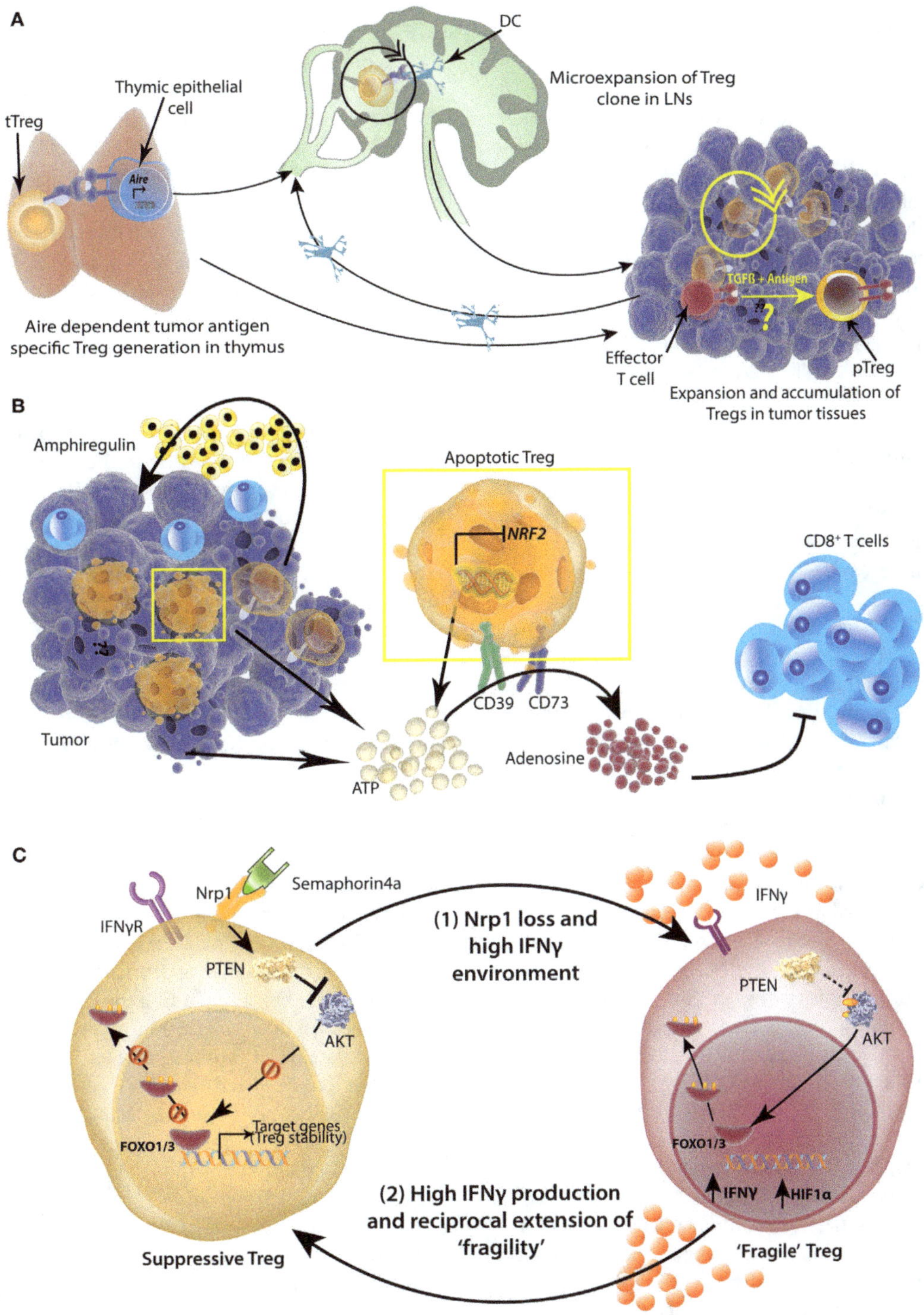

FIGURE 7 | Origin, accumulation, and functional potentiation of tumor-infiltrating regulatory T-cells (Tregs). **(A)** Tumor-specific antigens can be expressed by thymic epithelial cells in an *Aire*-dependent manner, which then select the tumor antigen-specific Tregs. These Tregs then expand in tumor draining lymph nodes (LNs) with the help of dendritic cells (DCs). Tregs can also be directly recruited to tumors and undergo expansion there. While intratumoral conversion of effector T-cells to pTregs is likely, the extent to which this occurs under physiological conditions is not completely understood. **(B)** A high number of TI-Tregs are apoptotic because of suppressed expression of *Nrf2*. These Tregs as well as dying tumor cells release copious amounts of ATP, which is converted to adenosine by Treg ectoenzymes CD39 and CD73 in a sequential manner. The resulting adenosine is highly suppressive to tumor-infiltrating CD8⁺ effector T-cells. Further, Tregs also produce Amphiregulin in certain tumor types, which help in tumor progression. **(C)** More than 50% of TI-Tregs express surface Neuropilin1 (Nrp1), which is a receptor for Semaphorin 4a. Upon ligation with Semaphorin4a, Nrp1 activates lipid phosphatase Phosphatase and tensin homolog (PTEN) which promptly dephosphorylates AKT rendering its sequestration in cytosol and nuclear retention of Foxo1/3 transcription factors which help in stabilization and survival of Tregs. A loss of Nrp1 renders Treg highly susceptible to IFNγ and such Tregs also produce high amount of IFNγ and HIF1α ("Fragile" Tregs). The resultant high IFNγ environment, reciprocally, can induce "fragility" in other Nrp1-sufficient Tregs as well, setting up a vicious cycle.

for Tregs, which were highly suppressive in a microsuppression assay and were highly proliferative based on increased expression of nuclear protein Ki67, a cellular marker for proliferation (223). Further transcriptome analysis of TI-Tregs from breast cancers and gastric cancers as well as brain metastases of NSCLC and liver metastasis of CRC, suggested a signature gene set for these cells (222). TI-Tregs expressed BATF, CCR8, CD30, IL1R2, IL21R, PDL1, and PDL2 along with FOXP3 and IL2Ra at a very high level (222). Recently, BATF was shown to be involved in context dependent gene set expression in tissue Tregs (224). In the IPEX patients, a gain-of-function mutation in FOXP3 locus (A384T) results in expanded DNA binding specificities of FOXP3. Its altered binding to *BATF* locus repressed BATF expression leading to repressed GATA3, ST2, and CCR4 expression in Tregs (224). These genes are significant in converting cTregs to eTregs, therefore, their decreased expression led to a widespread tissue-specific autoimmunity (224).

Genome-wide transcriptome analyses identified *MAGEH1*, Melanoma antigen family H1 gene, encoding a putative E3 ubiquitin ligase potentially regulating TI-Treg survival and function; Chemokine (C-C motif) receptor 8 (CCR8), known receptor for chemokines CCL1 (225), CCL8 (226), CCL16 (227), and CCL18 (228) in humans; CD177, a glycosyl-phosphatidylinositol-linked cell surface glycoprotein that can bind platelet endothelial cell adhesion molecule-1 and is known for neutrophil transmigration and survival (229); and *LAYN*, encoding a novel c-type lectin surface receptor layilin, a proposed receptor for Hyaluronan (230). However, subsequently, layilin has been found highly expressed on tumor-infiltrating cytotoxic $CD8^+$ T-cells as well, particularly those with an exhaustive (highly expressing *CTLA4*, *PDCD1*, and *HAVCR2*) phenotype (192). Enrichment of *LAYN*, *MAGEH1*, and *CCR8* in whole tumor samples correlated significantly with reduced 5-year survival rate of CRC and NSCLC patients (222). CCR8 expression was exclusively enriched on TI-Tregs, whereas CCR2, CCR4, and CCR5 expressions were found on other tumor-infiltrating and/or peripheral blood Tconv cells as well. Indeed, a CCR4 depleting antibody has been shown to deplete both Tregs and Tconv cells (231). Some Tregs in draining LNs also expressed high CCR8 which might be ones earmarked for tumor infiltration or Tregs in micrometastases inside LNs (217). As peripheral blood and/or LN Tregs do not express CCR8, its importance in recruitment of Tregs to tumors is not appreciated. It is possible that CCR8 is expressed to retain Tregs in tumors. Indeed, CCR8 ligands like CCL1 and CCL18 are highly transcribed in tumor-infiltrating myeloid cells (217). Whether, CCR8 expression is an indicator of highly suppressive TI-Tregs or it has further functional importance is not yet known. However, human Tregs exposed to CCR8 ligand CCL1 and not CCL8, CCL16, or CCL18 induce surface CCR8 expression *via* a STAT3-mediated pathway (232). Such cells, subsequently, upregulate their expression of FOXP3, CD39, Granzyme B, and IL10 and are functionally more suppressive in a microsuppression assay and in a mouse model of multiple sclerosis (232).

Function of TI-Tregs

There is a repertoire of known and yet unknown mechanisms which Tregs utilize to suppress an immune response. TI-Tregs also use similar mechanisms which include production of immunosuppressive cytokines like IL10 and TGFβ (233, 234); sequestration of IL2 (235); direct cytolysis of target lymphocytes using granzyme B and perforin (236); contact based immunosuppression using surface inhibitory molecules like CTLA4 (237), PD1 (238, 239), LAG3 (240), TIM3 (241), and CD39/CD73-generated adenosine-mediated T-cell suppression *via* adenosine receptor 2A (242, 243). However, how the TI-Tregs have highly accentuated suppressive response is not very well understood. A large accumulation of Tregs might help in a collective exaggerated suppression, but it cannot explain individual potentiation. Recently, it was shown that TI-Tregs are highly apoptotic on account of comparatively low expression of the transcription factor Nuclear factor like 2 (NRF2) (244). NRF2 regulates antioxidant defense system in macrophages and epithelial cells (245). A lack of NRF2 makes TI-Tregs more apoptotic in high oxidative stress tumor microenvironment. But, owing to increased release of ATP and high CD73/CD39 expression, apoptotic TI-Tregs generate large amount of adenosine and thus, become even more suppressive (244) (**Figure 7B**). It is to be noted though that earlier Imatinib induced apoptosis of TI-Tregs was shown to enhance antitumor immunity (246).

TI-Tregs in human breast cancers (217) and HCC (192) highly express *Il1r2* gene encoding a decoy IL1 receptor. Also, TI-Tregs are found to be highly stable owing to the enhanced expression of lipid phosphatase Phosphatase and tensin homolog (PTEN) and VEGF receptor Nrp1 (199, 238, 247). Binding of Nrp1 to its ligand Semaphorin4a increased Foxo1 and Foxo3 nuclear localization by inhibiting AKT phosphorylation which stabilized Treg signature genes and antiapoptotic genes (247) (**Figure 7C**). AKT dephosphorylation was achieved by activation of PTEN by Nrp1. Indeed, mice with Treg specific PTEN deletion generate an accentuated antitumor immune response (238). Nrp1 expression is primarily important for TI-Tregs as the loss of Nrp1 even from a fraction of Tregs under appropriate experimental conditions, rendered all the Tregs (including those that were Nrp1 sufficient) "fragile" (199). This observation emphasizes that Tregs can not only modulate other immune cells but can phenotypically influence other Tregs as well. The TI-Treg fragility was shown to be induced by IFNγ production by Nrp1-deficient Tregs and exogenous IFNγ (199) (**Figure 7C**). The authors further show that HIF1α was a major factor induced in Nrp1-deficient and fragile Tregs, and both HIF1α and IFNγ can be induced by hypoxia (199). However, as most of the solid tumors become progressively hypoxic (248, 249), whether this phenomenon is prevalent in progressive tumors and if so, whether it is efficient for a significant regeneration of antitumor immune response, remains to be seen. TI-Tregs have been shown to highly express receptor activator of nuclear factor κB ligand (RANKL), which upon binding to its receptor RANK expressed in mammary carcinoma cells increases lung metastasis (250). RANKL has also been implicated in renewal of breast cancer progenitor cells (251) and metastasis of prostate cancers (252) by modulating protein kinase inhibitor of nuclear factor κB kinase α (IKKα). Overall, these findings suggest that there is a specific phenotypic and functional identity to TI-Tregs and thus, it is possible to selectively target them for triggering efficient antitumor immunity.

OTHER Tregs IN TISSUE INFLAMMATION AND HOMEOSTASIS

As the diversity in characteristics and functions of tissue Tregs is being unraveled, several other interesting populations have been described which deserve more detailed phenotypic and functional characterization.

Regeneration Powerhouse

It was reported earlier that in a non-inflammatory model of regenerative alveologenesis, Tregs enhanced epithelial proliferation. A Treg coculture with type II alveolar cells (AT2) increased their proliferation in CD103-dependent manner (253). In accordance to these findings, a distinct population of Tregs expressing high levels of pro-inflammatory cytokine IL18 receptor (IL18R) and ST2 has been described in lungs (150). IL18R$^+$ Tregs expand early in the course of a lung injury and enhance tissue repair by producing a large amounts of tissue repair protein amphiregulin in an "innate" manner, independent of TCR engagement (150) (**Figure 8A**). In animals with Treg specific amphiregulin deficiency, a rapid decline in lung functions was observed upon intranasal influenza virus infection, while antiviral immune

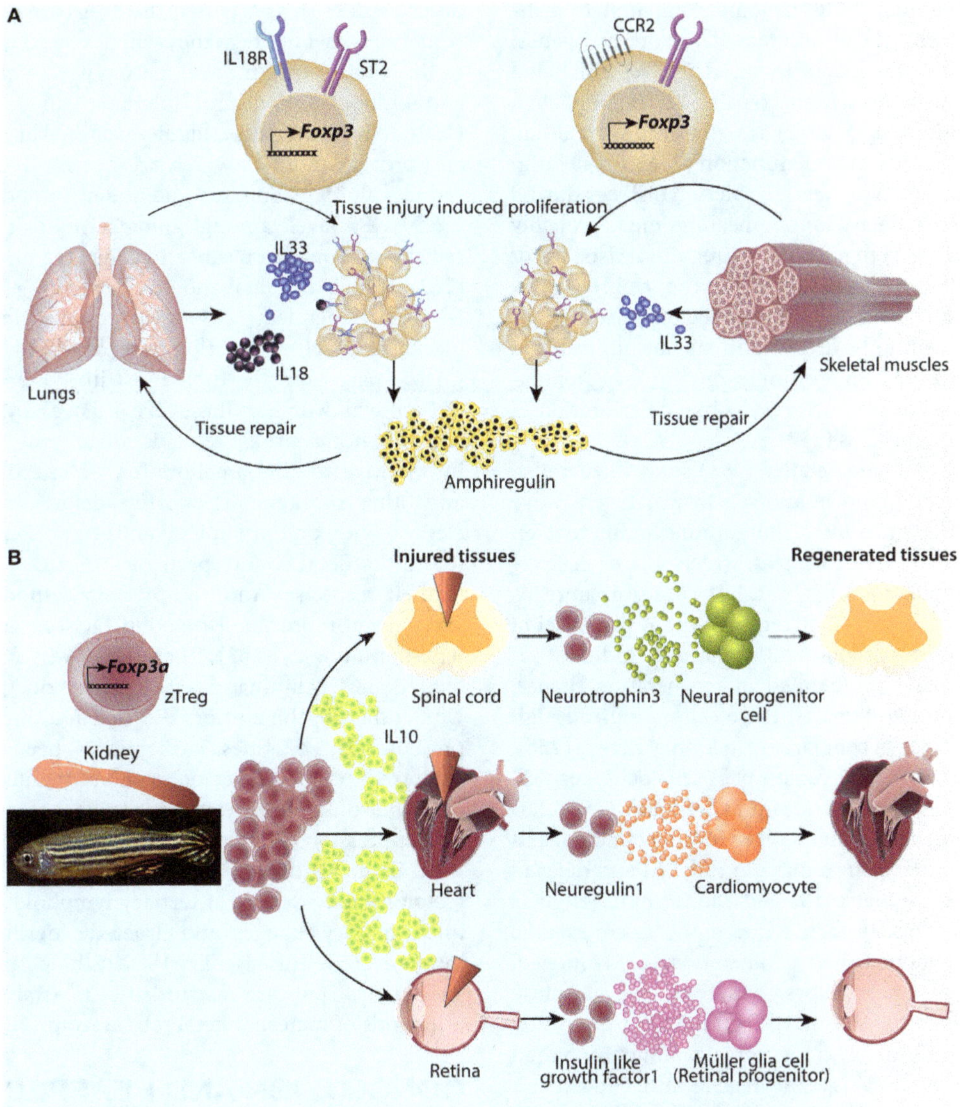

FIGURE 8 | Emerging evidences highlight a compulsory requirement of regulatory T-cells (Tregs) in tissue regeneration and repair. **(A)** Both lungs and muscles contain population of Tregs which proliferate vigorously upon tissue injury. Lung reparative Tregs respond to both inflammatory IL18 and alarmin IL33 and produce amphiregulin in a TCR-independent manner. Muscle Tregs respond to IL33 produced upon muscle damage and produce amphiregulin for subsequent repair. **(B)** In zebrafish, mammalian *Foxp3* ortholog *Foxp3a* expressing Tregs (zTregs) are primarily present in kidney. However, upon tissue injury, they soon accumulate at the site of the injury. Apart from anti-inflammatory IL10 production, zTregs co-localize with organ progenitor cells and provide tissue-specific growth factors to progenitors like neurotrophin3 for neural progenitors in spinal cord, neuregulin1 for cardiomyocytes in heart, and insulin-like growth factor1 to Müller glial cells in retina.

response was intact (150). Transcriptomic analysis revealed that these "repair Tregs" have a distinct gene expression pattern indicating their proficiency in extracellular matrix remodeling and tissue repair (150).

Another unique tissue Treg population has been found in skeletal muscles, where by virtue of amphiregulin secretion, they help in muscle regeneration and healing. These cells, usually accounting for 10% of muscle T-cells at a steady state, proliferate vigorously after an intramuscular administration of cardiotoxin, which induces hypercontraction and myofibril death induced acute injury (254), reaching close to 50% of muscle T-cell population (188). High expression of Nrp1 and Helios and a unique and restricted TCR repertoire suggests thymic origin of muscle Tregs and reactivity to a local muscle antigen (188). These Tregs have a unique transcriptome compared to lymphoid organ Tregs with several differentially expressed genes. They have upregulated transcripts involved in Treg mediated suppression (*Il10, Gzmb*, etc.), tissue repair (*Il1rl1, Areg*, etc.), and muscle regeneration (255) (*Ccr2*) as well as genes encoding proteins found in contractile muscle function (256) like nebulin and nebulin-like proteins (*Neb, Nebl*). Depletion of Tregs during a muscle injury episode delays muscle healing, most probably because of loss of Treg generated amphiregulin. Also, fibro/adipogenic progenitors in skeletal muscles produce high levels of IL33, whose receptor ST2 is highly expressed on muscle Tregs. Thus, muscle Tregs seem to be involved in an alarmin induced repair process (**Figure 8A**). Interestingly, muscle Treg population declines in old age mice which results in a deterioration of repair and regeneration process (257).

Recently, a very elegant and detailed (258) study in zebrafish has elaborated upon yet unknown and spectacular regenerative capabilities of Tregs (**Figure 8B**). The authors found that an ortholog of mammalian *Foxp3, Foxp3a*, which was exclusively expressed in a subpopulation of zebrafish T-cells, was upregulated most prominently in distinct regenerating organs. Zebra fish Tregs (zTregs) were predominantly found in kidneys but infiltrated and vigorously proliferated in regenerating tissues. As in the mammalian counterparts, these cells expressed high levels of *Nrp1a* and *Helios* in comparison to kidney zTregs (258). It has been reported that CNS1 region of *Foxp3* locus, responsible for pTreg generation, is not found in zebrafish (259). For identification of zTreg's role in organ regeneration, punctual and continuous deletion of *Foxp3a* resulted in reduced and delayed regeneration in heart, spinal cord, and retina injury models (258). Deletion of zTregs, in fact, reduced the tissue-specific precursor cells and subdued their proliferation (258). Indeed, zTregs were found near progenitors, sometimes even in close contact (258). However, the most striking finding of this study is that zTregs which presumably came from a common unbiased pool, became plastic in a tissue-specific regenerative context and produced tissue precursor cell specific regeneration factors like Neurotrophin 3 for neural progenitors in regenerating spinal cord, Neuregulin 1 for cardiomyocytes in injured heart and insulin-like growth factor 1 for retinal progenitor Müller glia cells (258) (**Figure 8B**). That zTregs are the primary source of these growth factors was confirmed by rescue of regeneration in zTreg depleted tissues by recombinant tissue-specific growth factors (258). The regeneration potential of zTregs was independent of their immunosuppressive potential or at least was not dependent on their IL10 production as IL10-deficient cells were fully capable of inducing precursor cell proliferation. However, regeneration potential was *Foxp3a*-dependent as regeneration process was significantly reduced in *Foxp3a*$^{-/-}$ tissues along with growth factor expression levels (258). On the other hand, *Areg* expression was not *Foxp3a* dependent and its role in regeneration was limited. It would be interesting to extrapolate and confirm similar findings in murine and human tissues.

Feto-Maternal Tolerance

An equally fascinating population of Tregs which accumulates in murine placenta to induce maternal tolerance to fetus has been described (259). To say that the Tregs are extremely important from the outset of pregnancy will not be an overshoot [reviewed in Ref. (260, 261)]. Indeed, mating itself expands uterine Tregs and induces a transient "tolerance" to paternal alloantigens (260). In both humans and mice, seminal plasma contains TGFβ and prostaglandin E, which are potent Treg inducers. In fact, seminal fluid in humans and rodents contains highest measured TGFβ levels among biological fluids (260). Women with recurrent spontaneous abortions have reduced Treg population (262). Female decidual and uterus draining LN Treg generation is CNS1 dependent (259) and increased fetal resorption and placental T-cell infiltration was observed in CNS1-deficient mice. Apart from the their most likely peripheral origin, it is not known whether these Tregs have a distinct phenotypic and functional profile, elucidation of which could come very informative toward amelioration of infertility, pre-eclampsia, and other spontaneous abortive disorders. Very recently, an elegant study on human fetal antigen presenting cells (263) has found that fetal counterparts of DCs are primarily tolerogenic in their response. And, the primary response is generation of Tregs, even more than the adult DCs, in an *in vitro* Treg differentiation assay (263). These DCs were found across several fetal tissues, including spleen, thymus, skin, gut, and lungs (263). Unfortunately, the authors did not describe if Tregs were also present in these tissues. Earlier, it has been shown that human fetal Tregs promote tolerance to non-inherited maternal antigens (264) but only recently, it came to light that Tregs are required for suppression of *in utero* autoimmunity as well. Two children with IPEX syndrome, who died soon after birth, presented histological evidences of tertiary lymphoid structures, chronic inflammatory changes, and targeted exocrine pancreas autoimmunity (265). This signifies that in the perplexing settings of a pregnancy, Tregs are instrumental in establishing tolerance at both ends of maternal–fetal relationship.

CONCLUSION AND PERSPECTIVES

Translational utility of many biological processes is marred by lack of specificity. A similar dilemma exists for Treg biologists as well; however, in case of Tregs selective therapeutic targeting appears to be achievable by virtue of harnessing their gradually established phenotypic and functional diversity. Recent studies have provided evidence that even for the organs like testes and eye, which are conventionally considered immune-privileged; there are populations of Tregs maintaining dominant tolerance and/or tissue homeostasis. While in testis, where otherwise privileged autoantigen escapes from the seminiferous tubules, only to generate systemic tolerance *via* Tregs (266), the retina actively recruits Tregs, which not only attenuate inflammation, but also repair the vasculature, saving blinding neovascular retinopathies (267). Another layer of specificity is added by discovery of tissue-resident Tregs and their unique characteristics. However, most of the information except the recent reports on skin resident Tregs and TI-Tregs are from mouse tissues. There are several differences in structure as well as physiology between mice and humans. For example, mouse skin contains a thin muscle layer *panniculus carnosus*, which is vestigial in humans (268). This helps in contraction, revascularization and healing of wounds without scar formation in mouse. Human skin on the other hand heals by secondary intention leaving scar tissues. Thus, it is important to identify human tissue Tregs for an informed effort toward therapeutic usage.

There is a need to conclusively establish the origin and accumulating factors for tissue Tregs. One of the most pressing questions about almost all the tissue Tregs is identification of their natural ligands or tissue antigens. Although it has been demonstrated that in certain cases Tregs do not need TCR stimulation for some of their functions (150), Tregs with a smaller subset of specific TCR repertoire populate various tissues as well as malignancies. Therefore, cognate ligands that help in survival and proliferation of Tregs in these tissues are likely to have significant contributions in catering tissue-specific modulations. Proof of concept studies provide evidence that Tregs with defined antigen specificity (chimeric antigen receptor Tregs, CAR-Tregs) have potent immunosuppressive functions along with advantage of not inducing generalized immunosuppression (269).

Question remains as to how Tregs communicate with specific tissue cells-like adipocytes to establish a channel of communication with the environment. Beyond adaptation to inflammatory context, there are peculiarities of Treg biology, which modulate their effect temporally in life as well. Such as, Treg accumulation in aging WAT induces insulin resistance (79), whereas its accumulation in young obese WAT ameliorates it (83). The mechanisms that drive such specific outcomes need to be studied in detail. This accentuated capability to adapt sometimes becomes counterproductive too as seen in tumors where the suppressive capacity is enhanced even in comparison to normal tissue-resident Tregs and is, in turn, utilized by tumors for their survival and immune escape. The mechanisms by which Tregs can push the limits of their functional capabilities are yet to be identified.

A major aspect of tissue adaptation is adjusting the cellular metabolism according to the tissue environment. There are huge gaps in our understanding of both lymphoid and tissue Treg metabolism. In *in vitro* differentiated Tregs (iTregs), it was shown that Foxp3 suppresses glycolysis by repression of Myc and helps in developing resistance to L-lactate (270). Similarly, Foxp3 counters PI(3)K-Akt-mTORC1 to diminish glycolysis in iTregs (271). Contrastingly, splenic and TI-Tregs were shown to uptake more 2NBDG, a fluorescent glucose analog, while intratumoral effector T cells showed glucose deprivation leading to reduced production of glycolytic metabolite phosphoenol pyruvate, resulting in compromised effector functions *via* reduced calcium-NFAT signaling (272). More recently, glycolysis was found to be instrumental in Treg trafficking and migration to inflamed tissues. The induction of the glycolytic enzyme glucokinase GCK and cytoskeletal rearrangement upon its association with actin was shown to be critical for the process (273). These findings underscore the need for extensive studies to delineate metabolic reprogramming in not only tissue Tregs but also lymphoid Tregs under steady state and activated conditions.

One can only be amazed by the diversity and functional plasticity of Tregs. A question, therefore, always comes up as to why Tregs are the chosen ones? Whether similar diversities among other immune cell types are still awaiting discoveries, or whether Foxp3 and presumably other unknown factors provide some degree of functional uniqueness to Tregs, remains to be seen. Nevertheless, looking at the diversity of responses ranging from maintaining immune tolerance to tissue repair, to becoming a major stakeholder in maintenance of physiological function of tissues, it would be apt to say that Tregs are the proverbial "Jack of all trades," and certainly, "master" of some.

AUTHOR CONTRIBUTIONS

AS and DR planned and wrote the manuscript.

FUNDING

This work was supported by Project IBS-R005 of the Institute for Basic Science, Korean Ministry of Science, Information/Communication Technology and Future Planning.

REFERENCES

1. Golub ES, Green DR. *Immunology*. Sunderland, MA: Sinauer Associates (1991).
2. Grignolio A, Mishto M, Faria AM, Garagnani P, Franceschi C, Tieri P. Towards a liquid self: how time, geography, and life experiences reshape the biological identity. *Front Immunol* (2014) 5:153. doi:10.3389/fimmu.2014.00153
3. Luo X, Miller SD, Shea LD. Immune tolerance for autoimmune disease and cell transplantation. *Annu Rev Biomed Eng* (2016) 18:181–205. doi:10.1146/annurev-bioeng-110315-020137
4. Steinman RM. Decisions about dendritic cells: past, present, and future. *Annu Rev Immunol* (2012) 30:1–22. doi:10.1146/annurev-immunol-100311-102839
5. Lewis KL, Reizis B. Dendritic cells: arbiters of immunity and immunological tolerance. *Cold Spring Harb Perspect Biol* (2012) 4(8):a007401. doi:10.1101/cshperspect.a007401
6. Liu J, Cao X. Regulatory dendritic cells in autoimmunity: a comprehensive review. *J Autoimmun* (2015) 63:1–12. doi:10.1016/j.jaut.2015.07.011
7. Mauri C, Menon M. Human regulatory B cells in health and disease: therapeutic potential. *J Clin Invest* (2017) 127(3):772–9. doi:10.1172/JCI85113
8. Dai YC, Zhong J, Xu JF. Regulatory B cells in infectious disease (review). *Mol Med Rep* (2017) 16(1):3–10. doi:10.3892/mmr.2017.6605
9. Wang S, Xia P, Chen Y, Qu Y, Xiong Z, Ye B, et al. Regulatory innate lymphoid cells control innate intestinal inflammation. *Cell* (2017) 171(1):201–16.e18. doi:10.1016/j.cell.2017.07.027

10. White AM, Wraith DC. Tr1-like T cells – an enigmatic regulatory T cell lineage. *Front Immunol* (2016) 7:355. doi:10.3389/fimmu.2016.00355
11. Wing JB, Sakaguchi S. Foxp3(+) T(reg) cells in humoral immunity. *Int Immunol* (2014) 26(2):61–9. doi:10.1093/intimm/dxt060
12. Lu L, Barbi J, Pan F. The regulation of immune tolerance by FOXP3. *Nat Rev Immunol* (2017) 17(11):703–17. doi:10.1038/nri.2017.75
13. Josefowicz SZ, Lu LF, Rudensky AY. Regulatory T cells: mechanisms of differentiation and function. *Annu Rev Immunol* (2012) 30:531–64. doi:10.1146/annurev.immunol.25.022106.141623
14. Xing Y, Hogquist KA. T-cell tolerance: central and peripheral. *Cold Spring Harb Perspect Biol* (2012) 4(6):1–15. doi:10.1101/cshperspect.a006957
15. Surh CD, Sprent J. T-cell apoptosis detected in situ during positive and negative selection in the thymus. *Nature* (1994) 372(6501):100–3. doi:10.1038/372100a0
16. Moran AE, Hogquist KA. T-cell receptor affinity in thymic development. *Immunology* (2012) 135(4):261–7. doi:10.1111/j.1365-2567.2011.03547.x
17. Nemazee D. Receptor editing in lymphocyte development and central tolerance. *Nat Rev Immunol* (2006) 6(10):728–40. doi:10.1038/nri1939
18. Cohen PL, Eisenberg RA. Lpr and gld: single gene models of systemic autoimmunity and lymphoproliferative disease. *Annu Rev Immunol* (1991) 9:243–69. doi:10.1146/annurev.iy.09.040191.001331
19. Sakaguchi S, Sakaguchi N, Asano M, Itoh M, Toda M. Immunologic self-tolerance maintained by activated T cells expressing IL-2 receptor alpha-chains (CD25). Breakdown of a single mechanism of self-tolerance causes various autoimmune diseases. *J Immunol* (1995) 155(3):1151–64.
20. Nishizuka Y, Sakakura T. Ovarian dysgenesis induced by neonatal thymectomy in the mouse. *Endocrinology* (1971) 89(3):886–93. doi:10.1210/endo-89-3-886
21. Taguchi O, Nishizuka Y, Sakakura T, Kojima A. Autoimmune oophoritis in thymectomized mice: detection of circulating antibodies against oocytes. *Clin Exp Immunol* (1980) 40(3):540–53.
22. Taguchi O, Nishizuka Y. Experimental autoimmune orchitis after neonatal thymectomy in the mouse. *Clin Exp Immunol* (1981) 46(2):425–34.
23. Kojima A, Tanaka-Kojima Y, Sakakura T, Nishizuka Y. Spontaneous development of autoimmune thyroiditis in neonatally thymectomized mice. *Lab Invest* (1976) 34(6):550–7.
24. Kojima A, Taguchi O, Nishizuka Y. Experimental production of possible autoimmune castritis followed by macrocytic anemia in athymic nude mice. *Lab Invest* (1980) 42(4):387–95.
25. Kojima A, Prehn RT. Genetic susceptibility to post-thymectomy autoimmune diseases in mice. *Immunogenetics* (1981) 14(1–2):15–27. doi:10.1007/BF00344296
26. Penhale WJ, Irvine WJ, Inglis JR, Farmer A. Thyroiditis in T cell-depleted rats: suppression of the autoallergic response by reconstitution with normal lymphoid cells. *Clin Exp Immunol* (1976) 25(1):6–16.
27. Sakaguchi S, Fukuma K, Kuribayashi K, Masuda T. Organ-specific autoimmune diseases induced in mice by elimination of T cell subset. I. Evidence for the active participation of T cells in natural self-tolerance; deficit of a T cell subset as a possible cause of autoimmune disease. *J Exp Med* (1985) 161(1):72–87. doi:10.1084/jem.161.1.72
28. Powrie F, Leach MW, Mauze S, Caddle LB, Coffman RL. Phenotypically distinct subsets of CD4+ T cells induce or protect from chronic intestinal inflammation in C. B-17 scid mice. *Int Immunol* (1993) 5(11):1461–71. doi:10.1093/intimm/5.11.1461
29. Morrissey PJ, Charrier K, Braddy S, Liggitt D, Watson JD. CD4+ T cells that express high levels of CD45RB induce wasting disease when transferred into congenic severe combined immunodeficient mice. Disease development is prevented by cotransfer of purified CD4+ T cells. *J Exp Med* (1993) 178(1):237–44. doi:10.1084/jem.178.1.237
30. Asano M, Toda M, Sakaguchi N, Sakaguchi S. Autoimmune disease as a consequence of developmental abnormality of a T cell subpopulation. *J Exp Med* (1996) 184(2):387–96. doi:10.1084/jem.184.2.387
31. Shevach EM. Regulatory T cells in autoimmmunity*. *Annu Rev Immunol* (2000) 18:423–49. doi:10.1146/annurev.immunol.18.1.423
32. Godfrey VL, Wilkinson JE, Rinchik EM, Russell LB. Fatal lymphoreticular disease in the scurfy (sf) mouse requires T cells that mature in a sf thymic environment: potential model for thymic education. *Proc Natl Acad Sci U S A* (1991) 88(13):5528–32. doi:10.1073/pnas.88.13.5528
33. Blair PJ, Bultman SJ, Haas JC, Rouse BT, Wilkinson JE, Godfrey VL. CD4+CD8- T cells are the effector cells in disease pathogenesis in the scurfy (sf) mouse. *J Immunol* (1994) 153(8):3764–74.
34. Kanangat S, Blair P, Reddy R, Daheshia M, Godfrey V, Rouse BT, et al. Disease in the scurfy (sf) mouse is associated with overexpression of cytokine genes. *Eur J Immunol* (1996) 26(1):161–5. doi:10.1002/eji.1830260125
35. Zahorsky-Reeves JL, Wilkinson JE. The murine mutation scurfy (sf) results in an antigen-dependent lymphoproliferative disease with altered T cell sensitivity. *Eur J Immunol* (2001) 31(1):196–204. doi:10.1002/1521-4141(200101)31:1<196::AID-IMMU196>3.0.CO;2-9
36. Tivol EA, Borriello F, Schweitzer AN, Lynch WP, Bluestone JA, Sharpe AH. Loss of CTLA-4 leads to massive lymphoproliferation and fatal multiorgan tissue destruction, revealing a critical negative regulatory role of CTLA-4. *Immunity* (1995) 3(5):541–7. doi:10.1016/1074-7613(95)90125-6
37. Kulkarni AB, Huh CG, Becker D, Geiser A, Lyght M, Flanders KC, et al. Transforming growth factor beta 1 null mutation in mice causes excessive inflammatory response and early death. *Proc Natl Acad Sci U S A* (1993) 90(2):770–4. doi:10.1073/pnas.90.2.770
38. Brunkow ME, Jeffery EW, Hjerrild KA, Paeper B, Clark LB, Yasayko SA, et al. Disruption of a new forkhead/winged-helix protein, scurfin, results in the fatal lymphoproliferative disorder of the scurfy mouse. *Nat Genet* (2001) 27(1):68–73. doi:10.1038/83784
39. Bennett CL, Christie J, Ramsdell F, Brunkow ME, Ferguson PJ, Whitesell L, et al. The immune dysregulation, polyendocrinopathy, enteropathy, X-linked syndrome (IPEX) is caused by mutations of FOXP3. *Nat Genet* (2001) 27(1):20–1. doi:10.1038/83713
40. Wildin RS, Ramsdell F, Peake J, Faravelli F, Casanova JL, Buist N, et al. X-linked neonatal diabetes mellitus, enteropathy and endocrinopathy syndrome is the human equivalent of mouse scurfy. *Nat Genet* (2001) 27(1):18–20. doi:10.1038/83707
41. Powell BR, Buist NR, Stenzel P. An X-linked syndrome of diarrhea, polyendocrinopathy, and fatal infection in infancy. *J Pediatr* (1982) 100(5):731–7. doi:10.1016/S0022-3476(82)80573-8
42. Khattri R, Cox T, Yasayko SA, Ramsdell F. An essential role for Scurfin in CD4+CD25+ T regulatory cells. *Nat Immunol* (2003) 4(4):337–42. doi:10.1038/ni909
43. Hori S, Nomura T, Sakaguchi S. Control of regulatory T cell development by the transcription factor Foxp3. *Science* (2003) 299(5609):1057–61. doi:10.1126/science.1079490
44. Fontenot JD, Gavin MA, Rudensky AY. Foxp3 programs the development and function of CD4+CD25+ regulatory T cells. *Nat Immunol* (2003) 4(4):330–6. doi:10.1038/ni904
45. Fontenot JD, Rasmussen JP, Williams LM, Dooley JL, Farr AG, Rudensky AY. Regulatory T cell lineage specification by the forkhead transcription factor foxp3. *Immunity* (2005) 22(3):329–41. doi:10.1016/j.immuni.2005.01.016
46. Zheng Y, Josefowicz S, Chaudhry A, Peng XP, Forbush K, Rudensky AY. Role of conserved non-coding DNA elements in the Foxp3 gene in regulatory T-cell fate. *Nature* (2010) 463(7282):808–12. doi:10.1038/nature08750
47. Rudra D, deRoos P, Chaudhry A, Niec RE, Arvey A, Samstein RM, et al. Transcription factor Foxp3 and its protein partners form a complex regulatory network. *Nat Immunol* (2012) 13(10):1010–9. doi:10.1038/ni.2402
48. Hsieh CS, Lee HM, Lio CW. Selection of regulatory T cells in the thymus. *Nat Rev Immunol* (2012) 12(3):157–67. doi:10.1038/nri3155
49. Li MO, Rudensky AY. T cell receptor signalling in the control of regulatory T cell differentiation and function. *Nat Rev Immunol* (2016) 16(4):220–33. doi:10.1038/nri.2016.26
50. Hsieh CS, Zheng Y, Liang Y, Fontenot JD, Rudensky AY. An intersection between the self-reactive regulatory and nonregulatory T cell receptor repertoires. *Nat Immunol* (2006) 7(4):401–10. doi:10.1038/ni1318
51. Moran AE, Holzapfel KL, Xing Y, Cunningham NR, Maltzman JS, Punt J, et al. T cell receptor signal strength in Treg and iNKT cell development demonstrated by a novel fluorescent reporter mouse. *J Exp Med* (2011) 208(6):1279–89. doi:10.1084/jem.20110308
52. Kitagawa Y, Ohkura N, Kidani Y, Vandenbon A, Hirota K, Kawakami R, et al. Guidance of regulatory T cell development by Satb1-dependent super-enhancer establishment. *Nat Immunol* (2017) 18(2):173–83. doi:10.1038/ni.3646

53. Zhang X, Izikson L, Liu L, Weiner HL. Activation of CD25(+)CD4(+) regulatory T cells by oral antigen administration. *J Immunol* (2001) 167(8): 4245–53. doi:10.4049/jimmunol.167.8.4245
54. Mucida D, Kutchukhidze N, Erazo A, Russo M, Lafaille JJ, Curotto de Lafaille MA. Oral tolerance in the absence of naturally occurring Tregs. *J Clin Invest* (2005) 115(7):1923–33. doi:10.1172/JCI24487
55. Apostolou I, Sarukhan A, Klein L, von Boehmer H. Origin of regulatory T cells with known specificity for antigen. *Nat Immunol* (2002) 3(8):756–63. doi:10.1038/ni816
56. Takimoto T, Wakabayashi Y, Sekiya T, Inoue N, Morita R, Ichiyama K, et al. Smad2 and Smad3 are redundantly essential for the TGF-beta-mediated regulation of regulatory T plasticity and Th1 development. *J Immunol* (2010) 185(2):842–55. doi:10.4049/jimmunol.0904100
57. Chen W, Konkel JE. Development of thymic Foxp3(+) regulatory T cells: TGF-beta matters. *Eur J Immunol* (2015) 45(4):958–65. doi:10.1002/eji.201444999
58. Ruan Q, Kameswaran V, Tone Y, Li L, Liou HC, Greene MI, et al. Development of Foxp3(+) regulatory t cells is driven by the c-Rel enhanceosome. *Immunity* (2009) 31(6):932–40. doi:10.1016/j.immuni.2009.10.006
59. Cretney E, Xin A, Shi W, Minnich M, Masson F, Miasari M, et al. The transcription factors Blimp-1 and IRF4 jointly control the differentiation and function of effector regulatory T cells. *Nat Immunol* (2011) 12(4):304–11. doi:10.1038/ni.2006
60. Smigiel KS, Richards E, Srivastava S, Thomas KR, Dudda JC, Klonowski KD, et al. CCR7 provides localized access to IL-2 and defines homeostatically distinct regulatory T cell subsets. *J Exp Med* (2014) 211(1):121–36. doi:10.1084/jem.20131142
61. Ito T, Hanabuchi S, Wang YH, Park WR, Arima K, Bover L, et al. Two functional subsets of FOXP3+ regulatory T cells in human thymus and periphery. *Immunity* (2008) 28(6):870–80. doi:10.1016/j.immuni.2008.03.018
62. Zheng Y, Chaudhry A, Kas A, deRoos P, Kim JM, Chu TT, et al. Regulatory T-cell suppressor program co-opts transcription factor IRF4 to control T(H)2 responses. *Nature* (2009) 458(7236):351–6. doi:10.1038/nature07674
63. Koch MA, Tucker-Heard G, Perdue NR, Killebrew JR, Urdahl KB, Campbell DJ. The transcription factor T-bet controls regulatory T cell homeostasis and function during type 1 inflammation. *Nat Immunol* (2009) 10(6):595–602. doi:10.1038/ni.1731
64. Chaudhry A, Rudra D, Treuting P, Samstein RM, Liang Y, Kas A, et al. CD4+ regulatory T cells control TH17 responses in a Stat3-dependent manner. *Science* (2009) 326(5955):986–91. doi:10.1126/science.1172702
65. Chaudhry A, Samstein RM, Treuting P, Liang Y, Pils MC, Heinrich JM, et al. Interleukin-10 signaling in regulatory T cells is required for suppression of Th17 cell-mediated inflammation. *Immunity* (2011) 34(4):566–78. doi:10.1016/j.immuni.2011.03.018
66. Chung Y, Tanaka S, Chu F, Nurieva RI, Martinez GJ, Rawal S, et al. Follicular regulatory T cells expressing Foxp3 and Bcl-6 suppress germinal center reactions. *Nat Med* (2011) 17(8):983–8. doi:10.1038/nm.2426
67. Linterman MA, Pierson W, Lee SK, Kallies A, Kawamoto S, Rayner TF, et al. Foxp3+ follicular regulatory T cells control the germinal center response. *Nat Med* (2011) 17(8):975–82. doi:10.1038/nm.2425
68. Virtanen KA, van Marken Lichtenbelt WD, Nuutila P. Brown adipose tissue functions in humans. *Biochim Biophys Acta* (2013) 1831(5):1004–8. doi:10.1016/j.bbalip.2012.12.011
69. Reue K. A thematic review series: lipid droplet storage and metabolism: from yeast to man. *J Lipid Res* (2011) 52(11):1865–8. doi:10.1194/jlr.E020602
70. Konige M, Wang H, Sztalryd C. Role of adipose specific lipid droplet proteins in maintaining whole body energy homeostasis. *Biochim Biophys Acta* (2014) 1842(3):393–401. doi:10.1016/j.bbadis.2013.05.007
71. Boutens L, Stienstra R. Adipose tissue macrophages: going off track during obesity. *Diabetologia* (2016) 59(5):879–94. doi:10.1007/s00125-016-3904-9
72. Trayhurn P. Hypoxia and adipose tissue function and dysfunction in obesity. *Physiol Rev* (2013) 93(1):1–21. doi:10.1152/physrev.00017.2012
73. Castoldi A, Naffah de Souza C, Camara NO, Moraes-Vieira PM. The macrophage switch in obesity development. *Front Immunol* (2015) 6:637. doi:10.3389/fimmu.2015.00637
74. O'Sullivan TE, Rapp M, Fan X, Weizman OE, Bhardwaj P, Adams NM, et al. Adipose-resident group 1 innate lymphoid cells promote obesity-associated insulin resistance. *Immunity* (2016) 45(2):428–41. doi:10.1016/j.immuni.2016.06.016
75. Nishimura S, Manabe I, Takaki S, Nagasaki M, Otsu M, Yamashita H, et al. Adipose natural regulatory B cells negatively control adipose tissue inflammation. *Cell Metab* (2013) 18:759–66. doi:10.1016/j.cmet.2013.09.017
76. Feuerer M, Herrero L, Cipolletta D, Naaz A, Wong J, Nayer A, et al. Lean, but not obese, fat is enriched for a unique population of regulatory T cells that affect metabolic parameters. *Nat Med* (2009) 15(8):930–9. doi:10.1038/nm.2002
77. Vasanthakumar A, Kallies A. The regulatory T cell: jack-of-all-trades. *Trends Immunol* (2015) 36(12):756–8. doi:10.1016/j.it.2015.10.002
78. Cipolletta D, Cohen P, Spiegelman BM, Benoist C, Mathis D. Appearance and disappearance of the mRNA signature characteristic of Treg cells in visceral adipose tissue: age, diet, and PPARgamma effects. *Proc Natl Acad Sci U S A* (2015) 112(2):482–7. doi:10.1073/pnas.1423486112
79. Bapat SP, Myoung Suh J, Fang S, Liu S, Zhang Y, Cheng A, et al. Depletion of fat-resident Treg cells prevents age-associated insulin resistance. *Nature* (2015) 528(7580):137–41. doi:10.1038/nature16151
80. Kolodin D, van Panhuys N, Li C, Magnuson AM, Cipolletta D, Miller CM, et al. Antigen- and cytokine-driven accumulation of regulatory T cells in visceral adipose tissue of lean mice. *Cell Metab* (2015) 21(4):543–57. doi:10.1016/j.cmet.2015.03.005
81. Correia-Neves M, Waltzinger C, Mathis D, Benoist C. The shaping of the T cell repertoire. *Immunity* (2001) 14(1):21–32. doi:10.1016/S1074-7613(01)00086-3
82. Kälin S, Becker M, Ott VB, Serr I, Hosp F, Mollah MMH, et al. A Stat6/Pten axis links regulatory T cells with adipose tissue function. *Cell Metab* (2017) 26(3):475–92.e7. doi:10.1016/j.cmet.2017.08.008
83. Cipolletta D, Feuerer M, Li A, Kamei N, Lee J, Shoelson SE, et al. PPAR-[ggr] is a major driver of the accumulation and phenotype of adipose tissue Treg cells. *Nature* (2012) 486(7404):549–53. doi:10.1038/nature11132
84. Vasanthakumar A, Moro K, Xin A, Liao Y, Gloury R, Kawamoto S, et al. The transcriptional regulators IRF4, BATF and IL-33 orchestrate development and maintenance of adipose tissue-resident regulatory T cells. *Nat Immunol* (2015) 16(3):276–85. doi:10.1038/ni.3085
85. Medrikova D, Sijmonsma TP, Sowodniok K, Richards DM, Delacher M, Sticht C, et al. Brown adipose tissue harbors a distinct sub-population of regulatory T cells. *PLoS One* (2015) 10(2):e0118534. doi:10.1371/journal.pone.0118534
86. Hotamisligil GS, Shargill NS, Spiegelman BM. Adipose expression of tumor necrosis factor-alpha: direct role in obesity-linked insulin resistance. *Science* (1993) 259(5091):87–91. doi:10.1126/science.7678183
87. Xu H, Barnes GT, Yang Q, Tan G, Yang D, Chou CJ, et al. Chronic inflammation in fat plays a crucial role in the development of obesity-related insulin resistance. *J Clin Invest* (2003) 112(12):1821–30. doi:10.1172/JCI200319451
88. Ganguly D. Do type I interferons link systemic autoimmunities and metabolic syndrome in a pathogenetic continuum? *Trends Immunol* (2018) 39(1):28–43. doi:10.1016/j.it.2017.07.001
89. Wagner NM, Brandhorst G, Czepluch F, Lankeit M, Eberle C, Herzberg S, et al. Circulating regulatory T cells are reduced in obesity and may identify subjects at increased metabolic and cardiovascular risk. *Obesity (Silver Spring)* (2013) 21(3):461–8. doi:10.1002/oby.20087
90. Kim JM, Rasmussen JP, Rudensky AY. Regulatory T cells prevent catastrophic autoimmunity throughout the lifespan of mice. *Nat Immunol* (2007) 8(2):191–7. doi:10.1038/ni1428
91. Smith U. Pioglitazone: mechanism of action. *Int J Clin Pract Suppl* (2001) (121):13–8.
92. Carobbio S, Pellegrinelli V, Vidal-Puig A. Adipose tissue function and expandability as determinants of lipotoxicity and the metabolic syndrome. *Adv Exp Med Biol* (2017) 960:161–96. doi:10.1007/978-3-319-48382-5_7
93. Wernstedt Asterholm I, Tao C, Morley TS, Wang QA, Delgado-Lopez F, Wang ZV, et al. Adipocyte inflammation is essential for healthy adipose tissue expansion and remodeling. *Cell Metab* (2014) 20(1):103–18. doi:10.1016/j.cmet.2014.05.005
94. Kim JY, van de Wall E, Laplante M, Azzara A, Trujillo ME, Hofmann SM, et al. Obesity-associated improvements in metabolic profile through expansion of adipose tissue. *J Clin Invest* (2007) 117(9):2621–37. doi:10.1172/JCI31021

95. Rothwell NJ, Stock MJ. A role for brown adipose tissue in diet-induced thermogenesis. *Nature* (1979) 281(5726):31–5. doi:10.1038/281031a0
96. Sender R, Fuchs S, Milo R. Are we really vastly outnumbered? Revisiting the ratio of bacterial to host cells in humans. *Cell* (2016) 164(3):337–40. doi:10.1016/j.cell.2016.01.013
97. Sender R, Fuchs S, Milo R. Revised estimates for the number of human and bacteria cells in the body. *PLoS Biol* (2016) 14(8):e1002533. doi:10.1371/journal.pbio.1002533
98. Shapira M. Gut microbiotas and host evolution: scaling up symbiosis. *Trends Ecol Evol* (2016) 31(7):539–49. doi:10.1016/j.tree.2016.03.006
99. Powell DW, Pinchuk IV, Saada JI, Chen X, Mifflin RC. Mesenchymal cells of the intestinal lamina propria. *Annu Rev Physiol* (2011) 73:213–37. doi:10.1146/annurev.physiol.70.113006.100646
100. Yang Y, Zhang Y, Cao Z, Ji H, Yang X, Iwamoto H, et al. Anti-VEGF- and anti-VEGF receptor-induced vascular alteration in mouse healthy tissues. *Proc Natl Acad Sci U S A* (2013) 110(29):12018–23. doi:10.1073/pnas.1301331110
101. Mowat AM, Agace WW. Regional specialization within the intestinal immune system. *Nat Rev Immunol* (2014) 14(10):667–85. doi:10.1038/nri3738
102. Johansson ME, Phillipson M, Petersson J, Velcich A, Holm L, Hansson GC. The inner of the two Muc2 mucin-dependent mucus layers in colon is devoid of bacteria. *Proc Natl Acad Sci U S A* (2008) 105(39):15064–9. doi:10.1073/pnas.0803124105
103. Li H, Limenitakis JP, Fuhrer T, Geuking MB, Lawson MA, Wyss M, et al. The outer mucus layer hosts a distinct intestinal microbial niche. *Nat Commun* (2015) 6:8292. doi:10.1038/ncomms9292
104. Bernier-Latmani J, Petrova TV. Intestinal lymphatic vasculature: structure, mechanisms and functions. *Nat Rev Gastroenterol Hepatol* (2017) 14(9):510–26. doi:10.1038/nrgastro.2017.79
105. Tanoue T, Atarashi K, Honda K. Development and maintenance of intestinal regulatory T cells. *Nat Rev Immunol* (2016) 16(5):295–309. doi:10.1038/nri.2016.36
106. Panduro M, Benoist C, Mathis D. Tissue Tregs. *Annu Rev Immunol* (2016) 34:609–33. doi:10.1146/annurev-immunol-032712-095948
107. Sefik E, Geva-Zatorsky N, Oh S, Konnikova L, Zemmour D, McGuire AM, et al. MUCOSAL IMMUNOLOGY. Individual intestinal symbionts induce a distinct population of RORgamma(+) regulatory T cells. *Science* (2015) 349(6251):993–7. doi:10.1126/science.aaa9420
108. Schiering C, Krausgruber T, Chomka A, Frohlich A, Adelmann K, Wohlfert EA, et al. The alarmin IL-33 promotes regulatory T-cell function in the intestine. *Nature* (2014) 513(7519):564–8. doi:10.1038/nature13577
109. Kim KS, Hong SW, Han D, Yi J, Jung J, Yang BG, et al. Dietary antigens limit mucosal immunity by inducing regulatory T cells in the small intestine. *Science* (2016) 351(6275):858–63. doi:10.1126/science.aac5560
110. Wohlfert EA, Grainger JR, Bouladoux N, Konkel JE, Oldenhove G, Ribeiro CH, et al. GATA3 controls Foxp3(+) regulatory T cell fate during inflammation in mice. *J Clin Invest* (2011) 121(11):4503–15. doi:10.1172/JCI57456
111. Atarashi K, Tanoue T, Shima T, Imaoka A, Kuwahara T, Momose Y, et al. Induction of colonic regulatory T cells by indigenous *Clostridium* species. *Science* (2011) 331(6015):337–41. doi:10.1126/science.1198469
112. Geuking MB, Cahenzli J, Lawson MA, Ng DC, Slack E, Hapfelmeier S, et al. Intestinal bacterial colonization induces mutualistic regulatory T cell responses. *Immunity* (2011) 34(5):794–806. doi:10.1016/j.immuni.2011.03.021
113. Lathrop SK, Bloom SM, Rao SM, Nutsch K, Lio CW, Santacruz N, et al. Peripheral education of the immune system by colonic commensal microbiota. *Nature* (2011) 478(7368):250–4. doi:10.1038/nature10434
114. Nutsch K, Chai JN, Ai TL, Russler-Germain E, Feehley T, Nagler CR, et al. Rapid and efficient generation of regulatory T cells to commensal antigens in the periphery. *Cell Rep* (2016) 17(1):206–20. doi:10.1016/j.celrep.2016.08.092
115. Thornton AM, Korty PE, Tran DQ, Wohlfert EA, Murray PE, Belkaid Y, et al. Expression of Helios, an Ikaros transcription factor family member, differentiates thymic-derived from peripherally induced Foxp3+ T regulatory cells. *J Immunol* (2010) 184(7):3433–41. doi:10.4049/jimmunol.0904028
116. Weiss JM, Bilate AM, Gobert M, Ding Y, Curotto de Lafaille MA, Parkhurst CN, et al. Neuropilin 1 is expressed on thymus-derived natural regulatory T cells, but not mucosa-generated induced Foxp3+ T reg cells. *J Exp Med* (2012) 209(10):1723–42, S1. doi:10.1084/jem.20120914
117. Yadav M, Louvet C, Davini D, Gardner JM, Martinez-Llordella M, Bailey-Bucktrout S, et al. Neuropilin-1 distinguishes natural and inducible regulatory T cells among regulatory T cell subsets in vivo. *J Exp Med* (2012) 209(10):1713–22, S1–19. doi:10.1084/jem.20120822
118. Gottschalk RA, Corse E, Allison JP. Expression of Helios in peripherally induced Foxp3+ regulatory T cells. *J Immunol* (2012) 188(3):976–80. doi:10.4049/jimmunol.1102964
119. Szurek E, Cebula A, Wojciech L, Pietrzak M, Rempala G, Kisielow P, et al. Differences in expression level of Helios and neuropilin-1 do not distinguish thymus-derived from extrathymically-induced CD4+Foxp3+ regulatory T cells. *PLoS One* (2015) 10(10):e0141161. doi:10.1371/journal.pone.0141161
120. Xu L, Kitani A, Stuelten C, McGrady G, Fuss I, Strober W. Positive and negative transcriptional regulation of the Foxp3 gene is mediated by access and binding of the Smad3 protein to enhancer I. *Immunity* (2010) 33(3):313–25. doi:10.1016/j.immuni.2010.09.001
121. Coombes JL, Siddiqui KR, Arancibia-Carcamo CV, Hall J, Sun CM, Belkaid Y, et al. A functionally specialized population of mucosal CD103+ DCs induces Foxp3+ regulatory T cells via a TGF-beta and retinoic acid-dependent mechanism. *J Exp Med* (2007) 204(8):1757–64. doi:10.1084/jem.20070590
122. Hill JA, Hall JA, Sun CM, Cai Q, Ghyselinck N, Chambon P, et al. Retinoic acid enhances Foxp3 induction indirectly by relieving inhibition from CD4+CD44hi Cells. *Immunity* (2008) 29(5):758–70. doi:10.1016/j.immuni.2008.09.018
123. Cebula A, Seweryn M, Rempala GA, Pabla SS, McIndoe RA, Denning TL, et al. Thymus-derived regulatory T cells contribute to tolerance to commensal microbiota. *Nature* (2013) 497(7448):258–62. doi:10.1038/nature12079
124. Korn LL, Hubbeling HG, Porrett PM, Yang Q, Barnett LG, Laufer TM. Regulatory T cells occupy an isolated niche in the intestine that is antigen independent. *Cell Rep* (2014) 9(5):1567–73. doi:10.1016/j.celrep.2014.11.006
125. Wang Y, Su MA, Wan YY. An essential role of the transcription factor GATA-3 for the function of regulatory T cells. *Immunity* (2011) 35(3):337–48. doi:10.1016/j.immuni.2011.08.012
126. Bertheloot D, Latz E. HMGB1, IL-1alpha, IL-33 and S100 proteins: dual-function alarmins. *Cell Mol Immunol* (2017) 14(1):43–64. doi:10.1038/cmi.2016.34
127. Chan JK, Roth J, Oppenheim JJ, Tracey KJ, Vogl T, Feldmann M, et al. Alarmins: awaiting a clinical response. *J Clin Invest* (2012) 122(8):2711–9. doi:10.1172/JCI62423
128. Siede J, Frohlich A, Datsi A, Hegazy AN, Varga DV, Holecska V, et al. IL-33 receptor-expressing regulatory T cells are highly activated, Th2 biased and suppress CD4 T cell proliferation through IL-10 and TGFbeta release. *PLoS One* (2016) 11(8):e0161507. doi:10.1371/journal.pone.0161507
129. Ohnmacht C, Park JH, Cording S, Wing JB, Atarashi K, Obata Y, et al. MUCOSAL IMMUNOLOGY. The microbiota regulates type 2 immunity through RORgammat(+) T cells. *Science* (2015) 349(6251):989–93. doi:10.1126/science.aac4263
130. Yang BH, Hagemann S, Mamareli P, Lauer U, Hoffmann U, Beckstette M, et al. Foxp3(+) T cells expressing RORgammat represent a stable regulatory T-cell effector lineage with enhanced suppressive capacity during intestinal inflammation. *Mucosal Immunol* (2016) 9(2):444–57. doi:10.1038/mi.2015.74
131. Li X, Liang Y, LeBlanc M, Benner C, Zheng Y. Function of a Foxp3 cis-element in protecting regulatory T cell identity. *Cell* (2014) 158(4):734–48. doi:10.1016/j.cell.2014.07.030
132. Davie JR. Inhibition of histone deacetylase activity by butyrate. *J Nutr* (2003) 133(7 Suppl):2485S–93S. doi:10.1093/jn/133.7.2485S
133. Arpaia N, Campbell C, Fan X, Dikiy S, van der Veeken J, deRoos P, et al. Metabolites produced by commensal bacteria promote peripheral regulatory T-cell generation. *Nature* (2013) 504(7480):451–5. doi:10.1038/nature12726
134. Furusawa Y, Obata Y, Fukuda S, Endo TA, Nakato G, Takahashi D, et al. Commensal microbe-derived butyrate induces the differentiation of colonic regulatory T cells. *Nature* (2013) 504(7480):446–50. doi:10.1038/nature12721
135. Zhu HC, Qiu T, Liu XH, Dong WC, Weng XD, Hu CH, et al. Tolerogenic dendritic cells generated by RelB silencing using shRNA prevent acute

rejection. *Cell Immunol* (2012) 274(1–2):12–8. doi:10.1016/j.cellimm.2012.02.012

136. Shih VF, Davis-Turak J, Macal M, Huang JQ, Ponomarenko J, Kearns JD, et al. Control of RelB during dendritic cell activation integrates canonical and noncanonical NF-kappaB pathways. *Nat Immunol* (2012) 13(12):1162–70. doi:10.1038/ni.2446
137. Frank DN, St Amand AL, Feldman RA, Boedeker EC, Harpaz N, Pace NR. Molecular-phylogenetic characterization of microbial community imbalances in human inflammatory bowel diseases. *Proc Natl Acad Sci U S A* (2007) 104(34):13780–5. doi:10.1073/pnas.0706625104
138. Thibault R, De Coppet P, Daly K, Bourreille A, Cuff M, Bonnet C, et al. Down-regulation of the monocarboxylate transporter 1 is involved in butyrate deficiency during intestinal inflammation. *Gastroenterology* (2007) 133(6):1916–27. doi:10.1053/j.gastro.2007.08.041
139. Xu M, Pokrovskii M, Ding Y, Yi R, Au C, Harrison OJ, et al. c-MAF-dependent regulatory T cells mediate immunological tolerance to a gut pathobiont. *Nature* (2018) 554:373–7. doi:10.1038/nature25500
140. Xu J, Yang Y, Qiu G, Lal G, Wu Z, Levy DE, et al. c-Maf regulates IL-10 expression during Th17 polarization. *J Immunol* (2009) 182(10):6226–36. doi:10.4049/jimmunol.0900123
141. Konkel JE, Zhang D, Zanvit P, Chia C, Zangarle-Murray T, Jin W, et al. Transforming growth factor-beta signaling in regulatory T cells controls T helper-17 cells and tissue-specific immune responses. *Immunity* (2017) 46(4):660–74. doi:10.1016/j.immuni.2017.03.015
142. Li MO, Flavell RA. TGF-beta: a master of all T cell trades. *Cell* (2008) 134(3):392–404. doi:10.1016/j.cell.2008.07.025
143. Rubtsov YP, Rudensky AY. TGFbeta signalling in control of T-cell-mediated self-reactivity. *Nat Rev Immunol* (2007) 7(6):443–53. doi:10.1038/nri2095
144. Zeng H, Chi H. Metabolic control of regulatory T cell development and function. *Trends Immunol* (2015) 36(1):3–12. doi:10.1016/j.it.2014.08.003
145. Sun CM, Hall JA, Blank RB, Bouladoux N, Oukka M, Mora JR, et al. Small intestine lamina propria dendritic cells promote de novo generation of Foxp3 T reg cells via retinoic acid. *J Exp Med* (2007) 204(8):1775–85. doi:10.1084/jem.20070602
146. Bakdash G, Vogelpoel LT, van Capel TM, Kapsenberg ML, de Jong EC. Retinoic acid primes human dendritic cells to induce gut-homing, IL-10-producing regulatory T cells. *Mucosal Immunol* (2015) 8(2):265–78. doi:10.1038/mi.2014.64
147. Kang SW, Kim SH, Lee N, Lee WW, Hwang KA, Shin MS, et al. 1,25-Dihyroxyvitamin D3 promotes FOXP3 expression via binding to vitamin D response elements in its conserved noncoding sequence region. *J Immunol* (2012) 188(11):5276–82. doi:10.4049/jimmunol.1101211
148. Lu D, Lan B, Din Z, Chen H, Chen G. A vitamin D receptor agonist converts CD4+ T cells to Foxp3+ regulatory T cells in patients with ulcerative colitis. *Oncotarget* (2017) 8(32):53552–62. doi:10.18632/oncotarget.18614
149. Zaiss DM, van Loosdregt J, Gorlani A, Bekker CP, Grone A, Sibilia M, et al. Amphiregulin enhances regulatory T cell-suppressive function via the epidermal growth factor receptor. *Immunity* (2013) 38(2):275–84. doi:10.1016/j.immuni.2012.09.023
150. Arpaia N, Green JA, Moltedo B, Arvey A, Hemmers S, Yuan S, et al. A distinct function of regulatory T cells in tissue protection. *Cell* (2015) 162(5):1078–89. doi:10.1016/j.cell.2015.08.021
151. Green JA, Arpaia N, Schizas M, Dobrin A, Rudensky AY. A nonimmune function of T cells in promoting lung tumor progression. *J Exp Med* (2017) 214(12):3565–75. doi:10.1084/jem.20170356
152. Sujino T, London M, Hoytema van Konijnenburg DP, Rendon T, Buch T, Silva HM, et al. Tissue adaptation of regulatory and intraepithelial CD4(+) T cells controls gut inflammation. *Science* (2016) 352(6293):1581–6. doi:10.1126/science.aaf3892
153. Hoytema van Konijnenburg DP, Mucida D. Intraepithelial lymphocytes. *Curr Biol* (2017) 27(15):R737–9. doi:10.1016/j.cub.2017.05.073
154. Di Meglio P, Perera GK, Nestle FO. The multitasking organ: recent insights into skin immune function. *Immunity* (2011) 35(6):857–69. doi:10.1016/j.immuni.2011.12.003
155. Kanitakis J. Anatomy, histology and immunohistochemistry of normal human skin. *Eur J Dermatol* (2002) 12(4):390–9.
156. Halabi-Tawil M, Ruemmele FM, Fraitag S, Rieux-Laucat F, Neven B, Brousse N, et al. Cutaneous manifestations of immune dysregulation, polyendocrinopathy, enteropathy, X-linked (IPEX) syndrome. *Br J Dermatol* (2009) 160(3):645–51. doi:10.1111/j.1365-2133.2008.08835.x
157. Sanchez Rodriguez R, Pauli ML, Neuhaus IM, Yu SS, Arron ST, Harris HW, et al. Memory regulatory T cells reside in human skin. *J Clin Invest* (2014) 124(3):1027–36. doi:10.1172/JCI72932
158. Ali N, Zirak B, Rodriguez RS, Pauli ML, Truong HA, Lai K, et al. Regulatory T cells in skin facilitate epithelial stem cell differentiation. *Cell* (2017) 169(6):1119–29.e11. doi:10.1016/j.cell.2017.05.002
159. Scharschmidt TC, Vasquez KS, Truong HA, Gearty SV, Pauli ML, Nosbaum A, et al. A wave of regulatory T cells into neonatal skin mediates tolerance to commensal microbes. *Immunity* (2015) 43(5):1011–21. doi:10.1016/j.immuni.2015.10.016
160. Povoleri GA, Scotta C, Nova-Lamperti EA, John S, Lombardi G, Afzali B. Thymic versus induced regulatory T cells – who regulates the regulators? *Front Immunol* (2013) 4:169. doi:10.3389/fimmu.2013.00169
161. Huehn J, Polansky JK, Hamann A. Epigenetic control of FOXP3 expression: the key to a stable regulatory T-cell lineage? *Nat Rev Immunol* (2009) 9(2):83–9. doi:10.1038/nri2474
162. Hadeiba H, Lahl K, Edalati A, Oderup C, Habtezion A, Pachynski R, et al. Plasmacytoid dendritic cells transport peripheral antigens to the thymus to promote central tolerance. *Immunity* (2012) 36(3):438–50. doi:10.1016/j.immuni.2012.01.017
163. Kohli K, Janssen A, Forster R. Plasmacytoid dendritic cells induce tolerance predominantly by cargoing antigen to lymph nodes. *Eur J Immunol* (2016) 46(11):2659–68. doi:10.1002/eji.201646359
164. Nestle FO, Conrad C, Tun-Kyi A, Homey B, Gombert M, Boyman O, et al. Plasmacytoid predendritic cells initiate psoriasis through interferon-alpha production. *J Exp Med* (2005) 202(1):135–43. doi:10.1084/jem.20050500
165. Gregorio J, Meller S, Conrad C, Di Nardo A, Homey B, Lauerma A, et al. Plasmacytoid dendritic cells sense skin injury and promote wound healing through type I interferons. *J Exp Med* (2010) 207(13):2921–30. doi:10.1084/jem.20101102
166. Rosenblum MD, Gratz IK, Paw JS, Lee K, Marshak-Rothstein A, Abbas AK. Response to self antigen imprints regulatory memory in tissues. *Nature* (2011) 480(7378):538–42. doi:10.1038/nature10664
167. van der Veeken J, Gonzalez AJ, Cho H, Arvey A, Hemmers S, Leslie CS, et al. Memory of inflammation in regulatory T cells. *Cell* (2016) 166:977–90. doi:10.1016/j.cell.2016.07.006
168. Sather BD, Treuting P, Perdue N, Miazgowicz M, Fontenot JD, Rudensky AY, et al. Altering the distribution of Foxp3(+) regulatory T cells results in tissue-specific inflammatory disease. *J Exp Med* (2007) 204(6):1335–47. doi:10.1084/jem.20070081
169. Campbell JJ, Haraldsen G, Pan J, Rottman J, Qin S, Ponath P, et al. The chemokine receptor CCR4 in vascular recognition by cutaneous but not intestinal memory T cells. *Nature* (1999) 400(6746):776–80. doi:10.1038/23495
170. Horikawa T, Nakayama T, Hikita I, Yamada H, Fujisawa R, Bito T, et al. IFN-gamma-inducible expression of thymus and activation-regulated chemokine/CCL17 and macrophage-derived chemokine/CCL22 in epidermal keratinocytes and their roles in atopic dermatitis. *Int Immunol* (2002) 14(7):767–73. doi:10.1093/intimm/dxf044
171. Yoshie O, Matsushima K. CCR4 and its ligands: from bench to bedside. *Int Immunol* (2015) 27(1):11–20. doi:10.1093/intimm/dxu079
172. Mariani M, Lang R, Binda E, Panina-Bordignon P, D'Ambrosio D. Dominance of CCL22 over CCL17 in induction of chemokine receptor CCR4 desensitization and internalization on human Th2 cells. *Eur J Immunol* (2004) 34(1):231–40. doi:10.1002/eji.200324429
173. Belkaid Y, Hand TW. Role of the microbiota in immunity and inflammation. *Cell* (2014) 157(1):121–41. doi:10.1016/j.cell.2014.03.011
174. Belkaid Y, Segre JA. Dialogue between skin microbiota and immunity. *Science* (2014) 346(6212):954–9. doi:10.1126/science.1260144
175. Yang S, Fujikado N, Kolodin D, Benoist C, Mathis D. Immune tolerance. Regulatory T cells generated early in life play a distinct role in maintaining self-tolerance. *Science* (2015) 348(6234):589–94. doi:10.1126/science.aaa7017
176. Sardella C, Winkler C, Quignodon L, Hardman JA, Toffoli B, Giordano Attianese GMP, et al. Delayed hair follicle morphogenesis and hair follicle dystrophy in a lipoatrophy mouse model of Pparg total deletion. *J Invest Dermatol* (2018) 138(3):500–10. doi:10.1016/j.jid.2017.09.024

177. Coulson-Thomas VJ, Gesteira TF, Esko J, Kao W. Heparan sulfate regulates hair follicle and sebaceous gland morphogenesis and homeostasis. *J Biol Chem* (2014) 289(36):25211–26. doi:10.1074/jbc.M114.572511
178. Nagao K, Kobayashi T, Moro K, Ohyama M, Adachi T, Kitashima DY, et al. Stress-induced production of chemokines by hair follicles regulates the trafficking of dendritic cells in skin. *Nat Immunol* (2012) 13(8):744–52. doi:10.1038/ni.2353
179. Scharschmidt TC, Vasquez KS, Pauli ML, Leitner EG, Chu K, Truong HA, et al. Commensal microbes and hair follicle morphogenesis coordinately drive Treg migration into neonatal skin. *Cell Host Microbe* (2017) 21(4): 467–77.e5. doi:10.1016/j.chom.2017.03.001
180. Naik S, Bouladoux N, Wilhelm C, Molloy MJ, Salcedo R, Kastenmuller W, et al. Compartmentalized control of skin immunity by resident commensals. *Science* (2012) 337(6098):1115–9. doi:10.1126/science.1225152
181. Yamazaki S, Nishioka A, Kasuya S, Ohkura N, Hemmi H, Kaisho T, et al. Homeostasis of thymus-derived Foxp3+ regulatory T cells is controlled by ultraviolet B exposure in the skin. *J Immunol* (2014) 193(11):5488–97. doi:10.4049/jimmunol.1400985
182. Bernard JJ, Cowing-Zitron C, Nakatsuji T, Muehleisen B, Muto J, Borkowski AW, et al. Ultraviolet radiation damages self noncoding RNA and is detected by TLR3. *Nat Med* (2012) 18(8):1286–90. doi:10.1038/nm.2861
183. Racz E, Prens EP. Phototherapy of psoriasis, a chronic inflammatory skin disease. *Adv Exp Med Biol* (2017) 996:287–94. doi:10.1007/978-3-319-56017-5_24
184. Davis DM, Borok J, Udkoff J, Lio P, Spergel J. Atopic dermatitis: phototherapy and systemic therapy. *Semin Cutan Med Surg* (2017) 36(3):118–23. doi:10.12788/j.sder.2017.027
185. Fujisaki J, Wu J, Carlson AL, Silberstein L, Putheti P, Larocca R, et al. In vivo imaging of Treg cells providing immune privilege to the haematopoietic stem-cell niche. *Nature* (2011) 474(7350):216–9. doi:10.1038/nature10160
186. Nosbaum A, Prevel N, Truong HA, Mehta P, Ettinger M, Scharschmidt TC, et al. Cutting edge: regulatory T cells facilitate cutaneous wound healing. *J Immunol* (2016) 196(5):2010–4. doi:10.4049/jimmunol.1502139
187. Bodnar RJ. Epidermal growth factor and epidermal growth factor receptor: the Yin and Yang in the treatment of cutaneous wounds and cancer. *Adv Wound Care (New Rochelle)* (2013) 2(1):24–9. doi:10.1089/wound.2011.0326
188. Burzyn D, Kuswanto W, Kolodin D, Shadrach JL, Cerletti M, Jang Y, et al. A special population of regulatory T cells potentiates muscle repair. *Cell* (2013) 155(6):1282–95. doi:10.1016/j.cell.2013.10.054
189. Dvorak HF. Tumors: wounds that do not heal. Similarities between tumor stroma generation and wound healing. *N Engl J Med* (1986) 315(26):1650–9. doi:10.1056/NEJM198612253152606
190. Dvorak HF. Tumors: wounds that do not heal-redux. *Cancer Immunol Res* (2015) 3(1):1–11. doi:10.1158/2326-6066.CIR-14-0209
191. Balkwill F, Mantovani A. Inflammation and cancer: back to Virchow? *Lancet* (2001) 357(9255):539–45. doi:10.1016/S0140-6736(00)04046-0
192. Zheng C, Zheng L, Yoo JK, Guo H, Zhang Y, Guo X, et al. Landscape of infiltrating T cells in liver cancer revealed by single-cell sequencing. *Cell* (2017) 169(7):1342–56.e16. doi:10.1016/j.cell.2017.05.035
193. Nagase H, Takeoka T, Urakawa S, Morimoto-Okazawa A, Kawashima A, Iwahori K, et al. ICOS(+) Foxp3(+) TILs in gastric cancer are prognostic markers and effector regulatory T cells associated with *Helicobacter pylori*. *Int J Cancer* (2017) 140(3):686–95. doi:10.1002/ijc.30475
194. Akimova T, Zhang T, Negorev D, Singhal S, Stadanlick J, Rao A, et al. Human lung tumor FOXP3+ Tregs upregulate four "Treg-locking" transcription factors. *JCI Insight* (2017) 2(16):1–20. doi:10.1172/jci.insight.94075
195. Loyher PL, Rochefort J, Baudesson de Chanville C, Hamon P, Lescaille G, Bertolus C, et al. CCR2 influences T regulatory cell migration to tumors and serves as a biomarker of cyclophosphamide sensitivity. *Cancer Res* (2016) 76(22):6483–94. doi:10.1158/0008-5472.CAN-16-0984
196. You Y, Li Y, Li M, Lei M, Wu M, Qu Y, et al. Ovarian cancer stem cells promote tumour immune privilege and invasion via CCL5 and regulatory T cells. *Clin Exp Immunol* (2018) 191(1):60–73. doi:10.1111/cei.13044
197. Tang Y, Xu X, Guo S, Zhang C, Tang Y, Tian Y, et al. An increased abundance of tumor-infiltrating regulatory T cells is correlated with the progression and prognosis of pancreatic ductal adenocarcinoma. *PLoS One* (2014) 9(3):e91551. doi:10.1371/journal.pone.0091551
198. Vence L, Palucka AK, Fay JW, Ito T, Liu YJ, Banchereau J, et al. Circulating tumor antigen-specific regulatory T cells in patients with metastatic melanoma. *Proc Natl Acad Sci U S A* (2007) 104(52):20884–9. doi:10.1073/pnas.0710557105
199. Overacre-Delgoffe AE, Chikina M, Dadey RE, Yano H, Brunazzi EA, Shayan G, et al. Interferon-gamma drives Treg fragility to promote antitumor immunity. *Cell* (2017) 169(6):1130–41.e11. doi:10.1016/j.cell.2017.05.005
200. Salama P, Phillips M, Grieu F, Morris M, Zeps N, Joseph D, et al. Tumor-infiltrating FOXP3+ T regulatory cells show strong prognostic significance in colorectal cancer. *J Clin Oncol* (2009) 27(2):186–92. doi:10.1200/JCO.2008.18.7229
201. Frey DM, Droeser RA, Viehl CT, Zlobec I, Lugli A, Zingg U, et al. High frequency of tumor-infiltrating FOXP3(+) regulatory T cells predicts improved survival in mismatch repair-proficient colorectal cancer patients. *Int J Cancer* (2010) 126(11):2635–43. doi:10.1002/ijc.24989
202. Sinicrope FA, Rego RL, Ansell SM, Knutson KL, Foster NR, Sargent DJ. Intraepithelial effector (CD3+)/regulatory (FoxP3+) T-cell ratio predicts a clinical outcome of human colon carcinoma. *Gastroenterology* (2009) 137(4): 1270–9. doi:10.1053/j.gastro.2009.06.053
203. Miyara M, Yoshioka Y, Kitoh A, Shima T, Wing K, Niwa A, et al. Functional delineation and differentiation dynamics of human CD4+ T cells expressing the FoxP3 transcription factor. *Immunity* (2009) 30(6):899–911. doi:10.1016/j.immuni.2009.03.019
204. Sakaguchi S, Miyara M, Costantino CM, Hafler DA. FOXP3+ regulatory T cells in the human immune system. *Nat Rev Immunol* (2010) 10(7):490–500. doi:10.1038/nri2785
205. Saito T, Nishikawa H, Wada H, Nagano Y, Sugiyama D, Atarashi K, et al. Two FOXP3(+)CD4(+) T cell subpopulations distinctly control the prognosis of colorectal cancers. *Nat Med* (2016) 22(6):679–84. doi:10.1038/nm.4086
206. Stover DG, Bierie B, Moses HL. A delicate balance: TGF-beta and the tumor microenvironment. *J Cell Biochem* (2007) 101(4):851–61. doi:10.1002/jcb.21149
207. Pickup M, Novitskiy S, Moses HL. The roles of TGFbeta in the tumour microenvironment. *Nat Rev Cancer* (2013) 13(11):788–99. doi:10.1038/nrc3603
208. Bilate AM, Lafaille JJ. Induced CD4+Foxp3+ regulatory T cells in immune tolerance. *Annu Rev Immunol* (2012) 30:733–58. doi:10.1146/annurev-immunol-020711-075043
209. Getnet D, Maris CH, Hipkiss EL, Grosso JF, Harris TJ, Yen HR, et al. Tumor recognition and self-recognition induce distinct transcriptional profiles in antigen-specific CD4 T cells. *J Immunol* (2009) 182(8):4675–85. doi:10.4049/jimmunol.0803400
210. Zhou G, Levitsky HI. Natural regulatory T cells and de novo-induced regulatory T cells contribute independently to tumor-specific tolerance. *J Immunol* (2007) 178(4):2155–62. doi:10.4049/jimmunol.178.4.2155
211. van Rooij N, van Buuren MM, Philips D, Velds A, Toebes M, Heemskerk B, et al. Tumor exome analysis reveals neoantigen-specific T-cell reactivity in an ipilimumab-responsive melanoma. *J Clin Oncol* (2013) 31(32):e439–42. doi:10.1200/JCO.2012.47.7521
212. Cohen CJ, Gartner JJ, Horovitz-Fried M, Shamalov K, Trebska-McGowan K, Bliskovsky VV, et al. Isolation of neoantigen-specific T cells from tumor and peripheral lymphocytes. *J Clin Invest* (2015) 125(10):3981–91. doi:10.1172/JCI82416
213. Johanns TM, Ward JP, Miller CA, Wilson C, Kobayashi DK, Bender D, et al. Endogenous neoantigen-specific CD8 T cells identified in two glioblastoma models using a cancer immunogenomics approach. *Cancer Immunol Res* (2016) 4(12):1007–15. doi:10.1158/2326-6066.CIR-16-0156
214. Malchow S, Leventhal DS, Nishi S, Fischer BI, Shen L, Paner GP, et al. Aire-dependent thymic development of tumor-associated regulatory T cells. *Science* (2013) 339(6124):1219–24. doi:10.1126/science.1233913
215. Hindley JP, Ferreira C, Jones E, Lauder SN, Ladell K, Wynn KK, et al. Analysis of the T-cell receptor repertoires of tumor-infiltrating conventional and regulatory T cells reveals no evidence for conversion in carcinogen-induced tumors. *Cancer Res* (2011) 71(3):736–46. doi:10.1158/0008-5472.CAN-10-1797
216. Sainz-Perez A, Lim A, Lemercier B, Leclerc C. The T-cell receptor repertoire of tumor-infiltrating regulatory T lymphocytes is skewed toward public sequences. *Cancer Res* (2012) 72(14):3557–69. doi:10.1158/0008-5472.CAN-12-0277
217. Plitas G, Konopacki C, Wu K, Bos PD, Morrow M, Putintseva EV, et al. Regulatory T cells exhibit distinct features in human breast cancer. *Immunity* (2016) 45(5):1122–34. doi:10.1016/j.immuni.2016.10.032

218. Leonard JD, Gilmore DC, Dileepan T, Nawrocka WI, Chao JL, Schoenbach MH, et al. Identification of natural regulatory T cell epitopes reveals convergence on a dominant autoantigen. *Immunity* (2017) 47(1):107–17.e8. doi:10.1016/j.immuni.2017.06.015
219. Waight JD, Takai S, Marelli B, Qin G, Hance KW, Zhang D, et al. Cutting edge: epigenetic regulation of Foxp3 defines a stable population of CD4+ regulatory T cells in tumors from mice and humans. *J Immunol* (2015) 194(3):878–82. doi:10.4049/jimmunol.1402725
220. Polansky JK, Kretschmer K, Freyer J, Floess S, Garbe A, Baron U, et al. DNA methylation controls Foxp3 gene expression. *Eur J Immunol* (2008) 38(6):1654–63. doi:10.1002/eji.200838105
221. Ohkura N, Hamaguchi M, Morikawa H, Sugimura K, Tanaka A, Ito Y, et al. T cell receptor stimulation-induced epigenetic changes and Foxp3 expression are independent and complementary events required for Treg cell development. *Immunity* (2012) 37(5):785–99. doi:10.1016/j.immuni.2012.09.010
222. De Simone M, Arrigoni A, Rossetti G, Gruarin P, Ranzani V, Politano C, et al. Transcriptional landscape of human tissue lymphocytes unveils uniqueness of tumor-infiltrating T regulatory cells. *Immunity* (2016) 45(5):1135–47. doi:10.1016/j.immuni.2016.10.021
223. Sobecki M, Mrouj K, Camasses A, Parisis N, Nicolas E, Lleres D, et al. The cell proliferation antigen Ki-67 organises heterochromatin. *Elife* (2016) 5:e13722. doi:10.7554/eLife.13722
224. Hayatsu N, Miyao T, Tachibana M, Murakami R, Kimura A, Kato T, et al. Analyses of a mutant Foxp3 allele reveal BATF as a critical transcription factor in the differentiation and accumulation of tissue regulatory T cells. *Immunity* (2017) 47(2):268–83.e9. doi:10.1016/j.immuni.2017.07.008
225. Soler D, Chapman TR, Poisson LR, Wang L, Cote-Sierra J, Ryan M, et al. CCR8 expression identifies CD4 memory T cells enriched for FOXP3+ regulatory and Th2 effector lymphocytes. *J Immunol* (2006) 177(10):6940–51. doi:10.4049/jimmunol.177.10.6940
226. Islam SA, Chang DS, Colvin RA, Byrne MH, McCully ML, Moser B, et al. Mouse CCL8, a CCR8 agonist, promotes atopic dermatitis by recruiting IL-5+ T(H)2 cells. *Nat Immunol* (2011) 12(2):167–77. doi:10.1038/ni.1984
227. Nakayama T, Kato Y, Hieshima K, Nagakubo D, Kunori Y, Fujisawa T, et al. Liver-expressed chemokine/CC chemokine ligand 16 attracts eosinophils by interacting with histamine H4 receptor. *J Immunol* (2004) 173(3):2078–83. doi:10.4049/jimmunol.173.3.2078
228. Islam SA, Ling MF, Leung J, Shreffler WG, Luster AD. Identification of human CCR8 as a CCL18 receptor. *J Exp Med* (2013) 210(10):1889–98. doi:10.1084/jem.20130240
229. Xie Q, Klesney-Tait J, Keck K, Parlet C, Borcherding N, Kolb R, et al. Characterization of a novel mouse model with genetic deletion of CD177. *Protein Cell* (2015) 6(2):117–26. doi:10.1007/s13238-014-0109-1
230. Murata M, Yudoh K, Shimizu H, Beppu M, Nakamura H, Kato T, et al. Layilin, a talin-binding hyaluronan receptor, is expressed in human articular chondrocytes and synoviocytes and is down-regulated by interleukin-1beta. *Mod Rheumatol* (2013) 23(3):478–88. doi:10.3109/s10165-012-0686-x
231. Kurose K, Ohue Y, Wada H, Iida S, Ishida T, Kojima T, et al. Phase Ia study of FoxP3+ CD4 Treg depletion by infusion of a humanized anti-CCR4 antibody, KW-0761, in cancer patients. *Clin Cancer Res* (2015) 21(19):4327–36. doi:10.1158/1078-0432.CCR-15-0357
232. Barsheshet Y, Wildbaum G, Levy E, Vitenshtein A, Akinseye C, Griggs J, et al. CCR8(+)FOXp3(+) Treg cells as master drivers of immune regulation. *Proc Natl Acad Sci U S A* (2017) 114(23):6086–91. doi:10.1073/pnas.1621280114
233. Liu C, Workman CJ, Vignali DA. Targeting regulatory T cells in tumors. *FEBS J* (2016) 283(14):2731–48. doi:10.1111/febs.13656
234. Campbell DJ, Koch MA. Phenotypical and functional specialization of FOXP3+ regulatory T cells. *Nat Rev Immunol* (2011) 11(2):119–30. doi:10.1038/nri2916
235. Chinen T, Kannan AK, Levine AG, Fan X, Klein U, Zheng Y, et al. An essential role for the IL-2 receptor in Treg cell function. *Nat Immunol* (2016) 17(11):1322–33. doi:10.1038/ni.3540
236. Cao X, Cai SF, Fehniger TA, Song J, Collins LI, Piwnica-Worms DR, et al. Granzyme B and perforin are important for regulatory T cell-mediated suppression of tumor clearance. *Immunity* (2007) 27(4):635–46. doi:10.1016/j.immuni.2007.08.014
237. Wing K, Onishi Y, Prieto-Martin P, Yamaguchi T, Miyara M, Fehervari Z, et al. CTLA-4 control over Foxp3+ regulatory T cell function. *Science* (2008) 322(5899):271–5. doi:10.1126/science.1160062
238. Sharma MD, Shinde R, McGaha TL, Huang L, Holmgaard RB, Wolchok JD, et al. The PTEN pathway in Tregs is a critical driver of the suppressive tumor microenvironment. *Sci Adv* (2015) 1(10):e1500845. doi:10.1126/sciadv.1500845
239. Jacobs JF, Idema AJ, Bol KF, Nierkens S, Grauer OM, Wesseling P, et al. Regulatory T cells and the PD-L1/PD-1 pathway mediate immune suppression in malignant human brain tumors. *Neuro Oncol* (2009) 11(4):394–402. doi:10.1215/15228517-2008-104
240. Liang B, Workman C, Lee J, Chew C, Dale BM, Colonna L, et al. Regulatory T cells inhibit dendritic cells by lymphocyte activation gene-3 engagement of MHC class II. *J Immunol* (2008) 180(9):5916–26. doi:10.4049/jimmunol.180.9.5916
241. Gautron AS, Dominguez-Villar M, de Marcken M, Hafler DA. Enhanced suppressor function of TIM-3+ FoxP3+ regulatory T cells. *Eur J Immunol* (2014) 44(9):2703–11. doi:10.1002/eji.201344392
242. Stagg J, Divisekera U, Duret H, Sparwasser T, Teng MW, Darcy PK, et al. CD73-deficient mice have increased antitumor immunity and are resistant to experimental metastasis. *Cancer Res* (2011) 71(8):2892–900. doi:10.1158/0008-5472.CAN-10-4246
243. Borsellino G, Kleinewietfeld M, Di Mitri D, Sternjak A, Diamantini A, Giometto R, et al. Expression of ectonucleotidase CD39 by Foxp3+ Treg cells: hydrolysis of extracellular ATP and immune suppression. *Blood* (2007) 110(4):1225–32. doi:10.1182/blood-2006-12-064527
244. Maj T, Wang W, Crespo J, Zhang H, Wang W, Wei S, et al. Oxidative stress controls regulatory T cell apoptosis and suppressor activity and PD-L1-blockade resistance in tumor. *Nat Immunol* (2017) 18(12):1332–41. doi:10.1038/ni.3868
245. Li N, Alam J, Venkatesan MI, Eiguren-Fernandez A, Schmitz D, Di Stefano E, et al. Nrf2 is a key transcription factor that regulates antioxidant defense in macrophages and epithelial cells: protecting against the proinflammatory and oxidizing effects of diesel exhaust chemicals. *J Immunol* (2004) 173(5):3467–81. doi:10.4049/jimmunol.173.5.3467
246. Balachandran VP, Cavnar MJ, Zeng S, Bamboat ZM, Ocuin LM, Obaid H, et al. Imatinib potentiates antitumor T cell responses in gastrointestinal stromal tumor through the inhibition of Ido. *Nat Med* (2011) 17(9):1094–100. doi:10.1038/nm.2438
247. Delgoffe GM, Woo SR, Turnis ME, Gravano DM, Guy C, Overacre AE, et al. Stability and function of regulatory T cells is maintained by a neuropilin-1-semaphorin-4a axis. *Nature* (2013) 501(7466):252–6. doi:10.1038/nature12428
248. Noman MZ, Hasmim M, Messai Y, Terry S, Kieda C, Janji B, et al. Hypoxia: a key player in antitumor immune response. A review in the theme: cellular responses to hypoxia. *Am J Physiol Cell Physiol* (2015) 309(9):C569–79. doi:10.1152/ajpcell.00207.2015
249. Wilson WR, Hay MP. Targeting hypoxia in cancer therapy. *Nat Rev Cancer* (2011) 11(6):393–410. doi:10.1038/nrc3064
250. Tan W, Zhang W, Strasner A, Grivennikov S, Cheng JQ, Hoffman RM, et al. Tumour-infiltrating regulatory T cells stimulate mammary cancer metastasis through RANKL-RANK signalling. *Nature* (2011) 470(7335):548–53. doi:10.1038/nature09707
251. Cao Y, Luo JL, Karin M. IkappaB kinase alpha kinase activity is required for self-renewal of ErbB2/Her2-transformed mammary tumor-initiating cells. *Proc Natl Acad Sci U S A* (2007) 104(40):15852–7. doi:10.1073/pnas.0706728104
252. Luo JL, Tan W, Ricono JM, Korchynskyi O, Zhang M, Gonias SL, et al. Nuclear cytokine-activated IKK alpha controls prostate cancer metastasis by repressing Maspin. *Nature* (2007) 446(7136):690–4. doi:10.1038/nature05656
253. Mock JR, Garibaldi BT, Aggarwal NR, Jenkins J, Limjunyawong N, Singer BD, et al. Foxp3+ regulatory T cells promote lung epithelial proliferation. *Mucosal Immunol* (2014) 7(6):1440–51. doi:10.1038/mi.2014.33
254. Le G, Lowe DA, Kyba M. Freeze injury of the tibialis anterior muscle. *Methods Mol Biol* (2016) 1460:33–41. doi:10.1007/978-1-4939-3810-0_3
255. Warren GL, Hulderman T, Mishra D, Gao X, Millecchia L, O'Farrell L, et al. Chemokine receptor CCR2 involvement in skeletal muscle regeneration. *FASEB J* (2005) 19(3):413–5. doi:10.1096/fj.04-2421fje

256. Chu M, Gregorio CC, Pappas CT. Nebulin, a multi-functional giant. *J Exp Biol* (2016) 219(Pt 2):146–52. doi:10.1242/jeb.126383
257. Kuswanto W, Burzyn D, Panduro M, Wang KK, Jang YC, Wagers AJ, et al. Poor repair of skeletal muscle in aging mice reflects a defect in local, interleukin-33-dependent accumulation of regulatory T cells. *Immunity* (2016) 44(2):355–67. doi:10.1016/j.immuni.2016.01.009
258. Hui SP, Sheng DZ, Sugimoto K, Gonzalez-Rajal A, Nakagawa S, Hesselson D, et al. Zebrafish regulatory T cells mediate organ-specific regenerative programs. *Dev Cell* (2017) 43(6):659–72.e5. doi:10.1016/j.devcel.2017.11.010
259. Samstein RM, Josefowicz SZ, Arvey A, Treuting PM, Rudensky AY. Extrathymic generation of regulatory T cells in placental mammals mitigates maternal-fetal conflict. *Cell* (2012) 150(1):29–38. doi:10.1016/j.cell.2012.05.031
260. Robertson SA, Prins JR, Sharkey DJ, Moldenhauer LM. Seminal fluid and the generation of regulatory T cells for embryo implantation. *Am J Reprod Immunol* (2013) 69(4):315–30. doi:10.1111/aji.12107
261. Ruocco MG, Chaouat G, Florez L, Bensussan A, Klatzmann D. Regulatory T-cells in pregnancy: historical perspective, state of the art, and burning questions. *Front Immunol* (2014) 5:389. doi:10.3389/fimmu.2014.00389
262. Arruvito L, Sanz M, Banham AH, Fainboim L. Expansion of CD4+CD25+and FOXP3+ regulatory T cells during the follicular phase of the menstrual cycle: implications for human reproduction. *J Immunol* (2007) 178(4):2572–8. doi:10.4049/jimmunol.178.4.2572
263. McGovern N, Shin A, Low G, Low D, Duan K, Yao LJ, et al. Human fetal dendritic cells promote prenatal T-cell immune suppression through arginase-2. *Nature* (2017) 546(7660):662–6. doi:10.1038/nature22795
264. Mold JE, Michaelsson J, Burt TD, Muench MO, Beckerman KP, Busch MP, et al. Maternal alloantigens promote the development of tolerogenic fetal regulatory T cells in utero. *Science* (2008) 322(5907):1562–5. doi:10.1126/science.1164511
265. Allenspach EJ, Finn LS, Rendi MH, Eken A, Singh AK, Oukka M, et al. Absence of functional fetal regulatory T cells in humans causes in utero organ-specific autoimmunity. *J Allergy Clin Immunol* (2017) 140(2):616–9.e7. doi:10.1016/j.jaci.2017.02.017
266. Tung KS, Harakal J, Qiao H, Rival C, Li JC, Paul AG, et al. Egress of sperm autoantigen from seminiferous tubules maintains systemic tolerance. *J Clin Invest* (2017) 127(3):1046–60. doi:10.1172/JCI89927
267. Deliyanti D, Talia DM, Zhu T, Maxwell MJ, Agrotis A, Jerome JR, et al. Foxp3(+) Tregs are recruited to the retina to repair pathological angiogenesis. *Nat Commun* (2017) 8(1):748. doi:10.1038/s41467-017-00751-w
268. Naldaiz-Gastesi N, Goicoechea M, Alonso-Martin S, Aiastui A, Lopez-Mayorga M, Garcia-Belda P, et al. Identification and characterization of the dermal panniculus carnosus muscle stem cells. *Stem Cell Reports* (2016) 7(3):411–24. doi:10.1016/j.stemcr.2016.08.002
269. MacDonald KG, Hoeppli RE, Huang Q, Gillies J, Luciani DS, Orban PC, et al. Alloantigen-specific regulatory T cells generated with a chimeric antigen receptor. *J Clin Invest* (2016) 126(4):1413–24. doi:10.1172/JCI82771
270. Angelin A, Gil-de-Gomez L, Dahiya S, Jiao J, Guo L, Levine MH, et al. Foxp3 reprograms T cell metabolism to function in low-glucose, high-lactate environments. *Cell Metab* (2017) 25:1282–93.e7. doi:10.1016/j.cmet.2016.12.018
271. Gerriets VA, Kishton RJ, Johnson MO, Cohen S, Siska PJ, Nichols AG, et al. Foxp3 and toll-like receptor signaling balance Treg cell anabolic metabolism for suppression. *Nat Immunol* (2016) 17:1459–66. doi:10.1038/ni.3577
272. Ho PC, Bihuniak JD, Macintyre AN, Staron M, Liu X, Amezquita R, et al. Phosphoenolpyruvate is a metabolic checkpoint of anti-tumor T cell responses. *Cell* (2015) 162(6):1217–28. doi:10.1016/j.cell.2015.08.012
273. Kishore M, Cheung KCP, Fu H, Bonacina F, Wang G, Coe D, et al. Regulatory T cell migration is dependent on glucokinase-mediated glycolysis. *Immunity* (2017) 47(5):875–89.e10. doi:10.1016/j.immuni.2017.10.017

10

Epigenetic codes programing class switch recombination

Bharat Vaidyanathan[1,2] and Jayanta Chaudhuri[1,2*]

[1] Immunology and Microbial Pathogenesis Program, Weill Cornell Graduate School, New York, NY, USA, [2] Immunology Program, Sloan Kettering Institute, New York, NY, USA

Edited by:
Paolo Casali,
The University of Texas Health Science Center at San Antonio, USA

Reviewed by:
Almudena R. Ramiro,
Centro Nacional de Investigaciones Cardiovasculares, Spain
Claude-Agnes Reynaud,
INSERM, France
Hong Zan,
The University of Texas Health Science Center at San Antonio, USA

***Correspondence:**
Jayanta Chaudhuri,
1275 York Avenue, New York, NY 10065, USA
chaudhuj@mskcc.org

Class switch recombination imparts B cells with a fitness-associated adaptive advantage during a humoral immune response by using a precision-tailored DNA excision and ligation process to swap the default constant region gene of the antibody with a new one that has unique effector functions. This secondary diversification of the antibody repertoire is a hallmark of the adaptability of B cells when confronted with environmental and pathogenic challenges. Given that the nucleotide sequence of genes during class switching remains unchanged (genetic constraints), it is logical and necessary therefore, to integrate the adaptability of B cells to an epigenetic state, which is dynamic and can be heritably modulated before, after, or even during an antibody-dependent immune response. Epigenetic regulation encompasses heritable changes that affect function (phenotype) without altering the sequence information embedded in a gene, and include histone, DNA and RNA modifications. Here, we review current literature on how B cells use an epigenetic code language as a means to ensure antibody plasticity in light of pathogenic insults.

Keywords: AID, DNA repair, DNA deamination, recombination, non-coding RNAs

Introduction

Genes are the basic molecular unit of heredity in all organisms since it is the gene (genotype) and not the trait (phenotype; except for imprinted genes) that is inherited. A gene usually refers to a particular sequence of nucleotides that has an annotated function. However, phenotypic manifestations can be governed by factors beyond (epi) genes (genetics), which too are hereditary. Epigenetic alterations are carried out by a repertoire of modifiers (writers and erasers) and readers, which can act on either proteins (histones) or nucleic acid (DNA/RNA) (1–3). Epigenetic regulation also includes non-coding RNAs (micro-RNA and long non-coding RNA), which can directly or indirectly (via recruitment of proteins) affect gene expression (4–6). This complex layer of gene regulation is a testament to the pliability that the system needs and possesses. The immune system exemplifies one such complex system that is geared to adapt to the environment, and B cells that make antibodies also need to reshape their antibody repertoire during antigenic challenges. Thus, it is not surprising that B cells overcome genetic constraints and integrate environmental cues into a complex network of gene regulation, which is both flexible and heritable. Dynamic epigenetic alterations engineered with spatiotemporal precision that expand the genetic code beyond A, G, C, and T, would be ideal for B cells in their quest to diversify the antibody repertoire during infection by an ever-evolving array of pathogens.

Class switch recombination (CSR) is one such secondary antibody diversification that occurs in peripheral lymphoid organs when B cells encounter antigen, and is dependent on cytokine/chemokine cues generated by T cells and stromal cells (7). The switching of the antibody isotype from IgM (or IgD)

to IgG, IgE, or IgA is necessary to impart distinct effector functions (8, 9). At the molecular level, CSR is a deletional-recombination reaction occurring between repetitive DNA elements, called switch (S) regions that precede each constant region (C_H) segment. Cytokine stimulation and/or antigen binding to B cells stimulate "germline" transcription through the S regions and promote accessibility of the DNA deaminase AID (activation-induced cytidine deaminase), whose activity leads to the generation of DNA double-strand breaks (DSBs) at S regions. End-joining of DSBs between donor (usually Sμ) and acceptor S (Sγ, Sε, or Sα) regions replaces Cμ for a different C_H gene segment downstream of the rearranged variable region segment to complete CSR (**Figure 1**). The drivers of germline transcription, AID expression, its target specificity and factors in end-joining have been extensively studied and reviewed elsewhere in Ref. (8, 10–13).

The role of histone modifications, DNA methylation, and non-coding RNAs during CSR has been recognized and appreciated significantly in the last decade (4, 14, 15). Given that B cells encounter an inflammatory milieu during an immune response and since the same cues can also program epigenetic changes, it suffices to say that there must be an underlying intricate chromatin network landscape, which is shaped to govern CSR. In this review, we will focus on recent advances that buttress the existence of epigenetic codes that orchestrate CSR.

Epigenetic Control of Switch (S) Region Locus Accessibility and Antibody Response

S regions are highly repetitive G-rich sequences that precede each constant region gene. Transcription through these regions is necessary for CSR. However, constitutive (donor S region) and inducible (acceptor S region) transcription is associated either with a poised and dynamic epigenetic state, respectively (4). Donor S region (Sμ) has a transcriptionally active state even in naïve B cells, suggesting that it is poised for participation in CSR. Histone modifications like H3K4me3 and H3K9ac are present at Sμ in naïve B cells and increases upon stimulation (16–19). These are marks associated with an open chromatin conformation that would favor accessibility of the CSR machinery including tethering AID to donor S region.

On the other hand, the acceptor S regions (Sγ1, Sγ3, Sγ2a, Sε, and Sα) are inaccessible to the CSR machinery at the basal state. When the B cell faces an antigenic challenge that provides CSR triggers including T cell help (CD40 ligation), pattern-recognition receptor ligation and the cytokine milieu (IL4, TGFβ, retinoic acid, BAFF, and IFNγ), the cognate S acceptor region accumulate histone modifications that are permissive to transcription and accessibility of only the particular S acceptor participating in CSR. The alterations include removal of repressive chromatin marks (H3K9me3 and H3K27me3) and also induction of H3K9ac and H3K4me3 (**Figure 2**) (17, 18). Knockdown of histone chaperone FACT complex components (SSRP1 and SPT16), Spt6, and methyl transferases (Ash2 and Wdr5) in CH12F3 cells have revealed the pertinence of the histone marks in regulating locus accessibility and S region cleavage, and thus CSR to IgA, a function which extends beyond germline transcript induction (20–22). If the same holds true in primary B cells and is it generalizable for CSR to other antibody isotypes remains to be determined. Additionally, H3K9me3 mark found at donor S region can recruit HP1γ-KAP1 complex, which facilitates AID tethering (17). The enzyme Suv39h1, which is probably the histone methyl transferase involved in the deposition of this histone mark, plays a positive role in inducing CSR to IgA, since deletion of the gene impairs IgA CSR in primary B cells without affecting GLT (23). It is not specifically clear as to why there is isotype specificity if H3K9me3 is a donor S region mark.

A word of caution in the interpretation of all these results is warranted since most of the studies show strong correlative but

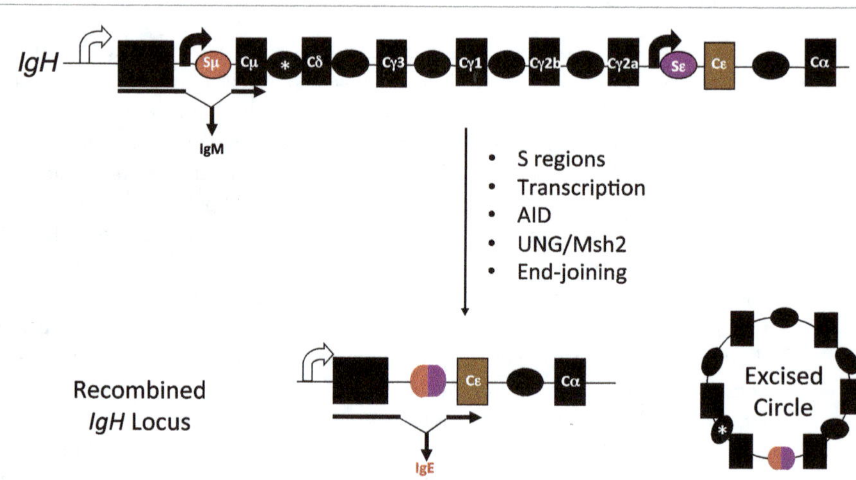

FIGURE 1 | Overview of CSR. Each of the CH genes is preceded by transcribed, repetitive DNA elements called switch (S) regions. AID mediated DNA deamination, followed by processing of deaminated cytidines by components of the base excision and mismatch repair machineries (UNG and Msh2, respectively) lead to the generation of DNA double-strand breaks. End-joining of double-strand breaks between donor and acceptor S regions completes CSR. Scheme for CSR to IgE is shown; block curved arrows indicate germline transcription from promoters upstream of Sμ and Sε; *represents a putative, but uncharacterized switch region upstream of Cδ.

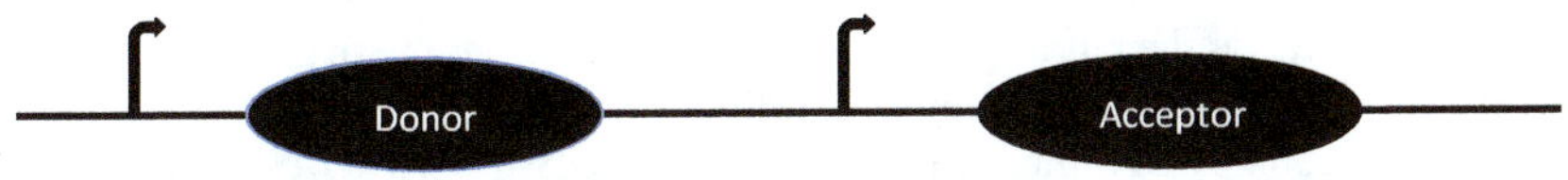

	Donor Naive	Donor Activated	Acceptor Naive	Acceptor Activated
H3K4me3	+	+++	-	+++
H3K9Ac	+	+++	-	+++
H3K9me3	+	-	+++	-
H3K27me3	-	-	+++	-

FIGURE 2 | The histone modifications on donor and acceptor S regions in naïve and activated B cells are shown.

not direct causative evidence; genetic models targeting the histone modifying enzymes would be required to unequivocally support the claims. Even the use of genetic or pharmacologic approach to manipulate histone modifications might not provide conclusive proof of their specific role in locus accessibility due to functional promiscuity/essentiality of the enzymes. Future studies are necessary to uncover the complex relationships that probably exist between multiple factors influenced by a single histone modification, and how an ensemble of spatiotemporal histone modifications orchestrates CSR.

The function of mixed-lineage leukemia (MLL)-like H3K4 methyl transferase complex in CSR was tested by deletion of a key component PTIP conditionally in B cells (24, 25). These studies revealed that compromised H3K4me and acetylation and global chromatin architectural changes associated with the loss of PTIP leads to decreased S region accessibility, germline transcription, and thus compromised CSR to multiple isotypes (24, 25).

The function of histone acetylation/deacetylation in B cells was uncovered by conditionally inactivating MOZ (H3K9 acetyl transferase) and HDAC-1 and -2 genes in mature B cells (26, 27). Stage-specific MOZ deletion suggested that it is required for optimal GC response (proper affinity maturation and memory formation) (26, 28). HDAC-1/2 were absolutely necessary for the proliferative burst that B cells undergo during stimulation for CSR, and double-deficient B cells fail to divide and die by apoptosis when challenged with LPS + IL4 (29). In contrast, pharmacological intervention with HDAC inhibitors, butyrate and valproic acid, *in vivo* during T-dependent/independent antibody response and *ex vivo*, did not affect B cell proliferation and viability (30). However, they did block CSR and plasma cell differentiation by upregulating cognate micro-RNAs that dampen AID and Blimp1, critical for CSR and plasma cell differentiation, respectively. Interestingly, the therapeutic potential of HDAC inhibitors in treating antibody-mediated lupus was highlighted by the finding that they ameliorated disease and prolonged survival in a mouse model of lupus (30). Discrepancies between genetic and pharmacological approaches can be due to milder effect of inhibitors or more broad effects on multiple HDACs beside HDAC-1/2.

Finally, the function of polycomb repressive complex (PRC)-2 component, Ezh2 (histone methyl transferase), which was shown to be necessary for B cell development (31), during GC response was tested by conditional inactivation of Ezh2 using Cγ1-cre (32, 33). Two independent studies provided compelling evidence that the germinal center (GC) formation and consequent cell-fate decisions including CSR, SHM, plasma cell differentiation and memory response are critically shaped by Ezh2 (32, 33). H3K27me3 and H3K4me3 ChIP-Seq in Ezh2-sufficient versus -deficient GC B cells revealed that Ezh2 negatively regulates terminal differentiation by epigenetically (via PRC2) regulating Blimp1, Xbp1, and Irf4, and thus promotes long-lasting immunity by sustaining antibody diversification and memory B cell differentiation (26, 33). Gain of function mutant Ezh2 alleles (found in lymphoma patients) cause GC hyperplasia in mice and cooperate with Bcl2 to accelerate and sustain malignant transformation of GC B cells (32). Combinational therapeutic targeting of Ezh2 for specific B cell malignancies (GC-DLBCL) will definitely be enticing (32, 33).

Epigenetic Control of AID Expression

AID is the key enzyme that is essential for CSR. It is probably one of the only proteins unique to stimulated mature B cells, and AID fate-mapping studies corroborate that physiologically functional levels of expression are largely restricted to B cells (34). It instigates DNA lesions in the form of deaminated deoxycytidine (dC), i.e., deoxyuridine (dU) at donor and acceptor S regions, which is subsequently processed by the general base excision repair, mismatch repair machineries, and DNA end-processing enzymes, such as, Mre11 and CtIP to generate DNA DSBs (10). Since it can induce DSBs, it is a potential mutator, and thus, AID expression is stringently controlled at the transcriptional and post-translational levels (8, 12). However, herein we review epigenetic factors modulating AID expression.

At the epigenetic level, AID expression is controlled by DNA methylation–demethylation and micro-RNAs. The AID locus, especially the promoter sites for cognate stimuli-induced transcriptional factors are hypermethylated in naïve B cells and the mark is reversibly modulated during different stages of B cell-fate program (35). Activated B cells or GC (GL7+Fas+) B cells acquire a permissive epigenetic landscape of hypomethylation that allows robust AID expression by STAT6, NF-κβ and Hox-C4 transcription factors (4). Besides, phylogenetic footprinting, histone acetylation, and DNase1 hypersensitivity site (DHS)-mapping revealed that the AID locus is dynamically shaped during an ongoing immune response (36). Histone H3 acetylation is increased at AID regulatory regions upon *in vitro* stimulation of naïve B cells and in GC B cells. In activated B cells, a conserved non-coding sequence 7kb downstream of the AID locus maps to a DHS and regulates AID expression positively, via the binding of a yet to be identified protein (36). However, AID is turned off epigenetically upon terminal differentiation, probably as a means to preserve antigen specificity of the antibody secreting B cells (36).

Post-transcriptional regulation of AID by micro-RNAs 155, 181b, 93, and 361, provides an additional layer of safeguard against a potent genome mutator (12). miR155, is the best studied one, which suppresses *aicda* expression by binding to a canonical site on the 3′-UTR of *aicda.* Although miR155 has functions way beyond suppressing AID in B cells undergoing CSR, as evidenced by compromised CSR in absence of miR155, yet its specific effect on regulating AID is significant. Mutation of the miR155-binding site on *aicda* 3′-UTR leads to increased AID levels that potentiate cMyc-IgH translocations (37, 38). Besides, miR155 and AID levels are inversely correlated in Burkitt's lymphoma, and an IL10/miR155 axis can potentially modulate AID expression during chronic inflammation and lymphomagenesis (39).

Epigenetic Control of AID Targeting

An enzyme like AID is a dual-edged sword; on one hand, it is mandatory for optimal humoral immunity but on the other, a threat to genomic integrity. Therefore, a normal B cell must delegate adequate layers of safeguard in addition to regulating AID expression, which would primarily target AID to the physiological targets. Genetic factors controlling AID targeting and function have been reviewed elsewhere in Ref. (12, 13, 40). Herein, we will focus on epigenetic guides of this potent mutator.

Histone Modifications

One way to limit the risk of collateral damage would be to sequester AID at hotspot target motifs. S regions are GC-rich and possess stretches of 5′-AGCT-3′, which are AID hotspots (13). These regions, when transcribed form stable R-loop structures that provide single-stranded DNA substrates for AID (10). An intriguing finding is that histone modifications, such as, H3S10 phosphorylation induced in CSR-activated B cells have also been linked to R-loop formation (41). Stable R-loops formed during CSR stimulation of B cells at S regions also accumulate H3K9AcS10ph modification. The classical adaptor protein 14-3-3, which has unique specificity for 5′-AGCT-3′ repeats and H3K9AcS10ph modification, also directly binds AID (42, 43). Thus, it is well poised to recruit AID to recombining S regions during CSR, thereby serving as transducers of the epigenetic code (4). It remains to be seen, however, if genome-wide occupancy of 14-3-3, H3K9AcS10ph, and AID overlap, or if 14-3-3 only functions during physiological AID targeting. Another study focused on the chromatin-bound AID-interactome to reveal that the RNA polymerase-associated factor (PAF) complex member LEO1 is required for efficient targeting of AID to Sμ in CH12F3A cells (44). It will be interesting to test if the function of LEO1 is also pertinent in B cells undergoing *ex vivo* CSR and more importantly in GC B cells. AID was also shown to bind the KAP1-HP1γ complex, the latter of which recognizes H3K9me3 (17). AID targeting was dependent on KAP1 and also on its association with HP1, since genetic manipulation studies clearly revealed that AID occupancy at Sμ was dampened due to loss of KAP1 alone or its interaction with HP1 (17).

Super-Enhancers and Regulatory Clusters

Enhancers are classically defined as a class of DNA elements that function in promoting transcription of gene from a distance, and irrespective of their orientation with respect to the target gene (45). Advance is sequencing techniques like DHS mapping (Dnase-seq), ChIP-seq and 3C-5C, Hi-Seq in the last decades has enabled genome-wide characterization of enhancers. Key features include presence of Dnasel hypersensitive sites, multiple transcription factor binding sites, histone modifications like H3K4me1 and H3K27Ac, and looping to contact promoter elements far apart in the genome (46). Essentially now, the presence of a chromatin profile as alluded to above is considered as a hallmark of enhancers, although to date these are strongly correlative yet not always functionally causative. A new class of regulatory DNA elements has been defined recently, termed super-enhancers or stretch-enhancers (47, 48). These are cell-type specific enhancers that play a key role in establishing lineage or cell identity (47, 48). They are defined as clusters of large regulatory domains that have remarkable enrichment for transcription factor and coactivator (Mediator) binding along with a characteristic chromatin landscape (nucleosome occupancy and histone modifications) (46). Since AID expression and CSR are unique to B cells, it would make sense to regulate this cell-type specific expression and targeting by integrating stimulation cues to topologically associated domains i.e., super-enhancers. Recent work from several laboratories has greatly advanced our understanding of AID targeting/mistargeting (49–51).

Using genome-wide sequencing approaches including GRO-seq, DNase-seq, and ChIP-seq, AID targets were found to be mostly unique in different cell-types (B cells, MEFs) although they shared common features of being transcriptionally active regions. However, transcription alone was not sufficient to explain the distinct set of hotspot in MEF versus B cells (49). Analysis of genes transcribed in both cell-types but only targeted in one, led to identification of a shared set of epigenetic attributes including H3K27Ac and H3K36me3, which typify enhancers (49). Deep sequencing techniques allowed uncovering a remarkable overlap of AID target sites to regions of the genome that constitute super-enhancers (50, 51). The AID off-targets like Cd83 in CSR-activated B cells map to regions enriched in chromatin marks, typical of super-enhancers, and lie within sites of convergent transcription (sense transcription from promoter of genes and anti-sense transcription from super-enhancer) (50, 51). A majority of AID-instigated lesions (irrespective of cell-type) occurred at transcription start sites, which were connected over long distances to multiple topologically active "regulatory clusters" (51). A central theme that came out from these elegant studies is that the nuclear microenvironment, which can vary from one cell type to another (even between *ex vivo* CSR-activated B cells and GC B cells), greatly influences AID target selection, yet the targets do share the following commonalities: (a) highly transcribed super-enhancers, (b) topologically interconnected clusters, and (c) sites of convergent transcription (50–52) (**Figure 3**). How these findings fit the available models of stalled Pol-II (Spt5), 14-3-3, RNA exosome, PTBP2-mediated AID targeting remains to be explored (8). Additionally, these strong correlative evidences should now be tested for causation using the CRISPR-Cas9 system by abrogating transcription or knocking out the eRNA transcripts, to query if it affects the mutational landscape in AID-expressing cells. Another open question is whether convergent transcription regulates physiological Ig locus targeting of AID during CSR. These exciting avenues remain to be explored and would be at the forefront of research of AID biology in the coming years.

Non-Coding RNA

AID, being a member of the APOBEC-family of enzymes, has long been known to be associated with RNA and RNA metabolism-associated factors, such as, RNA Pol-II, Spt5, RNA exosome, PTBP2, and CTNNBL1 (8). Since AID activity has been strongly linked to transcription, R-loop formation and anti-sense RNA processing, a recent study delved into the details of how non-coding RNA biology can impact AID targeting (14). Using a mouse model of conditional inactivation of an essential component of the RNA exosome (Exosc3), it was revealed that the RNA exosome shapes the non-coding transcriptome in B cells in a way that allows AID to access sites of anti-sense and divergent transcription (14). This was true for many of the well-characterized off-target sites of AID in B cells including Cd79b, Cd83, Pim1, IL4ra, and cMyc. However, the proposed model of divergently transcribed loci generating RNA exosome substrates facilitating single-stranded DNA access to AID is in contradiction with the convergent transcription model (14, 50), and future work is necessary to address the discrepancies.

Another elegant finding of Exosc3 and 10 conditional deletions in mature B cells was that it unraveled a novel role of this cellular RNA degradation factory in regulating enhancer (e) and super-enhancer (se) RNAs, which as discussed before might have a remarkable impact on AID mistargeting (14, 50, 51, 53). The genome-wide mapping of changes in non-coding RNA transcriptome in RNA exosome-deficient B cells undergoing CSR led to the identification of a distal divergent eRNA-transcribing element (lncRNA-CSR) (53). Ablation of transcription from this element profoundly impacted looping-dependent long-range DNA interactions with IgH 3′ regulatory region super-enhancer and compromised CSR. Additionally, the RNA exosome appears to promote genomic integrity in activated B cells by chewing up genome-destabilizing R-loop structures that emanate from active enhancers and also by regulating chromatin silencing (53). Questions come to mind as to how the CSR-promoting R-loop structures at S regions are preserved temporally, and how the RNA exosome function in facilitating template strand deamination by AID is in unison with its more global functions in genomic integrity (54). Nonetheless, these compelling studies have definitely united super-enhancer and ncRNA biology into B cell research, especially CSR, and will propel the field forward in coming years.

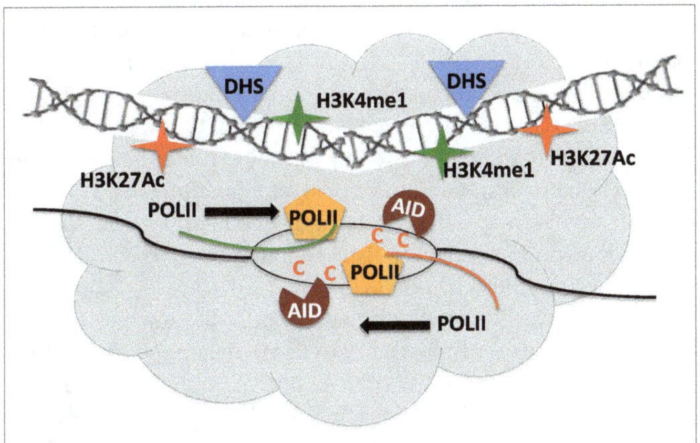

FIGURE 3 | Regulatory clusters containing super-enhancers modulate AID mistargeting. Convergent transcription between promoters of target gene and super-enhancers from topologically associated domains (TAD) allow access of AID to single-stranded DNA and promote off-target activity. DHS – Dnase1 hypersensitive sites.

Co-transcriptional processes and factors including RNA pol-II stalling, RNA exosomes, and even eRNA/seRNA appear to reinforce the transcription and R-loop dependent AID targeting model (12, 14, 16, 50, 51, 53, 54). It can be concluded that the requirement for transcription (convergent/divergent) for AID targeting/mistargeting has been testified. However, an intriguing finding predating the discovery of AID was that processing of switch transcripts by splicing was also necessary for CSR (55, 56). The role of transcript *per se* was elusive and post-transcriptional/splicing mechanisms regulating CSR have been understudied. To address if the sterile switch transcripts have a role in CSR, a mouse model of debranching enzyme (DBR1) haploinsufficiency and a knockdown approach in CH12F3A cells was used (15). These experiments revealed that if the generation of the transcript, post lariat debranching is abrogated, without affecting transcription or splicing, still, CSR is substantially impaired. The defect in CSR in DBR knockdown cells could be fully rescued by providing the switch RNA *in trans*, buttressing specificity of the phenotype (15). The defect in CSR was attributable to a failure to recruit AID to S regions, suggesting that the RNA might act *in trans* to guide AID back to the DNA locus due to sequence complementarity. This was indeed true, because provision of Sα transcripts *in trans* (in DBR1 knockdown CH12F3A cells) although could rescue AID recruitment to Sα but failed to target AID to Sμ, and thus failed to rescue CSR.

The structural basis of AID binding to RNA was due to the ability of the S region RNA to fold into G-quadruplex structures, which could be recognized by a recognition motif in AID that has a conserved G133 residue (15). Interestingly, this residue was also mutated (G133V) in human patients with hyper IgM syndrome (57). Indeed, G133V AID could not be recruited to S regions in B cells and failed completely to rescue CSR in AID-deficient cells, despite being catalytically active, expressed at similar levels and having similar subcellular localization as WT AID (15). The model proposed based on these findings is that following transcription of the S regions, the spliced out lariat is debranched by DBR1, the debranched RNA assumes G-quadruplex structures, which facilitates AID binding and allows sequence- and structure-specific recruitment of AID to DNA during CSR (**Figure 4**). This physiological targeting mechanism can have implications for off-target AID activity as well because primary transcripts of many off-target AID genes (compared to non-target ones) have the potential to form G-quadruplex structures (15).

This opens up the field with many questions: how does the hand-off of AID-RNA complex to the DNA take place, and how the co-transcriptional mechanisms of AID targeting are complemented by this post-splicing mechanism to ensure a coordinated system enabling efficient CSR.

Epigenetic Control of DNA Repair

The culmination of AID activity and lesion processing at recombining S regions during CSR is the generation of DNA DSBs, which constitute one of the most toxic lesions in a cell. Every cell in the body has evolved highly efficient and elaborate system dedicated to repair DSBs in order to promote survival and prevent translocations. However, a B cell faces a daunting challenge; not only does it have to repair the breaks to limit translocation potential, but it also has to time the process with such exquisite precision that it promotes long-range recombination. The non-homologous end-joining repair pathway is the most well-characterized one that is used during CSR (10). However, other pathways, such as, homologous recombination and alternative end-joining also play a role albeit to a lesser extent (8). The function of major players (genetic) in the AID-induced DNA damage response/repair phase that allow recombination including ATM, H2AX, Ligase IV, 53BP1, and Rif1 have been studied in-depth and reviewed elsewhere in Ref. (8, 10, 11, 13).

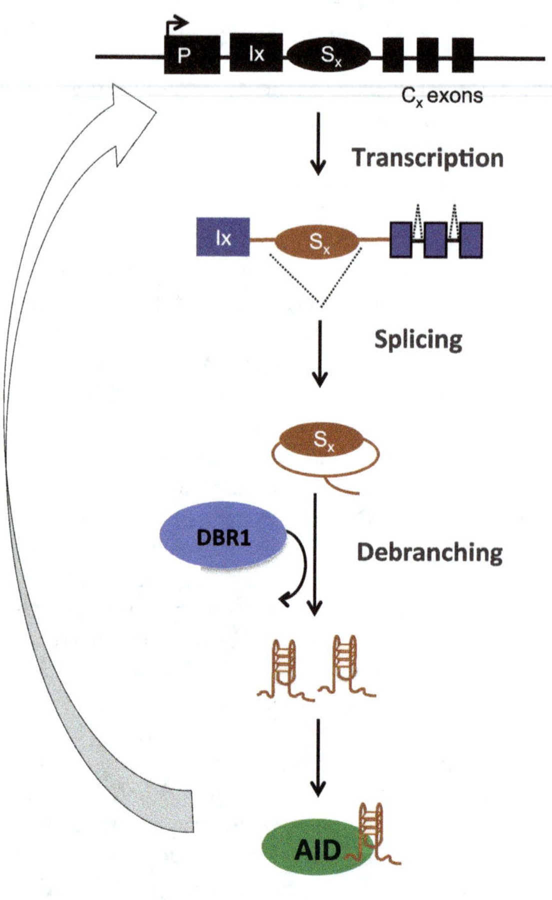

FIGURE 4 | Post-splicing RNA-dependent targeting mechanism of AID during CSR. Transcribed S region are spliced, debranched (by DBR1) and the switch RNA assumes G-quadruplex conformation that allows structure- and sequence-dependent AID targeting back to S region DNA

DNA insults have to be dealt within the context of a highly organized chromatin microenvironment and it is rational to assume that DNA DSB repair would be modulated significantly by epigenetic factors (58–60). Histones and many other DNA repair proteins undergo different post-translational modifications (PTMs) including phosphorylation, ubiquitylation, acetylation, methylation, sumoylation, and PARylation during an active repair response (61). These modifications can serve multiple purposes including serving as scaffold to recruit essential DNA repair factors, many of which harbor complementary domains to recognize the PTM. The histone variant H2AX gets phosphorylated at Ser 139 (γH2AX) in response to DNA damage by PI3K-like family of kinases (ATM, ATR, and DNA-PKcs), a classical DNA DSB marker. H2AX deficiency compromises CSR possibly due to defect in long-range chromatin remodeling and synapsis. BRCT domain containing proteins like MDC1 and 53BP1 also play an important role in the cascade of DNA repair events following DSB induction (62). MDC1, via its BRCT domain recognizes γH2AX and allows recruitment of E3 ubiquitin ligases RNF8 and RNF168, both of which are required for efficient CSR. The CSR defects are milder as compared to that in 53BP1-deficient B cells (63–65). 53BP1 functions mainly to prevent resection of DNA ends by recruiting Rif1 (66), and allows for timely persistence of breaks to be joined *in trans* (to acceptor S regions) rather than in cis (intra-switch recombination). 53BP1 recruitment to DNA is dependent on H4K20me2 mark, which is recognized via its tudor domain. Mutation in the tudor domain leads to compromised CSR, implying that reading the chromatin mark is important in potentiating its function (67). 53BP1 has been recently shown to recognize DNA damage-induced H2AK15 ubiquitylation (68), and it remains to be seen if this function also regulates CSR. The histone methyl transferase MMSET (WHSC1, implicated in Wolf-Hirschornn Syndrome) also functions during CSR, since knockdown of MMSET impairs 53BP1 recruitment to DNA damage site and compromises CSR (69). Lastly, the bromo-domain reader, Brd4, was also shown to function during CSR by providing an ideal chromatin platform during DNA repair phase (70). Brd4 inhibitor JQ1 perturbed CSR by affecting 53BP1 accumulation and end-joining pathway choice (70). JQ1 also compromised *in vivo* GC response during T-dependent Ag challenge, and this was suggested to be due to failure of NF-kappa B signaling and Bcl6 upregulation (71). However JQ1 can have non-specific effects, and genetic or domain-specific mutational approaches to test Brd4 function must be employed in the future to establish its role in CSR.

The methyl cytosine dioxygenase family of enzymes (TETs), has been in focus for their ability to demethylate specific regions of the genome (indirectly, via conversion of methylated cytidines to hydroxymethylated cytidines followed by engagement of base-excison repair) derepress genes (2). These TET enzymes have been found to be mutated or shut-off in many tumors, suggesting that they might have epigenetic tumor suppressive functions. Indeed, deletion of TET1 in mice was associated with increased propensity of development of B cell lymphomas (72). TET1 was required for maintenance of normal 5hmC levels and distribution across the genome, which allowed adequate expression of essential DNA repair genes (e.g., *lig1*, *ogg1*, *rad50*, and *rad51*). Absence of TET1 led to increased γH2AX foci and DNA damage sensitivity due to lack of repair and potentiated lymphomagenesis (pre-malignant B lymphomas at pro-B cell stage) (72). Outstanding questions about the role of other TET enzymes (TET2 and TET3), and even AID as a demethylase in B cell physiology and pathology remain to be explored (73, 74).

Lastly, chromatin remodeling complexes too have been implicated in reorganizing the chromatin during CSR. Defects in INO80 nucleosome remodeler in humans and in CH12F3A cells compromises CSR, likely due to improper loading of the cohesion complex and synaptic complex formation (75). Indeed, defects in cohesion loading proteins do cause abrogation of CSR (76, 77). These findings need to be introspected further because INO80 and cohesion complex have global cellular functions that extend beyond CSR.

Summary and Perspective

Taken together, a bevy of epigenetic factors including "histone codes", ncRNA, micro-RNAs, and super-enhancers communicate and coordinate to provide a dynamic chromatin landscape, which is geared for optimal diversification of the antibody repertoire.

Advances in sequencing-based techniques and data from the ENCODE project have greatly propelled research in the last decade (78). B cell biology, especially CSR has been investigated at depths like never before, and this has revealed the complexities that underlie this mechanistically counterintuitive process, which the B cell has to accommodate as a cost for co-evolution with pathogens. The smooth collisions of the chromatin and enhancer landscapes that facilitate CSR have been unraveled, however a multitude of questions lie ahead.

New modifications of histones continue to be identified. For example, crotonylation (79), which is thought to be similar to acetylation in being catalyzed by p300 in presence of intracellular crotonyl-CoA (79, 80), and even its erasers have been identified (81). Given that histone acetylation has functions in CSR, it remains to be seen if and how crotonylation can modulate CSR. DNA methylation has been extensively studied over the years and its role in locus accessibility and gene expression (epigenomic) is well characterized. But recently there has been identification of RNA methylation (N^6-methyl-adenosine) as an epitranscriptomic modification (1). Transcriptome-wide m^6A-mapping has provided great insight into the prevalence and relevance of this RNA modification, and how it impacts gene expression (82). Identification of m^6A "readers", "writers" and "erasers" has also propelled epitranscriptomic research (82). Given that CSR is impacted significantly by an integral non-coding RNA (eRNA, seRNA, lncRNA, and micro-RNA) component, and that RNA methylation is more prominent in non-coding RNAs, it will be unsurprising if this modification impacts CSR (83–85). Additionally, a very recent identification of N^6-methyl-deoxyadenosine modification in the DNA of lower eukaryotes as a new "epigenetic" mark also opens up the question whether the writers and erasers of this mark will impact CSR in higher eukaryotes (86–88).

Recent upsurge in research on the impact of microbiota on a multitude of processes in the immune system during health and disease has uncovered the significance of this symbiotic association over centuries of evolution (89). Given that microbes have been shown to produce metabolites that functionally impact the epigenetic status of the host (90), it is tempting to speculate that even antibody responses *in vivo* will be epigenetically shaped by commensal-derived metabolites.

Most research reviewed herein has focused on positive regulation of CSR. But, one aspect that has to be borne in mind is that *in vivo*, CSR is only one of the multiple cell-fates that a clonally expanding population of B cells undergoes. So, there has to be coordinated allocation to other cell-fates including plasma cell differentiation and memory B cell differentiation, possibly by negative modulation of CSR. There has to be active genetic and epigenetic modules that skew cell-fate decisions toward one versus another path. It is rational to presume that such fine-tuning would be necessary in order to achieve an overall humoral response encompassing all aspects of adaptive immunity (adaptability, specificity, and memory). Future research is warranted to understand molecular mechanisms of negative regulation of the individual modules of cell-fate decision programs in B cells during a GC response.

A programed DNA damage process, such as, CSR is rare and unique to B cells, the fundamental understanding of which will propel basic (understanding DNA repair, recombination, and immunity) and translational science (ontogeny of lymphomas and its therapies). Epigenetics undoubtedly has enormous influence on physiology (adaptive immunity) and pathology (autoimmunity and lymphomagenesis) (4). Thus, exciting times lie ahead for research in CSR due to the establishment of the solid framework of the epigenetic landscape governing CSR.

References

1. Fu Y, Dominissini D, Rechavi G, He C. Gene expression regulation mediated through reversible m(6)A RNA methylation. *Nat Rev Genet* (2014) **15**:293–306. doi:10.1038/nrg3724
2. Kohli RM, Zhang Y. TET enzymes, TDG and the dynamics of DNA demethylation. *Nature* (2013) **502**:472–9. doi:10.1038/nature12750
3. Musselman CA, Lalonde ME, Cote J, Kutateladze TG. Perceiving the epigenetic landscape through histone readers. *Nat Struct Mol Biol* (2012) **19**:1218–27. doi:10.1038/nsmb.2436
4. Li G, Zan H, Xu Z, Casali P. Epigenetics of the antibody response. *Trends Immunol* (2013) **34**:460–70. doi:10.1016/j.it.2013.03.006
5. Rinn JL, Chang HY. Genome regulation by long noncoding RNAs. *Annu Rev Biochem* (2012) **81**:145–66. doi:10.1146/annurev-biochem-051410-092902
6. Holoch D, Moazed D. RNA-mediated epigenetic regulation of gene expression. *Nat Rev Genet* (2015) **16**:71–84. doi:10.1038/nrg3863
7. Victora GD, Nussenzweig MC. Germinal centers. *Annu Rev Immunol* (2012) **30**:429–57. doi:10.1146/annurev-immunol-020711-075032
8. Matthews AJ, Zheng S, DiMenna LJ, Chaudhuri J. Regulation of immunoglobulin class-switch recombination: choreography of noncoding transcription, targeted DNA deamination, and long-range DNA repair. *Adv Immunol* (2014) **122**:1–57. doi:10.1016/B978-0-12-800267-4.00001-8
9. Rouaud P, Saintamand A, Saad F, Carrion C, Lecardeur S, Cogne M, et al. Elucidation of the enigmatic IgD class-switch recombination via germline deletion of the IgH 3′ regulatory region. *J Exp Med* (2014) **211**:975–85. doi:10.1084/jem.20131385
10. Stavnezer J, Guikema JE, Schrader CE. Mechanism and regulation of class switch recombination. *Annu Rev Immunol* (2008) **26**:261–92. doi:10.1146/annurev.immunol.26.021607.090248

11. Stavnezer J, Schrader CE. IgH chain class switch recombination: mechanism and regulation. *J Immunol* (2014) **193**:5370–8. doi:10.4049/jimmunol.1401849
12. Vaidyanathan B, Yen WF, Pucella JN, Chaudhuri J. AIDing chromatin and transcription-coupled orchestration of immunoglobulin class-switch recombination. *Front Immunol* (2014) **5**:120. doi:10.3389/fimmu.2014.00120
13. Xu Z, Zan H, Pone EJ, Mai T, Casali P. Immunoglobulin class-switch DNA recombination: induction, targeting and beyond. *Nat Rev Immunol* (2012) **12**:517–31. doi:10.1038/nri3216
14. Pefanis E, Wang J, Rothschild G, Lim J, Chao J, Rabadan R, et al. Noncoding RNA transcription targets AID to divergently transcribed loci in B cells. *Nature* (2014) **514**:389–93. doi:10.1038/nature13580
15. Zheng S, Vuong BQ, Vaidyanathan B, Lin JY, Huang FT, Chaudhuri J. Non-coding RNA generated following lariat debranching mediates targeting of AID to DNA. *Cell* (2015) **161**:762–73. doi:10.1016/j.cell.2015.03.020
16. Wang L, Wuerffel R, Feldman S, Khamlichi AA, Kenter AL. S region sequence, RNA polymerase II, and histone modifications create chromatin accessibility during class switch recombination. *J Exp Med* (2009) **206**:1817–30. doi:10.1084/jem.20081678
17. Jeevan-Raj BP, Robert I, Heyer V, Page A, Wang JH, Cammas F, et al. Epigenetic tethering of AID to the donor switch region during immunoglobulin class switch recombination. *J Exp Med* (2011) **208**:1649–60. doi:10.1084/jem.20110118
18. Chowdhury M, Forouhi O, Dayal S, McCloskey N, Gould HJ, Felsenfeld G, et al. Analysis of intergenic transcription and histone modification across the human immunoglobulin heavy-chain locus. *Proc Natl Acad Sci U S A* (2008) **105**:15872–7. doi:10.1073/pnas.0808462105
19. Kuang FL, Luo Z, Scharff MD. H3 trimethyl K9 and H3 acetyl K9 chromatin modifications are associated with class switch recombination. *Proc Natl Acad Sci U S A* (2009) **106**:5288–93. doi:10.1073/pnas.0901368106
20. Daniel JA, Nussenzweig A. Roles for histone H3K4 methyltransferase activities during immunoglobulin class-switch recombination. *Biochim Biophys Acta* (2012) **1819**:733–8. doi:10.1016/j.bbagrm.2012.01.019
21. Stanlie A, Aida M, Muramatsu M, Honjo T, Begum NA. Histone3 lysine4 trimethylation regulated by the facilitates chromatin transcription complex is critical for DNA cleavage in class switch recombination. *Proc Natl Acad Sci U S A* (2010) **107**:22190–5. doi:10.1073/pnas.1016923108
22. Begum NA, Stanlie A, Nakata M, Akiyama H, Honjo T. The histone chaperone Spt6 is required for activation-induced cytidine deaminase target determination through H3K4me3 regulation. *J Biol Chem* (2012) **287**:32415–29. doi:10.1074/jbc.M112.351569
23. Bradley SP, Kaminski DA, Peters AHFM, Jenuwein T, Stavnezer J. The histone methyltransferase Suv39h1 increases class switch recombination specifically to IgA. *J Immunol* (2006) **177**:1179–88. doi:10.4049/jimmunol.177.2.1179
24. Daniel JA, Santos MA, Wang Z, Zang C, Schwab KR, Jankovic M, et al. PTIP promotes chromatin changes critical for immunoglobulin class switch recombination. *Science* (2010) **329**:917–23. doi:10.1126/science.1187942
25. Schwab KR, Patel SR, Dressler GR. Role of PTIP in class switch recombination and long-range chromatin interactions at the immunoglobulin heavy chain locus. *Mol Cell Biol* (2011) **31**:1503–11. doi:10.1128/MCB.00990-10
26. Good-Jacobson KL. Regulation of germinal center, B-cell memory, and plasma cell formation by histone modifiers. *Front Immunol* (2014) **5**:596. doi:10.3389/fimmu.2014.00596
27. Good-Jacobson KL, Chen Y, Voss AK, Smyth GK, Thomas T, Tarlinton D. Regulation of germinal center responses and B-cell memory by the chromatin modifier MOZ. *Proc Natl Acad Sci U S A* (2014) **111**:9585–90. doi:10.1073/pnas.1402485111
28. Amieux PS, Cummings DE, Motamed K, Brandon EP, Wailes LA, Le K, et al. Compensatory regulation of RIalpha protein levels in protein kinase A mutant mice. *J Biol Chem* (1997) **272**:3993–8. doi:10.1074/jbc.272.7.3993
29. Yamaguchi T, Cubizolles F, Zhang Y, Reichert N, Kohler H, Seiser C, et al. Histone deacetylases 1 and 2 act in concert to promote the G1-to-S progression. *Genes Dev* (2010) **24**:455–69. doi:10.1101/gad.552310
30. White CA, Pone EJ, Lam T, Tat C, Hayama KL, Li G, et al. Histone deacetylase inhibitors upregulate B cell microRNAs that silence AID and blimp-1 expression for epigenetic modulation of antibody and autoantibody responses. *J Immunol* (2014) **193**:5933–50. doi:10.4049/jimmunol.1401702
31. Su IH, Basavaraj A, Krutchinsky AN, Hobert O, Ullrich A, Chait BT, et al. Ezh2 controls B cell development through histone H3 methylation and Igh rearrangement. *Nat Immunol* (2003) **4**:124–31. doi:10.1038/ni876
32. Beguelin W, Popovic R, Teater M, Jiang Y, Bunting KL, Rosen M, et al. EZH2 is required for germinal center formation and somatic EZH2 mutations promote lymphoid transformation. *Cancer Cell* (2013) **23**:677–92. doi:10.1016/j.ccr.2013.04.011
33. Caganova M, Carrisi C, Varano G, Mainoldi F, Zanardi F, Germain PL, et al. Germinal center dysregulation by histone methyltransferase EZH2 promotes lymphomagenesis. *J Clin Invest* (2013) **123**:5009–22. doi:10.1172/JCI70626
34. Rommel PC, Bosque D, Gitlin AD, Croft GF, Heintz N, Casellas R, et al. Fate mapping for activation-induced cytidine deaminase (AID) marks non-lymphoid cells during mouse development. *PLoS One* (2013) **8**:e69208. doi:10.1371/journal.pone.0069208
35. Fujimura S, Matsui T, Kuwahara K, Maeda K, Sakaguchi N. Germinal center B-cell-associated DNA hypomethylation at transcriptional regions of the AID gene. *Mol Immunol* (2008) **45**:1712–9. doi:10.1016/j.molimm.2007.09.023
36. Crouch EE, Li Z, Takizawa M, Fichtner-Feigl S, Gourzi P, Montano C, et al. Regulation of AID expression in the immune response. *J Exp Med* (2007) **204**:1145–56. doi:10.1084/jem.20061952
37. Teng G, Hakimpour P, Landgraf P, Rice A, Tuschl T, Casellas R, et al. MicroRNA-155 is a negative regulator of activation-induced cytidine deaminase. *Immunity* (2008) **28**:621–9. doi:10.1016/j.immuni.2008.03.015
38. Dorsett Y, McBride KM, Jankovic M, Gazumyan A, Thai TH, Robbiani DF, et al. MicroRNA-155 suppresses activation-induced cytidine deaminase-mediated Myc-Igh translocation. *Immunity* (2008) **28**:630–8. doi:10.1016/j.immuni.2008.04.002
39. Fairfax KA, Gantier MP, Mackay F, Williams BR, McCoy CE. IL-10 regulates Aicda expression through miR-155. *J Leukoc Biol* (2015) **97**:71–8. doi:10.1189/jlb.2A0314-178R
40. Vuong BQ, Chaudhuri J. Combinatorial mechanisms regulating AID-dependent DNA deamination: interacting proteins and post-translational modifications. *Semin Immunol* (2012) **24**:264–72. doi:10.1016/j.smim.2012.05.006
41. Castellano-Pozo M, Santos-Pereira JM, Rondon AG, Barroso S, Andujar E, Perez-Alegre M, et al. R loops are linked to histone H3 S10 phosphorylation and chromatin condensation. *Mol Cell* (2013) **52**:583–90. doi:10.1016/j.molcel.2013.10.006
42. Lam T, Thomas LM, White CA, Li G, Pone EJ, Xu Z, et al. Scaffold functions of 14-3-3 adaptors in B cell immunoglobulin class switch DNA recombination. *PLoS One* (2013) **8**:e80414. doi:10.1371/journal.pone.0080414
43. Li G, White CA, Lam T, Pone EJ, Tran DC, Hayama KL, et al. Combinatorial H3K9acS10ph histone modification in IgH locus S regions targets 14-3-3 adaptors and AID to specify antibody class-switch DNA recombination. *Cell Rep* (2013) **5**:702–14. doi:10.1016/j.celrep.2013.09.031
44. Willmann KL, Milosevic S, Pauklin S, Schmitz KM, Rangam G, Simon MT, et al. A role for the RNA pol II-associated PAF complex in AID-induced immune diversification. *J Exp Med* (2012) **209**:2099–111. doi:10.1084/jem.20112145
45. Banerji J, Rusconi S, Schaffner W. Expression of a beta-globin gene is enhanced by remote SV40 DNA sequences. *Cell* (1981) **27**:299–308. doi:10.1016/0092-8674(81)90413-X
46. Pott S, Lieb JD. What are super-enhancers? *Nat Genet* (2015) **47**:8–12. doi:10.1038/ng.3167
47. Parker SC, Stitzel ML, Taylor DL, Orozco JM, Erdos MR, Akiyama JA, et al. Chromatin stretch enhancer states drive cell-specific gene regulation and harbor human disease risk variants. *Proc Natl Acad Sci U S A* (2013) **110**:17921–6. doi:10.1073/pnas.1317023110
48. Hnisz D, Abraham BJ, Lee TI, Lau A, Saint-Andre V, Sigova AA, et al. Super-enhancers in the control of cell identity and disease. *Cell* (2013) **155**:934–47. doi:10.1016/j.cell.2013.09.053
49. Wang Q, Oliveira T, Jankovic M I, Silva T, Hakim O, Yao K, et al. Epigenetic targeting of activation-induced cytidine deaminase. *Proc Natl Acad Sci U S A* (2014) **111**:18667–72. doi:10.1073/pnas.1420575111
50. Meng FL, Du Z, Federation A, Hu J, Wang Q, Kieffer-Kwon KR, et al. Convergent transcription at intragenic super-enhancers targets AID-initiated genomic instability. *Cell* (2014) **159**:1538–48. doi:10.1016/j.cell.2014.11.014
51. Qian J, Wang Q, Dose M, Pruett N, Kieffer-Kwon KR, Resch W, et al. B cell super-enhancers and regulatory clusters recruit AID tumorigenic activity. *Cell* (2014) **159**:1524–37. doi:10.1016/j.cell.2014.11.013
52. Alinikula J, Schatz DG. Super-enhancer transcription converges on AID. *Cell* (2014) **159**:1490–2. doi:10.1016/j.cell.2014.12.007

53. Pefanis E, Wang J, Rothschild G, Lim J, Kazadi D, Sun J, et al. RNA exosome-regulated long non-coding RNA transcription controls super-enhancer activity. *Cell* (2015) **161**:774–89. doi:10.1016/j.cell.2015.04.034
54. Basu U, Meng FL, Keim C, Grinstein V, Pefanis E, Eccleston J, et al. The RNA exosome targets the AID cytidine deaminase to both strands of transcribed duplex DNA substrates. *Cell* (2011) **144**:353–63. doi:10.1016/j.cell.2011.01.001
55. Hein K, Lorenz MG, Siebenkotten G, Petry K, Christine R, Radbruch A. Processing of switch transcripts is required for targeting of antibody class switch recombination. *J Exp Med* (1998) **188**:2369–74. doi:10.1084/jem.188.12.2369
56. Lorenz M, Jung S, Radbruch A. Switch transcripts in immunoglobulin class switching. *Science* (1995) **267**:1825–8. doi:10.1126/science.7892607
57. Mahdaviani SA, Hirbod-Mobarakeh A, Wang N, Aghamohammadi A, Hammarstrom L, Masjedi MR, et al. Novel mutation of the activation-induced cytidine deaminase gene in a Tajik family: special review on hyper-immunoglobulin M syndrome. *Expert Rev Clin Immunol* (2012) **8**:539–46. doi:10.1586/eci.12.46
58. Alt FW, Zhang Y, Meng FL, Guo C, Schwer B. Mechanisms of programmed DNA lesions and genomic instability in the immune system. *Cell* (2013) **152**:417–29. doi:10.1016/j.cell.2013.01.007
59. Bunting SF, Nussenzweig A. End-joining, translocations and cancer. *Nat Rev Cancer* (2013) **13**:443–54. doi:10.1038/nrc3537
60. Price BD, D'Andrea AD. Chromatin remodeling at DNA double-strand breaks. *Cell* (2013) **152**:1344–54. doi:10.1016/j.cell.2013.02.011
61. Daniel JA, Nussenzweig A. The AID-induced DNA damage response in chromatin. *Mol Cell* (2013) **50**:309–21. doi:10.1016/j.molcel.2013.04.017
62. Lou Z, Minter-Dykhouse K, Franco S, Gostissa M, Rivera MA, Celeste A, et al. MDC1 maintains genomic stability by participating in the amplification of ATM-dependent DNA damage signals. *Mol Cell* (2006) **21**:187–200. doi:10.1016/j.molcel.2005.11.025
63. Santos MA, Huen MS, Jankovic M, Chen HT, Lopez-Contreras AJ I, Klein A, et al. Class switching and meiotic defects in mice lacking the E3 ubiquitin ligase RNF8. *J Exp Med* (2010) **207**:973–81. doi:10.1084/jem.20092308
64. Ramachandran S, Chahwan R, Nepal RM, Frieder D, Panier S, Roa S, et al. The RNF8/RNF168 ubiquitin ligase cascade facilitates class switch recombination. *Proc Natl Acad Sci U S A* (2010) **107**:809–14. doi:10.1073/pnas.0913790107
65. Ward IM, Reina-San-Martin B, Olaru A, Minn K, Tamada K, Lau JS, et al. 53BP1 is required for class switch recombination. *J Cell Biol* (2004) **165**:459–64. doi:10.1083/jcb.200403021
66. Alt FW. Antibody diversity. New mechanism revealed [news]. *Nature* (1986) **322**:772–3. doi:10.1038/322772a0
67. Bothmer A, Robbiani DF, Di Virgilio M, Bunting SF I, Klein A, Feldhahn N, et al. Regulation of DNA end joining, resection, and immunoglobulin class switch recombination by 53BP1. *Mol Cell* (2011) **42**:319–29. doi:10.1016/j.molcel.2011.03.019
68. Fradet-Turcotte A, Canny MD, Escribano-Diaz C, Orthwein A, Leung CC, Huang H, et al. 53BP1 is a reader of the DNA-damage-induced H2A Lys 15 ubiquitin mark. *Nature* (2013) **499**:50–4. doi:10.1038/nature12318
69. Pei H, Wu X, Liu T, Yu K, Jelinek DF, Lou Z. The histone methyltransferase MMSET regulates class switch recombination. *J Immunol* (2013) **190**:756–63. doi:10.4049/jimmunol.1201811
70. Stanlie A, Yousif AS, Akiyama H, Honjo T, Begum NA. Chromatin reader Brd4 functions in Ig class switching as a repair complex adaptor of nonhomologous end-joining. *Mol Cell* (2014) **55**:97–110. doi:10.1016/j.molcel.2014.05.018
71. Gao F, Yang Y, Wang Z, Gao X, Zheng B. BRAD4 plays a critical role in germinal center response by regulating Bcl-6 and NF-kappaB activation. *Cell Immunol* (2015) **294**:1–8. doi:10.1016/j.cellimm.2015.01.010
72. Cimmino L, Dawlaty MM, diaye-Lobry DN, Yap YS, Bakogianni S, Yu Y, et al. TET1 is a tumor suppressor of hematopoietic malignancy. *Nat Immunol* (2015) **16**:653–62. doi:10.1038/ni.3148
73. Kumar R, DiMenna L, Schrode N, Liu TC, Franck P, Munoz-Descalzo S, et al. AID stabilizes stem-cell phenotype by removing epigenetic memory of pluripotency genes. *Nature* (2013) **500**:89–92. doi:10.1038/nature12299
74. Fritz EL, Rosenberg BR, Lay K, Mihailovic A, Tuschl T, Papavasiliou FN. A comprehensive analysis of the effects of the deaminase AID on the transcriptome and methylome of activated B cells. *Nat Immunol* (2013) **14**:749–55. doi:10.1038/ni.2616
75. Kracker S, Di Virgilio M, Schwartzentruber J, Cuenin C, Forveille M, Deau MC, et al. An inherited immunoglobulin class-switch recombination deficiency associated with a defect in the INO80 chromatin remodeling complex. *J Allergy Clin Immunol* (2015) **135**(998–1007):e1006. doi:10.1016/j.jaci.2014.08.030
76. Enervald E, Du L, Visnes T, Bjorkman A, Lindgren E, Wincent J, et al. A regulatory role for the cohesin loader NIPBL in nonhomologous end joining during immunoglobulin class switch recombination. *J Exp Med* (2013) **210**:2503–13. doi:10.1084/jem.20130168
77. Thomas-Claudepierre AS, Schiavo E, Heyer V, Fournier M, Page A, Robert I, et al. The cohesin complex regulates immunoglobulin class switch recombination. *J Exp Med* (2013) **210**:2495–502. doi:10.1084/jem.20130166
78. Yue F, Cheng Y, Breschi A, Vierstra J, Wu W, Ryba T, et al. A comparative encyclopedia of DNA elements in the mouse genome. *Nature* (2014) **515**:355–64. doi:10.1038/nature13992
79. Tan M, Luo H, Lee S, Jin F, Yang JS, Montellier E, et al. Identification of 67 histone marks and histone lysine crotonylation as a new type of histone modification. *Cell* (2011) **146**:1016–28. doi:10.1016/j.cell.2011.08.008
80. Sabari BR, Tang Z, Huang H, Yong-Gonzalez V, Molina H, Kong HE, et al. Intracellular crotonyl-CoA stimulates transcription through p300-catalyzed histone crotonylation. *Mol Cell* (2015) **58**:203–15. doi:10.1016/j.molcel.2015.02.029
81. Bao X, Wang Y, Li X, Li XM, Liu Z, Yang T, et al. Identification of 'erasers' for lysine crotonylated histone marks using a chemical proteomics approach. *Elife* (2014) **3**:2999. doi:10.7554/eLife.02999
82. Meyer KD, Jaffrey SR. The dynamic epitranscriptome: N6-methyladenosine and gene expression control. *Nat Rev Mol Cell Biol* (2014) **15**:313–26. doi:10.1038/nrm3785
83. Alarcon CR, Lee H, Goodarzi H, Halberg N, Tavazoie SF. N6-methyladenosine marks primary microRNAs for processing. *Nature* (2015) **519**:482–5. doi:10.1038/nature14281
84. Liu N, Dai Q, Zheng G, He C, Parisien M, Pan T. N(6)-methyladenosine-dependent RNA structural switches regulate RNA-protein interactions. *Nature* (2015) **518**:560–4. doi:10.1038/nature14234
85. Wang X, Lu Z, Gomez A, Hon GC, Yue Y, Han D, et al. N6-methyladenosine-dependent regulation of messenger RNA stability. *Nature* (2014) **505**:117–20. doi:10.1038/nature12730
86. Zhang G, Huang H, Liu D, Cheng Y, Liu X, Zhang W, et al. N(6)-methyladenine DNA modification in *Drosophila*. *Cell* (2015) **161**:893–906. doi:10.1016/j.cell.2015.04.018
87. Greer EL, Blanco MA, Gu L, Sendinc E, Liu J, Aristizabal-Corrales D, et al. DNA methylation on N(6)-adenine in *C. elegans*. *Cell* (2015) **161**:868–78. doi:10.1016/j.cell.2015.04.005
88. Fu Y, Luo GZ, Chen K, Deng X, Yu M, Han D, et al. N(6)-methyldeoxyadenosine marks active transcription start sites in *Chlamydomonas*. *Cell* (2015) **161**:879–92. doi:10.1016/j.cell.2015.04.010
89. Round JL, Mazmanian SK. The gut microbiota shapes intestinal immune responses during health and disease. *Nat Rev Immunol* (2009) **9**:313–23. doi:10.1038/nri2515
90. Furusawa Y, Obata Y, Fukuda S, Endo TA, Nakato G, Takahashi D, et al. Commensal microbe-derived butyrate induces the differentiation of colonic regulatory T cells. *Nature* (2013) **504**:446–50. doi:10.1038/nature12721

11

Immunity to pathogens taught by specialized human dendritic cell subsets

Jens Geginat [1*]***, Giulia Nizzoli*** [1]***, Moira Paroni*** [1]***, Stefano Maglie*** [1]***, Paola Larghi*** [1]***,***
Steve Pascolo [2] ***and Sergio Abrignani*** [1,3]

[1] Istituto Nazionale di Genetica Molecolare "Romeo ed Enrica Invernizzi" (INGM), Milan, Italy, [2] Department of Dermatology, University Hospital of Zurich, Zurich, Switzerland, [3] DISCCO, Department of Clinical Sciences and Community Health, University of Milano, Milan, Italy

Edited by:
Elisabetta Padovan,
University of Basel, Switzerland

Reviewed by:
Marina Cella,
Washington University School of Medicine, USA
Shahram Salek-ardakani,
University of Florida, USA

****Correspondence:***
Jens Geginat
geginat@ingm.org

Dendritic cells (DCs) are specialized antigen-presenting cells (APCs) that have a key role in immune responses because they bridge the innate and adaptive arms of the immune system. They mature upon recognition of pathogens and upregulate MHC molecules and costimulatory receptors to activate antigen-specific $CD4^+$ and $CD8^+$ T cells. It is now well established that DCs are not a homogeneous population but are composed of different subsets with specialized functions in immune responses to specific pathogens. Upon viral infections, plasmacytoid DCs (pDCs) rapidly produce large amounts of IFN-α, which has potent antiviral functions and activates several other immune cells. However, pDCs are not particularly potent APCs and induce the tolerogenic cytokine IL-10 in $CD4^+$ T cells. In contrast, myeloid DCs (mDCs) are very potent APCs and possess the unique capacity to prime naive T cells and consequently to initiate a primary adaptive immune response. Different subsets of mDCs with specialized functions have been identified. In mice, $CD8\alpha^+$ mDCs capture antigenic material from necrotic cells, secrete high levels of IL-12, and prime Th1 and cytotoxic T-cell responses to control intracellular pathogens. Conversely, $CD8\alpha^-$ mDCs preferentially prime $CD4^+$ T cells and promote Th2 or Th17 differentiation. BDCA-3^+ mDC2 are the human homologue of $CD8\alpha^+$ mDCs, since they share the expression of several key molecules, the capacity to cross-present antigens to $CD8^+$ T-cells and to produce IFN-λ. However, although several features of the DC network are conserved between humans and mice, the expression of several toll-like receptors as well as the production of cytokines that regulate T-cell differentiation are different. Intriguingly, recent data suggest specific roles for human DC subsets in immune responses against individual pathogens. The biology of human DC subsets holds the promise to be exploitable in translational medicine, in particular for the development of vaccines against persistent infections or cancer.

Keywords: dendritic cells, cytokines, toll-like receptors, T-cell differentiation, cytotoxic T cells

INTRODUCTION

Human beings are constantly exposed to a myriad of pathogens, including bacteria, fungi, and viruses. These foreign invaders or cohabitants contain molecular structures that are sensed by the innate immune system, which mounts a first-line defense and also activates a pathogen-specific, adaptive immune response. The adaptive immune system is composed of B cells that produce specific antibodies, CD8$^+$ T cells that can kill pathogen-infected cells, and CD4$^+$ T cells that produce effector cytokines and coordinate the immune response. T cells express antigen receptors (T-cell antigen receptors, TCR) that recognize specific peptides presented on MHC molecules. CD8$^+$ T cells recognize peptides presented by MHC class-I molecules that are ubiquitously expressed, whereas CD4$^+$ T cells are activated by peptide-MHC class-II complexes, which are largely restricted to antigen-presenting cells (APCs). Dendritic cells (DCs) can express very high levels of MHC and costimulatory molecules, and it is generally accepted that they are the relevant cells to induce the activation ("priming") of antigen-specific "naive" T cells (1, 2) and induce their differentiation into various types of effector T cells.

The elimination or containment of different types of pathogens requires dedicated classes of adaptive immune responses (3). Thus, pathogens like viruses or intracellular bacteria require CD4$^+$ and CD8$^+$ T cells that produce IFN-γ and kill infected cells (Th1 and CTL, respectively). IL-12 is the critical cytokine that induces this type of response, but IL-12 production by DC is tightly controlled and requires several stimuli derived from pathogens and from CD4$^+$ helper T cells (4–9). Conversely, extracellular bacteria and fungi require a different type of response that can be mediated by Th17 cells (10–12). These effector cells are induced by proinflammatory cytokines produced by DC and macrophages (13) and attract neutrophils that in turn phagocytose extracellular bacteria (14). A third type of effector response is the Th2 response, which is required to expel extracellular parasites such as helminths by activating eosinophils and basophils and by inducing antibodies of the IgE class (15). IL-4 is the critical cytokine that induces this response (16), but IL-4 is normally not produced by DC (17, 18). Finally, these different effector responses have to be controlled by specialized regulatory T cells, in particular by IL-10-producing T cells ("Tr1 cells"), which are generated from effector cells and are important to avoid excessive tissue damage by adaptive immune responses (19–22). Cytokines that promote this type of regulatory T-cell response are IFN-α, IL-27, and IL-10 (23–25), and all these cytokines can be produced by DCs (26, 27).

DCs HAVE THE UNIQUE CAPACITY TO PRIME T-CELL RESPONSES

Professional APCs have to present pathogen-derived peptides on MHC molecules to activate antigen-specific T cells. DCs are phagocytic in the immature state, i.e., under steady-state conditions and upon initial pathogen encounter, and can take up antigenic material by pinocytosis or by surface receptor-mediated internalization (28). Proteins from pathogens are then shuttled to lysosomes where they are chopped to peptides and loaded on MHC class-II molecules (29, 30). These peptide–MHC complexes are then transported to the plasma membrane to activate specific CD4$^+$ T cells. The presentation of peptides derived from exogenous proteins on MHC class-I, a process called cross-presentation (31, 32), is a largely unique feature of DCs and is particularly important to activate CD8$^+$ T cells in viral infections. Virus-infected cells express viral proteins in the cytosol where they are degraded to peptides by the proteasome, translocated to the endoplasmic reticulum by TAP proteins, and loaded on MHC class-I molecules (31). However, since DCs are not necessarily infected by viruses, they must be able to process virus-derived proteins also from external sources, such as virus-infected cells, to activate CD8$^+$ T cells. The mechanism of cross-presentation is still incompletely understood, but two distinct pathways via vacuoles and peptide translocation from phagolysosomes to the cytosol have been described (32). It is believed that cross-presentation is the most important pathway leading to the induction of cytotoxic T-cell responses, and excellent reviews have been published on this relevant topic (31–33).

Naive T cells have a very high activation threshold (34), and only professional APCs that express high levels of MHC and costimulatory molecules such as DCs are able to induce proliferation of naive T cells (35). Several receptor–ligand interactions contribute to naive T-cell activation (36–38), but CD28 costimulation is particularly important to amplify the signal transduced by the TCR (39). Monocytes efficiently present peptides derived from extracellular proteins on MHC class-II to activate antigen-experienced CD4$^+$ T cells (34), and this capacity can be exploited to selectively expand antigen-specific memory T cells (40). However, monocytes have an approximately 1000-fold lower capacity to prime naive CD4$^+$ T cells as compared to DCs (Nizzoli et al., under review) and home to non-lymphoid tissues in the steady state. However, upon inflammation, they can differentiate to inflammatory DCs (41) and home to lymph nodes where they can activate T cells (42, 43). In addition, there is some evidence that CD16$^+$ subsets of human blood monocytes might contain DCs (27, 44, 45). Naive T cells constantly recirculate in the blood and migrate through secondary lymphoid organs (46), but are largely excluded from non-lymphoid tissues. In secondary lymphoid tissues, they migrate to the T-cell zone, where they encounter DCs (47). B cells are also present in secondary lymphoid organs and can potently present antigen to T cells when they internalize and process antigens that have specifically bound to their B-cell receptor (48). However, B cells are physically separated from naive T cells in lymph nodes and only following TCR activation naive T cells migrate to the B-cell zone where they interact with antigen-specific B cells to induce antibody production (49, 50). Thus, antigen presentation by B cells appears to be important for the activation of antigen-experienced T cells rather than for naive T-cell priming.

PATHOGEN-ASSOCIATED MOLECULAR PATTERNS INDUCE DC MATURATION

Dendritic cells are generated from committed precursors in the bone marrow that are released into the circulation to seed peripheral organs (51–55). Both monocytes and DCs can be derived from common myeloid progenitors (CMPs), but committed precursors that selectively give rise to monocytes or DCs (51) or even selected DC subsets (53, 54) have been identified in humans and mice. DCs are poorly stimulatory in the immature state and can induce a partial T-cell activation, leading to deletion of autoreactive CD8+ T cells (56–59). In addition, they promote self-tolerance by inducing Foxp3+ regulatory CD4+ T cells that suppress autoreactive T cells (60). Pathogens induce the maturation of DCs that consequently acquire the capacity to produce polarizing cytokines and to prime pathogen-specific effector T-cell responses. Pathogen-derived molecular patterns [PAMPs (61, 62)] are recognized by DCs and lead to the efficient presentation of antigens to T cells (63). There are different classes of pathogen-sensing receptors, including Toll-like receptors (62, 64), nucleotide-binding oligomerization domain (NOD)-like receptors (65), retinoic acid-inducible gene 1 (RIG-I)-like receptors (66), and C-type lectins (67). TLRs recognize different PAMPs, including nucleic acids or cell wall components such as proteins and lipoproteins (68, 69). In the case of viruses, nucleic acids are sensed not only by different TLRs in endosomes but also by cytosolic receptors like RIG-I (66, 70) and induce a potent activation of DCs. Importantly, subsets of DCs express different patterns of pathogen-sensing receptors and might thus preferentially respond to individual pathogens (71, 72). DNA viruses such as cytomegalovirus (CMV) and herpes simplex virus (HSV) and also bacteria can activate DCs via unmethylated CpG-containing DNA (69), which is sensed by TLR9. Double- and single-stranded RNAs, which are generated by both DNA and RNA viruses, are sensed by DCs via TLR3 (73) and TLR7/8 (74, 75), respectively. Of note, TLR3 is restricted to mDCs (71) and induces cross-presentation capacities (76). Viruses such as respiratory syncytial virus (RSV) and hepatitis C virus (HCV) can also activate DCs via TLR2 or TLR4, which are expressed on the plasma membrane and recognize viral proteins (77). TLR2 is also involved in immune responses to fungi (78) and Gram-positive bacteria (79, 80) while TLR4 recognizes lipopolysaccharide (LPS) (81), a cell membrane compound of Gram-negative bacteria. Many pathogens like viruses activate DCs via multiple TLRs (77). Moreover, other immune cells, including T cells themselves, feed-back on DCs to regulate the ongoing response. In particular, CD40 stimulation by CD4+ helper T cells is crucial for CD8+ T-cell stimulation and IL-12 production (4, 5). Moreover, IFN-γ (6) and paradoxically also IL-4 (7, 8) that can be provided by T cells further enhance IL-12 production (9).

Surface TLRs such as TLR2 and TLR4 signal via the adaptor protein Myd88 (82) to induce the activation of Map kinases and the nuclear translocation of the transcription factor NF-κB, which in turn induces the transcription of proinflammatory cytokines (62). Endosomal TLRs 7, 8, and 9 also signal via Myd88 but activate IRF7, which in turn induces type-1 interferon production (83, 84). TLR3 is an exception since it does not signal via Myd88 but utilizes TRIF (85) to activate IRF3 (86, 87) or IRF7 (88). How all these complex signaling pathways are integrated by DCs to induce the appropriate T-cell response is still incompletely understood (88–90).

SPECIALIZED DC SUBSETS INDUCE DIFFERENT CLASSES OF T-CELL RESPONSES IN MICE

Dendritic cells in mice can be subdivided into distinct subsets with specific functions. Some DCs are stably resident in lymph nodes while others are positioned in non-lymphoid tissues to sense tissue-invading pathogens, but are migratory and are recruited via the lymph following pathogen encounter in a CCR7-dependent manner (91, 92). In secondary lymphoid tissues, two major DC subsets are myeloid DCs (mDCs) and plasmacytoid DCs (pDCs; **Table 1**) (72, 93, 94). Both pDCs and mDCs upregulate MHC and costimulatory molecules like CD80 and CD86 upon maturation (72) that bind to CD28 and are required to induce full T-cell stimulation (39). However, pDCs are poorly phagocytic and have a different regulation of MHC class-II turnover upon maturation as compared to mDCs (95). Thus, mDCs stop phagocytosis and peptide loading on MHC upon pathogen recognition and stably present peptides from antigenic material they had acquired upon pathogen encounter (30, 96, 97). This maturation-induced stabilization of peptide–MHC complexes enhances the priming of pathogen-specific T cells by mDCs. In contrast, pDCs continue to present new peptides on MHC complexes even in the mature stage (95). On the one hand, this limits their capacity to stimulate pathogen-specific T cells; on the other hand, this enables them to present also late-expressed viral antigens when they are actively infected. This diverse regulation of MHC–peptide stability in mDCs and pDCs suggests that they present different antigens to T cells.

TABLE 1 | Surface markers expressed on human and mouse DC subsets.

Subsets	Mouse (spleen)			Human (blood)		
	CD8α−	CD8α+	pDC	mDC1	mDC2	pDC
CD11c	+	+	Low	++	+	−
CD11b	+	+/−	−	+	−	−
BDCA-1/CD1c	n/a	n/a	n/a	+	−	−
BDCA-2/CD303	−	−	+	−	−	+
BDCA-3/CD141	−	−	−	−	+	−
BDCA-4/CD304	−	−	−	−	−	+

This table summarizes the expression of widely used surface markers to identify DC subsets in humans and mice.

Plasmacytoid DCs are present in lymph nodes and are largely absent from non-lymphoid organs, but they can be recruited upon inflammation (98). The role of pDC in T-cell priming is still debated (99). There is consensus that they are poorly stimulatory in their resting state (100, 101), but while some groups proposed that they become potent APCs following TLR stimulation and prime CD4+ and cross-prime CD8+ T-cell responses (102–105), others concluded that also mature pDCs have only low priming and cross-priming capacities and might rather be tolerogenic (101). The rapid and abundant production of type-1 interferon by pDC suggests a pivotal role in viral infections, even if their capacity to prime virus-specific T cells directly appears to be limited. IFN-α can also be produced by other immune cells and by virus-infected cells, but the early and systemic IFN-α response is believed to depend on pDCs (101). Consistently, in the case of HSV infections, it was shown that pDCs were important for systemic but not local protection (106). However, in several other viral infections in mice, including vesicular stomatitis virus (VSV), lymphocytic choriomeningitis virus (LCMV), RSV, and mouse cytomegalovirus (MCMV), pDCs do not seem to play a major role (100). In marked contrast, in mouse hepatitis virus (MHV) infection, the antiviral response against this coronavirus was largely pDC dependent (107) (**Figure 1**). Finally, pDCs have been found by several groups to induce the production of the anti-inflammatory cytokine IL-10 by CD4+ T cells, suggesting that they might be important to inhibit excessive T-cell responses. Several proteins expressed by pDCs were found to promote IL-10 induction in T cells, including the Notch ligand Delta-like 4 (108), ICOSL (109, 110), as well as IFN-α (23, Nizzoli et al., under review).

Myeloid DCs are a heterogeneous population, and different mDC subsets can be identified that preferentially initiate different types of adaptive immune responses (**Figure 1**). In the spleen of mice, mDCs can be subdivided into CD8α+ and CD8α− subsets (**Table 1**). CD8α+ mDCs produce high levels of bioactive IL-12p70 and efficiently cross-prime CD8+ T-cell responses (111). They express CLEC9A, a C-type lectin, that enables them to take up antigenic material from dying cells, and their generation was shown to rely on the transcription factors BATF3 and IRF8 (112, 113). Moreover, they express the chemokine receptor XCR1 that favors their colocalization with CD8+ T cells (114). Altogether the present evidence indicates that CD8α+ DCs are specialized to induce Th1 and CTL responses in response to intracellular pathogens (115, 116). Notably, DCs in the gut that express CD103 have similar characteristics and are closely related to CD8α+ DC (117, 118). CD8α− DCs express CD11b and can be further subdivided into CD4+ and CD4−CD8− subsets. They preferentially prime CD4+ T-cell responses (119) and promote Th17 responses, but they can also induce Th2 cells (113, 120). Interestingly, CD11b+ DCs produce IL-23 in the gut and are required for protection against *Citrobacter rodentium* (121). Their generation depends on the transcription factor IRF4, while KLF4 expression is required for Th2, but not for Th17 induction (122). Notably, however, CD8α− DCs and also pDCs can cross-prime CD8+ T-cell responses under certain conditions (102–104, 123). Moreover, it was shown that upon appropriate microbial stimulation all mDC subsets have the potential to promote either Th1 or Th2 responses (124). Thus, although the proposed functional specialization of DC subsets is an intriguing and helpful concept, it might also be an oversimplification, since DC subsets have considerable plasticity and the induction of a specific type of immune response critically depends on the stimuli they receive from pathogens as well as from other immune cells (125).

DIFFERENT PATHOGEN SENSING BY DC SUBSETS IN HUMANS AND MICE

High numbers of human DCs can be generated *in vitro* by culturing monocytes with cytokines (41), and the large majority of studies on human DCs have been done with these monocyte-derived DCs. They are primary cells and show many behaviors of *in vivo* occurring DCs, including cytokine production as well as stable and potent antigen presentation upon maturation with TLR ligands (125). However, monocyte-derived DCs are not the appropriate model to study the role of specialized DC subsets in human immune responses.

Dendritic cells circulating at low frequency in human peripheral blood share several features with murine splenic DC subsets (126) (**Table 1**). Human pDCs have been identified more than 15 years ago as the natural IFN-α-producing cells (127, 128). They express TLR7 and TLR9 and produce large amounts of IFN-α in response to CpG DNA or influenza virus. Similar to their murine counterparts, they are poorly stimulatory (94), express the C-type lectin BDCA-2 (93), and induce IL-10 production in CD4+ T cells (129). In addition, subsets of mDCs can also be found in human blood and in tissues (130–133). As their murine homologues, they express CD11c and potently prime CD4+ and CD8+ T-cell responses. The expression of CD1c/BDCA-1 and CD141/BDCA-3 identifies two subsets among human mDCs in peripheral blood (93) and also in secondary lymphoid organs (105, 132, 134, 135). BDCA-3+ "mDC2" (**Table 1**) are rare, but it could recently be demonstrated that they represent the human counterpart of murine CD8α+ DCs (136–140). Thus, as CD8α+ DCs, they selectively express CLEC9A and XCR1 and are dependent on the transcription factor BATF3 (112, 136, 138, 140, 141). Importantly, they can cross-present exogenous antigens on MHC class-I to CD8+ T cells and produce IL-12 (134–136). CD1c+ "mDC1" (**Table 1**) are more frequent and share some features with CD8α− DC, including CD11b expression and IL-23 production (121, 142, Nizzoli et al., under review). Also TLR3 expression in DC subsets appears to be similar in humans and mice, since it is expressed at high levels on CD8α+ DCs and mDC2, at lower levels on CD8α− DCs and mDC1, and absent on pDC. Surprisingly, TLR3 in mice is not required for immune responses against several viruses, including LCMV, VSV, MCMV, and Reovirus, suggesting that TLR3 has not a pivotal role in antiviral immune defense (143). Consistently, TLR3 deficiency in humans selectively leads to uncontrolled HSV1 infections in the central nervous system (CNS) (144).

Different subsets of DC have also been identified in human non-lymphoid tissues where they are strategically positioned to recognize invading pathogens, in particular at barrier surfaces. These migratory DC subsets play a crucial role to transport antigenic material of pathogens that invade specific tissues to draining

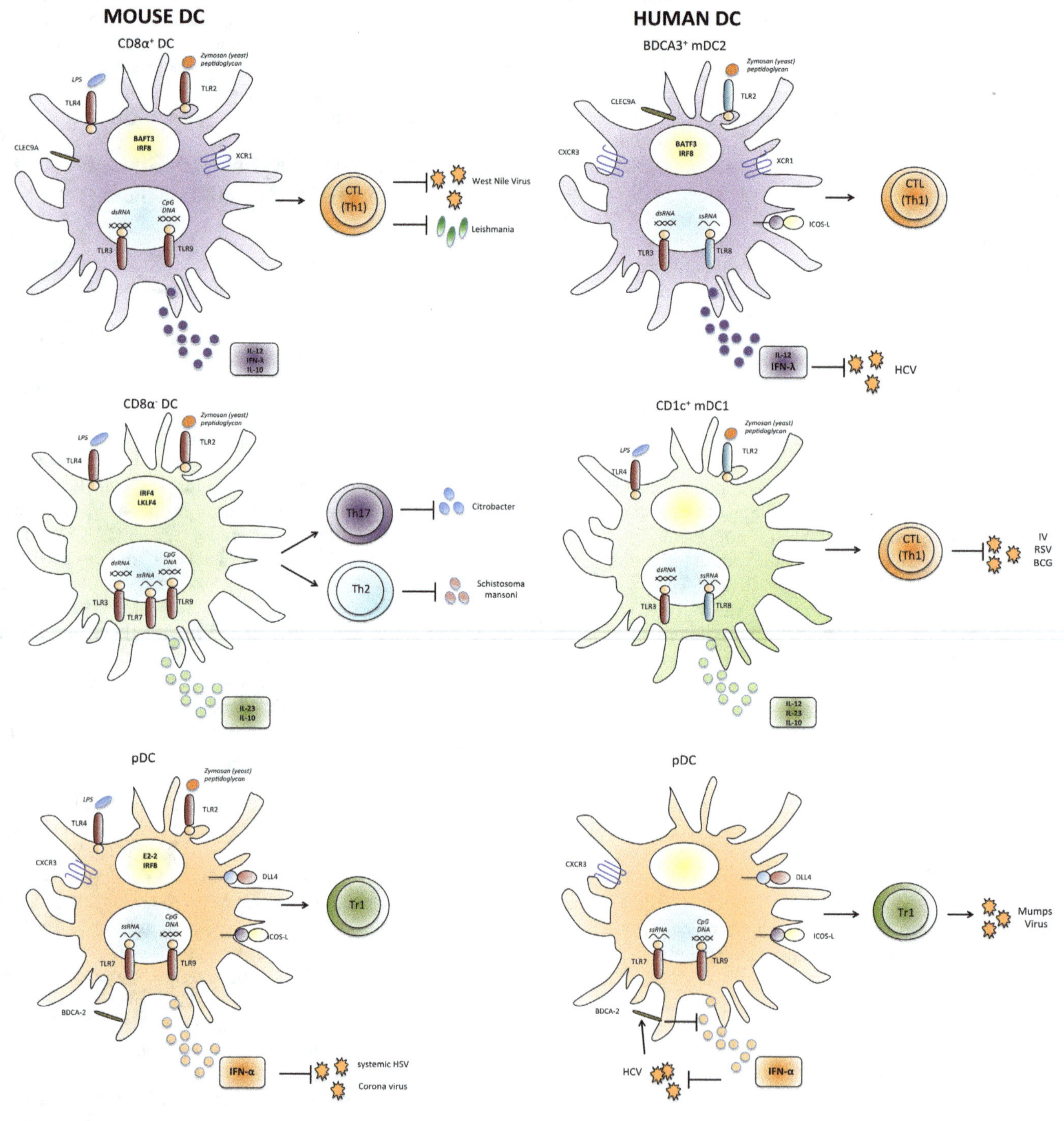

FIGURE 1 | Properties and functions of human and mouse DC subsets. Human and mouse mDC and pDC subsets express partially different patterns of pathogen-sensing receptors and cytokines and might thus have unique functions in inducing appropriate types of T-cell responses against individual pathogens. IV, influenza virus; HCV, hepatitis C virus; RSV, respiratory syncytial virus; HIV, human immunodeficiency virus; HSV, herpes simplex virus; BCG, Bacillus Calmette–Guérin.

lymph nodes and thus to initiate a tissue-specific T-cell response (130, 145, 146). Human Langerhans cells were first described more than a century ago and reside in the epidermis and are thus the first DCs that encounter skin-invading pathogens. Upon activation, they mature and migrate to draining lymph nodes to activate $CD4^+$ and $CD8^+$ T cells. In the dermis, different subsets of interstitial DCs are present and can be classified according to CD14, CD1a, and CD141 expression. Dermal $CD14^+$ cells might represent monocyte-derived macrophages rather then DCs (147), but $CD1a^+$ and $CD141^+$ DCs, respectively, resemble the

CD1c$^+$ and CD141$^+$ DC subsets in peripheral blood (148). Also in the lung and the liver, DC subsets that are related to CD1c$^+$ and CD141$^+$ DCs could be identified (133). Finally, in the human intestine, DC subsets that express CD11b and CD103 are similar to CD1c$^+$ and CD141$^+$ DCs, respectively, and these intestinal DC subsets are also largely conserved between humans and mice (149).

Although the similarities between human and mouse DC subsets are often emphasized, there are also some important differences in pathogen sensing by DCs in humans and mice (150). Importantly, the expression of several relevant TLRs is not conserved (**Figure 1**), presumably because humans and mice have evolved under the selective pressure of different pathogens. Thus, in mice, TLR7 and TLR9 are expressed by both pDC and mDC subsets (71), whereas in humans, they are restricted to pDCs (72). Also TLR4 expression is more restricted in human DCs, since it is expressed by mDC1 but not by mDC2 (136). Moreover, TLR8 is not expressed by human pDCs (72), and some agonists of human TLR8 such as the resiquimod R848 do not activate murine TLR8 (75, 151). Another relevant difference seems to be the role of the adaptor protein Myd88, which transduces signals from all TLRs with the notable exception of TLR3. Thus, mice deficient for Myd88 are highly susceptible to several infections by bacteria, viruses, parasites, and fungi. Conversely, Myd88-deficient patients are selectively affected by infections with pyogenic bacteria in childhood (152). Finally, human CD1c$^+$ DCs and also Langerhans cells seem to have superior capacities to cross-present antigens and to induce CTL responses as compared to their murine homologues (105, 134, 153, 154). Overall, these differences in pathogen sensing and T-cell activation between human and murine DCs are likely to have an important impact on their role in immune responses against specific pathogens.

SUBSET-SPECIFIC CYTOKINE PRODUCTION BY HUMAN DCs

Dendritic cell subsets in humans and mice express not only different patterns of toll-like receptors, but they have also partially distinct cytokine profiles (**Figure 1**). In particular, human mDC1 have a complex and quite unique regulation of cytokine production. Thus, while LPS triggers only low levels of cytokine production by mDC1, dual TLR stimulation with LPS or Poly-I:C (TLR3 ligand) in combination with R848 induces very high levels of a broad panel of cytokines, including TNF, IL-6, IL-10, IL-12, and IL-23 (Nizzoli et al., under review). The very potent cytokine-producing capacity of mDC1 has been missed in several studies where mDC1 were activated with single TLR ligands (45, 155, 156). Of note, single TLR stimulation is sufficient to induce antiviral cytokines by mDC2 and pDCs (see below) and proinflammatory cytokines by monocytes. Although mDC1 can secrete several proinflammatory cytokines that promote Th17 cell generation including IL-23 (142), it is unclear if they are the physiological inducers of Th17 cells or if monocyte-derived, inflammatory DCs do the job (12, 157). Also the identity of the DC subset that induces human Th2 responses is still enigmatic. It was originally proposed that mDCs induce Th1 polarization and pDCs Th2, but later it was shown that also pDCs can drive Th1 responses (158, 159). More recently, mDC2 but not mDC1 were found to induce Th2 cells in an aberrant response to influenza virus (160).

In apparent contrast to CD8α$^-$ DCs, mDC1 can produce high levels of IL-12 (134, 135), suggesting a relevant role in immune responses against intracellular pathogens. Moreover, the production of the anti-inflammatory cytokine IL-10, which can be produced by all mDCs in mice, is largely restricted to mDC1 in humans (Nizzoli et al., under review). Stimulation of mDC1 with the intestinal bacterium *Escherichia coli* or with LPS alone induces IL-10 and was proposed to induce a tolerogenic state in mDC1 (155). Although IL-10 is indeed a tolerogenic cytokine and a well-established negative regulator of DC maturation and cytokine production (161), it can paradoxically also have positive effects, in particular on CD8$^+$ T-cell responses (162, 163). Consistently, we found that IL-10 produced by mDC1 completely blocked the cross-priming of low-affinity CTL and enhanced the responsiveness of CD8$^+$ memory T cells to the homeostatic cytokine IL-15. Thus, mDC1-derived IL-10 appears to play an important positive role in CTL responses, since it selects high affinity cells upon priming and inhibits CTL memory attrition at the same time (Nizzoli et al., under review).

While mDC1 can secrete a broad panel of pro- and anti-inflammatory cytokines, mDC2 and pDC are largely dedicated to secrete high levels of antiviral cytokines. The subset specific production of IFN-α by pDC (128) and of IFN-λ by CD8α$^+$ and mDC2 (134, 137) appears to be largely conserved between humans and mice. The very potent IFN-λ-producing capacities of BDCA-3$^+$ DC (134, 137) suggest that analogous to pDCs they might be the relevant source of early and systemic IFN-λ in viral infections. Notably, IFN-λ has antiproliferative and antiviral activities similar to type-I interferon, but the expression of the IFN-λ receptor is much more restricted and found mainly on epithelial cells at barrier surfaces and in the liver (164). MDC2 can also secrete selected isoforms of IFN-α (165) and some IL-12 (134–136, 138), consistent with the view that they play an important role in antiviral immune responses. As previously mentioned for murine pDCs, IFN-α is not only a powerful antiviral cytokine that activates several different types of immune cells, but it also induces IL-10 production in CD4$^+$ T cells, suggesting that pDCs induce Tr1-like regulatory T cells also in humans (21, 23, 108, Nizzoli et al., under review).

SPECIFIC ROLES OF HUMAN DC SUBSETS IN RESPONSES TO INDIVIDUAL PATHOGENS

The more restricted expression of TLRs and the specific cytokine-producing capacities of human DC subset suggest that they play unique roles in immune responses against individual pathogens. The roles of human DC subsets in pathogen-specific immune response are however difficult to address directly because patients that selectively lack a DC subset of interest have not been identified so far. Nevertheless, some interesting findings were reported. In particular, mDC2 appear to be highly relevant in HCV infection. Single-nucleotide polymorphisms in the IFN-λ3 gene locus are strongly associated with spontaneous clearance and response to therapy in HCV patients (166). All DC subsets can secrete some IFN-λ1 (134, 167), but mDC2 produce much higher amounts. Moreover, IFN-λ2/3 are largely restricted to mDC2, and importantly HCV induces IFN-λ3 production by mDC2 (168, Nizzoli et al., under review). Thus, mDC2 appear to be a highly relevant source for protective IFN-λ3 in HCV infection (169). Interestingly, an important role for mDC1 rather than for mDC2 was recently proposed in tuberculosis (170, 171). Thus, mDC1 were more efficiently infected with the Bacillus Calmette–Guérin (BCG) vaccine than other DCs and induced the activation of pDCs and $CD8^+$ T cells. Notably, mDC1 could not be replaced by mDC2 in this system, suggesting that mDC1 could play a non-redundant role in the defense against selected intracellular pathogens. MDC1 and mDC2 have also been suggested to play different roles in RSV infection (172, 173). Thus, mDC subsets produced different cytokines in response to RSV, consistent with their different cytokine profiles upon stimulation with purified TLR ligands (134, Nizzoli et al., under review). Moreover, they induced different classes of T-cell responses, with mDC1 inducing preferentially Th1 cells and mDC2 inducing predominantly Th2 and T-regulatory cells. Similarly, mDC2, but not mDC1, were found to induce Th2 response to influenza virus (160). Also the capacity of pDCs to induce IL-10-producing regulatory T cells has been documented with a relevant pathogen, since pDCs were shown to induce IFN-γ and IL-10 production in antigen-experienced $CD4^+$ T cells specific for mumps virus (129). Conversely, $CD11c^+$ mDCs, which contain both mDC1 and mDC2, induced IFN-γ and, surprisingly, IL-5.

It is largely accepted that pDC-derived IFN-α is important to contain human viral infections. Thus, stabilized pegylated IFN-α is a widely used therapy for HCV patients. IFN-λ appears to be similar effective, but is less toxic presumably because of the more restricted expression of its receptor (164). Interestingly, the HCV glycoprotein E2 is a ligand for BDCA-2, which is specifically expressed on pDCs (**Table 1**) and inhibits IFN-α production (174, 175). In this way, HCV might inhibit IFN-α production to establish chronic infection. Finally, pDCs are also targeted by human immunodeficiency virus (HIV), but whether they play a protective or detrimental role is still unclear (176).

EXPLOITING DC BIOLOGY: VACCINES THAT INDUCE HUMORAL AND CELLULAR IMMUNE RESPONSES

Vaccines have been a major breakthrough for human health. Attenuated or killed pathogens are highly efficient to induce protective cellular and humoral immune responses, and the induced protective memory can last for a lifetime (177, 178). However, since these pathogen-based vaccines also have considerable side effects, proteins in combination with adjuvants that activate APCs are more often used. Protein vaccines induce $CD4^+$ T-cell responses and neutralizing antibodies, but they are poorly efficient in inducing cytotoxic T-cell responses and are also rather inefficient in inducing Th1 cells (179, 180). Frequently used adjuvants are alum, oil-in-water emulsions like MF59, and more recently also monophosphoryl lipid A (MPL), a detoxified form of LPS. In mice, different adjuvants were shown to induce different proinflammatory cytokines. Thus, alum acts via uric acid on inflammatory DCs (181), which leads to NOD-like receptor protein-3 (NALP3)-dependent IL-1β production (182). Conversely, MPL does not induce IL-1β (183) but induces specific antibodies through an IL-6-dependent mechanism (184), while MF-59 and alum act independently of IL-6 (185). However, the different TLR expression and cytokine production by human APC subsets should be considered when translating this knowledge from animal models to patients. A recent interesting report analyzed the response of APC subsets to 13 different vaccines and concluded that different vaccines activate indeed different APC populations (186). More direct information on the effect of DCs was obtained by vaccinations with peptide-pulsed monocyte-derived DCs in cancer patients, which can induce tumor-specific $CD8^+$ T cells (187), but the clinical responses were so far largely insufficient. MDCs might be more potent and are currently tested in clinical trials.

Nucleic acid-sensing TLRs are particularly potent to induce $CD8^+$ T-cell responses in mice (188) and have recently been employed as adjuvants in vaccines. Examples are CpG-DNA that stimulates TLR9 (189), and the TLR7 ligand imiquimod, which is used as a cream to stimulate DC locally in the skin, and was shown to induce $CD8^+$ T-cell responses *in situ* (190). Vaccines consisting of plasmid DNA coding for relevant protein antigens are a novel approach that efficiently induces humoral and cellular immune responses in animals. However, in humans, these DNA vaccines are often poorly immunogenic (191), presumably because they have only low adjuvant activity and stimulate mainly cytosolic DNA sensors rather than TLR9 (192), which in addition is restricted to pDCs and B cells in humans. An alternative promising approach is the vaccination with mRNA (193, 194), which delivers not only the antigenic protein directly to the cytosol, thereby bypassing the requirements for cross-presentation (195), but also induces mDC and pDC maturation and cytokine production via TLR7/8 at the same time (196). Indeed, intradermal injection of naked mRNA results in local uptake and translation of the nucleic acid (197) followed by the development of an adaptive immunity in mice (198) and in humans (199, 200). Since also lymph node-resident DCs are expected to be appropriate APCs to process antigens encoded by mRNA, direct injection of nucleic acid into lymph nodes has also been evaluated. In animal models, intra-lymph node injections of mRNA result in expression of the protein encoded by the mRNA in DCs. Furthermore, the injected mRNA activated lymph node-resident APCs and induced potent $CD4^+$ and $CD8^+$ T-cell responses as well as prophylactic and therapeutic antitumor immunity (201). The approach is currently being evaluated through two clinical studies exploring the efficacy of intra-lymph node mRNA vaccination in advanced melanoma patients. As a further development, systemic administration of a liposomal formulation of mRNA that delivers the nucleic acids to APCs present in secondary lymphoid organs is also being evaluated. Using the functional diversity of DCs *in vivo*, and their specific capabilities in generating appropriate adaptive immune responses, those systemic synthetic vaccines might recapitulate the natural mechanisms of immunity developed during pathogen infection and guarantee the development of therapeutically efficacious immune responses.

CONCLUSION AND PERSPECTIVE

Dendritic cells continue to attract much interest of immunologists because they are the most potent APCs in the immune system and are the principal inducers of naive T-cell differentiation. Intensive research in the last years has established that different subsets of DC exist in mice that have specialized functions and preferentially induce different types of immune responses. In humans, much has been learned from *in vitro* differentiated monocyte-derived DCs, and more recently, also different subsets of DC populating human tissues have been analyzed at the molecular and functional levels. It is fundamental to further define the biology of these *in vivo* occurring human DC subsets to understand and cure pathogenic immune-mediated processes in so different settings as autoimmunity, infections, and cancer. In particular, appropriate targeting of DC subsets by vaccines holds the promise to induce cytotoxic T-cell responses to eradicate persistent intracellular pathogens or tumors.

ACKNOWLEDGMENTS

JG, GN, and SA are supported by the CARIPLO foundation, SA is supported by the European Research Council, and the INGM is supported by the "Romeo ed Enrica Invernizzi" foundation.

REFERENCES

1. Steinman RM. The dendritic cell system and its role in immunogenicity. *Annu Rev Immunol* (1991) **9**:271–96. doi:10.1146/annurev.iy.09.040191.001415
2. Banchereau J, Briere F, Caux C, Davoust J, Lebecque S, Liu YJ, et al. Immunobiology of dendritic cells. *Annu Rev Immunol* (2000) **18**:767–811. doi:10.1146/annurev.immunol.18.1.767
3. Geginat J, Paroni M, Facciotti F, Gruarin P, Kastirr I, Caprioli F, et al. The CD4-centered universe of human T cell subsets. *Semin Immunol* (2013) **25**(4):252–62. doi:10.1016/j.smim.2013.10.012
4. Cella M, Scheidegger D, Palmer Lehmann K, Lane P, Lanzavecchia A, Alber G. Ligation of CD40 on dendritic cells triggers production of high levels of interleukin-12 and enhances T cell stimulatory capacity: T-T help via APC activation. *J Exp Med* (1996) **184**(2):747–52. doi:10.1084/jem.184.2.747
5. Koch F, Stanzl U, Jennewein P, Janke K, Heufler C, Kampgen E, et al. High level IL-12 production by murine dendritic cells: upregulation via MHC class II and CD40 molecules and downregulation by IL-4 and IL-10. *J Exp Med* (1996) **184**:741–6. doi:10.1084/jem.184.2.741
6. Ito T, Amakawa R, Inaba M, Ikehara S, Inaba K, Fukuhara S. Differential regulation of human blood dendritic cell subsets by IFNs. *J Immunol* (2001) **166**:2961–9. doi:10.4049/jimmunol.166.5.2961
7. Kalinski P, Smits HH, Schuitemaker JH, Vieira PL, van Eijk M, de Jong EC, et al. IL-4 is a mediator of IL-12p70 induction by human Th2 cells: reversal of polarized Th2 phenotype by dendritic cells. *J Immunol* (2000) **165**:1877–81. doi:10.4049/jimmunol.165.4.1877
8. Hochrein H, O'Keeffe M, Luft T, Vandenabeele S, Grumont RJ, Maraskovsky E, et al. Interleukin (IL)-4 is a major regulatory cytokine governing bioactive IL-12 production by mouse and human dendritic cells. *J Exp Med* (2000) **192**:823–34. doi:10.1084/jem.192.6.823
9. Hochrein H, Shortman K, Vremec D, Scott B, Hertzog P, O'Keeffe M. Differential production of IL-12, IFN-α, and IFN-γ by mouse dendritic cell subsets. *J Immunol* (2001) **166**(9):5448–55.
10. Liang SC, Tan XY, Luxenberg DP, Karim R, Dunussi-Joannopoulos K, Collins M, et al. Interleukin (IL)-22 and IL-17 are coexpressed by Th17 cells and cooperatively enhance expression of antimicrobial peptides. *J Exp Med* (2006) **203**(10):2271–9. doi:10.1084/jem.20061308
11. Ma CS, Chew GY, Simpson N, Priyadarshi A, Wong M, Grimbacher B, et al. Deficiency of Th17 cells in hyper IgE syndrome due to mutations in STAT3. *J Exp Med* (2008) **205**(7):1551–7. doi:10.1084/jem.20080218
12. Acosta-Rodriguez EV, Rivino L, Geginat J, Jarrossay D, Gattorno M, Lanzavecchia A, et al. Surface phenotype and antigenic specificity of human interleukin 17-producing T helper memory cells. *Nat Immunol* (2007) **8**(6):639–46. doi:10.1038/ni1467
13. Acosta-Rodriguez EV, Napolitani G, Lanzavecchia A, Sallusto F. Interleukins 1beta and 6 but not transforming growth factor-beta are essential for the differentiation of interleukin 17-producing human T helper cells. *Nat Immunol* (2007) **8**(9):942–9. doi:10.1038/ni1496
14. Mills KH. Induction, function and regulation of IL-17-producing T cells. *Eur J Immunol* (2008) **38**(10):2636–49. doi:10.1002/eji.200838535
15. Anderson GP, Coyle AJ. TH2 and 'TH2-like' cells in allergy and asthma: pharmacological perspectives. *Trends Pharmacol Sci* (1994) **15**(9):324–32. doi:10.1016/0165-6147(94)90027-2
16. Kopf M, Le Gros G, Bachmann M, Lamers MC, Bluethmann H, Kohler G. Disruption of the murine IL-4 gene blocks Th2 cytokine responses. *Nature* (1993) **362**:245–8. doi:10.1038/362245a0
17. Halim TY, Steer CA, Matha L, Gold MJ, Martinez-Gonzalez I, McNagny KM, et al. Group 2 innate lymphoid cells are critical for the initiation of adaptive T helper 2 cell-mediated allergic lung inflammation. *Immunity* (2014) **40**(3):425–35. doi:10.1016/j.immuni.2014.01.011
18. Licona-Limon P, Kim LK, Palm NW, Flavell RA. TH2, allergy and group 2 innate lymphoid cells. *Nat Immunol* (2013) **14**(6):536–42. doi:10.1038/ni.2617
19. Jankovic D, Kullberg MC, Feng CG, Goldszmid RS, Collazo CM, Wilson M, et al. Conventional T-bet(+)Foxp3(-) Th1 cells are the major source of host-protective regulatory IL-10 during intracellular protozoan infection. *J Exp Med* (2007) **204**(2):273–83. doi:10.1084/jem.20062175
20. Groux H, O'Garra A, Bigler M, Rouleau M, Antonenko S, de Vries JE, et al. A CD4+ T-cell subset inhibits antigen-specific T-cell responses and prevents colitis. *Nature* (1997) **389**(6652):737–42. doi:10.1038/39614
21. Haringer B, Lozza L, Steckel B, Geginat J. Identification and characterization of IL-10/IFN-gamma-producing effector-like T cells with regulatory function in human blood. *J Exp Med* (2009) **206**(5):1009–17. doi:10.1084/jem.20082238
22. Huber S, Gagliani N, Esplugues E, O'Connor W Jr, Huber FJ, Chaudhry A, et al. Th17 cells express interleukin-10 receptor and are controlled by Foxp3 and Foxp3+ regulatory CD4+ T cells in an interleukin-10-dependent manner. *Immunity* (2011) **34**(4):554–65. doi:10.1016/j.immuni.2011.01.020
23. Levings MK, Sangregorio R, Galbiati F, Squadrone S, de Waal Malefyt R, Roncarolo MG. IFN-alpha and IL-10 induce the differentiation of human type 1 T regulatory cells. *J Immunol* (2001) **166**(9):5530–9. doi:10.4049/jimmunol.166.9.5530
24. Murugaiyan G, Mittal A, Lopez-Diego R, Maier LM, Anderson DE, Weiner HL. IL-27 is a key regulator of IL-10 and IL-17 production by human CD4+ T cells. *J Immunol* (2009) **183**(4):2435–43. doi:10.4049/jimmunol.0900568
25. Le Buanec H, Gougeon ML, Mathian A, Lebon P, Dupont JM, Peltre G, et al. IFN-alpha and CD46 stimulation are associated with active lupus and skew natural T regulatory cell differentiation to type 1 regulatory T (Tr1) cells. *Proc Natl Acad Sci USA* (2011) **108**(47):18995–9000. doi:10.1073/pnas.1113301108
26. Shiokawa A, Tanabe K, Tsuji NM, Sato R, Hachimura S. IL-10 and IL-27 producing dendritic cells capable of enhancing IL-10 production of T cells are induced in oral tolerance. *Immunol Lett* (2009) **125**(1):7–14. doi:10.1016/j.imlet.2009.05.002

27. Gregori S, Tomasoni D, Pacciani V, Scirpoli M, Battaglia M, Magnani CF, et al. Differentiation of type 1 T regulatory cells (Tr1) by tolerogenic DC-10 requires the IL-10-dependent ILT4/HLA-G pathway. *Blood* (2010) **116**(6):935–44. doi:10.1182/blood-2009-07-234872
28. Sallusto F, Cella M, Danieli C, Lanzavecchia A. Dendritic cells use macropinocytosis and the mannose receptor to concentrate macromolecules in the major histocompatibility complex class II compartment: downregulation by cytokines and bacterial products. *J Exp Med* (1995) **182**:389–400. doi:10.1084/jem.182.2.389
29. Inaba K, Turley S, Iyoda T, Yamaide F, Shimoyama S, Reis e Sousa C, et al. The formation of immunogenic major histocompatibility complex class II-peptide ligands in lysosomal compartments of dendritic cells is regulated by inflammatory stimuli. *J Exp Med* (2000) **191**:927–36. doi:10.1084/jem.191.6.927
30. Turley SJ, Inaba K, Garrett WS, Ebersold M, Unternaehrer J, Steinman RM, et al. Transport of peptide-MHC class II complexes in developing dendritic cells. *Science* (2000) **288**:522–7. doi:10.1126/science.288.5465.522
31. Heath WR, Carbone FR. Cross-presentation in viral immunity and self-tolerance. *Nat Rev Immunol* (2001) **1**(2):126–34. doi:10.1038/35100512
32. Joffre OP, Segura E, Savina A, Amigorena S. Cross-presentation by dendritic cells. *Nat Rev Immunol* (2012) **12**(8):557–69. doi:10.1038/nri3254
33. Germain RN, Margulies DH. The biochemistry and cell biology of antigen processing and presentation. *Annu Rev Immunol* (1993) **11**:403–50. doi:10.1146/annurev.iy.11.040193.002155
34. Sanders ME, Makgoba MW, June CH, Young HA, Shaw S. Enhanced responsiveness of human memory T cells to CD2 and CD3 receptor-mediated activation. *Eur J Immunol* (1989) **19**(5):803–8. doi:10.1002/eji.1830190504
35. Mehta Damani A, Markowicz S, Engleman EG. Generation of antigen-specific CD4+ T cell lines from naive precursors. *Eur J Immunol* (1995) **25**(5):1206–11. doi:10.1002/eji.1830250511
36. Geginat J, Clissi B, Moro M, Dellabona P, Bender JR, Pardi R. CD28 and LFA-1 contribute to cyclosporin A-resistant T cell growth by stabilizing the IL-2 mRNA through distinct signaling pathways. *Eur J Immunol* (2000) **30**(4):1136–44. doi:10.1002/(SICI)1521-4141(200004)30:4<1136::AID-IMMU1136>3.0.CO;2-3
37. Ohshima Y, Yang LP, Uchiyama T, Tanaka Y, Baum P, Sergerie M, et al. OX40 costimulation enhances interleukin-4 (IL-4) expression at priming and promotes the differentiation of naive human CD4(+) T cells into high IL-4-producing effectors. *Blood* (1998) **92**(9):3338–45.
38. DeBenedette MA, Wen T, Bachmann MF, Ohashi PS, Barber BH, Stocking KL, et al. Analysis of 4-1BB ligand (4-1BBL)-deficient mice and of mice lacking both 4-1BBL and CD28 reveals a role for 4-1BBL in skin allograft rejection and in the cytotoxic T cell response to influenza virus. *J Immunol* (1999) **163**(9):4833–41.
39. Johnson JG, Jenkins MK. Accessory cell-derived signals required for T cell activation. *Immunol Res* (1993) **12**(1):48–64. doi:10.1007/BF02918368
40. Rivino L, Messi M, Jarrossay D, Lanzavecchia A, Sallusto F, Geginat J. Chemokine receptor expression identifies Pre-T helper (Th)1, Pre-Th2, and nonpolarized cells among human CD4+ central memory T cells. *J Exp Med* (2004) **200**(6):725–35. doi:10.1084/jem.20040774
41. Sallusto F, Lanzavecchia A. Efficient presentation of soluble antigen by cultured human dendritic cells is maintained by granulocyte/macrophage colony-stimulating factor plus interleukin 4 and downregulated by tumor necrosis factor alpha. *J Exp Med* (1994) **179**:1109–18. doi:10.1084/jem.179.4.1109
42. Cheong C, Matos I, Choi JH, Dandamudi DB, Shrestha E, Longhi MP, et al. Microbial stimulation fully differentiates monocytes to DC-SIGN/CD209(+) dendritic cells for immune T cell areas. *Cell* (2010) **143**(3):416–29. doi:10.1016/j.cell.2010.09.039
43. Nakano H, Lin KL, Yanagita M, Charbonneau C, Cook DN, Kakiuchi T, et al. Blood-derived inflammatory dendritic cells in lymph nodes stimulate acute T helper type 1 immune responses. *Nat Immunol* (2009) **10**(4):394–402. doi:10.1038/ni.1707
44. Schakel K, von Kietzell M, Hansel A, Ebling A, Schulze L, Haase M, et al. Human 6-sulfo LacNAc-expressing dendritic cells are principal producers of early interleukin-12 and are controlled by erythrocytes. *Immunity* (2006) **24**(6):767–77. doi:10.1016/j.immuni.2006.03.020
45. Piccioli D, Tavarini S, Borgogni E, Steri V, Nuti S, Sammicheli C, et al. Functional specialization of human circulating CD16 and CD1c myeloid dendritic-cell subsets. *Blood* (2007) **109**(12):5371–9. doi:10.1182/blood-2006-08-038422
46. Mackay CR, Marston WL, Dudler L. Naive and memory T cells show distinct pathways of lymphocyte recirculation. *J Exp Med* (1990) **171**:801–17. doi:10.1084/jem.171.3.801
47. Steinman RM, Pack M, Inaba K. Dendritic cells in the T-cell areas of lymphoid organs. *Immunol Rev* (1997) **156**:25–37. doi:10.1111/j.1600-065X.1997.tb00956.x
48. Lanzavecchia A. Antigen-specific interaction between T and B cells. *Nature* (1985) **314**(6011):537–9. doi:10.1038/314537a0
49. Breitfeld D, Ohl L, Kremmer E, Ellwart J, Sallusto F, Lipp M, et al. Follicular B helper T cells express CXC chemokine receptor 5, localize to B cell follicles, and support immunoglobulin production. *J Exp Med* (2000) **192**(11):1545–52. doi:10.1084/jem.192.11.1545
50. Muller G, Lipp M. Shaping up adaptive immunity: the impact of CCR7 and CXCR5 on lymphocyte trafficking. *Microcirculation* (2003) **10**(3–4):325–34. doi:10.1080/mic.10.3-4.325.334
51. Mildner A, Jung S. Development and function of dendritic cell subsets. *Immunity* (2014) **40**(5):642–56. doi:10.1016/j.immuni.2014.04.016
52. Liu K, Victora GD, Schwickert TA, Guermonprez P, Meredith MM, Yao K, et al. In vivo analysis of dendritic cell development and homeostasis. *Science* (2009) **324**(5925):392–7. doi:10.1126/science.1170540
53. Breton G, Lee J, Zhou YJ, Schreiber JJ, Keler T, Puhr S, et al. Circulating precursors of human CD1c+ and CD141+ dendritic cells. *J Exp Med* (2015) **212**(3):401–13. doi:10.1084/jem.20141441
54. Lee J, Breton G, Oliveira TY, Zhou YJ, Aljoufi A, Puhr S, et al. Restricted dendritic cell and monocyte progenitors in human cord blood and bone marrow. *J Exp Med* (2015) **212**(3):385–99. doi:10.1084/jem.20141442
55. Onai N, Obata-Onai A, Schmid MA, Ohteki T, Jarrossay D, Manz MG. Identification of clonogenic common Flt3+M-CSFR+ plasmacytoid and conventional dendritic cell progenitors in mouse bone marrow. *Nat Immunol* (2007) **8**(11):1207–16. doi:10.1038/ni1518
56. Steinman RM, Nussenzweig MC. Avoiding horror autotoxicus: the importance of dendritic cells in peripheral T cell tolerance. *Proc Natl Acad Sci U S A* (2002) **99**(1):351–8. doi:10.1073/pnas.231606698
57. Hawiger D, Inaba K, Dorsett Y, Guo M, Mahnke K, Rivera M, et al. Dendritic cells induce peripheral T cell unresponsiveness under steady state conditions in vivo. *J Exp Med* (2001) **194**(6):769–79. doi:10.1084/jem.194.6.769
58. Hernandez J, Aung S, Redmond WL, Sherman LA. Phenotypic and functional analysis of CD8(+) T cells undergoing peripheral deletion in response to cross-presentation of self-antigen. *J Exp Med* (2001) **194**(6):707–17. doi:10.1084/jem.194.6.707
59. Gett AV, Sallusto F, Lanzavecchia A, Geginat J. T cell fitness determined by signal strength. *Nat Immunol* (2003) **4**(4):355–60. doi:10.1038/ni908
60. Bacchetta R, Gregori S, Roncarolo MG. CD4+ regulatory T cells: mechanisms of induction and effector function. *Autoimmun Rev* (2005) **4**(8):491–6. doi:10.1016/j.autrev.2005.04.005
61. Janeway CA. The immune system evolved to discriminate infectious nonself from noninfectious self. *Immunol Today* (1992) **13**:11–6. doi:10.1016/0167-5699(92)90198-G
62. Medzhitov R, Preston-Hurlburt P, Janeway CA Jr. A human homologue of the *Drosophila* toll protein signals activation of adaptive immunity. *Nature* (1997) **388**(6640):394–7. doi:10.1038/41131
63. Cella M, Sallusto F, Lanzavecchia A. Origin, maturation and antigen presenting function of dendritic cells. *Curr Opin Immunol* (1997) **9**:10–6. doi:10.1016/S0952-7915(97)80153-7
64. Rock FL, Hardiman G, Timans JC, Kastelein RA, Bazan JF. A family of human receptors structurally related to *Drosophila* toll. *Proc Natl Acad Sci U S A* (1998) **95**(2):588–93. doi:10.1073/pnas.95.2.588
65. Motta V, Soares F, Sun T, Philpott DJ. NOD-like receptors: versatile cytosolic sentinels. *Physiol Rev* (2015) **95**(1):149–78. doi:10.1152/physrev.00009.2014
66. Bowie AG, Fitzgerald KA. RIG-I: tri-ing to discriminate between self and non-self RNA. *Trends Immunol* (2007) **28**(4):147–50. doi:10.1016/j.it.2007.02.002
67. Osorio F, Reis e Sousa C. Myeloid C-type lectin receptors in pathogen recognition and host defense. *Immunity* (2011) **34**(5):651–64. doi:10.1016/j.immuni.2011.05.001
68. Muzio M, Polentarutti N, Bosisio D, Prahladan MK, Mantovani A. Toll-like receptors: a growing family of immune receptors that are differentially

expressed and regulated by different leukocytes. *J Leukoc Biol* (2000) **67**(4):450–6.
69. Hemmi H, Takeuchi O, Kawai T, Kaisho T, Sato S, Sanjo H, et al. A toll-like receptor recognizes bacterial DNA. *Nature* (2000) **408**:740–5. doi:10.1038/35047123
70. Yang YL, Reis LF, Pavlovic J, Aguzzi A, Schafer R, Kumar A, et al. Deficient signaling in mice devoid of double-stranded RNA-dependent protein kinase. *EMBO J* (1995) **14**(24):6095–106.
71. Edwards AD, Diebold SS, Slack EM, Tomizawa H, Hemmi H, Kaisho T, et al. Toll-like receptor expression in murine DC subsets: lack of TLR7 expression by CD8 alpha+ DC correlates with unresponsiveness to imidazoquinolines. *Eur J Immunol* (2003) **33**(4):827–33. doi:10.1002/eji.200323797
72. Jarrossay D, Napolitani G, Colonna M, Sallusto F, Lanzavecchia A. Specialization and complementarity in microbial molecule recognition by human myeloid and plasmacytoid dendritic cells. *Eur J Immunol* (2001) **31**(11):3388–93. doi:10.1002/1521-4141(200111)31:11<3388::AID-IMMU3388>3.0.CO;2-Q
73. Alexopoulou L, Holt AC, Medzhitov R, Flavell RA. Recognition of double-stranded RNA and activation of NF-kappaB by toll-like receptor 3. *Nature* (2001) **413**(6857):732–8. doi:10.1038/35099560
74. Diebold SS, Kaisho T, Hemmi H, Akira S, Reis e Sousa C. Innate antiviral responses by means of TLR7-mediated recognition of single-stranded RNA. *Science* (2004) **303**(5663):1529–31. doi:10.1126/science.1093616
75. Heil F, Hemmi H, Hochrein H, Ampenberger F, Kirschning C, Akira S, et al. Species-specific recognition of single-stranded RNA via toll-like receptor 7 and 8. *Science* (2004) **303**(5663):1526–9. doi:10.1126/science.1093620
76. Schulz O, Diebold SS, Chen M, Naslund TI, Nolte MA, Alexopoulou L, et al. Toll-like receptor 3 promotes cross-priming to virus-infected cells. *Nature* (2005) **433**(7028):887–92. doi:10.1038/nature03326
77. Xagorari A, Chlichlia K. Toll-like receptors and viruses: induction of innate antiviral immune responses. *Open Microbiol J* (2008) **2**:49–59. doi:10.2174/1874285800802010049
78. Goodridge HS, Underhill DM. Fungal recognition by TLR2 and dectin-1. *Handb Exp Pharmacol* (2008) **183**:87–109. doi:10.1007/978-3-540-72167-3_5
79. Takeuchi O, Hoshino K, Kawai T, Sanjo H, Takada H, Ogawa T, et al. Differential roles of TLR2 and TLR4 in recognition of gram-negative and gram-positive bacterial cell wall components. *Immunity* (1999) **11**:443–51. doi:10.1016/S1074-7613(00)80119-3
80. Esen N, Tanga FY, DeLeo JA, Kielian T. Toll-like receptor 2 (TLR2) mediates astrocyte activation in response to the Gram-positive bacterium *Staphylococcus aureus*. *J Neurochem* (2004) **88**(3):746–58. doi:10.1046/j.1471-4159.2003.02202.x
81. Hoshino K, Takeuchi O, Kawai T, Sanjo H, Ogawa T, Takeda Y, et al. Cutting edge: toll-like receptor 4 (TLR4)-deficient mice are hyporesponsive to lipopolysaccharide: evidence for TLR4 as the Lps gene product. *J Immunol* (1999) **162**(7):3749–52.
82. Medzhitov R, Preston-Hurlburt P, Kopp E, Stadlen A, Chen C, Ghosh S, et al. MyD88 is an adaptor protein in the hToll/IL-1 receptor family signaling pathways. *Mol Cell* (1998) **2**(2):253–8. doi:10.1016/S1097-2765(00)80136-7
83. Honda K, Yanai H, Negishi H, Asagiri M, Sato M, Mizutani T, et al. IRF-7 is the master regulator of type-I interferon-dependent immune responses. *Nature* (2005) **434**(7034):772–7. doi:10.1038/nature03464
84. Kawai T, Sato S, Ishii KJ, Coban C, Hemmi H, Yamamoto M, et al. Interferon-alpha induction through toll-like receptors involves a direct interaction of IRF7 with MyD88 and TRAF6. *Nat Immunol* (2004) **5**(10):1061–8. doi:10.1038/ni1118
85. Yamamoto M, Sato S, Mori K, Hoshino K, Takeuchi O, Takeda K, et al. Cutting edge: a novel Toll/IL-1 receptor domain-containing adapter that preferentially activates the IFN-beta promoter in the toll-like receptor signaling. *J Immunol* (2002) **169**(12):6668–72. doi:10.4049/jimmunol.169.12.6668
86. Doyle S, Vaidya S, O'Connell R, Dadgostar H, Dempsey P, Wu T, et al. IRF3 mediates a TLR3/TLR4-specific antiviral gene program. *Immunity* (2002) **17**(3):251–63. doi:10.1016/S1074-7613(02)00390-4
87. Yamamoto M, Sato S, Hemmi H, Hoshino K, Kaisho T, Sanjo H, et al. Role of adaptor TRIF in the MyD88-independent toll-like receptor signaling pathway. *Science* (2003) **301**(5633):640–3. doi:10.1126/science.1087262
88. O'Neill LA. How toll-like receptors signal: what we know and what we don't know. *Curr Opin Immunol* (2006) **18**(1):3–9. doi:10.1016/j.coi.2005.11.012
89. Macagno A, Napolitani G, Lanzavecchia A, Sallusto F. Duration, combination and timing: the signal integration model of dendritic cell activation. *Trends Immunol* (2007) **28**(5):227–33. doi:10.1016/j.it.2007.03.008
90. Liu Q, Zhu Y, Yong WK, Sze NS, Tan NS, Ding JL. Cutting edge: synchronization of IRF1, JunB, and C/EBPbeta activities during TLR3-TLR7 cross-talk orchestrates timely cytokine synergy in the proinflammatory response. *J Immunol* (2015) **195**(3):801–5. doi:10.4049/jimmunol.1402358
91. Sozzani S, Allavena P, D'Amico G, Luini W, Bianchi G, Kataura M, et al. Differential regulation of chemokine receptors during dendritic cell maturation: a model for their trafficking properties. *J Immunol* (1998) **161**(3):1083–6.
92. Sallusto F, Schaerli P, Loetscher P, Schaniel C, Lenig D, Mackay CR, et al. Rapid and coordinated switch in chemokine receptor expression during dendritic cell maturation. *Eur J Immunol* (1998) **28**:2760–9. doi:10.1002/(SICI)1521-4141(199809)28:09<2760::AID-IMMU2760>3.0.CO;2-N
93. Dzionek A, Fuchs A, Schmidt P, Cremer S, Zysk M, Miltenyi S, et al. BDCA-2, BDCA-3, and BDCA-4: three markers for distinct subsets of dendritic cells in human peripheral blood. *J Immunol* (2000) **165**(11):6037–46. doi:10.4049/jimmunol.165.11.6037
94. MacDonald KP, Munster DJ, Clark GJ, Dzionek A, Schmitz J, Hart DN. Characterization of human blood dendritic cell subsets. *Blood* (2002) **100**(13):4512–20. doi:10.1182/blood-2001-11-0097
95. Sadaka C, Marloie-Provost MA, Soumelis V, Benaroch P. Developmental regulation of MHC II expression and transport in human plasmacytoid-derived dendritic cells. *Blood* (2009) **113**(10):2127–35. doi:10.1182/blood-2008-10-178152
96. Pierre P, Turley SJ, Gatti E, Hull M, Meltzer J, Mirza A, et al. Developmental regulation of MHC class II transport in mouse dendritic cells. *Nature* (1997) **388**:787–92. doi:10.1038/42039
97. Watts C. Capture and processing of exogenous antigens for presentation on MHC molecules. *Annu Rev Immunol* (1997) **15**:821–50. doi:10.1146/annurev.immunol.15.1.821
98. Yoneyama H, Matsuno K, Zhang Y, Nishiwaki T, Kitabatake M, Ueha S, et al. Evidence for recruitment of plasmacytoid dendritic cell precursors to inflamed lymph nodes through high endothelial venules. *Int Immunol* (2004) **16**(7):915–28. doi:10.1093/intimm/dxh093
99. Villadangos JA, Young L. Antigen-presentation properties of plasmacytoid dendritic cells. *Immunity* (2008) **29**(3):352–61. doi:10.1016/j.immuni.2008.09.002
100. Reizis B, Bunin A, Ghosh HS, Lewis KL, Sisirak V. Plasmacytoid dendritic cells: recent progress and open questions. *Annu Rev Immunol* (2011) **29**:163–83. doi:10.1146/annurev-immunol-031210-101345
101. Reizis B, Colonna M, Trinchieri G, Barrat F, Gilliet M. Plasmacytoid dendritic cells: one-trick ponies or workhorses of the immune system? *Nat Rev Immunol* (2011) **11**(8):558–65. doi:10.1038/nri3027
102. Mouries J, Moron G, Schlecht G, Escriou N, Dadaglio G, Leclerc C. Plasmacytoid dendritic cells efficiently cross-prime naive T cells in vivo after TLR activation. *Blood* (2008) **112**(9):3713–22. doi:10.1182/blood-2008-03-146290
103. Hoeffel G, Ripoche AC, Matheoud D, Nascimbeni M, Escriou N, Lebon P, et al. Antigen crosspresentation by human plasmacytoid dendritic cells. *Immunity* (2007) **27**(3):481–92. doi:10.1016/j.immuni.2007.07.021
104. Tel J, Schreibelt G, Sittig SP, Mathan TS, Buschow SI, Lambeck AJ, et al. Human plasmacytoid dendritic cells efficiently cross-present exogenous Ags to CD8+ T-cells, despite lower Ag uptake than myeloid dendritic cell subsets. *Blood* (2013) **121**(3):459–67. doi:10.1182/blood-2012-06-435644
105. Segura E, Durand M, Amigorena S. Similar antigen cross-presentation capacity and phagocytic functions in all freshly isolated human lymphoid organ-resident dendritic cells. *J Exp Med* (2013) **210**(5):1035–47. doi:10.1084/jem.20121103
106. Swiecki M, Wang Y, Gilfillan S, Colonna M. Plasmacytoid dendritic cells contribute to systemic but not local antiviral responses to HSV infections. *PLoS Pathog* (2013) **9**(10):e1003728. doi:10.1371/journal.ppat.1003728
107. Cervantes-Barragan L, Zust R, Weber F, Spiegel M, Lang KS, Akira S, et al. Control of coronavirus infection through plasmacytoid dendritic-cell-derived type I interferon. *Blood* (2007) **109**(3):1131–7. doi:10.1182/blood-2006-05-023770
108. Kassner N, Krueger M, Yagita H, Dzionek A, Hutloff A, Kroczek R, et al. Cutting edge: plasmacytoid dendritic cells induce IL-10 production in T cells

via the Delta-like-4/Notch axis. *J Immunol* (2010) **184**(2):550–4. doi:10.4049/jimmunol.0903152

109. Hutloff A, Dittrich AM, Beier KC, Eljaschewitsch B, Kraft R, Anagnostopoulos I, et al. ICOS is an inducible T-cell co-stimulator structurally and functionally related to CD28. *Nature* (1999) **397**:263–6. doi:10.1038/16717
110. Ito T, Yang M, Wang YH, Lande R, Gregorio J, Perng OA, et al. Plasmacytoid dendritic cells prime IL-10-producing T regulatory cells by inducible costimulator ligand. *J Exp Med* (2007) **204**(1):105–15. doi:10.1084/jem.20061660
111. Shortman K, Heath WR. The CD8+ dendritic cell subset. *Immunol Rev* (2010) **234**(1):18–31. doi:10.1111/j.0105-2896.2009.00870.x
112. Poulin LF, Reyal Y, Uronen-Hansson H, Schraml BU, Sancho D, Murphy KM, et al. DNGR-1 is a specific and universal marker of mouse and human Batf3-dependent dendritic cells in lymphoid and nonlymphoid tissues. *Blood* (2012) **119**(25):6052–62. doi:10.1182/blood-2012-01-406967
113. Murphy KM. Transcriptional control of dendritic cell development. *Adv Immunol* (2013) **120**:239–67. doi:10.1016/B978-0-12-417028-5.00009-0
114. Dorner BG, Dorner MB, Zhou X, Opitz C, Mora A, Guttler S, et al. Selective expression of the chemokine receptor XCR1 on cross-presenting dendritic cells determines cooperation with CD8+ T cells. *Immunity* (2009) **31**(5):823–33. doi:10.1016/j.immuni.2009.08.027
115. Maldonado-Lopez R, Maliszewski C, Urbain J, Moser M. Cytokines regulate the capacity of CD8alpha(+) and CD8alpha(-) dendritic cells to prime Th1/Th2 cells in vivo. *J Immunol* (2001) **167**(8):4345–50. doi:10.4049/jimmunol.167.8.4345
116. Ashok D, Schuster S, Ronet C, Rosa M, Mack V, Lavanchy C, et al. Cross-presenting dendritic cells are required for control of *Leishmania* major infection. *Eur J Immunol* (2014) **44**(5):1422–32. doi:10.1002/eji.201344242
117. Edelson BT, Kc W, Juang R, Kohyama M, Benoit LA, Klekotka PA, et al. Peripheral CD103+ dendritic cells form a unified subset developmentally related to CD8alpha+ conventional dendritic cells. *J Exp Med* (2010) **207**(4):823–36. doi:10.1084/jem.20091627
118. Rescigno M, Di Sabatino A. Dendritic cells in intestinal homeostasis and disease. *J Clin Invest* (2009) **119**(9):2441–50. doi:10.1172/JCI39134
119. Dudziak D, Kamphorst AO, Heidkamp GF, Buchholz VR, Trumpfheller C, Yamazaki S, et al. Differential antigen processing by dendritic cell subsets in vivo. *Science* (2007) **315**(5808):107–11. doi:10.1126/science.1136080
120. Maldonado-Lopez R, De Smedt T, Michel P, Godfroid J, Pajak B, Heirman C, et al. CD8alpha+ and CD8alpha− subclasses of dendritic cells direct the development of distinct T helper cells in vivo. *J Exp Med* (1999) **189**:587–92. doi:10.1084/jem.189.3.587
121. Satpathy AT, Briseno CG, Lee JS, Ng D, Manieri NA, Kc W, et al. Notch2-dependent classical dendritic cells orchestrate intestinal immunity to attaching-and-effacing bacterial pathogens. *Nat Immunol* (2013) **14**(9):937–48. doi:10.1038/ni.2679
122. Tussiwand R, Everts B, Grajales-Reyes GE, Kretzer NM, Iwata A, Bagaitkar J, et al. Klf4 expression in conventional dendritic cells is required for T helper 2 cell responses. *Immunity* (2015) **42**(5):916–28. doi:10.1016/j.immuni.2015.04.017
123. den Haan JM, Bevan MJ. Constitutive versus activation-dependent cross-presentation of immune complexes by CD8(+) and CD8(-) dendritic cells in vivo. *J Exp Med* (2002) **196**(6):817–27. doi:10.1084/jem.20020295
124. Manickasingham SP, Edwards AD, Schulz O, Reis e Sousa C. The ability of murine dendritic cell subsets to direct T helper cell differentiation is dependent on microbial signals. *Eur J Immunol* (2003) **33**(1):101–7. doi:10.1002/immu.200390001
125. Sallusto F, Lanzavecchia A. The instructive role of dendritic cells on T-cell responses. *Arthritis Res* (2002) **4**(Suppl 3):S127–32. doi:10.1186/ar567
126. O'Doherty U, Peng M, Gezelter S, Swiggard WJ, Betjes M, Bhardwaj N, et al. Human blood contains two subsets of dendritic cells, one immunologically mature and the other immature. *Immunology* (1994) **82**(3):487–93.
127. Siegal FP, Kadowaki N, Shodell M, Fitzgerald-Bocarsly PA, Shah K, Ho S, et al. The nature of the principal type 1 interferon-producing cells in human blood. *Science* (1999) **284**:1835–7. doi:10.1126/science.284.5421.1835
128. Cella M, Jarrossay D, Facchetti F, Alebardi O, Nakajima H, Lanzavecchia A, et al. Plasmacytoid monocytes migrate to inflamed lymph nodes and produce large amounts of type I interferon. *Nat Med* (1999) **5**:919–23. doi:10.1038/11360
129. Farkas L, Kvale EO, Lund-Johansen F, Jahnsen FL. Plasmacytoid dendritic cells induce a distinct cytokine pattern in virus-specific CD4+ memory T cells that is modulated by CpG oligodeoxynucleotides. *Scand J Immunol* (2006) **64**(4):404–11. doi:10.1111/j.1365-3083.2006.01792.x
130. Segura E, Valladeau-Guilemond J, Donnadieu MH, Sastre-Garau X, Soumelis V, Amigorena S. Characterization of resident and migratory dendritic cells in human lymph nodes. *J Exp Med* (2012) **209**(4):653–60. doi:10.1084/jem.20111457
131. Narbutt J, Lesiak A, Sysa-Jedrzejowska A, Smolewski P, Robak T, Zalewska A. The number and distribution of blood dendritic cells in the epidermis and dermis of healthy human subjects. *Folia Histochem Cytobiol* (2006) **44**(1):61–3.
132. Tabarkiewicz J, Rybojad P, Jablonka A, Rolinski J. CD1c+ and CD303+ dendritic cells in peripheral blood, lymph nodes and tumor tissue of patients with non-small cell lung cancer. *Oncol Rep* (2008) **19**(1):237–43.
133. Haniffa M, Shin A, Bigley V, McGovern N, Teo P, See P, et al. Human tissues contain CD141hi cross-presenting dendritic cells with functional homology to mouse CD103+ nonlymphoid dendritic cells. *Immunity* (2012) **37**(1):60–73. doi:10.1016/j.immuni.2012.04.012
134. Nizzoli G, Krietsch J, Weick A, Steinfelder S, Facciotti F, Gruarin P, et al. Human CD1c+ dendritic cells secrete high levels of IL-12 and potently prime cytotoxic T cell responses. *Blood* (2013) **122**(6):932–42. doi:10.1182/blood-2013-04-495424
135. Mittag D, Proietto AI, Loudovaris T, Mannering SI, Vremec D, Shortman K, et al. Human dendritic cell subsets from spleen and blood are similar in phenotype and function but modified by donor health status. *J Immunol* (2011) **186**(11):6207–17. doi:10.4049/jimmunol.1002632
136. Jongbloed SL, Kassianos AJ, McDonald KJ, Clark GJ, Ju X, Angel CE, et al. Human CD141+ (BDCA-3)+ dendritic cells (DCs) represent a unique myeloid DC subset that cross-presents necrotic cell antigens. *J Exp Med* (2010) **207**(6):1247–60. doi:10.1084/jem.20092140
137. Lauterbach H, Bathke B, Gilles S, Traidl-Hoffmann C, Luber CA, Fejer G, et al. Mouse CD8alpha+ DCs and human BDCA3+ DCs are major producers of IFN-lambda in response to poly IC. *J Exp Med* (2010) **207**(12):2703–17. doi:10.1084/jem.20092720
138. Poulin LF, Salio M, Griessinger E, Anjos-Afonso F, Craciun L, Chen JL, et al. Characterization of human DNGR-1+ BDCA3+ leukocytes as putative equivalents of mouse CD8alpha+ dendritic cells. *J Exp Med* (2010) **207**(6):1261–71. doi:10.1084/jem.20092618
139. Villadangos JA, Shortman K. Found in translation: the human equivalent of mouse CD8+ dendritic cells. *J Exp Med* (2010) **207**(6):1131–4. doi:10.1084/jem.20100985
140. Crozat K, Guiton R, Contreras V, Feuillet V, Dutertre CA, Ventre E, et al. The XC chemokine receptor 1 is a conserved selective marker of mammalian cells homologous to mouse CD8alpha+ dendritic cells. *J Exp Med* (2010) **207**(6):1283–92. doi:10.1084/jem.20100223
141. Bachem A, Guttler S, Hartung E, Ebstein F, Schaefer M, Tannert A, et al. Superior antigen cross-presentation and XCR1 expression define human CD11c+CD141+ cells as homologues of mouse CD8+ dendritic cells. *J Exp Med* (2010) **207**(6):1273–81. doi:10.1084/jem.20100348
142. Dillon SM, Rogers LM, Howe R, Hostetler LA, Buhrman J, McCarter MD, et al. Human intestinal lamina propria CD1c+ dendritic cells display an activated phenotype at steady state and produce IL-23 in response to TLR7/8 stimulation. *J Immunol* (2010) **184**(12):6612–21. doi:10.4049/jimmunol.1000041
143. Edelmann KH, Richardson-Burns S, Alexopoulou L, Tyler KL, Flavell RA, Oldstone MB. Does toll-like receptor 3 play a biological role in virus infections? *Virology* (2004) **322**(2):231–8. doi:10.1016/j.virol.2004.01.033
144. Zhang SY, Jouanguy E, Ugolini S, Smahi A, Elain G, Romero P, et al. TLR3 deficiency in patients with herpes simplex encephalitis. *Science* (2007) **317**(5844):1522–7. doi:10.1126/science.1139522
145. Klechevsky E. Human dendritic cells – stars in the skin. *Eur J Immunol* (2013) **43**(12):3147–55. doi:10.1002/eji.201343790
146. Henri S, Poulin LF, Tamoutounour S, Ardouin L, Guilliams M, de Bovis B, et al. CD207+ CD103+ dermal dendritic cells cross-present keratinocyte-derived

antigens irrespective of the presence of Langerhans cells. *J Exp Med* (2010) **207**(1):189–206. doi:10.1084/jem.20091964

147. McGovern N, Schlitzer A, Gunawan M, Jardine L, Shin A, Poyner E, et al. Human dermal CD14(+) cells are a transient population of monocyte-derived macrophages. *Immunity* (2014) **41**(3):465–77. doi:10.1016/j.immuni.2014.08.006
148. Said A, Weindl G. Regulation of dendritic cell function in inflammation. *J Immunol Res* (2015) **2015**:743169. doi:10.1155/2015/743169
149. Watchmaker PB, Lahl K, Lee M, Baumjohann D, Morton J, Kim SJ, et al. Comparative transcriptional and functional profiling defines conserved programs of intestinal DC differentiation in humans and mice. *Nat Immunol* (2014) **15**(1):98–108. doi:10.1038/ni.2768
150. von Bernuth H, Picard C, Puel A, Casanova JL. Experimental and natural infections in MyD88- and IRAK-4-deficient mice and humans. *Eur J Immunol* (2012) **42**(12):3126–35. doi:10.1002/eji.201242683
151. Bauer S, Pigisch S, Hangel D, Kaufmann A, Hamm S. Recognition of nucleic acid and nucleic acid analogs by toll-like receptors 7, 8 and 9. *Immunobiology* (2008) **213**(3–4):315–28. doi:10.1016/j.imbio.2007.10.010
152. von Bernuth H, Picard C, Jin Z, Pankla R, Xiao H, Ku CL, et al. Pyogenic bacterial infections in humans with MyD88 deficiency. *Science* (2008) **321**(5889):691–6. doi:10.1126/science.1158298
153. Artyomov MN, Munk A, Gorvel L, Korenfeld D, Cella M, Tung T, et al. Modular expression analysis reveals functional conservation between human Langerhans cells and mouse cross-priming dendritic cells. *J Exp Med* (2015) **212**(5):743–57. doi:10.1084/jem.20131675
154. Cohn L, Chatterjee B, Esselborn F, Smed-Sorensen A, Nakamura N, Chalouni C, et al. Antigen delivery to early endosomes eliminates the superiority of human blood BDCA3+ dendritic cells at cross presentation. *J Exp Med* (2013) **210**(5):1049–63. doi:10.1084/jem.20121251
155. Kassianos AJ, Hardy MY, Ju X, Vijayan D, Ding Y, Vulink AJ, et al. Human CD1c (BDCA-1)+ myeloid dendritic cells secrete IL-10 and display an immuno-regulatory phenotype and function in response to *Escherichia coli*. *Eur J Immunol* (2012) **42**(6):1512–22. doi:10.1002/eji.201142098
156. Napolitani G, Rinaldi A, Bertoni F, Sallusto F, Lanzavecchia A. Selected toll-like receptor agonist combinations synergistically trigger a T helper type 1-polarizing program in dendritic cells. *Nat Immunol* (2005) **6**(8):769–76. doi:10.1038/ni1223
157. Segura E, Touzot M, Bohineust A, Cappuccio A, Chiocchia G, Hosmalin A, et al. Human inflammatory dendritic cells induce Th17 cell differentiation. *Immunity* (2013) **38**(2):336–48. doi:10.1016/j.immuni.2012.10.018
158. Rissoan MC, Soumelis V, Kadowaki N, Grouard G, Briere F, de Waal Malefyt R, et al. Reciprocal control of T helper cell and dendritic cell differentiation. *Science* (1999) **283**:1183–6. doi:10.1126/science.283.5405.1183
159. Cella M, Facchetti F, Lanzavecchia A, Colonna M. Plasmacytoid dendritic cells activated by influenza virus and CD40L drive a potent Th1 polarization. *Nat Immunol* (2000) **1**:305–10. doi:10.1038/79747
160. Yu CI, Becker C, Metang P, Marches F, Wang Y, Toshiyuki H, et al. Human CD141+ dendritic cells induce CD4+ T cells to produce type 2 cytokines. *J Immunol* (2014) **193**(9):4335–43. doi:10.4049/jimmunol.1401159
161. Sabat R, Grutz G, Warszawska K, Kirsch S, Witte E, Wolk K, et al. Biology of interleukin-10. *Cytokine Growth Factor Rev* (2010) **21**(5):331–44. doi:10.1016/j.cytogfr.2010.09.002
162. Groux H, Bigler M, de Vries JE, Roncarolo MG. Inhibitory and stimulatory effects of IL-10 on human CD8+ T cells. *J Immunol* (1998) **160**(7):3188–93.
163. Cui W, Liu Y, Weinstein JS, Craft J, Kaech SM. An interleukin-21-interleukin-10-STAT3 pathway is critical for functional maturation of memory CD8+ T cells. *Immunity* (2011) **35**(5):792–805. doi:10.1016/j.immuni.2011.09.017
164. Donnelly RP, Dickensheets H, O'Brien TR. Interferon-lambda and therapy for chronic hepatitis C virus infection. *Trends Immunol* (2011) **32**(9):443–50. doi:10.1016/j.it.2011.07.002
165. Meixlsperger S, Leung CS, Ramer PC, Pack M, Vanoaica LD, Breton G, et al. CD141+ dendritic cells produce prominent amounts of IFN-alpha after dsRNA recognition and can be targeted via DEC-205 in humanized mice. *Blood* (2013) **121**(25):5034–44. doi:10.1182/blood-2012-12-473413
166. Ge D, Fellay J, Thompson AJ, Simon JS, Shianna KV, Urban TJ, et al. Genetic variation in IL28B predicts hepatitis C treatment-induced viral clearance. *Nature* (2009) **461**(7262):399–401. doi:10.1038/nature08309
167. Megjugorac NJ, Gallagher GE, Gallagher G. IL-4 enhances IFN-lambda1 (IL-29) production by plasmacytoid DCs via monocyte secretion of IL-1Ra. *Blood* (2010) **115**(21):4185–90. doi:10.1182/blood-2009-09-246157
168. Zhang S, Kodys K, Li K, Szabo G. Human type 2 myeloid dendritic cells produce interferon-lambda and amplify interferon-alpha in response to hepatitis C virus infection. *Gastroenterology* (2013) **144**(2):414.e–25.e. doi:10.1053/j.gastro.2012.10.034
169. Yoshio S, Kanto T, Kuroda S, Matsubara T, Higashitani K, Kakita N, et al. Human blood dendritic cell antigen 3 (BDCA3)(+) dendritic cells are a potent producer of interferon-lambda in response to hepatitis C virus. *Hepatology* (2013) **57**(5):1705–15. doi:10.1002/hep.26182
170. Lozza L, Farinacci M, Bechtle M, Staber M, Zedler U, Baiocchini A, et al. Communication between human dendritic cell subsets in tuberculosis: requirements for naive CD4(+) T cell stimulation. *Front Immunol* (2014) **5**:324. doi:10.3389/fimmu.2014.00324
171. Lozza L, Farinacci M, Fae K, Bechtle M, Staber M, Dorhoi A, et al. Crosstalk between human DC subsets promotes antibacterial activity and CD8+ T-cell stimulation in response to bacille Calmette-Guerin. *Eur J Immunol* (2014) **44**(1):80–92. doi:10.1002/eji.201343797
172. Gupta MR, Kolli D, Garofalo RP. Differential response of BDCA-1+ and BDCA-3+ myeloid dendritic cells to respiratory syncytial virus infection. *Respir Res* (2013) **14**:71. doi:10.1186/1465-9921-14-71
173. Gupta MR, Kolli D, Molteni C, Casola A, Garofalo RP. Paramyxovirus infection regulates T cell responses by BDCA-1+ and BDCA-3+ myeloid dendritic cells. *PLoS One* (2014) **9**(6):e99227. doi:10.1371/journal.pone.0099227
174. Florentin J, Aouar B, Dental C, Thumann C, Firaguay G, Gondois-Rey F, et al. HCV glycoprotein E2 is a novel BDCA-2 ligand and acts as an inhibitor of IFN production by plasmacytoid dendritic cells. *Blood* (2012) **120**(23):4544–51. doi:10.1182/blood-2012-02-413286
175. Dzionek A, Sohma Y, Nagafune J, Cella M, Colonna M, Facchetti F, et al. BDCA-2, a novel plasmacytoid dendritic cell-specific type II C-type lectin, mediates antigen capture and is a potent inhibitor of interferon alpha/beta induction. *J Exp Med* (2001) **194**(12):1823–34. doi:10.1084/jem.194.12.1823
176. O'Brien M, Manches O, Bhardwaj N. Plasmacytoid dendritic cells in HIV infection. *Adv Exp Med Biol* (2013) **762**:71–107. doi:10.1007/978-1-4614-4433-6_3
177. Hammarlund E, Lewis MW, Hansen SG, Strelow LI, Nelson JA, Sexton GJ, et al. Duration of antiviral immunity after smallpox vaccination. *Nat Med* (2003) **9**(9):1131–7. doi:10.1038/nm917
178. Monath TP. Yellow fever vaccine. *Expert Rev Vaccines* (2005) **4**(4):553–74. doi:10.1586/14760584.4.4.553
179. Divekar AA, Zaiss DM, Lee FE, Liu D, Topham DJ, Sijts AJ, et al. Protein vaccines induce uncommitted IL-2-secreting human and mouse CD4 T cells, whereas infections induce more IFN-gamma-secreting cells. *J Immunol* (2006) **176**(3):1465–73. doi:10.4049/jimmunol.176.3.1465
180. Parvanova I, Rettig L, Knuth A, Pascolo S. The form of NY-ESO-1 antigen has an impact on the clinical efficacy of anti-tumor vaccination. *Vaccine* (2011) **29**(22):3832–6. doi:10.1016/j.vaccine.2011.03.073
181. Kool M, Soullie T, van Nimwegen M, Willart MA, Muskens F, Jung S, et al. Alum adjuvant boosts adaptive immunity by inducing uric acid and activating inflammatory dendritic cells. *J Exp Med* (2008) **205**(4):869–82. doi:10.1084/jem.20071087
182. Martinon F, Petrilli V, Mayor A, Tardivel A, Tschopp J. Gout-associated uric acid crystals activate the NALP3 inflammasome. *Nature* (2006) **440**(7081):237–41. doi:10.1038/nature04516
183. Okemoto K, Kawasaki K, Hanada K, Miura M, Nishijima M. A potent adjuvant monophosphoryl lipid A triggers various immune responses, but not secretion of IL-1beta or activation of caspase-1. *J Immunol* (2006) **176**(2):1203–8. doi:10.4049/jimmunol.176.2.1203
184. Hui G, Hashimoto C. Interleukin-6 has differential influence on the ability of adjuvant formulations to potentiate antibody responses to a *Plasmodium falciparum* blood-stage vaccine. *Vaccine* (2007) **25**(36):6598–603. doi:10.1016/j.vaccine.2007.10.010
185. Brewer JM, Conacher M, Gaffney M, Douglas M, Bluethmann H, Alexander J. Neither interleukin-6 nor signalling via tumour necrosis factor receptor-1 contribute to the adjuvant activity of Alum and Freund's adjuvant. *Immunology* (1998) **93**(1):41–8. doi:10.1046/j.1365-2567.1998.00399.x
186. Banchereau R, Baldwin N, Cepika AM, Athale S, Xue Y, Yu CI, et al. Transcriptional specialization of human dendritic cell subsets in response to microbial vaccines. *Nat Commun* (2014) **5**:5283. doi:10.1038/ncomms6283

187. Palucka K, Ueno H, Fay J, Banchereau J. Harnessing dendritic cells to generate cancer vaccines. *Ann N Y Acad Sci* (2009) **1174**:88–98. doi:10.1111/j.1749-6632.2009.05000.x
188. Mandraju R, Murray S, Forman J, Pasare C. Differential ability of surface and endosomal TLRs to induce CD8 T cell responses in vivo. *J Immunol* (2014) **192**(9):4303–15. doi:10.4049/jimmunol.1302244
189. Scheiermann J, Klinman DM. Clinical evaluation of CpG oligonucleotides as adjuvants for vaccines targeting infectious diseases and cancer. *Vaccine* (2014) **32**(48):6377–89. doi:10.1016/j.vaccine.2014.06.065
190. Fehres CM, Bruijns SC, van Beelen AJ, Kalay H, Ambrosini M, Hooijberg E, et al. Topical rather than intradermal application of the TLR7 ligand imiquimod leads to human dermal dendritic cell maturation and CD8+ T-cell cross-priming. *Eur J Immunol* (2014) **44**(8):2415–24. doi:10.1002/eji.201344094
191. Vandepapeliere P, Horsmans Y, Moris P, Van Mechelen M, Janssens M, Koutsoukos M, et al. Vaccine adjuvant systems containing monophosphoryl lipid A and QS21 induce strong and persistent humoral and T cell responses against hepatitis B surface antigen in healthy adult volunteers. *Vaccine* (2008) **26**(10):1375–86. doi:10.1016/j.vaccine.2007.12.038
192. Coban C, Kobiyama K, Jounai N, Tozuka M, Ishii KJ. DNA vaccines: a simple DNA sensing matter? *Hum Vaccin Immunother* (2013) **9**(10):2216–21. doi:10.4161/hv.25893
193. Pascolo S. Messenger RNA-based vaccines. *Expert Opin Biol Ther* (2004) **4**(8):1285–94. doi:10.1517/14712598.4.8.1285
194. Pascolo S. The messenger's great message for vaccination. *Expert Rev Vaccines* (2015) **14**(2):153–6. doi:10.1586/14760584.2015.1000871
195. Teufel R, Carralot JP, Scheel B, Probst J, Walter S, Jung G, et al. Human peripheral blood mononuclear cells transfected with messenger RNA stimulate antigen-specific cytotoxic T-lymphocytes in vitro. *Cell Mol Life Sci* (2005) **62**(15):1755–62. doi:10.1007/s00018-005-5067-6
196. Scheel B, Teufel R, Probst J, Carralot JP, Geginat J, Radsak M, et al. Toll-like receptor-dependent activation of several human blood cell types by protamine-condensed mRNA. *Eur J Immunol* (2005) **35**(5):1557–66. doi:10.1002/eji.200425656
197. Probst J, Weide B, Scheel B, Pichler BJ, Hoerr I, Rammensee HG, et al. Spontaneous cellular uptake of exogenous messenger RNA in vivo is nucleic acid-specific, saturable and ion dependent. *Gene Ther* (2007) **14**(15):1175–80. doi:10.1038/sj.gt.3302964
198. Hoerr I, Obst R, Rammensee HG, Jung G. In vivo application of RNA leads to induction of specific cytotoxic T lymphocytes and antibodies. *Eur J Immunol* (2000) **30**(1):1–7. doi:10.1002/1521-4141(200001)30:1<1::AID-IMMU1>3.0.CO;2-#
199. Weide B, Carralot JP, Reese A, Scheel B, Eigentler TK, Hoerr I, et al. Results of the first phase I/II clinical vaccination trial with direct injection of mRNA. *J Immunother* (2008) **31**(2):180–8. doi:10.1097/CJI.0b013e31815ce501
200. Rittig SM, Haentschel M, Weimer KJ, Heine A, Muller MR, Brugger W, et al. Intradermal vaccinations with RNA coding for TAA generate CD8+ and CD4+ immune responses and induce clinical benefit in vaccinated patients. *Mol Ther* (2011) **19**(5):990–9. doi:10.1038/mt.2010.289
201. Kreiter S, Selmi A, Diken M, Koslowski M, Britten CM, Huber C, et al. Intranodal vaccination with naked antigen-encoding RNA elicits potent prophylactic and therapeutic antitumoral immunity. *Cancer Res* (2010) **70**(22):9031–40. doi:10.1158/0008-5472.CAN-10-0699

12

The interplay between monocytes/ macrophages and CD4$^+$ T Cell subsets in rheumatoid arthritis

*Ceri A. Roberts, Abigail K. Dickinson and Leonie S. Taams**

Centre for Molecular and Cellular Biology of Inflammation (CMCBI), Division of Immunology, Infection and Inflammatory Disease, King's College London, London, UK

Edited by:
Elisabetta Padovan, Basel University Hospital and University of Basel, Switzerland

Reviewed by:
Paul Garside, University of Glasgow, UK
Florent Ginhoux, Singapore Immunology Network, Singapore

***Correspondence:**
Leonie S. Taams
leonie.taams@kcl.ac.uk

Rheumatoid arthritis (RA) is a chronic inflammatory disease characterized by inflammation of the synovial lining (synovitis). The inflammation in the RA joint is associated with and driven by immune cell infiltration, synovial hyperproliferation, and excessive production of proinflammatory mediators, such as tumor necrosis factor α (TNFα), interferon γ (IFNγ), interleukin (IL)-1β, IL-6, and IL-17, eventually resulting in damage to the cartilage and underlying bone. The RA joint harbors a wide range of immune cell types, including monocytes, macrophages, and CD4$^+$ T cells (both proinflammatory and regulatory). The interplay between CD14$^+$ myeloid cells and CD4$^+$ T cells can significantly influence CD4$^+$ T cell function, and conversely, effector vs. regulatory CD4$^+$ T cell subsets can exert profound effects on monocyte/macrophage function. In this review, we will discuss how the interplay between CD4$^+$ T cells and monocytes/macrophages may contribute to the immunopathology of RA.

Keywords: rheumatoid arthritis, inflammation, immune regulation, cell polarization, myeloid cell, T helper cell, Treg

RHEUMATOID ARTHRITIS

Rheumatoid arthritis (RA) is a chronic inflammatory and debilitating disease, characterized by inflammation of the lining of the joint (synovitis), eventually leading to the destruction of cartilage and the underlying bone. RA affects between 0.5 and 1% of the Western adult population with a female:male ratio of 3:1. The exact etiology of RA is still unknown, but it is widely accepted that RA is a multifactorial disease with genetic, environmental (e.g., smoking), gender and age-associated factors contributing to the disease process (1–3).

Typical hallmarks of RA are pannus formation and synovial hyperplasia, caused by proliferating fibroblasts and infiltrating immune cells. These events promote leukocyte recruitment, immune cell activation, and production of inflammatory mediators and proteinases, all of which eventually contribute to joint damage. A wide range of immune cells has been detected in the RA joint, including CD4$^+$ T cells, CD8$^+$ T cells, B cells, NK cells, γδ T cells, mast cells and myeloid cells. Various soluble mediators produced by these immune cells have been shown to correlate with disease progression and/or severity in RA, e.g., rheumatoid factor, anti-citrullinated peptide antibodies, tumor necrosis factor (TNF)α, interleukin (IL)-6, IL-1, and IL-17A (2, 4). The importance of the immune system in disease pathogenesis is illustrated by the recent success of biologic therapies that target key inflammatory cytokines (e.g., TNFα blockade and anti-IL-6R therapy), immune molecules (e.g., CTLA4-Ig leading to blockade of CD80/CD86-mediated costimulation), and immune cells (e.g., B cell depletion).

MONOCYTES AND MACROPHAGES IN RHEUMATOID ARTHRITIS

Monocytes/macrophages are a potent source of proinflammatory cytokines, in particular TNFα, IL-6 and IL-1, and matrix metalloproteinases (MMPs), leading to endothelial cell activation, acute phase reactions, and cartilage damage. These cells can also produce a wide range of chemokines, which help recruit additional leukocytes to the inflamed joint. In addition, monocytes have the ability to polarize $CD4^+$ T cells and can differentiate into osteoclasts, which may further contribute to their role in RA pathogenesis. As such, monocytes and macrophages are viewed as relevant therapeutic targets in RA (5–7).

Myeloid cells with a monocyte/macrophage phenotype (i.e., $CD14^+CD68^+$) are present in large numbers in the rheumatoid joint. Several studies have shown that these cells produce proinflammatory cytokines (8, 9) and have an activated phenotype with increased expression of HLA-DR (involved in antigen presentation to $CD4^+$ T cells), costimulatory molecules (e.g., CD80, CD86, and CD40), adhesion molecules (e.g., CD54), and some chemokine receptors (10–18). The importance of synovial $CD68^+$ macrophages in RA pathogenesis is underlined by the findings that the presence of these cells correlates with disease activity markers (19, 20) and that a change in their presence has been reported to be a reliable biomarker for response to treatment (21). An early, small study in patients with RA ($n = 10$) noted that synovial $CD68^+$ cells were reduced in the perivascular and connective tissue areas 12 weeks after treatment with gold (22). Sublining macrophage count was also shown to correlate significantly with radiologic outcome and radiologic progression in patients with RA ($n = 23$–27) (20). An elegant study by Haringman et al. investigating arthroscopic synovial tissue biopsies from patients with RA ($n = 88$) participating in various clinical trials, showed that a reduction in the number of synovial sublining $CD68^+$ macrophages correlated significantly with clinical improvement independently of the therapeutic strategy (23). Importantly, the number of sublining macrophages did not change after placebo or ineffective treatment, supporting its use as a predictive biomarker for response to treatment (21, 23).

A growing number of studies have reported on the frequencies and phenotype of peripheral blood monocyte subsets in RA. Phenotypically, peripheral $CD14^+$ monocytes in patients with RA show some signs of altered activation with studies reporting increased expression of CD14, FcγRs, CD54, CD11b, and/or HLA-DR (18, 24–27), although not all studies agree on increased HLA-DR expression (24, 27). Peripheral blood monocytes from RA patients are also reported to express increased levels of transmembrane TNF (tmTNF) (28). Human monocytes can be divided into subpopulations based on expression of CD14 [lipopolysaccharide (LPS) coreceptor] and CD16 (FcγRIII). $CD14^{++}CD16^-$ "classical" monocytes are the most prevalent subset, representing ~90% of blood monocytes in healthy individuals. CD16-expressing cells are less frequent among circulating monocytes but are expanded in infection and inflammatory conditions (29). $CD16^+$ monocytes can be further subdivided into $CD14^{++/bright}$ (also called "intermediate") and $CD14^{dim}$ ("non-classical" or "patrolling") subsets (29, 30). Earlier studies, which did not necessarily discriminate between $CD14^{++/bright}CD16^+$ and $CD14^{dim}CD16^+$ cells, showed an increase in the percentage of $CD14^+CD16^+$ monocytes in RA blood (31–33). $CD14^+CD16^+$ monocytes in RA express high levels of CCR1, CCR5, ICAM-1, or TLR2 (27, 32, 33). Higher frequencies of $CD14^+CD16^+$ blood monocytes were associated with clinical parameters of active disease (31, 33). More recent data suggest that only the frequency of $CD14^{++/bright}CD16^+$ intermediate cells is increased in peripheral blood of patients with chronic RA compared to sex- and age-matched healthy donors, while the frequency of non-classical $CD14^{dim}CD16^+$ monocytes does not differ between patients and controls (27, 34, 35). The frequency of $CD14^{++/bright}CD16^+$ cells at baseline was found to negatively correlate with response to methotrexate treatment (34). However, another study reported, using absolute cell counts, that both $CD14^{++/bright}CD16^+$ and $CD14^{dim}CD16^+$ monocyte populations are increased in RA blood (36). Ligation of CD16 using immune complexes or FcγRIII-specific mAb enhances proinflammatory TNFα production, suggesting that the expression of CD16 could be functional (32, 34, 37).

Recently, Krasselt et al. showed that $CD14^{bright}CD56^+$ monocytes, which are predominantly composed of classical $CD14^{bright}CD16^-$ cells, produce more TNFα, IL-10, and IL-23 in response to LPS and demonstrate increased spontaneous production of reactive oxygen intermediates [reactive oxygen species (ROS)] compared to $CD14^{bright}CD56^-$ monocytes (38). $CD14^{bright}CD56^+$ frequencies were positively correlated with age in healthy controls and were expanded in the blood of young RA patients compared to age-matched healthy controls. The $CD14^{bright}CD56^+$ subpopulation was reduced in a longitudinal study of 16 RA patients following anti-TNF treatment. Additional studies are required to further elucidate the role of $CD14^{bright}CD56^+$ monocytes in RA.

In RA synovial fluid, it appears to be the intermediate $CD14^{++/bright}CD16^+$ monocyte population that is increased in frequency compared to matched peripheral blood (31, 33, 35). One explanation for the increased frequency of CD16 expressing synovial monocytes is that there is a specific expansion of the $CD14^{++/bright}CD16^+$ monocyte population. Another non-mutually exclusive explanation is that there is *de novo* expression of CD16 triggered by the inflammatory milieu. It was shown that *in vitro* stimulation of healthy monocytes with recombinant transforming growth factor β (TGFβ) or RA synovial fluid induced elevated CD16 expression, an effect that was inhibited by TGFβ signaling blockade (35).

Table 1 summarizes the reported phenotypic features of $CD14^+$ cells derived from RA peripheral blood or synovial fluid, and cells with a macrophage phenotype in synovial tissue. It should be noted that studies on synovial fluid or synovial tissue generally involve the whole $CD14^+$ and/or $CD68^+$ population (which may contain monocytes and macrophages), rather than sorted subsets. Therefore, **Table 1** represents a summary of relevant literature reports on monocyte/macrophage cell phenotypes

TABLE 1 | Phenotypic features of monocytes/macrophages from RA peripheral blood, synovial fluid, and synovial tissue.

Compartment	Phenotype	Reference
(a) Peripheral blood	↑ HLA-DR, CD14, CD40, CD54, CD11b	(18, 24–26)
	↑ Fcγ receptors (including CD16)	(18, 24, 26, 27, 31–36)
	↑ CCR3, CCR4, CCR5	(15)
	↑ tmTNFα	(28)
	↑ Spontaneous IL-1β production	(25, 28)
	↑ Resistance to apoptosis	(28, 39)
(b) Synovial fluid	↑ HLA-DR, CD40, CD54, CD80, CD86, CD276	(11, 13, 14, 16–18, 35)
	↑ CD16$^+$	(18, 31, 33, 35)
	↓ CCR1, CCR2, CCR4, ↑CCR3, CCR5	(15)
	↑ Resistance to apoptosis	(39, 40)
(c) Synovial tissue	HLA-DR$^+$	(10, 14)
	CD68$^+$	(15, 19–23)
	CD163$^+$	(12)
	IL-1$^+$, TNFα$^+$, IL-6$^+$, GM-CSF$^+$, TGFβ$^+$	(8, 9, 14)

Arrows indicate phenotypic alterations observed in CD14$^+$ cells from the peripheral blood of rheumatoid arthritis (RA) patients in comparison to healthy donor peripheral blood CD14$^+$ cells (a), or in CD14$^+$ cells from RA synovial fluid compared to RA peripheral blood CD14$^+$ cells (b). Phenotypic markers that are expressed on cells with a macrophage phenotype from RA synovial tissue (c).

within different anatomical compartments rather than a direct comparison of these cells *between* different compartments.

EFFECT OF MONOCYTES/ MACROPHAGES ON CD4$^+$ T CELL SUBSETS

In addition to the innate effector functions of monocytes/macrophages in terms of proinflammatory cytokine and chemokine production, their inflammatory role in RA pathogenesis may stem from their function as a bridge to the adaptive immune system. Colocalization of CD14$^+$ cells with clusters of CD4$^+$ effector T cells at sites of inflammation has been reported in inflamed rheumatoid synovium, as well as in inflamed tonsil, and psoriatic or atopic dermatitis skin (41, 42), suggesting that CD4$^+$ T cells and monocytes/macrophages can interact *in vivo* at sites of inflammation.

CD4$^+$ T Helper Cell Polarization by Monocytes/Macrophages

Dendritic cells (DCs) are classically considered to be the major drivers of CD4$^+$ T helper cell polarization; however, evidence is accumulating that monocytes/macrophages can also play a role in this process. Monocytes and/or macrophages can be major sources of IL-1β, IL-6, IL-12, and IL-23, cytokines known to be present in the RA joint (4, 8, 9, 43, 44). IL-12 is involved in driving CD4$^+$ T helper 1 (Th1) cell polarization, while IL-1β, IL-6, and IL-23 can drive and maintain Th17 polarization. Interferon γ (IFNγ)$^+$CD4$^+$ T cells (indicative of Th1 cells) and IL-17$^+$ CD4$^+$ T cells (indicative of Th17 cells) are readily detectable in the RA joint, in both the tissue and the fluid (45–47). Th1 cells were originally thought to be one of the major contributors in RA pathogenesis, based on their abundance in RA synovial fluid, their key role in certain experimental models of arthritis, as well as the inflammatory function of IFNγ particularly on macrophage activation. However, studies have shown that IFNγ may also have a protective, rather than an exacerbating role in RA (48–50), which may be due to its antagonistic effects on Th17 induction (51) or on VEGF production (46, 52), thereby possibly inhibiting angiogenesis.

In recent years, IL-17 and Th17 cells have gained attention as critical mediators in RA pathogenesis. IL-17 is a potent proinflammatory cytokine that works in synergy with TNFα to induce the inflammatory events and joint damage that are characteristic of RA (53, 54). The receptors for IL-17 (IL-17RA and IL-17RC) are expressed in RA synovium, including on CD14$^+$ monocytes/macrophages (55) and stimulation of RA synovium with IL-17 leads to production of IL-6, MMPs, and joint degradation (56–58). Blood CD14$^+$ monocytes can be potent inducers of human Th17 responses depending on their activation status. Human blood monocytes activated by peptidoglycan or LPS were shown to efficiently promote Th17 responses from cocultured naive CD4$^+$ T cells in the presence of anti-CD3 mAb (59). Our own lab found that following *in vitro* activation with LPS, peripheral blood CD14$^+$ monocytes from either healthy donors or RA patients promoted Th17 responses in an IL-1β- and TNFα-dependent manner (17, 60). It was also shown that human monocytes stimulated *in vitro* with heat-killed pneumococci triggered a Th17 response which was dependent on TLR2 signaling (61). In contrast, stimulation with live pneumococci led to a mixed Th1/Th17 response due to monocyte production of IL-12p40. In a non-infectious setting, peripheral blood monocytes from patients with type 1 diabetes spontaneously secreted the proinflammatory cytokines IL-1β and IL-6. These cells induced higher frequencies of Th17 cells from memory T cells *in vitro* compared with monocytes from healthy control subjects, which was reduced by a combination of an IL-6-blocking Ab and IL-1R antagonist (62). Finally, healthy peripheral blood monocytes that were treated with RA synovial fluid prior to coculture with anti-CD3/CD28-stimulated CD4$^+$ T cells were shown to promote Th17 differentiation, which was attributed to a TNFα-mediated increase in monocytic production of IL-6 and IL-1β (63).

Additional studies in mice and human show that monocytes/macrophages from the synovial fluid of the inflamed arthritic joint, which may contain extravasated monocytes as well as tissue-resident macrophages, can promote IL-17 production in CD4$^+$ T cells (17, 35, 64). These data suggest that newly recruited CD4$^+$ T cells in the rheumatoid joint might be steered toward a Th17 response by local monocytes/macrophages. The ensuing positive feedback loop between Th17 cells and monocytes/macrophages may then perpetuate inflammation (42). In our own work, the induction of Th17 responses by *in vivo* activated monocytes isolated from RA synovial fluid was found to be independent of TNFα, IL-1β, IL-6, and IL-23, and to involve cell contact (17). In line with our observations, Yoon et al. found increased Th17 responses when stimulated autologous peripheral blood memory CD4$^+$ T cells were cocultured with RA synovial fluid monocytes, compared to responses elicited by circulating monocytes. In contrast to our finding that Th1 polarization was not strongly affected by the anatomical origin of monocytes (17), Yoon et al. found that intracellular IFNγ expression (and in most donors tested, the level of IFNγ in culture supernatants), was also significantly increased by coculture with synovial monocytes compared to blood monocytes (35). Thus, synovial monocytes/macrophages may promote both Th17 and Th1 responses.

It is currently unclear whether the capacity of monocytes to promote Th17 responses resides in a particular monocyte subset. Rossol et al. found that circulating intermediate $CD14^{++/bright}CD16^{+}$ monocytes in the presence of LPS promoted Th17 cell expansion from peripheral blood memory $CD4^{+}$ T cells *in vitro*, and that the frequency of $CD14^{++/bright}CD16^{+}$ monocytes in peripheral blood of RA patients correlated closely with *ex vivo* Th17 cell frequencies (27). Traunecker et al. reported that non-classical ($CD14^{dim}CD16^{+}$) monocytes from healthy donors when cocultured with autologous $CD4^{+}$ T cells and specific superantigens in the absence of pathogen-recognition receptor (PRR) stimuli were more efficient stimulators of IL-17-producing T cells; however, in the presence of PRR stimuli, Th17 expansion was mostly observed in cocultures with classical ($CD14^{++/bright}CD16^{-}$) or intermediate ($CD14^{++/bright}CD16^{+}$) monocytes (65). Blocking of LFA-1/ICAM-1 interaction increased the frequency of IL-17-producing T cells expanded from non-classical monocyte/$CD4^{+}$ T cell/superantigen cocultures. However, no significant differences in capacity to promote Th17 responses were observed in experiments assessing peripheral blood monocyte subsets from 11 RA patients. In contrast to the above studies, Smeekens et al. found that only $CD14^{++/bright}CD16^{-}$ classical monocytes and not $CD16^{+}$ monocytes could induce a protective Th17 response in response to *Candida albicans,* due to increased IL-1β and prostaglandin E2 production (66). It is crucial to achieve high degree purity separation for functional characterization of cell subpopulations and the use of magnetic bead separation to isolate $CD16^{+}$ vs. $CD16^{-}$ monocytes rather than high purity FACS-based cell sorting in the study by Smeekens et al. may therefore limit interpretation of the results. Nonetheless, a recent study by Liu et al. also found that after coculturing autologous memory $CD4^{+}$ T cells with FACS-purified monocyte subsets and anti-CD3, classical $CD14^{++/bright}CD16^{-}$ monocytes most potently expanded $IL\text{-}17^{+}$ memory $CD4^{+}$ T cells (67). Non-classical $CD14^{+}CD16^{++}$ monocytes were the strongest inducers of IFNγ expression in naive $CD4^{+}$ T cell cocultures. The above *in vitro* experiments employ different modes of T cell activation with or without PRR stimulation of monocytes, which may contribute to the heterogeneity of the results obtained. Activation of T cells via crosslinking of soluble anti-CD3 (67) triggers MHC-independent T cell activation, whereas stimulation via superantigen (65) crosslinks MHC on monocytes and TCR on T cells, more closely representing an MHC-restricted antigen-specific stimulation. Altering the activation state of monocyte subsets via PRR agonists (27, 65, 66) may also affect their capacity to polarize $CD4^{+}$ T cells. Any conclusions drawn from these and future studies regarding the contribution of different monocyte subsets to $CD4^{+}$ T cell polarization should take into account the choice of *in vitro* stimulation and ideally should be confirmed in multiple systems.

Monocytes/macrophages are also a major source of IL-15 (68), a pleiotropic cytokine which mediates several important proinflammatory effects on both monocytes/macrophages and $CD4^{+}$ T cells. The IL-15Rα is overexpressed on blood-derived lymphocytes and monocytes in RA patients (69), and IL-15 is found at high levels in RA SF (70). IL-15 plays an important role in regulating T cell migration and was shown *in vivo* to facilitate accumulation of adoptively transferred T cells in RA synovial tissues engrafted into immune deficient SCID mice (71). IL-15 also promotes TNFα production by synovial T cells (72), and IL-15-activated blood-derived or synovial T cells can induce TNFα in a macrophage cell line and in RA blood- or synovium-derived monocytes/macrophages in a cell-contact-dependent manner (72). IL-15 may also promote IL-17 production by synovial T cells (73), although in mice a fine-tuning effect of IL-15 on Th17 differentiation was reported (74). IL-18 is another proinflammatory cytokine expressed in RA synovium, most prominently in $CD68^{+}$ macrophages (75). IL-18 acts in synergy with other cytokines, including IL-12 and IL-15, to stimulate T cell production of IFNγ and synovial macrophage release of TNFα (75). In the RA joint, IL-18 also acts as a chemoattractant for synovial $CD4^{+}$ T cells (76) and monocytes (77). Together, these data indicate that production of IL-15 and IL-18 by monocytes and/or macrophages may also be relevant in driving or polarizing inflammatory $CD4^{+}$ T cell responses in the RA joint.

In addition to their role as antigen-presenting and cytokine-producing cells, macrophages can efficiently generate ROS, an important antimicrobial defense mechanism that occurs via activation of the phagocytic NADPH oxidase complex. Rats and mice with genetic variation in the neutrophil cytosolic factor *Ncf1* (encoding p47phox, an activating protein in this complex) demonstrate reduced capacity to exert oxidative burst and increased incidence and severity of T cell-dependent arthritis (78, 79). When efficient ROS production was restored specifically in macrophages, T cell-dependent arthritis development was ameliorated (80). *In vitro*, T cells from mice lacking functional macrophage *Ncf1* demonstrated increased proliferation and cytokine production in response to antigenic stimulation, as compared to T cells from mice with ROS-competent macrophages. Coculturing T cells from ROS-deficient mice with ROS-competent macrophages led to suppressed T cell IL-2 production and proliferative responses to antigen, suggesting that macrophage ROS production affects antigen presentation *in vitro*. However, irrespective of whether macrophages used in the coculture could produce ROS, IFNγ production was increased when $CD4^{+}$ T cells were derived from ROS-deficient mice, indicating that *in vivo* exposure to macrophage ROS production may suppress Th1 responses. In agreement with these findings, King et al. found that human T cells stimulated with anti-CD3/CD28 in the presence of ROS demonstrated an increase in type 2 cytokines with no alteration in type 1 cytokine production, even in culture conditions polarizing toward a Th1 phenotype, and which could be reversed by concomitant antioxidant exposure (81). Together, these findings suggest that ROS production by macrophages may have the potential to downregulate or modulate T helper cell responses.

It is well known that certain inbred mouse strains show a bias toward either Th1 or Th2 responses, e.g., C57BL/6 and BALB/c, respectively. The bias in Th1- or Th2-like cytokine profiles is maintained in NUDE or SCID mice lacking an adaptive immune system, suggesting a role for the innate immune system in driving this polarization and giving rise to the concept of M1 and M2 macrophages (82). Studies of transgenic (Tg) mice have provided *in vivo* evidence that inflammatory macrophage subpopulations can polarize $CD4^+$ T cell responses in mouse models of arthritis. Li et al. crossed a *Floxed* STOP-human/mouse DR5 Tg mouse with the LysM.Cre mouse, to express the Tg human/mouse-chimeric death receptor 5 (DR5) restrictively in myeloid lineage cells. Treatment of these mice with an antihuman DR5 agonistic antibody led to targeted depletion of $CD11b^{high}Ly6C^+$ inflammatory macrophages and reduced development and severity of collagen-induced arthritis (83). Interestingly, the depletion of this macrophage subpopulation also significantly reduced protein levels of IL-6 and IL-17A in sera, reduced synovial *Il17a*, *Il6*, *Tnfa*, and *Il23a(p19)* mRNA expression and reduced the frequency of IL-17A$^+$ and IFNγ$^+$CD4$^+$ T cells while increasing CD4$^+$Foxp3$^+$ cells in draining lymph nodes. These data support the notion that macrophages may be important contributors to $CD4^+$ T cell polarization.

Dissecting the precise role of monocytes/macrophages in initiating adaptive immune responses can be challenging due to overlapping function and lineage marker expression with DCs. DCs are professional antigen-presenting cells that play a key role in promoting an effective immune response. A multitude of pattern recognition receptors allows DCs to sense invading pathogens and present both exogenous and endogenous antigens to naive and memory T cells. Different subsets of DC exist, including conventional or classical DC (cDC) type 1, cDC type 2, plasmacytoid DC, and monocyte-derived DC (mo-DC). cDC develop independently from monocytes and originate from a common DC progenitor which expresses flt3 (84). It can be difficult to distinguish monocytes or macrophages from mo-DCs or cDC type 2, due to overlap in certain markers (e.g., CD14, CD11b, CD11c, and CX3CR1) (85). CD64 has been identified as a marker that can be used to distinguish mo-DCs from cDCs in mice; however, these cells remain difficult to distinguish from cDCs in humans (86). Recently, researchers have taken a genetic approach to ablate monocytes and macrophages while sparing cDCs and lymphocytes by depleting M-CSF-R$^+$LysM$^+$ cells. Although neither monocytes nor macrophages were required to initiate immunity, when both cell types were depleted during infection with the intestinal pathogens *Citrobacter rodentium* or *Listeria monocytogenes*, IFNγ$^+$CD4$^+$ T cells were reduced in the lamina propria, demonstrating the capacity of monocytes/macrophages to influence T cell polarization (87). In contrast, the IL-17 response was not altered by monocyte and macrophage depletion but was significantly impaired upon selective depletion of cDCs, indicating that this cell population is necessary for mucosal Th17 responses. Macrophage depletion has also been shown to reduce type 2-dependent immune responses in the lung and gut. Depletion of $CD11b^+$ F4/80$^+$ macrophages led to a significant reduction in recruitment and cytokine expression of Th2 cells in affected tissues of three models of IL-13-dependent inflammation, fibrosis, and immunity, without any such reduction in the draining lymph nodes (88). Since $CD11b^+$ DCs might also be susceptible to depletion, studies of CD11c-DTR and CD11b/c-DTR double Tg mice confirmed that macrophages but not $CD11c^+$ DCs were critical for the maintenance of type 2-dependent responses. Reduced expression of the Th2 cell chemoattractants CCL1 and CCL22 may be one mechanism through which Th2 cell recruitment is impaired in a *Schistosoma mansoni* egg-induced lung granuloma model following macrophage depletion (88). Macrophage production of the chemokine CCL5 was recently shown to be important for the maintenance of stable tissue-resident memory IFNγ-producing $CD4^+$ T cell (T_{RM}) populations in memory lymphocyte clusters in a mouse model of genital herpes (89). Further studies are needed to investigate the presence of T_{RM} in RA synovial tissue and the requirement for monocytes/macrophages in maintaining these populations.

T Helper Cell Recruitment by Monocytes/ Macrophages

As alluded to the previous section, monocytes/macrophages can play an important role in recruiting or maintaining $CD4^+$ T cells in the arthritic joint. The C–X–C motif chemokine receptor CXCR6$^+$ is abundantly expressed on type 1 polarized effector memory T cells in RA synovial fluid (90, 91). Expression of CXCR6 on synovial T cells is reported to coincide with elevated expression of CXCL16 (the ligand for CXCR6) by synovial macrophages, endothelial cells, and fibroblast-like synoviocytes (FLS) in hypertrophic RA synovium (90). Significantly increased levels of cleaved CXCL16 have been demonstrated in RA SF compared to control samples (90, 92), and RA synovial tissue macrophages express both CXCL16 and CXCR6 (92). *In vitro* migration experiments demonstrate that healthy PBMC or CXCR6$^+$ T cells isolated from RA SF can migrate in response to exogenous CXCL16 or CXCL16 present in SF (90, 92). Together, these data suggest that increased CXCL16 expression in RA synovium, either due to increased expression by macrophages (90) or due to increased influx of monocytes (93), promotes recruitment of CXCR6$^+$ T cells and may thereby contribute to synovial inflammation and immunopathology. CXCL16 expression can be differentially regulated by cytokines: the Th2-like cytokines IL-4, IL-10, and IL-13 suppress secretion of CXCL16 by monocytes/macrophages, while the Th1-associated cytokine IFNγ slightly enhances CXCL16 secretion (93). No modulation of CXCL16 levels was observed upon addition of IL-15, IL-18, or TNFα to monocytes/macrophages. In contrast, earlier work found that exposure of monocytes to TNFα upregulated transmembrane expression and secretion of CXCL16 (90) suggesting that a reduction in synovial TNFα levels might impact on recruitment of CXCR6$^+$ T cells to the joint. In a small study of three patients responding to anti-TNF treatment, *in situ* immunohistochemistry demonstrated significantly reduced synovial CXCL16 expression compared to the high expression levels observed pretreatment (90). This observation may be due to reduced monocyte numbers in the joint following treatment, since synovial cellularity is known to be reduced soon after anti-TNF infusion (94–96). Conversely, in three non-responder patients, CXCL16 expression remained high. In accordance with reduced CXCL16 expression in the joint following successful anti-TNF therapy, serum levels of CXCL16 were also decreased after anti-TNF treatment in two cohorts of 23 and 44 RA patients, respectively (97, 98). Thus far, these studies suggest that monocyte infiltration and/or type 1 cytokine production in the RA joint may enhance local production of soluble CXCL16, which may exacerbate local inflammation via recruitment of CXCR6$^+$ T cells.

Another chemokine receptor interaction of increasing interest in RA is the C–C chemokine ligand CCL20 [also known as macrophage inflammatory protein-3 alpha (MIP-3α)] and its C–C chemokine receptor CCR6 [recently reviewed in Ref. (99)]. CCR6 expression is commonly associated with Th17 cells (100), but this receptor is also expressed on memory T cells (101), including CD4$^+$ T cells expressing IFNγ with or without IL-17 (102), as well as DC, B cells, and regulatory T cell (Treg) (99). In the SKG mouse model of T cell-mediated autoimmune arthritis, the CCL20–CCR6 axis is implicated in recruiting Th17 cells to the joint, via spontaneous CCL20 production from adherent FLS (103). The authors found that dispersed monocytes from mouse synovial tissue did not produce CCL20 unless stimulated. Others found that unstimulated FLS from RA patients did not produce CCL20, but that stimulation with either IL-1β or TNFα led to the production of CCL20 at levels sufficient to promote CCR6-specific recruitment of mononuclear cells, and which could be increased by IL-17 and decreased by IL-4 (104). In patients with juvenile idiopathic arthritis, CCL20 mRNA was shown to be constitutively expressed by synovial monocytic cells (105). In addition, *in vitro* exposure to plasmin, a component of the fibrinolytic cascade which is generated in inflamed tissues, can trigger production of CCL20 by human macrophages and lead to chemotactic migration of CCR6$^+$ Th17 cells *in vitro* (106). A role for plasmin in RA has been suggested by observations from collagen-induced arthritis (107) but has yet to be confirmed in the human setting. In summary, there is a potential role for monocytes in influencing the CCL20–CCR6 axis in RA.

Modulation of CD4$^+$ Treg Function by Monocytes/Macrophages

In addition to effects on T helper cell polarization, activated monocytes and macrophages can also positively or negatively influence the function of CD4$^+$ Tregs through production of soluble mediators. IL-1β has been shown by several groups to drive IL-17 expression by CD4$^+$CD25$^+$ Tregs [reviewed in Ref. (108)]. Excessive production of IL-6 *in vivo* inhibited inducible Treg generation from naive T cells but did not affect the development and function of natural Tregs (109). A recent study showed that IL-6 negatively affected FOXP3 protein expression by reducing expression of USP7 and disrupting USP7–FOXP3 association. USP7 is a deubiquitinase that prevents proteasomal degradation of FOXP3, thereby increasing FOXP3 expression levels and enhancing Treg function (110). TNFα has also been shown to decrease FOXP3 expression and reduce Treg function (111, 112). Additionally, anti-TNF therapy was shown to induce the differentiation of a suppressive CD4$^+$CD25^{hi}FOXP3$^+$CD62L$^-$ Treg subpopulation through conversion of CD4$^+$CD25$^-$ T cells in RA patients (113).

Contrastingly, TNFα has also been shown to boost Treg expansion and/or function (114, 115). Our lab recently showed that monocytes, activated *in vitro* with LPS or with cytokines known to be present in the RA joint, can induce expression of proinflammatory cytokines (IL-17 and IFNγ) in CD4$^+$CD25$^+$CD127^{low} Tregs in an IL-6-, TNFα-, and IL-1β-dependent manner (18). However, despite the increase in proinflammatory cytokine expression, these Tregs maintained and even enhanced their suppressive capacity, indicating that acquisition of proinflammatory cytokine expression does not necessarily imply loss of suppressive function (18). Conversely, it has been shown that TNFα and IL-6 can alter the susceptibility of effector T cells to Treg-mediated regulation, making them resistant to suppression (116–118).

Monocytes/macrophages can also boost Treg function directly by producing soluble mediators that are immunoregulatory in nature. A population of CD11b$^+$F4/80$^+$CD11c$^-$ macrophages has been identified in the lamina propria which can induce Foxp3$^+$ Treg differentiation through a mechanism dependent on IL-10, retinoic acid, and TGFβ in the local milieu (119). As discussed above, macrophage-derived ROS might play a role in modulating effector T cell responses (80); however, it has also been suggested that ROS can promote Treg-mediated immune regulation (120–122). Using both human and rat systems, macrophages were shown to suppress T cell responses by inducing FOXP3$^+$ Tregs in a ROS-dependent manner (120). This was confirmed using macrophages from patients with chronic granulomatous disease (CGD) that are defective in ROS production; CGD macrophages allowed significantly more T cell activation and expansion and induced fewer FOXP3$^+$ cells than did macrophages from control subjects. T cells primed by CGD macrophages showed reduced inhibition of responder T cell proliferation and IFNγ or IL-17 production than did cells primed by control macrophages. Similar results were observed using rats with defective ROS production due to a SNP in *Ncf1*.

It was shown that monocyte subsets and their cytokines may have differential effects on subsets of Treg cells. In both humans and mice, ~70% of Tregs express the transcription factor Helios (123). CD16$^+$ monocytes have been described to inhibit proliferation of Helios$^+$ Tregs through a mechanism dependent on IL-12. In contrast, Tregs lacking Helios expression were suppressed by CD16$^-$ monocytes via TNFα, while TNFα blockade specifically expanded the Helios$^-$ Treg subset (124).

Figure 1 summarizes data from existing reports on the proposed mechanisms via which monocytes/macrophages may affect the function of CD4$^+$ effector vs. Tregs subsets. It should be noted that much of the reported evidence comes from *in vitro* studies, which indicate the potential involvement of these mechanisms but do not demonstrate conclusively if or where these events occur at the site of inflammation.

EFFECTS OF CD4$^+$ T CELL SUBSETS ON MONOCYTE/MACROPHAGE ACTIVATION AND FUNCTION

Monocyte/Macrophage Activation and Polarization by CD4$^+$ Effector T Cells

Monocytes and macrophages are capable of responding to a wide range of stimuli and environmental cues, which in turn

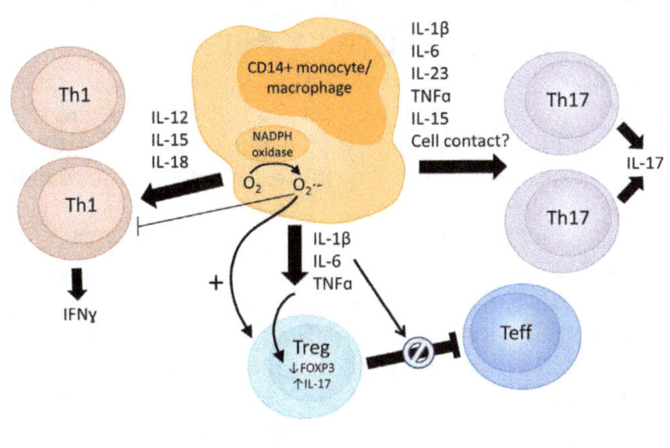

FIGURE 1 | Proposed mechanisms via which monocytes/macrophages in the inflamed RA joint can modulate CD4+ T cell responses. The arrow thickness reflects the evidence base to support the proposed mechanism. Monocyte/macrophage-derived cytokines, such as IL-1β, IL-6, TNFα, IL-12, IL-15, IL-18, and IL-23, are present in the RA joint (4, 8, 9, 43, 44, 70, 75). These cytokines can promote Th1 (IL-12, IL-15, and IL-18) and Th17 (IL-1β, IL-6, IL-15, IL-23, and TNFα) responses, and both Th1 and Th17 cells are detectable in synovial tissue and fluid (45–47). *In vitro* and *in vivo* data indicate that activated CD14+ blood monocytes or synovial monocytes/macrophages can potently induce Th17 (17, 35, 59–64) and/or Th1 (35, 61, 87) responses. Further studies are required to clarify whether different monocyte subsets preferentially promote specific Th responses. Activated monocytes/macrophages can also have profound effects on the phenotype and function of regulatory T cells (Tregs). Several groups have reported that IL-1β can drive IL-17 expression by CD4+CD25+ Tregs [reviewed in Ref. (108)], but these cells may retain suppressive capacity (18). Others have reported that TNFα and IL-6 lead to reduced FOXP3 expression in Tregs (110–112) or render effector T cells resistant to Treg-mediated suppression (116–118). Macrophage production of reactive oxygen species (ROS) may play a role in suppressing Th1 responses (80) and inducing FOXP3+ Tregs (120–122).

can determine their phenotype. Macrophages can be polarized into diverse subtypes often termed M1 and M2; however, these phenotypes represent extremes on a spectrum of functional states (125). A recent transcriptomics study provided elegant evidence to support the latter concept (126). In this study, gene expression profiling was performed on 299 macrophage samples stimulated with 28 different conditions. Monocytes were differentiated into macrophages using either GM-CSF or M-CSF. The macrophages were subsequently activated using typical M1 (e.g., IFNγ, LPS, and TNF) or M2 (e.g., IL-4 and IL-13) stimuli, and standardized microarrays were performed. Analysis of the transcriptomes using coregulation analysis generated two groups of samples positioned at either end of a bimodal axis, representing M1/M2 states. However, when the effect of other activation factors not associated with typical M1/M2 states was included in the analysis (e.g., high-density lipoprotein and free fatty acids), the spectrum expanded away from the axis to account for these dissimilar states. These data confirm that while it is possible to polarize macrophages into distinct M1/M2 populations, not all activators will generate populations that fit into or in between these states. It is therefore important to keep in mind that although in this review we refer to M1/M2 macrophages, a spectrum of activation outside of these phenotypes exists. Outside of stringent M1/M2 phenotypes, it has become increasingly difficult to determine the exact nature of macrophages within published work. A recent review has highlighted a lack of coherently used markers used to define macrophage populations within the field (127). The authors discuss that incomplete descriptions of how macrophages have been isolated, stimulated, and analyzed can lead to confusion between laboratories. Therefore, they propose a new nomenclature system, based on the macrophage activator and markers used to define the population. In this way, the anticipation is that we can better define and understand the distinct macrophage populations generated in different labs under different conditions and avoid confusion when attempting to place macrophages on a spectrum of activation.

Bearing in mind the limitations of the M1/M2 classification, cytokines that are typically associated with Th1 and Th2 cells have been used to polarize monocytes or macrophages *in vitro* with the Th1 cytokine IFNγ driving the M1 (classically activated) phenotype and the Th2 cytokines IL-4/IL-13 driving an M2 (alternatively activated) phenotype (128). Three further M2 subtypes have since been described; M2a, M2b, and M2c, all with different functional capabilities to those seen in an M1 phenotype (127, 129). M1 macrophages typically release high levels of proinflammatory cytokines, such as IL-1, IL-6, IL-12, and TNFα, have high production of reactive oxygen intermediates and metabolize arginine to nitric oxide. Typical M1 chemokines include CXCL5, CXCL8, CXCL9, CXCL10, and CXCL13. M2 macrophages are characterized by a switch in arginine metabolism from the iNOS pathway seen in M1 cells to the arginase pathway, releasing orthonine and polyamines. M2 cells release IL-10 and some IL-12 and express CD163, CD206, scavenger receptors A and B, and Dectin-1. M2 macrophages are generally considered to be involved in wound healing and to promote tissue remodeling through release of growth factors VEGF and TGFβ (129, 130).

In addition to Th1 and Th2 cytokines, it has been shown that the Th17-associated cytokine IL-17A has direct effects on macrophages leading to an increase in IL-1β, TNFα, and IL-6 (131, 132). Silencing of IL-17RA using siRNA reduced the upregulation of IL-1β, TNFα, and IL-6 by macrophages, thus showing that IL-17 signaling through IL-17RA can influence cytokine release of macrophages (132). IL-17 has been shown to be directly chemotactic for monocytes *in vitro* at concentrations found in RA synovial fluid, via ligation of IL-17RA and IL-17RC on monocytes and p38 MAPK activation (133). *In vivo*, human monocytes injected intravenously into SCID mice were recruited into subcutaneously implanted sponges which had been soaked with human IL-17 or the positive control CCL2 [also called monocyte chemoattractant protein-1 (MCP-1)] but not sponges soaked with IL-8 or IL-10 (133). Tissue-infiltrating Th17 cells (unlike Th1 and Th2 cells) also secrete CCL20 (45), which has been shown to be chemotactic for monocytes (134). IL-17 may also have indirect effects on monocyte chemotaxis through the induction of chemokine expression by other cell types present in the RA joint. *In vitro* addition of IL-17 to RA synovial fibroblasts or normal blood-derived macrophages effectively induced expression of CCL2 and CCL20 (135). However, *in vivo* only CCL2 was secreted following adenovirus-mediated intraperitoneal (i.p.) expression of IL-17. The increase in peritoneal CCL2 levels contributed to increased monocyte recruitment, which was reduced by i.p. injection of neutralizing anti-CCL2 (135). Local IL-17 expression in ankle joints was also associated with increased F4/80 staining and CCL2 levels. The IL-17-mediated induction of CCL2 appeared to involve the PI3K, ERK, and (at least in RA synovial fibroblasts) JNK pathways.

There is good evidence that TCR- or cytokine-activated T cells can activate monocytes, resulting in inflammatory cytokine and MMP production by monocytes in a cell-contact-dependent manner (39, 136–138). The $CD4^{+}CD45RO^{+}CCR7^{-}$ effector memory T cell subset of cytokine-activated T cells has been suggested to be a main driver of this stimulation (139). One study showed that distinct $CD4^{+}$ T cell subsets (Th1, Th2, or Th17) may differentially affect monocyte differentiation into distinct mo-DC subsets in a cell-contact- and cytokine-dependent manner (42). Cocultures of sorted Th1, Th2, and Th17 cells with isolated $CD14^{+}$ monocytes led to the generation of three distinct mo-DC subsets, as defined by typical DC markers. The monocytes cultured with Th1 cells formed DCs that secreted IL-12 and expressed CD86 and CD274 (DCth1), whereas those generated through culture with Th2 cells expressed increased levels of IL-10, CD275, and DC-SIGN (DCth2). Monocytes cultured with Th17 cells developed into DCs that secreted IL-1β, IL-6, and IL-23 but not IL-12 (DCth17). The DCs generated through coculture were then used as stimulators in a mixed leukocyte reaction; IFNγ and IL-17A were released from responding $CD4^{+}$ T cells when cultured with DCth1 and DCth17, respectively. These data are in line with the results described above on how different Th-related cytokines affect macrophage polarization.

$CD4^{+}$ T cells can also drive differentiation of monocytes into osteoclasts. Bone resorption by osteoclasts is of pathological significance in RA, causing "erosion sites" which can be used as a measure of disease severity and outcome. Studies have shown that $IFN\gamma^{+}$ human T cells cultured with peripheral blood monocytes in the presence of M-CSF can induce osteoclast formation via expression of the cytokine receptor activator of NF-κB ligand (RANKL) (140). IFNγ may, however, also disrupt the formation of osteoclasts by rapidly degrading the RANK adaptor protein TRAF6 (141), suggesting that the $IFN\gamma^{+}$ T cells can both contribute to and hinder the formation of osteoclasts. Th17 cells are often implicated in promoting osteoclastogenesis; Th17-associated cytokines were shown to upregulate RANKL on RA FLS and to directly induce monocyte-to-osteoclast differentiation (142, 143). In addition, RANKL-expressing Th17 cells were recently shown to convert mature osteoclasts to a bone resorptive state (144). T cells in the synovial fluid have been shown to express RANKL (145), and high levels of RANKL-expressing $CD3^{+}$ cells have been found in the synovial tissue of patients with RA (146), thus potentially contributing to osteoclast formation and therefore higher levels of bone resorption.

Together, these data indicate that prototypical T helper cell-associated cytokines can polarize, recruit, activate, or differentiate monocytes and/or macrophages. *In vivo*, the phenotype and function of monocytes and macrophages is likely to be dependent on many soluble factors and cellular interactions acting in concert.

Induction of Apoptosis in Monocytes and Macrophages by CD4+ T Cells

In addition to activating monocytes or macrophages, several reports have shown that activated $CD4^{+}$ T cells can kill these cells (147, 148). Later studies assigned this killing to $CD4^{+}CD25^{+}$ Tregs (149, 150) as well as to activated effector T cells, defined as Treg-depleted $CD4^{+}CD25^{-}$ T cells or cloned antigen-specific $CD4^{+}$ T cells (39, 148). A recent study showed that $CD4^{+}$ (and $CD8^{+}$) T cells from the BAL fluid of C57BL/6 mice express FASL and that these T cell populations can induce apoptosis in autologous alveolar macrophages. Although apoptosis by $CD8^{+}$ T cells was more prevalent, killing by $CD4^{+}$ T cells was observed (151). Evidence from our lab has shown that activated $CD4^{+}CD25^{-}$ effector T (Teff) cells upregulate FASL, and upon coculture with human monocytes, activate, and then kill the monocytes in a FAS/FASL-dependent manner (39). Blocking the FAS/FASL interactions reduced monocyte apoptosis but did not affect the expression of FAS, CD14, or HLA-DR on the monocytes, indicating that the monocytes still became activated by the T cells. T cells may also kill monocytes/macrophages in a FAS-independent mechanism, as TRAIL and TWEAK death receptor pathways have been implicated in macrophage killing by $CD4^{+}$ T cells (152).

Modulation of Monocyte/Macrophage Function by CD4+ Regulatory T Cells

Regulatory T cells are generally defined as $CD4^{+}CD25^{+}CD127^{low}$ $FOXP3^{+}$ cells. The suppressive effects of Tregs on immune cells have been documented widely, in particular on cells from the adaptive immune system ($CD4^{+}$ and $CD8^{+}$ T cells) [reviewed in Ref. (153–155)]. Tregs can employ several mechanisms of suppression including release of the inhibitory cytokines IL-10 and TGFβ, cytolysis via release of granzymes A and B, metabolic disruption via IL-2 consumption or through degradation of ATP to AMP/ADP, and eventually adenosine via the ectonucleotidases CD39 and CD73. There is ample evidence that Tregs can also interact directly with antigen-presenting cells, including monocytes and macrophages [reviewed in Ref. (156)].

Modulation of monocyte function *in vitro* has been shown by a series of experiments from our lab. The first study compared monocytes from the peripheral blood of healthy human donors cultured alone, or cocultured with autologous effector T cells or Tregs. Coculture with anti-CD3 mAb and effector T cells induced an activated phenotype in the monocytes, with increased levels of CD80, CD40, and HLA II compared to monocytes cultured alone (157). When monocytes were cocultured with Tregs, levels of CD40, CD80, and HLA II on monocytes were not increased compared to the monocyte only culture, while CD86 expression was significantly reduced. These monocytes were impaired in their ability to induce T cell proliferation in subsequent T cell stimulation assays. In a following study, we demonstrated that upon coculture with Tregs, monocytes expressed increased levels of the mannose receptor CD206 and hemoglobin/haptoglobin scavenger receptor CD163 (158), markers which are associated with M2-like macrophages (127, 129). In support of these phenotypic changes, we found that phagocytosis of FITC-zymosan/latex beads was increased in Treg cocultured monocytes, although the number of monocytes that phagocytosed the beads did not change significantly (158). Furthermore, LPS-induced NFκB activation and secretion of TNFα and IL-6 were decreased in monocytes cocultured with Tregs, compared to those cultured alone or with effector T cells. Using flow cytometry, it was shown that the frequencies of LPS-induced IL-6 and TNFα expressing monocytes were also reduced upon coculture with Tregs as compared to monocytes cultured alone or with Teffs, indicating that the observed differences in cytokine secretion were due to changes within cytokine-expressing monocytes (39). This was not due to cell death, as in contrast to $CD4^+CD25^-$ Teff, Tregs did not kill the monocytes upon interaction (39). The decreased production of IL-6 and TNFα in response to LPS was still observed when monocytes were re-purified after coculture (158), indicating that Tregs imprint changes in the monocytes, suggestive of "trained immunity." Immune memory has traditionally been associated with cells of the adaptive immune system; recently, the term "trained immunity" has been used to define the memory capacity within innate immune cells (159). Induction of trained immunity in monocytes has been shown in studies whereby exposure to beta-glucan led to epigenetic modifications in monocytes, resulting in phenotypic changes and altered function (160). Further investigation is required to determine whether the effects of Tregs on monocytes are reflective of a state of "trained immunity" in these cells.

The modulation of monocytes by Tregs was shown to be dependent in part on soluble factors (IL-10 and IL-4/IL-13) as well as cell-contact (158). A different group showed that cocultures of human $CD14^+$ monocytes with sorted Tregs led to increased levels of secreted IL-10 and higher levels of B7-H4 receptor on the monocytes. These monocytes were less capable of stimulating a T cell proliferative response, which was due in part to the expression of IL-10 and B7-H4 (161). Notably, work from the same group showed that the expression of B7-H4 was a marker for immunosuppressive tumor-associated macrophages in ovarian carcinoma (162), and that the presence of Tregs and macrophage-associated B7-H4 at the tumor site was negatively associated with patient outcome (163, 164). Together, these data indicate that modulation of monocytes and macrophages by Tregs may have functional consequences in disease.

Modulation of macrophage function by Tregs has also been shown *in vivo*. Adoptive transfer of syngeneic $CD4^+CD25^+$ Tregs into the peritoneal cavity of SCID mice revealed both phenotypic and functional changes in peritoneal macrophages (165). In this study, SCID mice were adoptively transferred with either no T cells, $CD4^+CD25^+$ Tregs, $CD4^+CD25^-$ T cells, or both $CD4^+CD25^+$ Treg and $CD4^+CD25^-$ T cells at a 1:1 ratio. The percentages of F4/80$^+$ macrophages expressing CD54, CD80, CD86, or I-A^d were significantly decreased in SCID mice transferred with Tregs compared to the control mice and were increased in mice receiving $CD4^+CD25^-$ T cells. The latter increase was inhibited when both T cell types were cotransferred. The group also showed that macrophages from mice transferred with Tregs had an enhanced phagocytic capacity compared to those transferred with $CD4^+CD25^-$ T cells or no T cells. The enhanced phagocytic capacity was reversed by transfer with both cell types. Upon LPS stimulation, macrophages from SCID mice transferred with $CD4^+CD25^+$ Treg cells produced more IL-10 and less IL-12 than those from mice transferred with $CD4^+CD25^-$ T cells. The macrophages from mice receiving Tregs were also impaired in their antigen-presenting capacity and showed higher arginase activity and lower nitric oxide production compared to those from mice transferred with $CD4^+CD25^-$ T cells or no T cells. Together, this work suggests that Tregs modulate macrophages toward an "M2" phenotype, with the functional and phenotypic characteristics of the modulated cells closely resembling those seen in the previously mentioned *in vitro* studies of human Tregs and monocytes.

Figure 2 summarizes existing evidence on the cellular and molecular mechanisms via which $CD4^+$ effector vs. regulatory T cell subsets can affect the phenotype or function of monocytes and macrophages. As indicated in **Figure 1**, since much of the reported evidence comes from *in vitro* studies, some caution should be exerted when extrapolating these findings to an *in vivo* situation.

DYSREGULATED MONOCYTE/ MACROPHAGE HOMEOSTASIS IN THE RHEUMATOID JOINT

The abundance of $CD14^+/CD68^+$ monocytes/macrophages in the rheumatoid joint suggests that these cells are recruited at a high rate, are long-lived or proliferative, and/or resistant to apoptosis. Evidence exists to support all these scenarios. Chemokines involved in monocyte recruitment, such as CCL2/MCP-1, CCL3/MIP-1α, and CCL5/RANTES, are readily detectable at the site of inflammation (96, 166), and blood monocytes from patients with RA express the corresponding chemokine receptors CCR1, CCR2, CCR3, and CCR5 (15). One study investigated the migration of labeled autologous $CD14^+$ blood monocytes, isolated by CliniMACS procedure, in RA patients using single photon emission computer tomography. A very small but specific fraction of 0.003% of re-infused monocytes was found to migrate to the inflamed joints, being detectable within 1 h after re-infusion (167). Interestingly, monocyte influx into the inflamed joint was not altered early after anti-TNF treatment (2 weeks post-treatment) even though disease activity was significantly reduced (168). The authors concluded that monocytes migrate continuously into the inflamed synovial tissue of RA, but at a slow macrophage-replacement rate, and that the rapid decrease in synovial macrophage numbers observed after anti-TNF treatment (23) cannot be explained by an immediate effect on monocyte influx.

Another contributing factor to the persistently high monocyte/macrophage presence in the rheumatoid joint is apoptosis resistance. Both RA peripheral blood monocytes and RA synovial monocytes/macrophages have been shown to be resistant to spontaneous cell death, agonistic Fas-antibody induced apoptosis, or responder T cell-mediated killing (28, 39, 40). Proposed underlying mechanisms include the enhanced expression of antiapoptotic molecules, such as FLIP and Mcl-1 in RA synovial

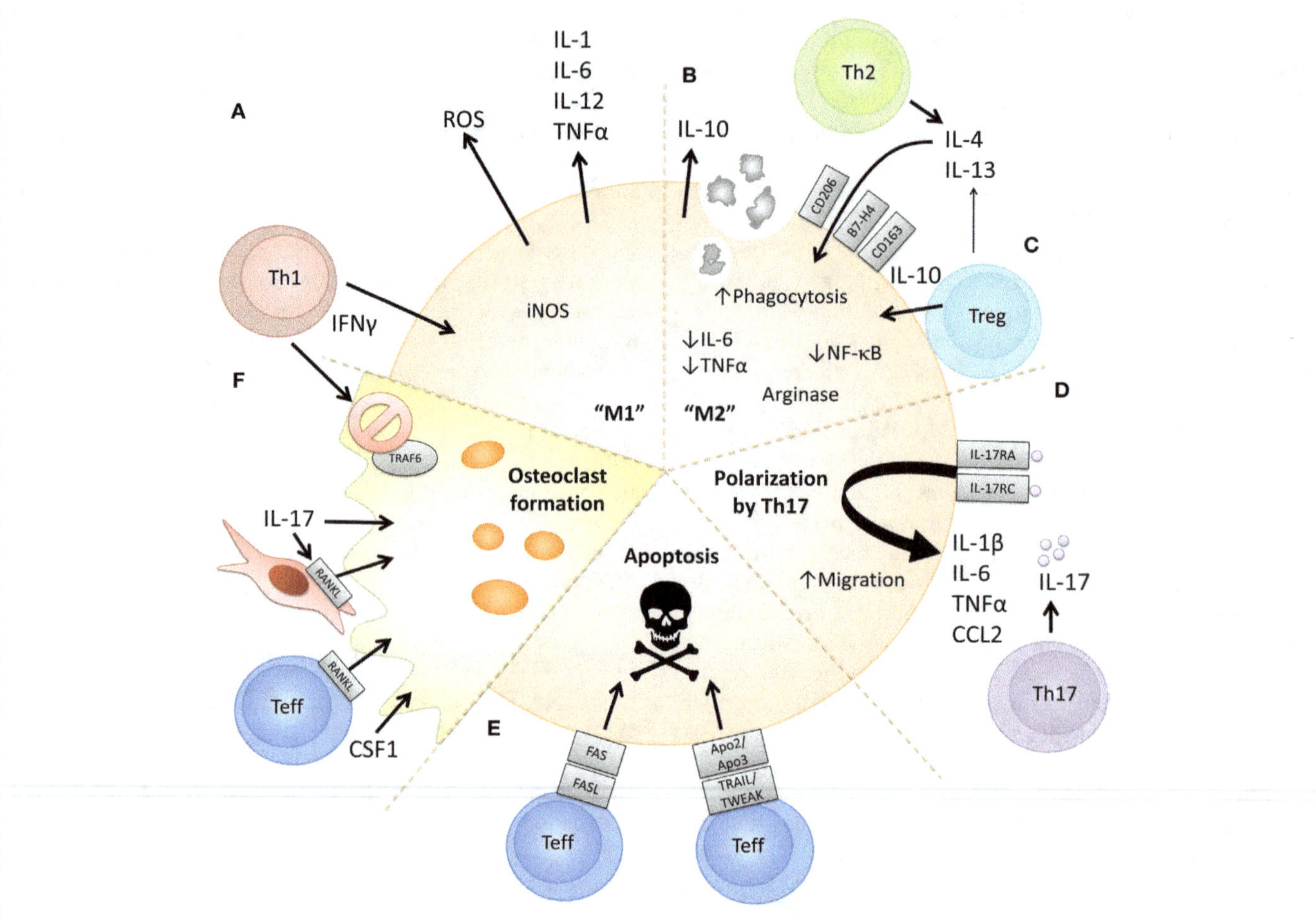

FIGURE 2 | Proposed cellular and molecular mechanisms via which CD4⁺ T cell subsets can polarize or modulate monocyte/macrophage function. **(A)** The prototypical Th1 cytokine IFNγ can polarize monocytes to an "M1" phenotype, promoting proinflammatory cytokine release, reactive oxygen species (ROS) production, and metabolism of arginine to nitric oxide [reviewed in Ref. (125, 127)]. **(B)** Prototypical Th2 cytokines IL-4 and IL-13 can polarize monocytes to an "M2" phenotype, characterized by expression of anti-inflammatory cytokines such as IL-10, expression of CD206, increased phagocytosis, and metabolism of arginine to orthonine and polyamine intermediates [reviewed in Ref. (125, 127)]. **(C)** $CD4^+CD25^+$ Tregs have also been shown to induce an alternatively activated or anti-inflammatory phenotype in monocytes in a cell-contact and soluble factor (IL-4, IL-13, and IL-10) dependent manner leading to reduced IL-6 and TNFα production, decreased NFκB activation and increased expression of IL-10, CD163, and B7-H4 (157, 158, 164, 165). **(D)** The prototypical Th17-associated cytokine IL-17 has been shown to increase levels of IL-1β, TNFα, and IL-6 released by macrophages (131, 132). IL-17 has also been suggested to be chemotactic for monocytes via ligation of IL-17RA/RC (133). **(E)** Evidence shows that activated $CD4^+CD25^-$ T cells can activate but also induce apoptosis in monocytes/macrophages. Both FAS/FASL- and TRAIL/TWEAK-dependent mechanisms have been proposed (39, 147, 148, 151, 152). **(F)** Activated RANKL-expressing Teff can drive osteoclast formation from monocytes when cultured in the presence of M-CSF (140). Th17-associated cytokines can upregulate RANKL on RA fibroblast-like synoviocytes and also directly induce monocyte-to-osteoclast differentiation (142, 143), while IFNγ has been shown to suppress osteoclast formation (141).

tissue (169, 170), the reduced expression of the proapoptotic Bcl-2 homology 3 (BH3)-only protein Bim (171), the increased production of TNFα and IL-1 which have antiapoptotic effects (172), and the increased presence of Tregs in the RA joint (173), which do not exert apoptotic effects on monocytes (39). Incubation with the anti-TNF drugs infliximab or adalimumab has been shown to increase apoptosis in healthy or RA peripheral blood monocytes, lending support to the role of TNF in regulating this process (28, 174). Conversely, defects in apoptosis pathway-associated molecules, such as occur in Fas-deficient (*lpr/lpr*) mice, lead to an increase in the number of circulating monocytes and an increase in the proinflammatory activity of peritoneal macrophages and the development of systemic autoimmune disease including lupus-like disease and inflammatory arthritis (175). A recent study showed that selective loss of Fas in myeloid cells was sufficient to induce SLE-like disease in mice (176). Together, these data illustrate that a dysregulation in monocyte/macrophage homeostasis may be an important contributing factor to chronic inflammatory joint disease.

In addition, recent advances in genetics have revealed an increasing number of susceptibility loci for RA (177), several of which may have relevance to monocyte/macrophage function or homeostasis, e.g., *CD40*, *TNFAIP3*, *IRAK1*, *TRAF1/TRAF6*, *IRF5* (178), and *RBPJ* (179). Future functional genomic studies may elucidate the exact role of these genes in RA and in monocytes/macrophages in particular.

Although knowledge regarding the phenotype and function of synovial macrophages is continuing to grow, it is much less clear what the origin of these cells is. Fate-mapping experiments in mice demonstrate that tissue-resident yolk sac-derived macrophages develop in a Myb-independent manner and can persist in adult mice independently of hematopoietic stem cells (180, 181). However, other work suggests that Myb-dependent fetal liver-derived monocytes also contribute to the pool of tissue-resident cells (182, 183). In addition, although self-renewing tissue-resident macrophage populations have been described (182–185), evidence suggests that recruited blood monocytes may play a role in replenishing the macrophage population during inflammation (186–188). The investigation of the origin and homeostasis of tissue macrophages remains an active field of research, and future work may be able to determine whether RA synovial macrophages are equivalent to these long-lived cells, or are continuously replaced by newly recruited peripheral monocytes.

TARGETING MONOCYTES/ MACROPHAGES IN RA

The findings discussed in this review indicate that selective targeting of monocytes/macrophages could have therapeutic benefit in RA [also reviewed in Ref. (5)]. This is supported by older data showing that treatment of severe RA with leukapheresis efficiently removed blood monocytes concomitant with a clinical response (189), and that depleting CCR2^{+} monocytes using anti-CCR2 mAb could ameliorate collagen-induced arthritis, although the effects were dependent on the dose of mAb used (190). *In vitro*, selective elimination of human macrophages using toxin-conjugated Abs against CD64 resulted in reduced T cell proliferation and reduced TNFα production by synovial fluid mononuclear cells and synovial tissue explants (191). Bim-BH3 mimetic therapy could induce apoptosis in myeloid cells and suppress clinical severity of experimental arthritis (171). siRNA-based therapeutic approaches are also being developed in order to selectively target certain genes or pathways (192).

Additionally, given the importance of T cell-monocyte crosstalk in promoting inflammation (17, 137, 193), approaches that target T cell-monocyte interactions may have therapeutic benefit. Indeed, this may be one way via which drugs like abatacept (CTLA4-Ig) exert their clinical effect. Previously underappreciated mechanisms of existing therapeutics may contribute to their efficacy by (in)directly targeting monocytes/ macrophages. For example, multiple studies have shown that blockade of IL-6 signaling via monoclonal antibody to the IL-6 receptor (tocilizumab) can boost Treg frequencies (194–198), but additional mechanisms of action may include reduction in CD69^{+}CD14^{+} and CD16^{+}CD14^{+} monocyte frequencies (197), induction of monocyte apoptosis, and inhibition of monocytic IL-6 mRNA expression (199). Despite the widespread uptake and high efficacy of TNFα inhibitor drugs in RA, the underlying mechanisms of action are not firmly established [reviewed in Ref. (200)]. TNF inhibitor drugs block signaling of the key monocyte/ macrophage-derived cytokine TNFα but can also reduce production of other proinflammatory mediators, such as IL-1β, GM-CSF, IL-6 and IL-8, in synovial membrane (201–203). Furthermore, it has been reported that Treg function can be restored or enhanced following TNFα inhibitor therapy (111, 204), and we and others recently demonstrated that TNFα blockade in cocultures of antigen presenting cells and CD4^{+} T cells favors development of an immunoregulatory phenotype in effector CD4^{+} T cells by promoting expression of IL-10 (205, 206). We showed that following TNF blockade, a significant proportion of IL-17 expressing CD4^{+} T cells coexpressed IL-10, which was biologically active and was able to modulate the phenotype of monocytes leading to reduced HLA-DR and CD40 expression and increased CD163 expression (205). Another postulated mechanism of anti-TNF drugs is via interaction with tmTNFα (28, 207). It was recently shown that production of cytokines and decoy receptors triggered by monocyte tmTNF crosslinking might provide a prognostic parameter for predicting therapeutic response to etanercept, suggesting a role for monocytic reverse signaling in the clinical efficacy of TNF inhibitors (208).

As previously discussed, monocytes/macrophages contribute to bone erosion in RA via differentiation into osteoclasts. Inhibiting osteoclastogenesis therefore presents a key target for therapeutic intervention, since the presence of bone erosions represents irreversible structural damage, associated with loss of joint function and poor quality of life. TNFα inhibitor drugs inhibit radiological progression, even in the absence of clinical response, via direct inhibitory effects on osteoclast differentiation and activity (209). Binding of CTLA4 to CD80/86 on monocytes provides a potent signal to inhibit differentiation into osteoclasts; accordingly abatacept was recently shown to inhibit osteoclastogenesis in human peripheral monocytes (210). A phase II clinical trial found that twice-yearly injections of the anti-RANKL drug denosumab inhibited progression of bone erosion in RA patients with active erosive disease but demonstrated no effect on disease activity (211). Similarly, RANKL knockout mice are protected from bone erosion in a serum transfer model of arthritis but display inflammation that is clinically and histologically similar to wild type (212). These data suggest that targeting osteoclastogenesis may have the potential to reduce structural joint damage, but that RANKL blockade alone may be ineffective at controlling the underlying inflammatory process. As an alternative strategy to inhibit osteoclastogenesis, targeting M-CSF receptor (M-CSFR, also known as CSF1R, c-FMS, and CD115) has been shown in various animal models of autoimmune arthritis to reduce both joint inflammation and bone destruction (213–216) However, in some models, while bone erosion is reduced, inflammation is unaffected by M-CSFR antibody blockade (215) or c-FMS kinase inhibition (217). Effective targeting of the M-CSFR pathway in RA may require blocking signaling of both its ligands, M-CSF and IL-34. Several clinical trials are currently investigating antibodies or small molecules targeting the M-CSFR pathway in RA and other indications [reviewed in Ref. (218)].

Epigenetic control of immune-mediated processes is a growing field of study with the potential to unveil mechanisms of immune regulation which may be amenable to therapeutic intervention. Bromodomain and extraterminal (BET) inhibitors have recently emerged as a promising approach to treat cancer but are also being investigated in the context of inflammatory disease. Blocking the recruitment of BET proteins to acetylated histones inhibits BET-mediated transcriptional activity. BET inhibitors have been shown to suppress expression of proinflammatory cytokines and chemokines in LPS-stimulated bone marrow-derived macrophages *in vitro* (219, 220). *In vivo* BET inhibition resulted in reduced Th17 differentiation, suppression of established Th17 responses, and protection against pathology in collagen-induced arthritis (221). A recent study found that BET inhibition suppressed cytokine-induced transcription in primary human monocytes in a gene-specific manner, without affecting JAK-STAT signaling. Instead, BET inhibition reduced recruitment of transcriptional machinery to the CXCL10 promoter and an upstream enhancer (222). In future studies, global approaches, such as genome-wide profiling, may identify additional functional pathways that are amenable to BET-mediated transcriptional regulation in monocytes/macrophages.

Additional therapeutic approaches under development for RA include proteasome inhibitors, such as bortezomib (223). Conflicting data on the effects of bortezomib on bone resorption are reported in different animal models of RA (224, 225). In human cells, bortezomib appears to inhibit osteoclastogenesis (226, 227). Selective inhibition of a subunit of the immunoproteasome (a class of proteasome primarily found in monocytes and lymphocytes) was shown to inhibit production of IL-23, TNFα, and IL-6 by LPS-activated monocytes and to reduce IFNγ and IL-2 production from anti-CD3/CD28-activated T cells (228). These data were generated using cells from healthy donors, but similar results were observed using PBMC from three RA patients. In mouse models of RA, immunoproteasome inhibition ameliorated disease and also blocked IL-23 production from activated monocytes.

Protein kinase inhibitors are another class of small molecule therapeutics gaining attention for the treatment of immune-mediated diseases. Tofacitinib, the first Janus kinase (JAK) inhibitor to be developed for RA was approved by the FDA in 2012. To date, most studies have focused on the effects of JAK inhibition in T cells

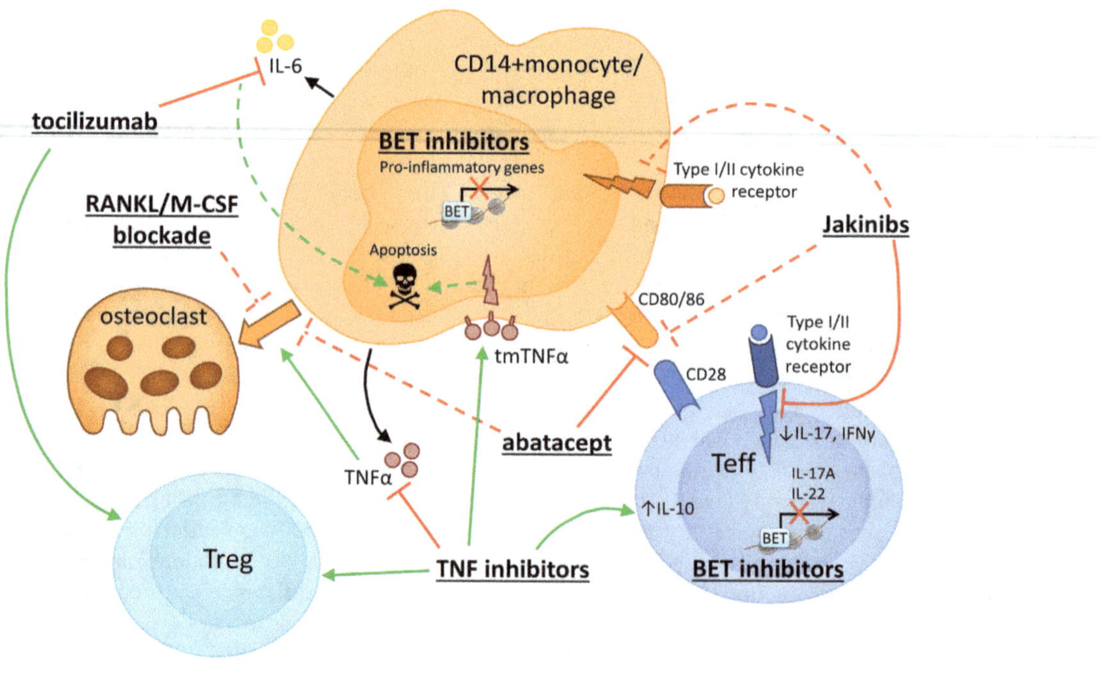

FIGURE 3 | Therapeutic strategies to target monocytes/macrophages in RA. Several novel strategies for drug intervention in RA, as well as currently used therapeutics, have potential mechanisms of action that target monocyte/macrophages or their interaction with CD4+ T cells. Selected therapies are presented with particular reference to their reported effects on monocyte/macrophage function and CD4+ T cell interactions. Red and green lines indicate inhibition and promotion, respectively, while dashed lines indicate novel or putative mechanisms that may require further confirmation. TNF inhibitor drugs block signaling of the key monocyte/macrophage-derived cytokine TNFα and have been shown to promote increased IL-10 expression in CD4+ T cells (205, 206), enhanced or restored Treg function (111, 204) and anti-osteoclast effects (209), and may also exert anti-inflammatory/proapoptotic effects on monocytes via "reverse signaling" through tmTNFα (28, 208). Blockade of IL-6 signaling (via monoclonal antibody to the IL-6 receptor, tocilizumab) reportedly boosts Treg frequencies (194–198) and has been suggested to inhibit monocyte IL-6 mRNA expression and induce monocyte apoptosis (199). Another widely used RA drug, abatacept (CTLA4-Ig), targets the interaction between monocytes and T cells, specifically impairing T cell costimulatory signals via CD80/CD86. Abatacept has also been reported to inhibit monocyte differentiation into osteoclasts (210). Several other approaches are currently under development to specifically target osteoclastogenesis, including blockade of RANKL (211) or M-CSF (218). Janus Kinase (JAK) inhibitors (Jakinibs) target JAK/STAT-mediated cytokine signaling in T cells and possibly also in macrophages (231, 232) and may reduce monocyte-derived DC costimulatory capacity (230). Bromodomain and extraterminal (BET) inhibitors are also under consideration for the treatment of inflammatory disease. Efficacy has been shown in collagen-induced arthritis where BET inhibition reduced Th17 responses (221). Reduced transcription of proinflammatory genes has been described in human monocytes (222) and mouse macrophages (219, 220) following *in vitro* exposure to BET inhibitors.

with relatively few data on the consequences in monocytes/macrophages. A recent report found that tofacitinib did not directly affect RA synovial monocytes, but that tofacitinib-exposed $CD4^+$ T cells demonstrated reduced proliferation, impaired IL-17 and IFNγ expression, and generated conditioned medium that when added to $CD14^+$ monocytes could inhibit IL-8 production (229). Others showed that tofacitinib reduced CD80/CD86 expression and therefore the T cell costimulatory capacity of human mo-DCs (230). In addition, tofacitinib and ruxolitinib, another JAK inhibitor drug, were shown to effectively suppress inflammatory responses of blood-derived and RA synovial macrophages (231). Tofacitinib also efficiently suppressed development of arthritis in a K/BxN serum transfer model. A cautionary observation was that JAK inhibition could enhance osteoclast differentiation *in vitro*. Also, in isolated mouse macrophages, both tofacitinib and ruxolitinib were found to block the IL-10-mediated feedback inhibition of cytokine transcription, thereby increasing LPS-induced cytokine production (232). These data indicate that JAK inhibitor drugs do have the capacity to modulate monocyte/macrophage function, but the exact cellular mechanisms that mediate the clinical efficacy of these therapeutics are still under investigation.

Figure 3 shows an overview of how drugs currently used to treat RA, as well as therapeutics under development, may target monocytes/macrophages or their interaction with $CD4^+$ T cells, to intervene in the underlying inflammatory and erosive disease processes.

SUMMARIZING CONCLUSION

In summary, there is strong evidence for a contributing role of both monocytes/macrophages and $CD4^+$ T cells in RA. In addition to directly promoting local inflammation by secreting proinflammatory mediators, synovial monocytes/macrophages secrete chemokines that can attract and maintain $CD4^+$ T cells in the joint. A growing evidence base suggests that activated (subsets of) monocytes can influence $CD4^+$ T helper cell polarization toward Th1/Th17. Through their cytokine production monocytes/macrophages may also impact on frequencies and function of regulatory $CD4^+$ T cells. Conversely, $CD4^+$ effector T cells can activate, polarize, as well as kill monocytes and macrophages and may influence monocyte chemotaxis, while $CD4^+$ Tregs can exert immunomodulatory effects on these cells, thereby enhancing their survival and inducing an anti-inflammatory state in monocytes/macrophages. To inform future research, refining the phenotypic characterization of monocyte/macrophage subpopulations by validating additional phenotypic markers would facilitate further investigation of their involvement in inflammatory conditions, such as RA. Given that the complexity of monocyte/macrophage phenotypes is not well understood or necessarily reflected in animal models or immortalized cell lines, studies of human primary monocytes and macrophages are essential to understand the contribution of these cells to RA pathogenesis. Improved knowledge regarding the origin of synovial monocyte/macrophages could lead to a better understanding of the roles of tissue-resident macrophages in the RA joint. Finally, further investigation into the direct interactions between tissue-resident $CD4^+$ T cell subsets and macrophages may elucidate how effector T cell responses are generated *in situ* as well as how macrophage responses can be regulated differentially by $CD4^+$ effector and Tregs. Several existing RA therapeutics are known to impact on the crosstalk between monocytes and $CD4^+$ T cells. An increased understanding of how the interactions between these cell types may contribute to immune pathology will benefit the development of new and improved therapeutic strategies.

ACKNOWLEDGMENTS

CR is supported by the King's Bioscience Institute and the Guy's and St Thomas' Charity Prize PhD Program in Biomedical and Translational Science, and AD is supported by a BBSRC CASE studentship (BB/L014165/1). The authors would like to thank Dr. Pierre Guermonprez (King's College London) for critical discussions.

REFERENCES

1. Klareskog L, Padyukov L, Rönnelid J, Alfredsson L. Genes, environment and immunity in the development of rheumatoid arthritis. *Curr Opin Immunol* (2006) **18**:650–5. doi:10.1016/j.coi.2006.06.004
2. McInnes IB, Schett G. The pathogenesis of rheumatoid arthritis. *New Engl J Med* (2011) **365**:2205–19. doi:10.1056/NEJMra1004965
3. Viatte S, Plant D, Raychaudhuri S. Genetics and epigenetics of rheumatoid arthritis. *Nat Rev Rheumatol* (2013) **9**:141–53. doi:10.1038/nrrheum.2012.237
4. McInnes IB, Schett G. Cytokines in the pathogenesis of rheumatoid arthritis. *Nat Rev Immunol* (2007) **7**:429–42. doi:10.1038/nri2094
5. Davignon J-L, Hayder M, Baron M, Boyer J-F, Constantin A, Apparailly F, et al. Targeting monocytes/macrophages in the treatment of rheumatoid arthritis. *Rheumatology* (2013) **52**:590–8. doi:10.1093/rheumatology/kes304
6. Li J, Hsu H-C, Mountz JD. Managing macrophages in rheumatoid arthritis by reform or removal. *Curr Rheumatol Rep* (2012) **14**:445–54. doi:10.1007/s11926-012-0272-4
7. Kinne RW, Stuhlmüller B, Burmester G-R. Cells of the synovium in rheumatoid arthritis. Macrophages. *Arthritis Res Ther* (2007) **9**:224–. doi:10.1186/ar2333
8. Chu CQ, Field M, Allard S, Abney E, Feldmann M, Maini RN. Detection of cytokines at the cartilage/pannus junction in patients with rheumatoid arthritis: implications for the role of cytokines in cartilage destruction and repair. *Br J Rheumatol* (1992) **31**:653–61. doi:10.1093/rheumatology/31.10.653
9. Firestein G, Alvaro-Gracia J, Maki R. Quantitative analysis of cytokine gene expression in rheumatoid arthritis. *J Immunol* (1990) **144**:3347–53.
10. Iguchi T, Kurosaka M, Ziff M. Electron microscopic study of HLA-DR and monocyte/macrophage staining cells in the rheumatoid synovial membrane. *Arthritis Rheum* (1986) **29**:600–13. doi:10.1002/art.1780290504
11. Ridley MG, Kingsley G, Pitzalis C, Panayi GS. Monocyte activation in rheumatoid arthritis: evidence for in situ activation and differentiation in joints. *Rheumatology* (1990) **29**:84–8. doi:10.1093/rheumatology/29.2.84
12. Cauli A, Yanni G, Panayi GS. Interleukin-1, interleukin-1 receptor antagonist and macrophage populations in rheumatoid arthritis synovial membrane. *Rheumatology* (1997) **36**:935–40. doi:10.1093/rheumatology/36.9.935
13. Koller M, Aringer M, Kiener H, Erlacher L, Machold K, Eberl G, et al. Expression of adhesion molecules on synovial fluid and peripheral blood monocytes in patients with inflammatory joint disease and osteoarthritis. *Ann Rheum Dis* (1999) **58**:709–12. doi:10.1136/ard.58.11.709

14. Kinne RW, Brauer R, Stuhlmuller B, Palombo-Kinne E, Burmester G-R. Macrophages in rheumatoid arthritis. *Arthritis Res* (2000) **2**:189–202. doi:10.1186/ar86
15. Katschke KJ, Rottman JB, Ruth JH, Qin S, Wu L, LaRosa G, et al. Differential expression of chemokine receptors on peripheral blood, synovial fluid, and synovial tissue monocytes/macrophages in rheumatoid arthritis. *Arthritis Rheum* (2001) **44**:1022–32. doi:10.1002/1529-0131(200105)44:5<1022:aid-anr181>3.0.co;2-n
16. van Amelsfort JMR, van Roon JAG, Noordegraaf M, Jacobs KMG, Bijlsma JWJ, Lafeber FPJG, et al. Proinflammatory mediator-induced reversal of CD4+,CD25+ regulatory T cell-mediated suppression in rheumatoid arthritis. *Arthritis Rheum* (2007) **56**:732–42. doi:10.1002/art.22414
17. Evans HG, Gullick NG, Kelly S, Pitzalis C, Lord GM, Kirkham BW, et al. *In vivo* activated monocytes from the site of inflammation in humans specifically promote Th17 responses. *Proc Natl Acad Sci U S A* (2009) **106**:6232–7. doi:10.1073/pnas.0808144106
18. Walter GJ, Evans HG, Menon B, Gullick NJ, Kirkham BW, Cope AP, et al. Interaction with activated monocytes enhances cytokine expression and suppressive activity of human CD4+CD45RO+CD25+CD127low regulatory T cells. *Arthritis Rheum* (2013) **65**:627–38. doi:10.1002/art.37832
19. Tak PP, Smeets TJM, Daha MR, Kluin PM, Meijers KAE, Brand R, et al. Analysis of the synovial cell infiltrate in early rheumatoid synovial tissue in relation to local disease activity. *Arthritis Rheum* (1997) **40**:217–25. doi:10.1002/art.1780400206
20. Mulherin D, Fitzgerald O, Bresnihan B. Synovial tissue macrophage populations and articular damage in rheumatoid arthritis. *Arthritis Rheum* (1996) **39**:115–24. doi:10.1002/art.1780390116
21. Bresnihan B, Gerlag DM, Rooney T, Smeets TJM, Wijbrandts CA, Boyle D, et al. Synovial macrophages as a biomarker of response to therapeutic intervention in rheumatoid arthritis: standardization and consistency across centers. *J Rheumatol* (2007) **34**:620–2.
22. Yanni G, Nabil M, Farahat MR, Poston RN, Panayi GS. Intramuscular gold decreases cytokine expression and macrophage numbers in the rheumatoid synovial membrane. *Ann Rheum Dis* (1994) **53**:315–22. doi:10.1136/ard.53.5.315
23. Haringman JJ, Gerlag DM, Zwinderman AH, Smeets TJM, Kraan MC, Baeten D, et al. Synovial tissue macrophages: a sensitive biomarker for response to treatment in patients with rheumatoid arthritis. *Ann Rheum Dis* (2005) **64**:834–8. doi:10.1136/ard.2004.029751
24. Shinohara S, Hirohata S, Inoue T, Ito K. Phenotypic analysis of peripheral blood monocytes isolated from patients with rheumatoid arthritis. *J Rheumatol* (1992) **19**:211–5.
25. Lioté F, Boval-Boizard B, Weill D, Kuntz D, Wautier JL. Blood monocyte activation in rheumatoid arthritis: increased monocyte adhesiveness, integrin expression, and cytokine release. *Clin Exp Immunol* (1996) **106**:13–9. doi:10.1046/j.1365-2249.1996.d01-820.x
26. Torsteinsdottir I, Arvidson N-G, Hällgren R, Håkansson L. Monocyte activation in rheumatoid arthritis (RA): increased integrin, Fcγ and complement receptor expression and the effect of glucocorticoids. *Clin Exp Immunol* (1999) **115**(3):554–60. doi:10.1046/j.1365-2249.1999.00817.x
27. Rossol M, Kraus S, Pierer M, Baerwald C, Wagner U. The CD14brightCD16+ monocyte subset is expanded in rheumatoid arthritis and promotes expansion of the Th17 cell population. *Arthritis Rheum* (2012) **64**:671–7. doi:10.1002/art.33418
28. Meusch U, Rossol M, Baerwald C, Hauschildt S, Wagner U. Outside-to-inside signaling through transmembrane tumor necrosis factor reverses pathologic interleukin-1β production and deficient apoptosis of rheumatoid arthritis monocytes. *Arthritis Rheum* (2009) **60**:2612–21. doi:10.1002/art.24778
29. Ziegler-Heitbrock L, Ancuta P, Crowe S, Dalod M, Grau V, Hart DN, et al. Nomenclature of monocytes and dendritic cells in blood. *Blood* (2010) **116**:e74–80. doi:10.1182/blood-2010-02-258558
30. Cros J, Cagnard N, Woollard K, Patey N, Zhang S-Y, Senechal B, et al. Human CD14dim monocytes patrol and sense nucleic acids and viruses via TLR7 and TLR8 receptors. *Immunity* (2010) **33**:375–86. doi:10.1016/j.immuni.2010.08.012
31. Wijngaarden S, van Roon JAG, Bijlsma JWJ, van de Winkel JGJ, Lafeber FPJG. Fc{gamma} receptor expression levels on monocytes are elevated in rheumatoid arthritis patients with high erythrocyte sedimentation rate who do not use anti-rheumatic drugs. *Rheumatology* (2003) **42**:681–8. doi:10.1093/rheumatology/keg174
32. Iwahashi M, Yamamura M, Aita T, Okamoto A, Ueno A, Ogawa N, et al. Expression of toll-like receptor 2 on CD16+ blood monocytes and synovial tissue macrophages in rheumatoid arthritis. *Arthritis Rheum* (2004) **50**:1457–67. doi:10.1002/art.20219
33. Kawanaka N, Yamamura M, Aita T, Morita Y, Okamoto A, Kawashima M, et al. CD14+,CD16+ blood monocytes and joint inflammation in rheumatoid arthritis. *Arthritis Rheum* (2002) **46**:2578–86. doi:10.1002/art.10545
34. Cooper DL, Martin SG, Robinson JI, Mackie SL, Charles CJ, Nam J, et al. FcgRIIIa expression on monocytes in rheumatoid arthritis: role in immune-complex stimulated TNF production and non-response to methotrexate therapy. *PLoS One* (2012) **7**:e28918. doi:10.1371/journal.pone.0028918
35. Yoon BR, Yoo S-J, Choi Yh, Chung Y-H, Kim J, Yoo IS, et al. Functional phenotype of synovial monocytes modulating inflammatory T-cell responses in rheumatoid arthritis (RA). *PLoS One* (2014) **9**:e109775. doi:10.1371/journal.pone.0109775
36. Coulthard LR, Geiler J, Mathews RJ, Church LD, Dickie LJ, Cooper DL, et al. Differential effects of infliximab on absolute circulating blood leucocyte counts of innate immune cells in early and late rheumatoid arthritis patients. *Clin Exp Immunol* (2012) **170**:36–46. doi:10.1111/j.1365-2249.2012.04626.x
37. Abrahams VM, Cambridge G, Lydyard PM, Edwards JCW. Induction of tumor necrosis factor α production by adhered human monocytes: a key role for Fcγ receptor type IIIA in rheumatoid arthritis. *Arthritis Rheum* (2000) **43**:608–16. doi:10.1002/1529-0131(200003)43:3<608:aid-anr18>3.0.co;2-g
38. Krasselt M, Baerwald C, Wagner U, Rossol M. CD56+ monocytes have a dysregulated cytokine response to lipopolysaccharide and accumulate in rheumatoid arthritis and immunosenescence. *Arthritis Res Ther* (2013) **15**:R139. doi:10.1186/ar4321
39. Jagger AL, Evans HG, Walter GJ, Gullick NJ, Menon B, Ballantine LE, et al. FAS/FAS-L dependent killing of activated human monocytes and macrophages by CD4+CD25- responder T cells, but not CD4+CD25+ regulatory T cells. *J Autoimmun* (2012) **38**:29–38. doi:10.1016/j.jaut.2011.11.015
40. Perlman H, Pagliari LJ, Liu H, Koch AE, Haines GK, Pope RM. Rheumatoid arthritis synovial macrophages express the Fas-associated death domain-like interleukin-1β-converting enzyme-inhibitory protein and are refractory to Fas-mediated apoptosis. *Arthritis Rheum* (2001) **44**:21–30. doi:10.1002/1529-0131(200101)44:1<21:aid-anr4>3.0.co;2-8
41. Fonseca JE, Edwards JCW, Blades S, Goulding NJ. Macrophage subpopulations in rheumatoid synovium: reduced CD163 expression in CD4+ T lymphocyte-rich microenvironments. *Arthritis Rheum* (2002) **46**:1210–6. doi:10.1002/art.10207
42. Alonso MN, Wong MT, Zhang AL, Winer D, Suhoski MM, Tolentino LL, et al. TH1, TH2, and TH17 cells instruct monocytes to differentiate into specialized dendritic cell subsets. *Blood* (2011) **118**:3311–20. doi:10.1182/blood-2011-03-341065
43. Hillyer P, Larche MJ, Bowman EP, McClanahan TK, de Waal Malefyt R, Schewitz LP, et al. Investigating the role of the interleukin-23/-17A axis in rheumatoid arthritis. *Rheumatology* (2009) **48**:1581–9. doi:10.1093/rheumatology/kep293
44. Stamp LK, Easson A, Pettersson L, Highton J, Hessian PA. Monocyte derived interleukin (IL)-23 is an important determinant of synovial IL-17A expression in rheumatoid arthritis. *J Rheumatol* (2009) **36**:2403–8. doi:10.3899/jrheum.081304
45. Pene J, Chevalier S, Preisser L, Venereau E, Guilleux M-H, Ghannam S, et al. Chronically inflamed human tissues are infiltrated by highly differentiated Th17 lymphocytes. *J Immunol* (2008) **180**:7423–30. doi:10.4049/jimmunol.180.11.7423
46. Gullick NJ, Evans HG, Church LD, Jayaraj DM, Filer A, Kirkham BW, et al. Linking power Doppler ultrasound to the presence of Th17 cells in the rheumatoid arthritis joint. *PLoS One* (2010) **5**:e12516. doi:10.1371/journal.pone.0012516
47. Leipe J, Grunke M, Dechant C, Reindl C, Kerzendorf U, Schulze-Koops H, et al. Role of Th17 cells in human autoimmune arthritis. *Arthritis Rheum* (2010) **62**:2876–85. doi:10.1002/art.27622
48. Kirkham BW, Lassere MN, Edmonds JP, Juhasz KM, Bird PA, Lee CS, et al. Synovial membrane cytokine expression is predictive of joint

damage progression in rheumatoid arthritis: a two-year prospective study (the DAMAGE study cohort). *Arthritis Rheum* (2006) **54**:1122–31. doi:10.1002/art.21749

49. Page CE, Smale S, Carty SM, Amos N, Lauder SN, Goodfellow RM, et al. Interferon-gamma inhibits interleukin-1beta-induced matrix metalloproteinase production by synovial fibroblasts and protects articular cartilage in early arthritis. *Arthritis Res Ther* (2010) **12**:R49. doi:10.1186/ar2960
50. Manoury-Schwartz B, Chiocchia G, Bessis N, Abehsira-Amar O, Batteux F, Muller S, et al. High susceptibility to collagen-induced arthritis in mice lacking IFN-gamma receptors. *J Immunol* (1997) **158**(11):5501–6.
51. Harrington LE, Hatton RD, Mangan PR, Turner H, Murphy TL, Murphy KM, et al. Interleukin 17-producing CD4+ effector T cells develop via a lineage distinct from the T helper type 1 and 2 lineages. *Nat Immunol* (2005) **6**:1123–32. doi:10.1038/ni1254
52. Kommineni VK, Nagineni CN, William A, Detrick B, Hooks JJ. IFN-γ acts as anti-angiogenic cytokine in the human cornea by regulating the expression of VEGF-A and sVEGF-R1. *Biochem Biophys Res Commun* (2008) **374**(3):479–84. doi:10.1016/j.bbrc.2008.07.042
53. Miossec P, Korn T, Kuchroo VK. Interleukin-17 and type 17 helper T cells. *N Engl J Med* (2009) **361**:888–98. doi:10.1056/NEJMra0707449
54. Lubberts E, Koenders M, van den Berg W. The role of T-cell interleukin-17 in conducting destructive arthritis: lessons from animal models. *Arthritis Res Ther* (2005) **7**:29–37. doi:10.1186/ar1478
55. Zrioual S, Toh M-L, Tournadre A, Zhou Y, Cazalis M-A, Pachot A, et al. IL-17RA and IL-17RC receptors are essential for IL-17A-induced ELR+ CXC chemokine expression in synoviocytes and are overexpressed in rheumatoid blood. *J Immunol* (2008) **180**:655–63. doi:10.4049/jimmunol.180.1.655
56. Chabaud M, Lubberts E, Joosten L, van den Berg WB, Miossec P. IL-17 derived from juxta-articular bone and synovium contributes to joint degradation in rheumatoid arthritis. *Arthritis Res* (2001) **3**:168–77. doi:10.1186/ar294
57. Miossec P. Interleukin-17 in rheumatoid arthritis: if T cells were to contribute to inflammation and destruction through synergy. *Arthritis Rheum* (2003) **48**:594–601. doi:10.1002/art.10816
58. Miossec P. Interleukin-17 in fashion, at last: ten years after its description, its cellular source has been identified. *Arthritis Rheum* (2007) **56**:2111–5. doi:10.1002/art.22733
59. Acosta-Rodriguez EV, Napolitani G, Lanzavecchia A, Sallusto F. Interleukins 1[beta] and 6 but not transforming growth factor-[beta] are essential for the differentiation of interleukin 17-producing human T helper cells. *Nat Immunol* (2007) **8**:942–9. doi:10.1038/ni1496
60. Evans HG, Suddason T, Jackson I, Taams LS, Lord GM. Optimal induction of T helper 17 cells in humans requires T cell receptor ligation in the context of toll-like receptor-activated monocytes. *Proc Natl Acad Sci U S A* (2007) **104**:17034–9. doi:10.1073/pnas.0708426104
61. Olliver M, Hiew J, Mellroth P, Henriques-Normark B, Bergman P. Human monocytes promote Th1 and Th17 responses to *Streptococcus pneumoniae*. *Infect Immun* (2011) **79**:4210–7. doi:10.1128/iai.05286-11
62. Bradshaw EM, Raddassi K, Elyaman W, Orban T, Gottlieb PA, Kent SC, et al. Monocytes from patients with type 1 diabetes spontaneously secrete proinflammatory cytokines inducing Th17 cells. *J Immunol* (2009) **183**:4432–9. doi:10.4049/jimmunol.0900576
63. Zheng Y, Sun L, Jiang T, Zhang D, He D, Nie H. TNFalpha promotes Th17 cell differentiation through IL-6 and IL-1beta produced by monocytes in rheumatoid arthritis. *J Immunol Res* (2014) **2014**:385352. doi:10.1155/2014/385352
64. Egan PJ, van Nieuwenhuijze A, Campbell IA, Wicks IP. Promotion of the local differentiation of murine Th17 cells by synovial macrophages during acute inflammatory arthritis. *Arthritis Rheum* (2008) **58**:3720–9. doi:10.1002/art.24075
65. Traunecker E, Gardner R, Fonseca JE, Polido-Pereira J, Seitz M, Villiger PM, et al. Blocking of LFA-1 enhances expansion of Th17 cells induced by human CD14+CD16++ nonclassical monocytes. *Eur J Immunol* (2015) **45**:1414–25. doi:10.1002/eji.201445100
66. Smeekens SP, van de Veerdonk FL, Joosten LAB, Jacobs L, Jansen T, Williams DL, et al. The classical CD14++CD16- monocytes, but not the patrolling CD14+CD16+ monocytes, promote Th17 responses to *Candida albicans*. *Eur J Immunol* (2011) **41**:2915–24. doi:10.1002/eji.201141418
67. Liu B, Dhanda A, Hirani S, Williams EL, Sen HN, Martinez Estrada F, et al. CD14++CD16+ monocytes are enriched by glucocorticoid treatment and are functionally attenuated in driving effector T cell responses. *J Immunol* (2015) **194**:5150–60. doi:10.4049/jimmunol.1402409
68. Doherty TM, Seder RA, Sher A. Induction and regulation of IL-15 expression in murine macrophages. *J Immunol* (1996) **156**:735–41.
69. Rückert R, Brandt K, Ernst M, Marienfeld K, Csernok E, Metzler C, et al. Interleukin-15 stimulates macrophages to activate CD4+ T cells: a role in the pathogenesis of rheumatoid arthritis? *Immunology* (2009) **126**:63–73. doi:10.1111/j.1365-2567.2008.02878.x
70. McInnes IB, al-Mughales J, Field M, Leung BP, Huang FP, Dixon R, et al. The role of interleukin-15 in T-cell migration and activation in rheumatoid arthritis. *Nat Med* (1996) **2**:175–82. doi:10.1038/nm0296-175
71. Oppenheimer-Marks N, Brezinschek RI, Mohamadzadeh M, Vita R, Lipsky PE. Interleukin 15 is produced by endothelial cells and increases the transendothelial migration of T cells In vitro and in the SCID mouse-human rheumatoid arthritis model In vivo. *J Clin Invest* (1998) **101**:1261–72. doi:10.1172/JCI1986
72. McInnes IB, Leung BP, Sturrock RD, Field M, Liew FY. Interleukin-15 mediates T cell-dependent regulation of tumor necrosis factor-α production in rheumatoid arthritis. *Nat Med* (1997) **3**:189–95. doi:10.1038/nm0297-189
73. Halvorsen EH, Strønen E, Hammer HB, Goll GL, Sollid LM, Molberg Ø. Interleukin-15 induces interleukin-17 production by synovial T cell lines from patients with rheumatoid arthritis. *Scand J Immunol* (2011) **73**:243–9. doi:10.1111/j.1365-3083.2010.02498.x
74. Pandiyan P, Yang X-P, Saravanamuthu SS, Zheng L, Ishihara S, O'Shea JJ, et al. The role of IL-15 in activating STAT5 and fine-tuning IL-17A production in CD4 T lymphocytes. *J Immunol* (2012) **189**:4237–46. doi:10.4049/jimmunol.1201476
75. Gracie JA, Forsey RJ, Chan WL, Gilmour A, Leung BP, Greer MR, et al. A proinflammatory role for IL-18 in rheumatoid arthritis. *J Clin Invest* (1999) **104**:1393–401. doi:10.1172/JCI7317
76. Komai-Koma M, Gracie JA, Wei X-Q, Xu D, Thomson N, McInnes IB, et al. Chemoattraction of human T cells by IL-18. *J Immunol* (2003) **170**:1084–90. doi:10.4049/jimmunol.170.2.1084
77. Ruth JH, Park CC, Amin MA, Lesch C, Marotte H, Shahrara S, et al. Interleukin-18 as an in vivo mediator of monocyte recruitment in rodent models of rheumatoid arthritis. *Arthritis Res Ther* (2010) **12**:R118. doi:10.1186/ar3055
78. Hultqvist M, Olofsson P, Holmberg J, Backstrom BT, Tordsson J, Holmdahl R. Enhanced autoimmunity, arthritis, and encephalomyelitis in mice with a reduced oxidative burst due to a mutation in the Ncf1 gene. *Proc Natl Acad Sci U S A* (2004) **101**:12646–51. doi:10.1073/pnas.0403831101
79. Olofsson P, Holmberg J, Tordsson J, Lu S, Akerstrom B, Holmdahl R. Positional identification of Ncf1 as a gene that regulates arthritis severity in rats. *Nat Genet* (2003) **33**:25–32. doi:10.1038/ng1058
80. Gelderman KA, Hultqvist M, Pizzolla A, Zhao M, Nandakumar KS, Mattsson R, et al. Macrophages suppress T cell responses and arthritis development in mice by producing reactive oxygen species. *J Clin Invest* (2007) **117**:3020–8. doi:10.1172/JCI31935
81. King MR, Ismail AS, Davis LS, Karp DR. Oxidative stress promotes polarization of human T cell differentiation toward a T helper 2 phenotype. *J Immunol* (2006) **176**:2765–72. doi:10.4049/jimmunol.176.5.2765
82. Mills CD, Kincaid K, Alt JM, Heilman MJ, Hill AM. M-1/M-2 macrophages and the Th1/Th2 paradigm. *J Immunol* (2000) **164**:6166–73. doi:10.4049/jimmunol.164.12.6166
83. Li J, Hsu H-C, Yang P, Wu Q, Li H, Edgington LE, et al. Treatment of arthritis by macrophage depletion and immunomodulation: testing an apoptosis-mediated therapy in a humanized death receptor mouse model. *Arthritis Rheum* (2012) **64**:1098–109. doi:10.1002/art.33423
84. Merad M, Sathe P, Helft J, Miller J, Mortha A. The dendritic cell lineage: ontogeny and function of dendritic cells and their subsets in the steady state and the inflamed setting. *Annu Rev Immunol* (2013) **31**:563–604. doi:10.1146/annurev-immunol-020711-074950
85. Guilliams M, Ginhoux F, Jakubzick C, Naik SH, Onai N, Schraml BU, et al. Dendritic cells, monocytes and macrophages: a unified nomenclature based on ontogeny. *Nat Rev Immunol* (2014) **14**:571–8. doi:10.1038/nri3712
86. Langlet C, Tamoutounour S, Henri S, Luche H, Ardouin L, Grégoire C, et al. CD64 expression distinguishes monocyte-derived and conventional

dendritic cells and reveals their distinct role during intramuscular immunization. *J Immunol* (2012) **188**:1751–60. doi:10.4049/jimmunol.1102744

87. Schreiber HA, Loschko J, Karssemeijer RA, Escolano A, Meredith MM, Mucida D, et al. Intestinal monocytes and macrophages are required for T cell polarization in response to *Citrobacter rodentium*. *J Exp Med* (2013) **210**:2025–39. doi:10.1084/jem.20130903
88. Borthwick LA, Barron L, Hart KM, Vannella KM, Thompson RW, Oland S, et al. Macrophages are critical to the maintenance of IL-13-dependent lung inflammation and fibrosis. *Mucosal Immunol* (2015). doi:10.1038/mi.2015.34
89. Iijima N, Iwasaki A. A local macrophage chemokine network sustains protective tissue-resident memory CD4 T cells. *Science* (2014) **346**:93–8. doi:10.1126/science.1257530
90. Van Der Voort R, Van Lieshout AWT, Toonen LWJ, Slöetjes AW, Van Den Berg WB, Figdor CG, et al. Elevated CXCL16 expression by synovial macrophages recruits memory T cells into rheumatoid joints. *Arthritis Rheum* (2005) **52**:1381–91. doi:10.1002/art.21004
91. Kim CH, Rott L, Kunkel EJ, Genovese MC, Andrew DP, Wu L, et al. Rules of chemokine receptor association with T cell polarization in vivo. *J Clin Invest* (2001) **108**:1331–9. doi:10.1172/JCI13543
92. Ruth JH, Haas CS, Park CC, Amin MA, Martinez RJ, Haines GK, et al. CXCL16-mediated cell recruitment to rheumatoid arthritis synovial tissue and murine lymph nodes is dependent upon the MAPK pathway. *Arthritis Rheum* (2006) **54**:765–78. doi:10.1002/art.21662
93. van Lieshout AWT, van der Voort R, Toonen LWJ, van Helden SFG, Figdor CG, van Riel PLCM, et al. Regulation of CXCL16 expression and secretion by myeloid cells is not altered in rheumatoid arthritis. *Ann Rheum Dis* (2009) **68**:1036–43. doi:10.1136/ard.2007.086611
94. van Kerckhove C, Melin-Aldana H, Elam MS, Luyrink L, Donnelly P, Taylor J, et al. A distinct HLA-DRw8 haplotype characterizes patients with juvenile rheumatoid arthritis. *Immunogenetics* (1990) **32**:304–8. doi:10.1007/BF00211643
95. Smeets TJ, Kraan MC, van Loon ME, Tak PP. Tumor necrosis factor alpha blockade reduces the synovial cell infiltrate early after initiation of treatment, but apparently not by induction of apoptosis in synovial tissue. *Arthritis Rheum* (2003) **48**:2155–62. doi:10.1002/art.11098
96. Taylor PC, Peters AM, Paleolog E, Chapman PT, Elliott MJ, McCloskey R, et al. Reduction of chemokine levels and leukocyte traffic to joints by tumor necrosis factor alpha blockade in patients with rheumatoid arthritis. *Arthritis Rheum* (2000) **43**:38–47. doi:10.1002/1529-0131(200001)43:1<38:AID-ANR6>3.0.CO;2-L
97. van Lieshout AW, Fransen J, Flendrie M, Eijsbouts AM, van den Hoogen FH, van Riel PL, et al. Circulating levels of the chemokine CCL18 but not CXCL16 are elevated and correlate with disease activity in rheumatoid arthritis. *Ann Rheum Dis* (2007) **66**:1334–8. doi:10.1136/ard.2006.066084
98. Kageyama Y, Torikai E, Nagano A. Anti-tumor necrosis factor-alpha antibody treatment reduces serum CXCL16 levels in patients with rheumatoid arthritis. *Rheumatol Int* (2007) **27**:467–72. doi:10.1007/s00296-006-0241-1
99. Lee AY, Körner H. CCR6 and CCL20: emerging players in the pathogenesis of rheumatoid arthritis. *Immunol Cell Biol* (2014) **92**:354–8. doi:10.1038/icb.2013.97
100. Annunziato F, Cosmi L, Santarlasci V, Maggi L, Liotta F, Mazzinghi B, et al. Phenotypic and functional features of human Th17 cells. *J Exp Med* (2007) **204**:1849–61. doi:10.1084/jem.20070663
101. Liao F, Rabin RL, Smith CS, Sharma G, Nutman TB, Farber JM. CC-chemokine receptor 6 is expressed on diverse memory subsets of T cells and determines responsiveness to macrophage inflammatory protein 3α. *J Immunol* (1999) **162**:186–94.
102. Acosta-Rodriguez EV, Rivino L, Geginat J, Jarrossay D, Gattorno M, Lanzavecchia A, et al. Surface phenotype and antigenic specificity of human interleukin 17-producing T helper memory cells. *Nat Immunol* (2007) **8**:639–46. doi:10.1038/ni1467
103. Hirota K, Yoshitomi H, Hashimoto M, Maeda S, Teradaira S, Sugimoto N, et al. Preferential recruitment of CCR6-expressing Th17 cells to inflamed joints via CCL20 in rheumatoid arthritis and its animal model. *J Exp Med* (2007) **204**:2803–12. doi:10.1084/jem.20071397
104. Tanida S, Yoshitomi H, Nishitani K, Ishikawa M, Kitaori T, Ito H, et al. CCL20 produced in the cytokine network of rheumatoid arthritis recruits CCR6+ mononuclear cells and enhances the production of IL-6. *Cytokine* (2009) **47**:112–8. doi:10.1016/j.cyto.2009.05.009
105. Bosco MC, Delfino S, Ferlito F, Battaglia F, Puppo M, Gregorio A, et al. Hypoxic synovial environment and expression of macrophage inflammatory protein 3γ/CCL20 in juvenile idiopathic arthritis. *Arthritis Rheum* (2008) **58**:1833–8. doi:10.1002/art.23516
106. Li Q, Laumonnier Y, Syrovets T, Simmet T. Recruitment of CCR6-expressing Th17 cells by CCL20 secreted from plasmin-stimulated macrophages. *Acta Biochim Biophys Sin* (2013) **45**:593–600. doi:10.1093/abbs/gmt049
107. Li J, Ny A, Leonardsson G, Nandakumar KS, Holmdahl R, Ny T. The plasminogen activator/plasmin system is essential for development of the joint inflammatory phase of collagen type II-induced arthritis. *Am J Pathol* (2005) **166**:783–92. doi:10.1016/S0002-9440(10)62299-7
108. Afzali B, Mitchell P, Lechler RI, John S, Lombardi G. Translational mini-review series on Th17 cells: induction of interleukin-17 production by regulatory T cells. *Clin Exp Immunol* (2010) **159**:120–30. doi:10.1111/j.1365-2249.2009.04038.x
109. Fujimoto M, Nakano M, Terabe F, Kawahata H, Ohkawara T, Han Y, et al. The influence of excessive IL-6 production in vivo on the development and function of Foxp3+ regulatory T cells. *J Immunol* (2011) **186**:32–40. doi:10.4049/jimmunol.0903314
110. van Loosdregt J, Fleskens V, Fu J, Brenkman AB, Bekker CP, Pals CE, et al. Stabilization of the transcription factor Foxp3 by the deubiquitinase USP7 increases Treg-cell-suppressive capacity. *Immunity* (2013) **39**:259–71. doi:10.1016/j.immuni.2013.05.018
111. Valencia X, Stephens G, Goldbach-Mansky R, Wilson M, Shevach EM, Lipsky PE. TNF down-modulates the function of human CD4+CD25hi T regulatory cells. *Blood* (2006) **108**:253–61. doi:10.1182/blood-2005-11-4567
112. Nie H, Zheng Y, Li R, Guo TB, He D, Fang L, et al. Phosphorylation of FOXP3 controls regulatory T cell function and is inhibited by TNF-[alpha] in rheumatoid arthritis. *Nat Med* (2013) **19**:322–8. doi:10.1038/nm.3085
113. Nadkarni S, Mauri C, Ehrenstein MR. Anti-TNF-alpha therapy induces a distinct regulatory T cell population in patients with rheumatoid arthritis via TGF-beta. *J Exp Med* (2007) **204**:33–9. doi:10.1084/jem.20061531
114. Grinberg-Bleyer Y, Saadoun D, Baeyens A, Billiard F, Goldstein JD, Gregoire S, et al. Pathogenic T cells have a paradoxical protective effect in murine autoimmune diabetes by boosting Tregs. *J Clin Invest* (2011) **120**:4558–68. doi:10.1172/JCI42945
115. Chen X, Baumel M, Mannel DN, Howard OM, Oppenheim JJ. Interaction of TNF with TNF receptor type 2 promotes expansion and function of mouse CD4+CD25+ T regulatory cells. *J Immunol* (2007) **179**:154–61. doi:10.4049/jimmunol.179.1.154
116. Wehrens EJ, Mijnheer G, Duurland CL, Klein M, Meerding J, van Loosdregt J, et al. Functional human regulatory T cells fail to control autoimmune inflammation due to PKB/c-akt hyperactivation in effector cells. *Blood* (2011) **118**:3538–48. doi:10.1182/blood-2010-12-328187
117. Herrath J, Müller M, Amoudruz P, Janson P, Michaëlsson J, Larsson PT, et al. The inflammatory milieu in the rheumatic joint reduces regulatory T cell function. *Eur J Immunol* (2011) **41**:2279–90. doi:10.1002/eji.201041004
118. Wehrens EJ, Prakken BJ, van Wijk F. T cells out of control-impaired immune regulation in the inflamed joint. *Nat Rev Rheumatol* (2012) **9**:34–42. doi:10.1038/nrrheum.2012.149
119. Denning TL, Wang Y-C, Patel SR, Williams IR, Pulendran B. Lamina propria macrophages and dendritic cells differentially induce regulatory and interleukin 17-producing T cell responses. *Nat Immunol* (2007) **8**(10):1086–94. doi:10.1038/ni1511
120. Kraaij MD, Savage ND, van der Kooij SW, Koekkoek K, Wang J, van den Berg JM, et al. Induction of regulatory T cells by macrophages is dependent on production of reactive oxygen species. *Proc Natl Acad Sci U S A* (2010) **107**:17686–91. doi:10.1073/pnas.1012016107
121. Kim H-R, Lee A, Choi E-J, Hong M-P, Kie J-H, Lim W, et al. Reactive oxygen species prevent imiquimod-induced psoriatic dermatitis through enhancing regulatory T cell function. *PLoS One* (2014) **9**:e91146. doi:10.1371/journal.pone.0091146
122. Efimova O, Szankasi P, Kelley TW. Ncf1 (p47phox) is essential for direct regulatory T cell mediated suppression of CD4+ effector T cells. *PLoS One* (2011) **6**:e16013. doi:10.1371/journal.pone.0016013
123. Thornton AM, Korty PE, Tran DQ, Wohlfert EA, Murray PE, Belkaid Y, et al. Expression of Helios, an Ikaros transcription factor family member, differentiates thymic-derived from peripherally induced Foxp3+ T regulatory cells. *J Immunol* (2010) **184**:3433–41. doi:10.4049/jimmunol.0904028

124. Zhong H, Yazdanbakhsh K. Differential control of Helios(±) Treg development by monocyte subsets through disparate inflammatory cytokines. *Blood* (2013) **121**:2494–502. doi:10.1182/blood-2012-11-469122
125. Mantovani A, Sica A, Sozzani S, Allavena P, Vecchi A, Locati M. The chemokine system in diverse forms of macrophage activation and polarization. *Trends Immunol* (2004) **25**:677–86. doi:10.1016/j.it.2004.09.015
126. Xue J, Schmidt Susanne V, Sander J, Draffehn A, Krebs W, Quester I, et al. Transcriptome-based network analysis reveals a spectrum model of human macrophage activation. *Immunity* (2014) **40**:274–88. doi:10.1016/j.immuni.2014.01.006
127. Murray PJ, Allen JE, Biswas SK, Fisher EA, Gilroy DW, Goerdt S, et al. Macrophage activation and polarization: nomenclature and experimental guidelines. *Immunity* (2014) **41**:14–20. doi:10.1016/j.immuni.2014.06.008
128. Gordon S, Taylor PR. Monocyte and macrophage heterogeneity. *Nat Rev Immunol* (2005) **5**:953–64. doi:10.1038/nri1733
129. Wang N, Liang H, Zen K. Molecular mechanisms that influence the macrophage M1-M2 polarization balance. *Front Immunol* (2014) **5**:614. doi:10.3389/fimmu.2014.00614
130. Koh TJ, DiPietro LA. Inflammation and wound healing: the role of the macrophage. *Expert Rev Mol Med* (2011) **13**:e23. doi:10.1017/S1462399411001943
131. Jovanovic DV, Di Battista JA, Martel-Pelletier J, Jolicoeur FC, He Y, Zhang M, et al. IL-17 stimulates the production and expression of proinflammatory cytokines, IL-β and TNF-α, by human macrophages. *J Immunol* (1998) **160**(7):3513–21.
132. Chen J, Liao MY, Gao XL, Zhong Q, Tang TT, Yu X, et al. IL-17A induces pro-inflammatory cytokines production in macrophages via MAPKinases, NF-kappaB and AP-1. *Cell Physiol Biochem* (2013) **32**:1265–74. doi:10.1159/000354525
133. Shahrara S, Pickens SR, Dorfleutner A, Pope RM. IL-17 induces monocyte migration in rheumatoid arthritis. *J Immunol* (2009) **182**:3884–91. doi:10.4049/jimmunol.0802246
134. Ruth JH, Shahrara S, Park CC, Morel JC, Kumar P, Qin S, et al. Role of macrophage inflammatory protein-3alpha and its ligand CCR6 in rheumatoid arthritis. *Lab Invest* (2003) **83**:579–88. doi:10.1097/01.LAB.0000062854.30195.52
135. Shahrara S, Pickens SR, Mandelin AM II, Karpus WJ, Huang Q, Kolls JK, et al. IL-17-mediated monocyte migration occurs partially through CC chemokine ligand 2/monocyte chemoattractant protein-1 induction. *J Immunol* (2010) **184**:4479–87. doi:10.4049/jimmunol.0901942
136. Sebbag M, Parry SL, Brennan FM, Feldmann M. Cytokine stimulation of T lymphocytes regulates their capacity to induce monocyte production of tumor necrosis factor-α, but not interleukin-10: possible relevance to pathophysiology of rheumatoid arthritis. *Eur J Immunol* (1997) **27**:624–32. doi:10.1002/eji.1830270308
137. Burger D, Dayer J. The role of human T-lymphocyte-monocyte contact in inflammation and tissue destruction. *Arthritis Res* (2002) **4**(Suppl 3):S169–76. doi:10.1186/ar558
138. Scanu A, Molnarfi N, Brandt KJ, Gruaz L, Dayer J-M, Burger D. Stimulated T cells generate microparticles, which mimic cellular contact activation of human monocytes: differential regulation of pro- and anti-inflammatory cytokine production by high-density lipoproteins. *J Leukoc Biol* (2008) **83**:921–7. doi:10.1189/jlb.0807551
139. Brennan F, Smith N, Owen S, Li C, Amjadi P, Green P, et al. Resting CD4+ effector memory T cells are precursors of bystander-activated effectors: a surrogate model of rheumatoid arthritis synovial T-cell function. *Arthritis Res Ther* (2008) **10**:R36. doi:10.1186/ar2390
140. Kotake S, Nanke Y, Mogi M, Kawamoto M, Furuya T, Yago T, et al. IFN-γ-producing human T cells directly induce osteoclastogenesis from human monocytes via the expression of RANKL. *Eur J Immunol* (2005) **35**:3353–63. doi:10.1002/eji.200526141
141. Takayanagi H, Ogasawara K, Hida S, Chiba T, Murata S, Sato K, et al. T-cell-mediated regulation of osteoclastogenesis by signalling cross-talk between RANKL and IFN-[gamma]. *Nature* (2000) **408**:600–5. doi:10.1038/35046102
142. Kim KW, Kim HR, Kim BM, Cho ML, Lee SH. Th17 cytokines regulate osteoclastogenesis in rheumatoid arthritis. *Am J Pathol* (2015) **185**:3011–24. doi:10.1016/j.ajpath.2015.07.017
143. Yago T, Nanke Y, Ichikawa N, Kobashigawa T, Mogi M, Kamatani N, et al. IL-17 induces osteoclastogenesis from human monocytes alone in the absence of osteoblasts, which is potently inhibited by anti-TNF-α antibody: a novel mechanism of osteoclastogenesis by IL-17. *J Cell Biochem* (2009) **108**:947–55. doi:10.1002/jcb.22326
144. Kikuta J, Wada Y, Kowada T, Wang Z, Sun-Wada GH, Nishiyama I, et al. Dynamic visualization of RANKL and Th17-mediated osteoclast function. *J Clin Invest* (2013) **123**:866–73. doi:10.1172/JCI65054
145. Miranda-Carus ME, Benito-Miguel M, Balsa A, Cobo-Ibanez T, Perez de Ayala C, Pascual-Salcedo D, et al. Peripheral blood T lymphocytes from patients with early rheumatoid arthritis express RANKL and interleukin-15 on the cell surface and promote osteoclastogenesis in autologous monocytes. *Arthritis Rheum* (2006) **54**:1151–64. doi:10.1002/art.21731
146. Kotake S, Udagawa N, Hakoda M, Mogi M, Yano K, Tsuda E, et al. Activated human T cells directly induce osteoclastogenesis from human monocytes: possible role of T cells in bone destruction in rheumatoid arthritis patients. *Arthritis Rheum* (2001) **44**:1003–12. doi:10.1002/1529-0131(200105)44:5<1003:AID-ANR179>3.0.CO;2-#
147. Pryjma J, Zembala M, Pituch-Noworolska A, Ernst M, Van der Bosch J, Flad HD. Monocyte-T-cell interactions in pokeweed mitogen-activated cultures. *Immunology* (1990) **71**:397–403.
148. Richardson BC, Buckmaster T, Keren DF, Johnson KJ. Evidence that macrophages are programmed to die after activating autologous, cloned, antigen-specific, CD4+ T cells. *Eur J Immunol* (1993) **23**:1450–5. doi:10.1002/eji.1830230708
149. Grossman WJ, Verbsky JW, Barchet W, Colonna M, Atkinson JP, Ley TJ. Human T regulatory cells can use the perforin pathway to cause autologous target cell death. *Immunity* (2004) **21**:589–601. doi:10.1016/j.immuni.2004.09.002
150. Venet F, Pachot A, Debard A-L, Bohe J, Bienvenu J, Lepape A, et al. Human CD4+CD25+ regulatory T lymphocytes inhibit lipopolysaccharide-induced monocyte survival through a Fas/Fas ligand-dependent mechanism. *J Immunol* (2006) **177**:6540–7. doi:10.4049/jimmunol.177.9.6540
151. Kearns MT, Barthel L, Bednarek JM, Yunt ZX, Henson PM, Janssen WJ. Fas ligand-expressing lymphocytes enhance alveolar macrophage apoptosis in the resolution of acute pulmonary inflammation. *Am J Physiol Lung Cell Mol Physiol* (2014) **307**:L62–70. doi:10.1152/ajplung.00273.2013
152. Kaplan MJ, Ray D, Mo R-R, Yung RL, Richardson BC. TRAIL (Apo2 Ligand) and TWEAK (Apo3 Ligand) mediate CD4+ T cell killing of antigen-presenting macrophages. *J Immunol* (2000) **164**:2897–904. doi:10.4049/jimmunol.164.6.2897
153. Shevach EM. Mechanisms of Foxp3+ T regulatory cell-mediated suppression. *Immunity* (2009) **30**:636–45. doi:10.1016/j.immuni.2009.04.010
154. Vignali DAA, Collison LW, Workman CJ. How regulatory T cells work. *Nat Rev Immunol* (2008) **8**:523–32. doi:10.1038/nri2343
155. Sakaguchi S, Wing K, Onishi Y, Prieto-Martin P, Yamaguchi T. Regulatory T cells: how do they suppress immune responses? *Int Immunol* (2009) **21**:1105–11. doi:10.1093/intimm/dxp095
156. Andre S, Tough DF, Lacroix-Desmazes S, Kaveri SV, Bayry J. Surveillance of antigen-presenting cells by CD4+CD25+ regulatory T cells in autoimmunity: immunopathogenesis and therapeutic implications. *Am J Pathol* (2009) **174**:1575–87. doi:10.2353/ajpath.2009.080987
157. Taams LS, van Amelsfort JMR, Tiemessen MM, Jacobs KMG, de Jong EC, Akbar AN, et al. Modulation of monocyte/macrophage function by human CD4+CD25+ regulatory T cells. *Hum Immunol* (2005) **66**:222–30. doi:10.1016/j.humimm.2004.12.006
158. Tiemessen MM, Jagger AJ, Evans HG, van Herwijnen MJC, John S, Taams LS. CD4+CD25+Foxp3+ regulatory T cells induce alternative activation of human monocytes/macrophages. *Proc Natl Acad Sci U S A* (2007) **104**:19446–51. doi:10.1073/pnas.0706832104
159. Netea Mihai G, Quintin J, van der Meer Jos WM. Trained immunity: a memory for innate host defense. *Cell Host Microbe* (2011) **9**:355–61. doi:10.1016/j.chom.2011.04.006
160. Saeed S, Quintin J, Kerstens HH, Rao NA, Aghajanirefah A, Matarese F, et al. Epigenetic programming of monocyte-to-macrophage differentiation and trained innate immunity. *Science* (2014) **345**:1251086. doi:10.1126/science.1251086
161. Kryczek I, Wei S, Zou L, Zhu G, Mottram P, Xu H, et al. Cutting edge: induction of B7-H4 on APCs through IL-10: novel suppressive mode for regulatory T cells. *J Immunol* (2006) **177**:40–4. doi:10.4049/jimmunol.177.1.40

162. Kryczek I, Zou L, Rodriguez P, Zhu G, Wei S, Mottram P, et al. B7-H4 expression identifies a novel suppressive macrophage population in human ovarian carcinoma. *J Exp Med* (2006) **203**:871–81. doi:10.1084/jem.20050930
163. Curiel T, Coukos G, Zou L, Alvarez X, Cheng P, Mottram P, et al. Specific recruitment of regulatory T cells in ovarian carcinoma fosters immune privilege and predicts reduced survival. *Nat Med* (2004) **10**:942–9. doi:10.1038/nm1093
164. Kryczek I, Wei S, Zhu G, Myers L, Mottram P, Cheng P, et al. Relationship between B7-H4, regulatory T cells, and patient outcome in human ovarian carcinoma. *Cancer Res* (2007) **67**:8900–5. doi:10.1158/0008-5472.can-07-1866
165. Liu G, Ma H, Qiu L, Li L, Cao Y, Ma J, et al. Phenotypic and functional switch of macrophages induced by regulatory CD4+CD25+ T cells in mice. *Immunol Cell Biol* (2011) **89**:130–42. doi:10.1038/icb.2010.70
166. Lebre MC, Vergunst CE, Choi IY, Aarrass S, Oliveira AS, Wyant T, et al. Why CCR2 and CCR5 blockade failed and why CCR1 blockade might still be effective in the treatment of rheumatoid arthritis. *PLoS One* (2011) **6**:e21772. doi:10.1371/journal.pone.0021772
167. Thurlings RM, Wijbrandts CA, Bennink RJ, Dohmen SE, Voermans C, Wouters D, et al. Monocyte scintigraphy in rheumatoid arthritis: the dynamics of monocyte migration in immune-mediated inflammatory disease. *PLoS One* (2009) **4**:e7865. doi:10.1371/journal.pone.0007865
168. Herenius MMJ, Thurlings RM, Wijbrandts CA, Bennink RJ, Dohmen SE, Voermans C, et al. Monocyte migration to the synovium in rheumatoid arthritis patients treated with adalimumab. *Ann Rheum Dis* (2011) **70**:1160–2. doi:10.1136/ard.2010.141549
169. Liu H, Eksarko P, Temkin V, Haines GK, Perlman H, Koch AE, et al. Mcl-1 is essential for the survival of synovial fibroblasts in rheumatoid arthritis. *J Immunol* (2005) **175**:8337–45. doi:10.4049/jimmunol.175.12.8337
170. Perlman H, Pagliari LJ, Georganas C, Mano T, Walsh K, Pope RM. FLICE-inhibitory protein expression during macrophage differentiation confers resistance to Fas-mediated apoptosis. *J Exp Med* (1999) **190**:1679–88. doi:10.1084/jem.190.11.1679
171. Scatizzi JC, Hutcheson J, Pope RM, Firestein GS, Koch AE, Mavers M, et al. Bim–Bcl-2 homology 3 mimetic therapy is effective at suppressing inflammatory arthritis through the activation of myeloid cell apoptosis. *Arthritis Rheum* (2010) **62**:441–51. doi:10.1002/art.27198
172. Wakisaka S, Suzuki N, Takeba Y, Shimoyama Y, Nagafuchi H, Takeno M, et al. Modulation by proinflammatory cytokines of Fas/Fas ligand-mediated apoptotic cell death of synovial cells in patients with rheumatoid arthritis (RA). *Clin Exp Immunol* (1998) **114**:119–28. doi:10.1046/j.1365-2249.1998.00701.x
173. van Amelsfort JMR, Jacobs KMG, Bijlsma JWJ, Lafeber FPJG, Taams LS. CD4+CD25+ regulatory T cells in rheumatoid arthritis: differences in presence, phenotype and function between peripheral blood and synovial fluid. *Arthritis Rheum* (2004) **50**:2775–85. doi:10.1002/art.20499
174. Shen C, Assche GV, Colpaert S, Maerten P, Geboes K, Rutgeerts P, et al. Adalimumab induces apoptosis of human monocytes: a comparative study with infliximab and etanercept. *Aliment Pharmacol Ther* (2005) **21**:251–8. doi:10.1111/j.1365-2036.2005.02309.x
175. Brown NJ, Hutcheson J, Bickel E, Scatizzi JC, Albee LD, Haines GK III, et al. Fas death receptor signaling represses monocyte numbers and macrophage activation in vivo. *J Immunol* (2004) **173**:7584–93. doi:10.4049/jimmunol.173.12.7584
176. Cuda CM, Agrawal H, Misharin AV, Haines GK, Hutcheson J, Weber E, et al. Requirement of myeloid cell-specific Fas expression for prevention of systemic autoimmunity in mice. *Arthritis Rheum* (2012) **64**:808–20. doi:10.1002/art.34317
177. Eyre S, Bowes J, Diogo D, Lee A, Barton A, Martin P, et al. High-density genetic mapping identifies new susceptibility loci for rheumatoid arthritis. *Nat Genet* (2012) **44**:1336–40. doi:10.1038/ng.2462
178. Krausgruber T, Blazek K, Smallie T, Alzabin S, Lockstone H, Sahgal N, et al. IRF5 promotes inflammatory macrophage polarization and TH1-TH17 responses. *Nat Immunol* (2011) **12**:231–8. doi:10.1038/ni.1990
179. Zhao B, Grimes SN, Li S, Hu X, Ivashkiv LB. TNF-induced osteoclastogenesis and inflammatory bone resorption are inhibited by transcription factor RBP-J. *J Exp Med* (2012) **209**:319–34. doi:10.1084/jem.20111566
180. Gomez Perdiguero E, Klapproth K, Schulz C, Busch K, Azzoni E, Crozet L, et al. Tissue-resident macrophages originate from yolk-sac-derived erythro-myeloid progenitors. *Nature* (2015) **518**:547–51. doi:10.1038/nature13989
181. Schulz C, Perdiguero EG, Chorro L, Szabo-Rogers H, Cagnard N, Kierdorf K, et al. A lineage of myeloid cells independent of Myb and hematopoietic stem cells. *Science* (2012) **336**:86–90. doi:10.1126/science.1219179
182. Hoeffel G, Wang Y, Greter M, See P, Teo P, Malleret B, et al. Adult Langerhans cells derive predominantly from embryonic fetal liver monocytes with a minor contribution of yolk sac-derived macrophages. *J Exp Med* (2012) **209**:1167–81. doi:10.1084/jem.20120340
183. Guilliams M, De Kleer I, Henri S, Post S, Vanhoutte L, De Prijck S, et al. Alveolar macrophages develop from fetal monocytes that differentiate into long-lived cells in the first week of life via GM-CSF. *J Exp Med* (2013) **210**:1977–92. doi:10.1084/jem.20131199
184. Yona S, Kim K-W, Wolf Y, Mildner A, Varol D, Breker M, et al. Fate mapping reveals origins and dynamics of monocytes and tissue macrophages under homeostasis. *Immunity* (2013) **38**:79–91. doi:10.1016/j.immuni.2012.12.001
185. Hashimoto D, Chow A, Noizat C, Teo P, Beasley Mary B, Leboeuf M, et al. Tissue-resident macrophages self-maintain locally throughout adult life with minimal contribution from circulating monocytes. *Immunity* (2013) **38**(4):792–804. doi:10.1016/j.immuni.2013.04.004
186. Bain CC, Bravo-Blas A, Scott CL, Gomez Perdiguero E, Geissmann F, Henri S, et al. Constant replenishment from circulating monocytes maintains the macrophage pool in the intestine of adult mice. *Nat Immunol* (2014) **15**:929–37. doi:10.1038/ni.2967
187. Molawi K, Wolf Y, Kandalla PK, Favret J, Hagemeyer N, Frenzel K, et al. Progressive replacement of embryo-derived cardiac macrophages with age. *J Exp Med* (2014) **211**:2151–8. doi:10.1084/jem.20140639
188. Epelman S, Lavine Kory J, Beaudin Anna E, Sojka Dorothy K, Carrero Javier A, Calderon B, et al. Embryonic and adult-derived resident cardiac macrophages are maintained through distinct mechanisms at steady state and during inflammation. *Immunity* (2014) **40**:91–104. doi:10.1016/j.immuni.2013.11.019
189. Hahn G, Stuhlmuller B, Hain N, Kalden JR, Pfizenmaier K, Burmester GR. Modulation of monocyte activation in patients with rheumatoid arthritis by leukapheresis therapy. *J Clin Invest* (1993) **91**:862–70. doi:10.1172/jci116307
190. Brühl H, Cihak J, Plachý J, Kunz-Schughart L, Niedermeier M, Denzel A, et al. Targeting of Gr-1+,CCR2+ monocytes in collagen-induced arthritis. *Arthritis Rheum* (2007) **56**:2975–85. doi:10.1002/art.22854
191. Van Roon JAG, Van Vuuren AJ, Wijngaarden S, Jacobs KMG, Bijlsma JWJ, Lafeber FPJG, et al. Selective elimination of synovial inflammatory macrophages in rheumatoid arthritis by an Fcγ receptor I-directed immunotoxin. *Arthritis Rheum* (2003) **48**:1229–38. doi:10.1002/art.10940
192. Apparailly F, Jorgensen C. siRNA-based therapeutic approaches for rheumatic diseases. *Nat Rev Rheumatol* (2013) **9**:56–62. doi:10.1038/nrrheum.2012.176
193. Brennan FM, Foey AD, Feldmann M. The importance of T cell interactions with macrophages in rheumatoid cytokine production. *Curr Top Microbiol Immunol* (2006) **305**:177–94. doi:10.1007/3-540-29714-6_9
194. Samson M, Audia S, Janikashvili N, Ciudad M, Trad M, Fraszczak J, et al. Inhibition of IL-6 function corrects Th17/Treg imbalance in rheumatoid arthritis patients. *Arthritis Rheum* (2012) **64**:2499–503. doi:10.1002/art.34477
195. Pesce B, Soto L, Sabugo F, Wurmann P, Cuchacovich M, López MN, et al. Effect of interleukin-6 receptor blockade on the balance between regulatory T cells and T helper type 17 cells in rheumatoid arthritis patients. *Clin Exp Immunol* (2013) **171**:237–42. doi:10.1111/cei.12017
196. Thiolat A, Semerano L, Pers YM, Biton J, Lemeiter D, Portales P, et al. Interleukin-6 receptor blockade enhances CD39+ regulatory T cell development in rheumatoid arthritis and in experimental arthritis. *Arthritis Rheumatol* (2014) **66**:273–83. doi:10.1002/art.38246
197. Kikuchi J, Hashizume M, Kaneko Y, Yoshimoto K, Nishina N, Takeuchi T. Peripheral blood CD4(+)CD25(+)CD127(low) regulatory T cells are significantly increased by tocilizumab treatment in patients with rheumatoid arthritis: increase in regulatory T cells correlates with clinical response. *Arthritis Res Ther* (2015) **17**:10. doi:10.1186/s13075-015-0526-4
198. Sarantopoulos A, Tselios K, Gkougkourelas I, Pantoura M, Georgiadou A-M, Boura P. Tocilizumab treatment leads to a rapid and sustained increase in Treg cell levels in rheumatoid arthritis patients: comment on the article by Thiolat et al. *Arthritis Rheumatol* (2014) **66**:2638. doi:10.1002/art.38714
199. Tono T, Aihara S, Hoshiyama T, Arinuma Y, Nagai T, Hirohata S. Effects of anti-IL-6 receptor antibody on human monocytes. *Mod Rheumatol* (2015) **25**:79–84. doi:10.3109/14397595.2014.914016

200. Tracey D, Klareskog L, Sasso EH, Salfeld JG, Tak PP. Tumor necrosis factor antagonist mechanisms of action: a comprehensive review. *Pharmacol Ther* (2008) **117**:244–79. doi:10.1016/j.pharmthera.2007.10.001
201. Brennan FM, Chantry D, Jackson A, Maini R, Feldmann M. Inhibitory effect of TNF alpha antibodies on synovial cell interleukin-1 production in rheumatoid arthritis. *Lancet* (1989) **2**:244–7. doi:10.1016/S0140-6736(89)90430-3
202. Haworth C, Brennan FM, Chantry D, Turner M, Maini RN, Feldmann M. Expression of granulocyte-macrophage colony-stimulating factor in rheumatoid arthritis: regulation by tumor necrosis factor-α. *Eur J Immunol* (1991) **21**:2575–9. doi:10.1002/eji.1830211039
203. Butler DM, Maini RN, Feldmann M, Brennan FM. Modulation of proinflammatory cytokine release in rheumatoid synovial membrane cell cultures. Comparison of monoclonal anti TNF-alpha antibody with the interleukin-1 receptor antagonist. *Eur Cytokine Netw* (1995) **6**:225–30.
204. Ehrenstein MR, Evans JG, Singh A, Moore S, Warnes G, Isenberg DA, et al. Compromised function of regulatory T cells in rheumatoid arthritis and reversal by anti-TNF{alpha} therapy. *J Exp Med* (2004) **200**:277–85. doi:10.1084/jem.20040165
205. Evans HG, Roostalu U, Walter GJ, Gullick NJ, Frederiksen KS, Roberts CA, et al. TNF-α blockade induces IL-10 expression in human CD4+ T cells. *Nat Commun* (2014) **5**:3199. doi:10.1038/ncomms4199
206. Boks MA, Kager-Groenland JR, Mousset CM, van Ham SM, ten Brinke A. Inhibition of TNF receptor signaling by anti-TNFα biologicals primes naïve CD4+ T cells towards IL-10+ T cells with a regulatory phenotype and function. *Clin Immunol* (2014) **151**:136–45. doi:10.1016/j.clim.2014.02.008
207. Mitoma H, Horiuchi T, Tsukamoto H, Tamimoto Y, Kimoto Y, Uchino A, et al. Mechanisms for cytotoxic effects of anti-tumor necrosis factor agents on transmembrane tumor necrosis factor α-expressing cells: comparison among infliximab, etanercept, and adalimumab. *Arthritis Rheum* (2008) **58**:1248–57. doi:10.1002/art.23447
208. Meusch U, Krasselt M, Rossol M, Baerwald C, Klingner M, Wagner U. In vitro response pattern of monocytes after tmTNF reverse signaling predicts response to anti-TNF therapy in rheumatoid arthritis. *J Transl Med* (2015) **13**:256. doi:10.1186/s12967-015-0620-z
209. Smolen JS, Han C, Bala M, Maini RN, Kalden JR, van der Heijde D, et al. Evidence of radiographic benefit of treatment with infliximab plus methotrexate in rheumatoid arthritis patients who had no clinical improvement: a detailed subanalysis of data from the anti-tumor necrosis factor trial in rheumatoid arthritis with concomitant therapy study. *Arthritis Rheum* (2005) **52**:1020–30. doi:10.1002/art.20982
210. Bozec A, Zaiss MM, Kagwiria R, Voll R, Rauh M, Chen Z, et al. T cell costimulation molecules CD80/86 inhibit osteoclast differentiation by inducing the IDO/tryptophan pathway. *Sci Transl Med* (2014) **6**:ra60–60. doi:10.1126/scitranslmed.3007764
211. Cohen SB, Dore RK, Lane NE, Ory PA, Peterfy CG, Sharp JT, et al. Denosumab treatment effects on structural damage, bone mineral density, and bone turnover in rheumatoid arthritis: a twelve-month, multicenter, randomized, double-blind, placebo-controlled, phase II clinical trial. *Arthritis Rheum* (2008) **58**:1299–309. doi:10.1002/art.23417
212. Pettit AR, Ji H, von Stechow D, Müller R, Goldring SR, Choi Y, et al. TRANCE/RANKL knockout mice are protected from bone erosion in a serum transfer model of arthritis. *Am J Pathol* (2001) **159**:1689–99. doi:10.1016/S0002-9440(10)63016-7
213. Ohno H, Uemura Y, Murooka H, Takanashi H, Tokieda T, Ohzeki Y, et al. The oral*ly-active* and selective c-Fms tyrosine kinase inhibitor Ki20227 inhibits disease progression in a collagen-induced arthritis mouse model. *Eur J Immunol* (2008) **38**:283–91. doi:10.1002/eji.200737199
214. Paniagua RT, Chang A, Mariano MM, Stein EA, Wang Q, Lindstrom TM, et al. c-Fms-mediated differentiation and priming of monocyte lineage cells play a central role in autoimmune arthritis. *Arthritis Res Ther* (2010) **12**:R32. doi:10.1186/ar2940
215. Toh M-L, Bonnefoy J-Y, Accart N, Cochin S, Pohle S, Haegel H, et al. Bone- and cartilage-protective effects of a monoclonal antibody against colony-stimulating factor 1 receptor in experimental arthritis. *Arthritis Rheumatol* (2014) **66**:2989–3000. doi:10.1002/art.38624
216. Hayder M, Poupot M, Baron M, Nigon D, Turrin C-O, Caminade A-M, et al. A phosphorus-based dendrimer targets inflammation and osteoclastogenesis in experimental arthritis. *Sci Transl Med* (2011) **3**:ra35–81. doi:10.1126/scitranslmed.3002212
217. Ando W, Hashimoto J, Nampei A, Tsuboi H, Tateishi K, Ono T, et al. Imatinib mesylate inhibits osteoclastogenesis and joint destruction in rats with collagen-induced arthritis (CIA). *J Bone Miner Metab* (2006) **24**:274–82. doi:10.1007/s00774-006-0684-1
218. Masteller EL, Wong BR. Targeting IL-34 in chronic inflammation. *Drug Discov Today* (2014) **19**:1212–6. doi:10.1016/j.drudis.2014.05.016
219. Nicodeme E, Jeffrey KL, Schaefer U, Beinke S, Dewell S, Chung C-W, et al. Suppression of inflammation by a synthetic histone mimic. *Nature* (2010) **468**:1119–23. doi:10.1038/nature09589
220. Belkina AC, Nikolajczyk BS, Denis GV. BET protein function is required for inflammation: Brd2 genetic disruption and BET inhibitor JQ1 impair mouse macrophage inflammatory responses. *J Immunol* (2013) **190**:3670–8. doi:10.4049/jimmunol.1202838
221. Mele DA, Salmeron A, Ghosh S, Huang H-R, Bryant BM, Lora JM. BET bromodomain inhibition suppresses TH17-mediated pathology. *J Exp Med* (2013) **210**:2181–90. doi:10.1084/jem.20130376
222. Chan CH, Fang C, Qiao Y, Yarilina A, Prinjha RK, Ivashkiv LB. BET bromodomain inhibition suppresses transcriptional responses to cytokine-Jak-STAT signaling in a gene-specific manner in human monocytes. *Eur J Immunol* (2015) **45**(1):287–97. doi:10.1002/eji.201444862
223. Verbrugge SE, Scheper RJ, Lems WF, de Gruijl TD, Jansen G. Proteasome inhibitors as experimental therapeutics of autoimmune diseases. *Arthritis Res Ther* (2015) **17**:17. doi:10.1186/s13075-015-0529-1
224. Polzer K, Neubert K, Meister S, Frey B, Baum W, Distler JH, et al. Proteasome inhibition aggravates tumor necrosis factor-mediated bone resorption in a mouse model of inflammatory arthritis. *Arthritis Rheum* (2011) **63**:670–80. doi:10.1002/art.30177
225. Yannaki E, Papadopoulou A, Athanasiou E, Kaloyannidis P, Paraskeva A, Bougiouklis D, et al. The proteasome inhibitor bortezomib drastically affects inflammation and bone disease in adjuvant-induced arthritis in rats. *Arthritis Rheum* (2010) **62**:3277–88. doi:10.1002/art.27690
226. von Metzler I, Krebbel H, Hecht M, Manz RA, Fleissner C, Mieth M, et al. Bortezomib inhibits human osteoclastogenesis. *Leukemia* (2007) **21**(9):2025–34. doi:10.1038/sj.leu.2404806
227. Kim Y-G, Kang JH, Kim HJ, Kim HJ, Kim H-H, Kim J-Y, et al. Bortezomib inhibits osteoclastogenesis and porphyromonas gingivalis lipopolysaccharide-induced alveolar bone resorption. *J Dent Res* (2015) **94**:1243–50. doi:10.1177/0022034515592592
228. Muchamuel T, Basler M, Aujay MA, Suzuki E, Kalim KW, Lauer C, et al. A selective inhibitor of the immunoproteasome subunit LMP7 blocks cytokine production and attenuates progression of experimental arthritis. *Nat Med* (2009) **15**:781–7. doi:10.1038/nm.1978
229. Tanaka Y. Recent progress and perspective in JAK inhibitors for rheumatoid arthritis: from bench to bedside. *J Biochem* (2015) **158**:173–9. doi:10.1093/jb/mvv069
230. Kubo S, Yamaoka K, Kondo M, Yamagata K, Zhao J, Iwata S, et al. The JAK inhibitor, tofacitinib, reduces the T cell stimulatory capacity of human monocyte-derived dendritic cells. *Ann Rheum Dis* (2013) **73**:2192–8. doi:10.1136/annrheumdis-2013-203756
231. Yarilina A, Xu K, Chan C, Ivashkiv LB. Regulation of inflammatory responses in tumor necrosis factor-activated and rheumatoid arthritis synovial macrophages by JAK inhibitors. *Arthritis Rheum* (2012) **64**:3856–66. doi:10.1002/art.37691
232. Pattison MJ, MacKenzie KF, Arthur JSC. Inhibition of JAKs in macrophages increases lipopolysaccharide-induced cytokine production by blocking IL-10-mediated feedback. *J Immunol* (2012) **189**:2784–92. doi:10.4049/jimmunol.1200310

13

Conventional treatment for multiple myeloma drives premature aging phenotypes and metabolic dysfunction in T Cells

Rachel Elizabeth Cooke[1,2], Kylie Margaret Quinn[3], Hang Quach[2,4], Simon Harrison[2,4], Henry Miles Prince[2,4], Rachel Koldej[1,2] and David Ritchie[1,2,4]*

[1] Australian Cancer Research Foundation Translational Research Laboratory, Royal Melbourne Hospital, Melbourne, VIC, Australia, [2] Department of Medicine, University of Melbourne, Melbourne, VIC, Australia, [3] School of Health and Biomedical Sciences, RMIT University, Melbourne, VIC, Australia, [4] Peter MacCallum Cancer Centre, Melbourne, VIC, Australia

Edited by:
Slavica Vuckovic,
Royal Prince Alfred Hospital, Australia

Reviewed by:
Anne Marit Sponaas,
Norwegian University of Science and Technology, Norway
Tuna Mutis,
Amsterdam University Medical Center, Netherlands
Taxiarchis Kourelis,
Mayo Clinic, United States

***Correspondence:**
Rachel Elizabeth Cooke
Rachel.Cooke@mh.org.au;
rachel.cooke@nh.org.au

New diagnoses of multiple myeloma (MM) tend to occur after the age of 60, by which time thymic output is severely reduced. As a consequence, lymphocyte recovery after lymphopenia-inducing anti-MM therapies relies on homeostatic proliferation of peripheral T cells rather than replenishment by new thymic emigrants. To assess lymphocyte recovery and phenotype in patients with newly diagnosed MM (NDMM) and relapsed/refractory MM (RRMM), we tracked CD4$^+$ and CD8$^+$ T cell populations at serial time points throughout treatment and compared them to age-matched healthy donors (HD). Anti-MM therapies and autologous stem cell transplant (ASCT) caused a permanent reduction in the CD4:8 ratio, a decrease in naïve CD4$^+$ T cells, and an increase in effector memory T cells and PD1-expressing CD4$^+$ T cells. Transcriptional profiling highlighted that genes associated with fatty acid β-oxidation were upregulated in T cells in RRMM, suggesting increased reliance on mitochondrial respiration. High mitochondrial mass was seen in all T cell subsets in RRMM but with relatively suppressed reactive oxygen species and mitochondrial membrane potential, indicating mitochondrial dysfunction. These findings highlight that anti-MM and ASCT therapies perturb the composition of the T cell compartment and drive substantial metabolic remodeling, which may affect the fitness of T cells for immunotherapies. This is particularly pertinent to chimeric antigen receptor (CAR)-T therapy, which might be more efficacious if T cells were stored prior to ASCT rather than at relapse.

Keywords: myeloma, T cell, metabolism, aging, autologous stem cell transplant

INTRODUCTION

Multiple myeloma (MM) is a malignancy of plasma cells within the bone marrow (BM) (1, 2) that is typically diagnosed in patients over the age of 60 years old (3). Treatment for MM has evolved over the last 10 years with the introduction of immune modulatory drugs (IMiDs) and proteasome inhibitors. This has led to a significant increase in life expectancy (2, 4), which is most pronounced in patients under 60 years old (5). However, it is notable that the typical age of onset for MM coincides with marked decline in immune function during normal biological aging driven by thymic involution and immunosenescence.

From 60 years old, both the number and repertoire diversity of T_N cells declines substantially due to a process known as thymic involution (6, 7). Thymic involution refers to a loss of thymic stromal tissue and function, which limits *de novo* production of naïve T (T_N) cells. With this decline in *de novo* T_N cell production, homeostatic proliferation of peripheral T cells appears to compensate and increases with age (8). As a result, in the event of a sudden decline in the number of lymphocytes (such as might occur during high dose chemotherapy), the aged thymus has limited capacity for T_N cell output (9, 10). Instead, repopulation of the peripheral T cell population is predominantly driven by lymphopenia-induced proliferation, mediated by the increased availability of γc cytokines, such as IL-7 and IL-15. Lymphopenia-induced proliferation favors expansion of $CD8^+$ memory T cells, because $CD8^+$ memory T cells express higher levels of a component of the IL-15 receptor (CD122) (11) and $CD4^+$ T cell homeostatic expansion is limited by IL-7-dependent STAT-1 activation (12). More recently, signaling from γc cytokines has been seen to drive metabolic remodeling in T cells in mouse models of aging, inflammation, and lymphopenia (13–15), but the impact of lymphopenia-inducing therapies on T cell metabolism in aged humans has not been defined.

Immunosenescence refers to a loss of intrinsic function in immune cells, which can undermine responses to vaccines, infections, and cancer (16). Chronic age-related inflammation and metabolic stress are thought to be significant drivers of immunosenescence for a variety of immune cells, including $CD4^+$ and $CD8^+$ T cells (17, 18). During MM disease, it is well established that MM cells can create a microenvironment of chronic inflammation in the BM, characterized by increased production of IL-6 in particular (19). IL-6 sustains tumor survival, but it also drives production of senescent cells that exhibit a senescence-associated secretory phenotype (20, 21), all of which are predicted to augment dysfunction in $CD4^+$ and $CD8^+$ T cells. Inflammation-associated cytokine stimulation is also known to drive metabolic changes in a variety of immune cells, including T cells (13–15). Given the complex relationship between T cell homeostasis, inflammation, and aging, understanding the shifts in the immune system that result from normal aging, MM disease and MM therapies will be critical for implementing immune therapies in MM patients (22).

Previously, we demonstrated a loss of T_N cells in the peripheral blood (PB) of MM patients, with a reciprocal expansion of effector memory (T_{EM}) cells (23). In the $CD8^+$ T cell population, a loss of T_N cells is already observed at diagnosis and is equivalent to the loss of T_N cells seen in elderly healthy donors (HD). In contrast, in the $CD4^+$ T cell population, T_N cells are relatively preserved in the elderly and newly diagnosed MM (NDMM), with significant loss of T_N cells only observed in relapsed/refractory MM (RRMM) (24). This also leads to a decrease in CD4:8 ratio, which is a characteristic finding in MM with disease progression (23, 25). While prior studies of patients with NDMM and RRMM concluded that changes in NK and T cell populations were corticosteroid-induced and/or disease-driven (23, 24, 26–28), autologous stem cell transplant (ASCT) and T cell-depleting therapies form the backbone of treatment for medically fit MM patients, and their long-term impact on T cell function has not been well-described.

In this study, we demonstrate that ASCT and/or MM disease does irreversibly change the composition of T cell populations, with a dramatic loss of $CD4^+$ T_N cells and reciprocal increase in $CD8^+$ effector memory T cells, and an increase in PD1-expressing $CD4^+$ T cells. We also observe metabolic changes in T cells from RRMM patients, with increased expression of transcripts for mitochondrial respiration, increased mitochondrial load, and decreased reactive oxygen species (ROS), which suggests a loss of metabolic fitness. We propose a model where ASCT and/or MM disease-derived inflammation drives increased inflammatory and γc cytokine signaling and lymphopenia-induced proliferation and accelerated immunosenescence, which would mediate the dramatic loss of T_N cells in MM patients and metabolic remodeling in the remaining T cells. These findings inform our current treatment protocols for MM and will guide integration of new immune-based therapies for MM. While lymphopenia may drive $CD4^+$ T_N cell loss, we may be able to intervene with dendritic cell (DC) vaccination, checkpoint blockade, or metabolic interventions during post-ASCT lymphopenia to better support the recovering T cell population. Furthermore, the collection of T cells prior to ASCT (as opposed to at the time of relapse) would likely provide a more efficacious chimeric antigen receptor (CAR)-T product.

MATERIALS AND METHODS

Human Samples and Cells

All research was conducted in full compliance with principles of the "Declaration of Helsinki," Good Clinical Practice, and within the laws and regulations of Australia. Cryopreserved peripheral blood mononuclear cells (PBMCs) were analyzed from MM patients enrolled on two historical clinical trials: LITVACC (ACTRN12613000344796) that recruited NDMM patients and REVLITE (NCT00482261) that recruited RRMM patients, which are illustrated in **Figure 1A**.

Newly diagnosed MM patients received four induction cycles of lenalidomide and dexamethasone (LEN/DEX) followed by ASCT, and they were then partitioned into one of two study arms, with either (i) monthly DC vaccines + LEN or (ii) LEN ± DEX maintenance therapy. Both study arms have been combined in this analysis as sample numbers were underpowered to detect any small variances. Paired patient PBMC samples (where available) were analyzed at three consecutive time points: cycle 4 of induction (Pre-ASCT, $n = 29$), at maintenance cycle 4 after ASCT (Post-ASCT, $n = 21$), and at last follow-up [end of treatment (EOT), $n = 21$]. The mean time to last follow-up was well over 2 years at 1069 days (range: 397–1780 days), to ensure maximal peripheral leukocyte reconstitution.

Relapsed/refractory MM patients were also treated with successive cycles of LEN/DEX and evaluated for stable disease, and for those who had stable disease, we analyzed PBMC samples

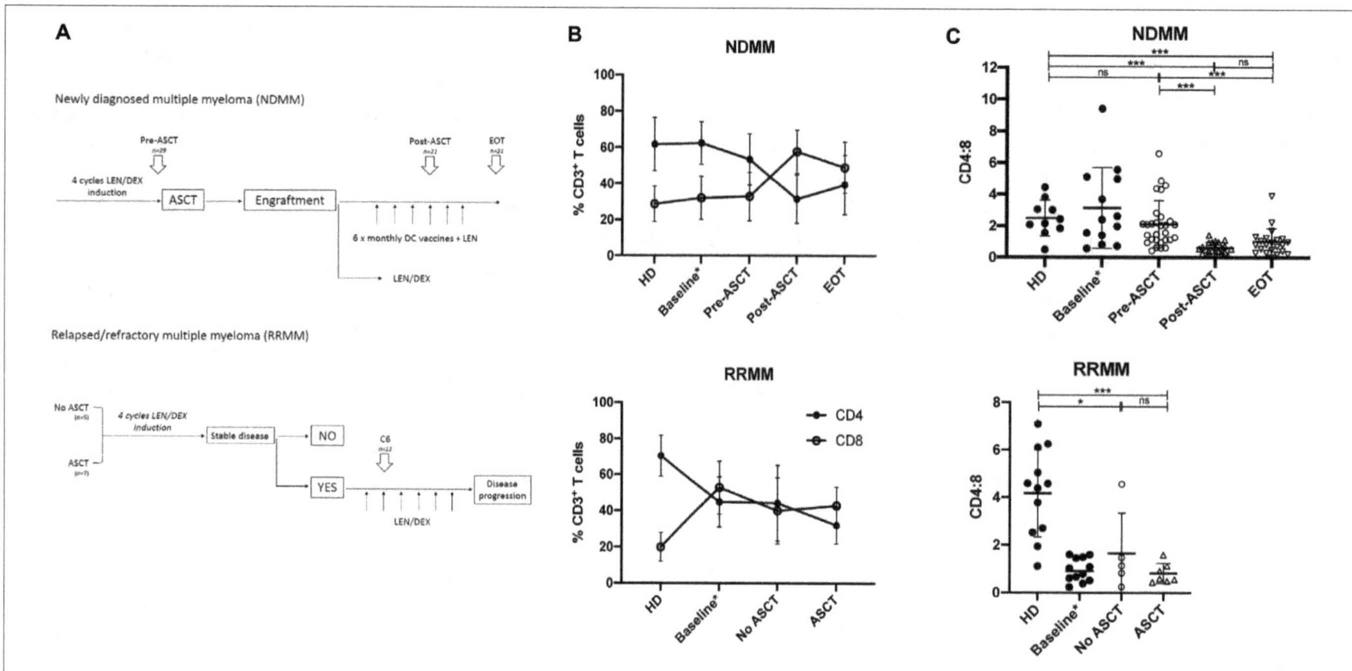

FIGURE 1 | CD4:8 is reduced post-ASCT and in RRMM. **(A)** Time points analyzed by flow cytometry (described in section "Materials and Methods"). In newly diagnosed MM (NDMM), paired samples (where available) were analyzed prior to autologous stem cell transplant (pre-ASCT, $n = 29$), post-ASCT ($n = 21$) and at end of treatment (EOT, $n = 21$). In relapsed/refractory MM (RRMM), samples were analyzed after six cycles LEN/DEX and subdivided into those patients who had not had a prior ASCT ($n = 5$) and those with prior ASCT ($n = 7$). **(B)** The proportion of $CD3^+$ T cells that are $CD4^+$ (black circle) or $CD8^+$ (clear circle) at serial time points in NDMM (top) and in RRMM (bottom) compared with HD. Baseline samples (NDMM $n = 21$, RRMM $n = 10$) analyzed in a prior study (23) are incorporated for interest. **(C)** CD4:8 ratio in NDMM (top) and in RRMM (bottom) compared with HD. Baseline samples (NDMM $n = 21$, RRMM $n = 10$) analyzed in a prior study (23) are incorporated for interest but are not included in statistical analysis. Statistical significance was determined using the Mann–Whitney test ($^*p < 0.05$, $^{***}p < 0.001$).

after six cycles of LEN/DEX. We retrospectively subdivided this group for analysis into those patients who had not received prior ASCT (No ASCT, $n = 5$) and those who had (ASCT, $n = 7$).

Peripheral blood mononuclear cells from age-matched HD were used as a control group and were collected via the Australian Red Cross Blood Service and the Victorian Blood Donor Registry.

T Cell Flow Cytometric Analysis

Flow cytometry was performed using Fixable viability stain 700 (BD Horizon) and directly conjugated anti-human antibodies: CD3 (SK7, BD Biosciences), CD4 (RPA-T4, BD Pharmingen or SK3, BD Horizon), CD8 (RPA-T8, BD Pharmingen), CD45RA (H100, eBiosciences), CD197 (CCR7) (3D12, eBiosciences) and CD279 (PD1) (EH12, BD Horizon). Cell surface staining was performed with 5×10^6 to 1×10^7 PBMCs in a 100-μl cell suspension of FACS buffer and antibody master mix for 30 min at 4°C. Cells were washed and resuspended in FACS buffer or complete RPMI containing mitochondrial fluorescent dyes for mitochondrial assessment. Lymphocytes were gated using forward and side scatter, followed by doublet and dead cell removal. BD Anti-Mouse or Anti-Goat Comp Beads were used to optimize fluorescence compensation settings for analysis. Fluorescence minus one (FMO) controls were used to assist with gating. Analysis was performed on a BD LSR Fortessa and analyzed using FlowJo software (Version 10). T cell differentiation subsets were defined as the following: Naïve (TN): CD3+CD4+/8^+CD45RA^+CC$R7^+$, central memory (T_{CM}): $CD3^+CD4^+/8^+CD45RA^-CCR7^+$, effector memory ($T_{EM}$): $CD3^+CD4^+/8^+CD45RA^-CCR7^-$, and effector memory $CD45RA^+$ (T_{EMRA}): $CD3^+CD4^+/8^+CD45RA^+CCR7^-$.

RNA Sequencing

$CD4^+$ T cells were enriched from PBMCs using the MACS® human $CD4^+$ T cell isolation kit, as per the manufacturer's instructions. $CD4^+$ T cell purity was >80%. RNA was extracted with Trizol, and cDNA library creation and RNA sequencing were performed by the Australian Genome Research Facility at the Walter and Eliza Hall Institute. Because there was significant RNA degradation in the sample set, the SMARTer Stranded Total RNA-Seq Kit—Pico Input Mammalian (Takara Bio USA) protocol was used, which incorporates a ribosomal RNA depletion. Genes needed to pass a 20 read threshold in >80% of samples in order to be analyzed. Bioinformatic analysis was performed at Melbourne Bioinformatics, University of Melbourne, utilizing the Limma linear model (29).

Real-Time qPCR

$CD4^+$ and $CD8^+$ T cells were enriched from PBMCs using the MACS® human $CD4^+$ T cell isolation kit or MACS® human $CD8^+$ Microbeads (Miltenyi Biotec), as per the manufacturer's instructions. RNA was extracted with Trizol and cDNA was synthesized using the Superscript VILO cDNA kit (Thermo

Fisher Scientific), as per the manufacturer's instructions. Target genes were analyzed using TaqMan gene expression assays with TaqMan Fast Universal master mix on the QuantStudio 7 Flex Real-Time PCR system (Thermo Fisher Scientific), as per the manufacturer's instructions. The housekeeping gene TBP was used as the endogenous control to calculate relative gene expression.

Mitochondrial Staining

After cell surface staining, cells were incubated at 37°C for 30 min in complete RPMI containing mitochondrial fluorescent dyes (Thermo Fisher Scientific), using a combination of MitoTracker deep red FM (MTdr) at 1:20,000 and either CellRox® Orange reagent (CellRoxO) at 1:1000 or tetramethylrhodamine, methyl ester (TMRM) at 1:3000. Cell suspensions were washed and resuspended in T cell media for flow cytometric analysis.

Statistical Analysis

Data were analyzed using GraphPad Prism software (version 7).

RESULTS

Phenotypic Changes in the Composition of T Cell Subsets

To track changes in T cell populations throughout the course of MM disease and treatment, we analyzed PBMCs from patients with NDMM and RRMM collected at serial time points throughout their treatment and compared with age-matched HD. Study design and analysis time points are described in section "Materials and Methods" and in **Figure 1A**, and patient characteristics are shown in **Supplementary Tables 1, 2.** Unfortunately, baseline samples from patients prior to any treatment were not available for this analysis, but they have been described in previous work (23), which we include for interest but do not include in statistical analysis as these are not matched samples and it should be noted that different fluorochromes and gating strategies were used in the prior analysis.

In NDMM, the CD4:8 ratio was similar to HD in patients at baseline and pre-ASCT after four induction cycles of LEN/DEX, but it was significantly reduced post-ASCT and did not recover to baseline by EOT (**Figures 1B,C**, left). Prolonged $CD4^+$ T cell depletion has been described after ASCT in children and young adults (10), but the CD4:8 ratio recovers to baseline levels by 1 year post-ASCT (30). Our results in an older population differ in this regard, and support findings by Chung et al. (30), who also demonstrated a reduction in the CD4:8 ratio in MM patients after ASCT up to 1 year post-ASCT. Subanalysis of the population that received DC vaccines (n = 8) suggested a trend toward expansion of the $CD8^+$ T cell population (and further reduction of CD4:8) compared with those receiving LEN/DEX therapy (n = 13) at the post-ASCT time point; however, this did not reach statistical significance and was indistinguishable by EOT (**Supplementary Figure 1**).

In RRMM (at baseline and after LEN/DEX treatment, irrespective of prior ASCT), the CD4:8 ratio was also significantly reduced compared with HD (**Figures 1B,C**, right), although we note that the mean CD4:8 ratio in the this HD group is higher than that used for the NDMM comparison that may reflect heterogeneity in the normal population and/or minor differences in the fluorochromes used. The CD4:8 ratio is likely reduced in RRMM patients as a whole as they were probably treated previously with cyclophosphamide (commonly used in induction regimens in Australia), which is known to induce lymphopenia.

We next observed the differentiation status of $CD4^+$ and $CD8^+$ T cell populations over the course of treatment. In NDMM pre-ACST, phenotypic composition was similar to HD, but post-ASCT, there was a significant decrease in the proportion of $CD4^+$ that were T_N and T_{CM} cells and a reciprocal increase in T_{EM} cells, which persisted to EOT (**Figures 2A,B**, left). In RRMM (at baseline and with treatment), there was also a significant decrease in the proportion of $CD4^+$ T_N cells but, unlike in NDMM, both the $CD4^+$ T_{CM} and T_{EM} populations had reciprocally expanded (**Figure 2C**, left). These shifts in phenotypic composition were not evident in $CD8^+$ T cells, because T_{EMRA} cells are already an established subset in older HD (**Figures 2B,C**, right).

There Are Temporal and Compartmental Differences in PD-1 Expression Between $CD4^+$ and $CD8^+$ T Cells

In the Vk*MYC murine model of MM, PD1 expression was shown to transiently increase on T cells 30 days post-transplant (31). PD-L1 blockade also increased the efficacy of hematopoietic stem cell transplant, adoptive T cell transfer, and a post-transplant DC vaccine (31), and increased survival when administered during the homeostatic proliferation phase after non-myeloablative total body irradiation (32). This suggests that PD1/PD-L1 monoclonal antibodies may be beneficial post-ASCT, but human studies have not demonstrated significantly altered PD1 expression post-ASCT (30). We wanted to further dissect PD1 expression in $CD4^+$ and $CD8^+$ T cell subsets during MM treatment.

In $CD4^+$ T cells, the proportion expressing PD1 was increased in both NDMM and RRMM patients compared with HD and was highest post-ASCT in NDMM (**Figures 3B,C**, left). In $CD8^+$ T cells, there was no statistically significant change but there did appear to be two populations post-ASCT: one with and one without PD1 expression (**Figures 3B,C**, right). Subanalysis shows a trend toward increased % $PD1^+$ in the group receiving DC vaccine but this does not reach statistical significance (**Supplementary Figure 3**). PD1 expression remained high in $CD4^+$ T cells at EOT, while it returned to normal in $CD8^+$ T cells (**Figure 3B**). The latter finding was also described in the post-allogeneic stem cell transplant setting, where PD1 facilitated apoptosis of alloreactive $CD8^+$ T cells by increasing ROS (33).

$PD1^+$ events were then backgated to define the phenotypic distribution of PD1 expression (**Supplementary Figure 2**).

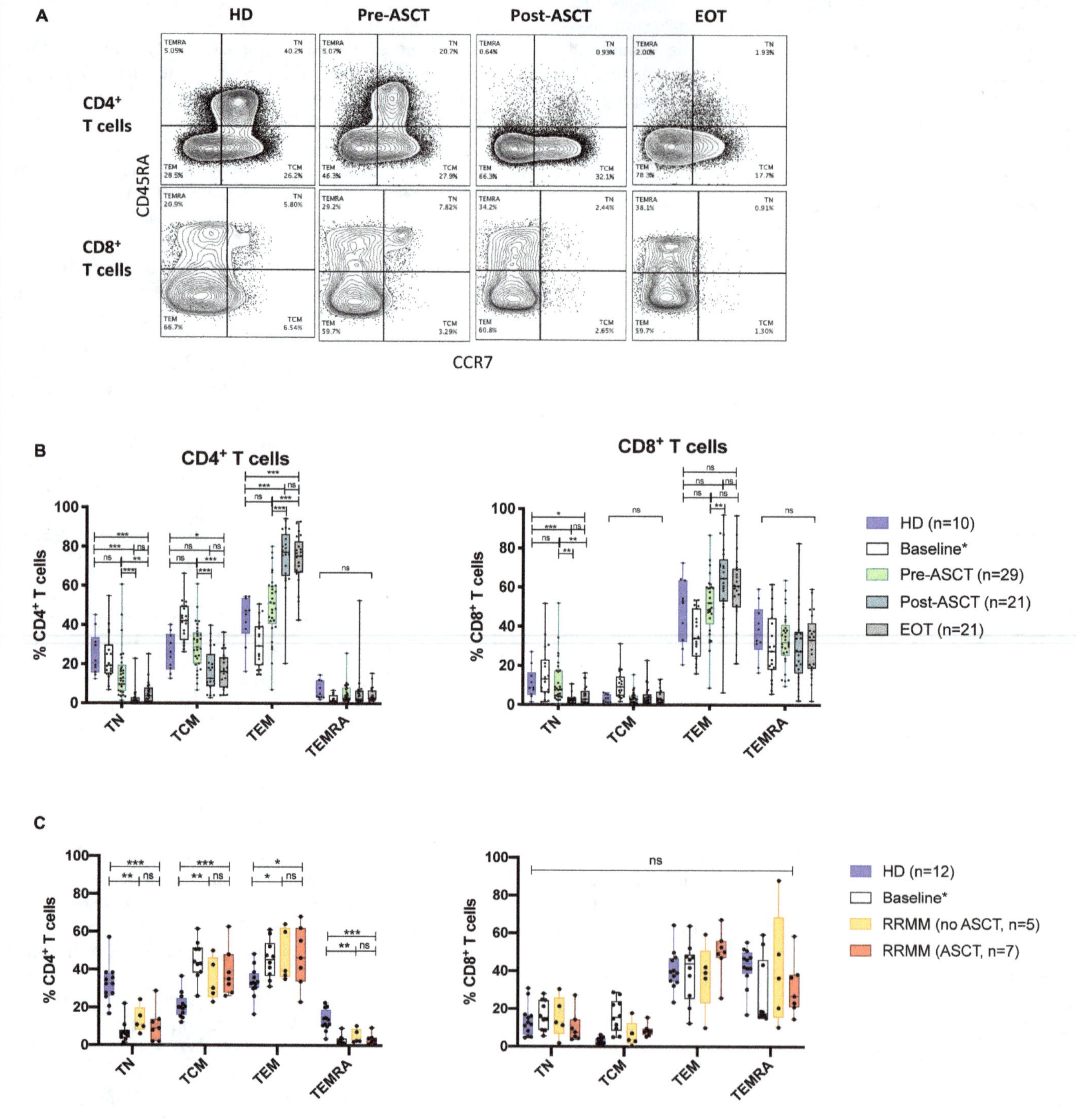

FIGURE 2 | Phenotypic composition of T cell populations with MM. **(A)** Representative flow plots of CD4$^+$ and CD8$^+$ T cells from serial time points in NDMM samples, defining T_N, T_{CM}, T_{EM}, and T_{EMRA} subsets. **(B,C)** The proportion of CD4$^+$ (left) and CD8$^+$ (right) T cells of each phenotype subsets at serial time points in **(B)** NDMM and **(C)** RRMM patient samples. Baseline samples analyzed in a prior study (23) are incorporated for interest but are not included in statistical analysis. Statistical significance was determined using multiple Student's *t*-tests with the Holm–Sidak method applied (*$p < 0.05$, **$p < 0.01$, ***$p < 0.001$).

In HD, most PD1$^+$ cells were T_{EM} phenotype, with minor proportions of T_N, T_{CM}, and T_{EMRA} phenotypes; however, there were significant proportions of T_{CM} and T_{EMRA} in CD4$^+$ and CD8$^+$ PD1$^+$ populations, respectively. We then assessed PD1 expression in T cell differentiation subsets (**Figure 3D**). In CD4$^+$ T cells, the proportion of T_N, T_{CM}, and T_{EMRA} that were PD1$^+$ increased significantly in NDMM post-ASCT and in RRMM with prior ASCT, compared with HD (**Figures 3E,F**, left). The proportion of CD4$^+$ T_{CM} that were PD1$^+$ also remained elevated at EOT in NDMM. In CD8 T cell subsets, differences in PD1

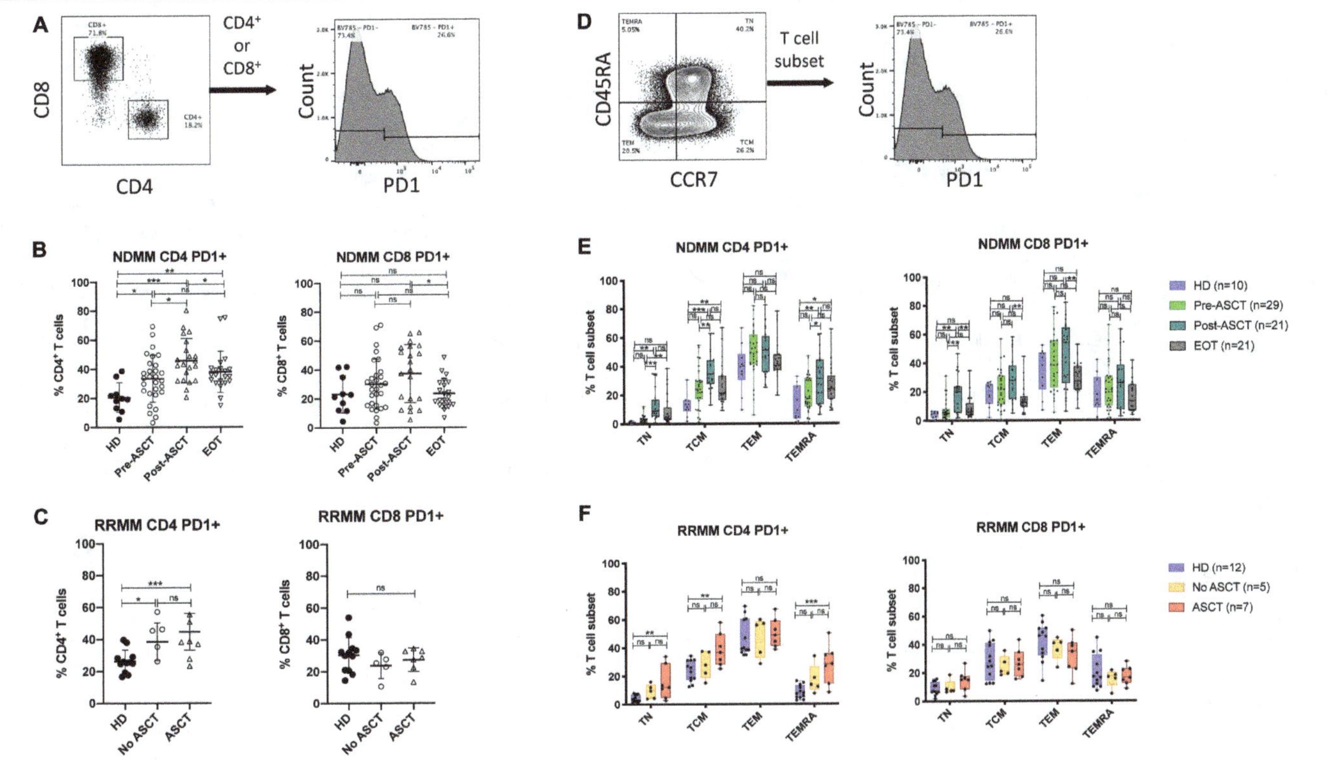

FIGURE 3 | PD1 expression on T cell subsets after ASCT. **(A–C)** PD1 expression in CD4⁺ and CD8⁺ T cells. **(A)** Representative gating strategy. **(B,C)** Scatter plots showing PD1⁺ events as% of CD4⁺ T cells (left) and CD8⁺ T cells (right) in **(B)** NDMM at serial time points and **(C)** RRMM, compared to HD. Statistical significance was determined using the Mann–Whitney test (*$p < 0.05$, **$p < 0.01$, ***$p < 0.001$). **(D–F)** PD1 expression in T cell differentiation subsets. **(D)** Representative gating strategy. **(E,F)** Box and whisker plots showing PD1⁺ events as% of T cell subset (T_N, T_{CM}, T_{EM}, and T_{EMRA}) for CD4⁺ T cells (left) and CD8⁺ T cells (right) in **(E)** NDMM at serial time points and **(F)** RRMM, compared to HD. Statistical significance was determined using the Student's *t*-test with the Holm–Sidak method applied (*$p < 0.05$, **$p < 0.01$, ***$p < 0.001$).

expression were modest (**Figures 3E,F**, right), in keeping with prior observations (30).

Fatty Acid β-Oxidation Is Increased in T Cells From RRMM Compared With HD

T cell function and survival are supported by the selective use of distinct metabolic pathways (34–36). For example, effector T cell activation and proliferation is supported by a shift toward aerobic glycolysis, while memory T cells utilize fatty acid oxidation (FAO) to fuel mitochondrial respiration. Furthermore, as previously mentioned, animal models demonstrate that aging, inflammation, and lymphopenia can all alter the metabolic capacity of T cells to promote mitochondrial respiration (13–15).

We performed preliminary RNA-Seq analysis on CD4⁺ T cells from HD ($n = 2$) and RRMM ($n = 2$) samples to identify differentially expressed genes (DEGs). When lists of DEGs were interrogated for significant enrichment of specific biological pathways in the KEGG databases, the top upregulated pathways included RAP1, PI3K-AKT, cAMP, calcium, and PPAR signaling pathways (**Supplementary Figure 4**), which can augment specific metabolic responses, particularly in relation to FAO and mitochondrial respiration.

To further explore this, we evaluated the expression of key genes for glycolysis and FAO (**Table 1**) in CD4⁺ and CD8⁺ T cells with a larger cohort of RRMM and HD samples by using quantitative PCR; sample characteristics are described in **Supplementary Table 3**. There was no difference in relative RNA quantitation (RQ) between RRMM and HD for nearly all of the glycolysis genes analyzed; the one exception was *PKM* (pyruvate kinase), which was increased in RRMM compared with HD (**Figure 4A**). While pyruvate kinase is in the glycolytic pathway, it generates pyruvate that can either undergo aerobic glycolysis or be converted into acetyl CoA to provide substrate for mitochondrial respiration. In contrast, the expression of nearly all of the FAO genes were significantly higher in both CD4⁺ and CD8⁺ T cells in RRMM compared to HD (**Figure 4B**). These results suggest that FAO and mitochondrial respiration is upregulated in T cells in RRMM compared with HD.

Mitochondrial Mass Is Significantly Increased in T Cell in RRMM

Given that genes associated with FAO and mitochondrial respiration were upregulated in T cells in RRMM, we then assessed mitochondrial mass using the MitoTracker™ Deep Red FM dye (MTdr). MTdr staining was significantly increased in

TABLE 1 | Genes analyzed by qPCR to assess glycolysis and fatty acid β-oxidation in T cells.

Mode of metabolism	Gene	Abbreviation	Function
Glycolysis	Hexokinase 1	HK1	Hexokinases phosphorylate glucose to produce glucose-6-phosphate, the first step of glycolysis. This gene encodes a ubiquitous form that localizes to the outer membrane of mitochondria.
	Pyruvate kinase, muscle	PKM	Enzyme involved in the production of pyruvate that can either undergo aerobic glycolysis or be converted to acetyl CoA (a substrate of the TCA cycle)
	Lactate dehydrogenase, A and B subunits	LDHA, LDHB	Catalyze the interconversion of pyruvate and lactate in the last step of aerobic glycolysis
Fatty acid β-oxidation	Carnitine palmitoyl transferase 1A	CPT1A	Rate-limiting enzyme in the transport of fatty acids across the mitochondrial inner membrane
	Acyl-CoA dehydrogenase, very long chain	ACADVL	Catalyzes the first step of the mitochondrial fatty acid β-oxidation pathway
	Acetyl-CoA acyltransferase 2	AACA2	Catalyzes the last step of the mitochondrial fatty acid β-oxidation pathway

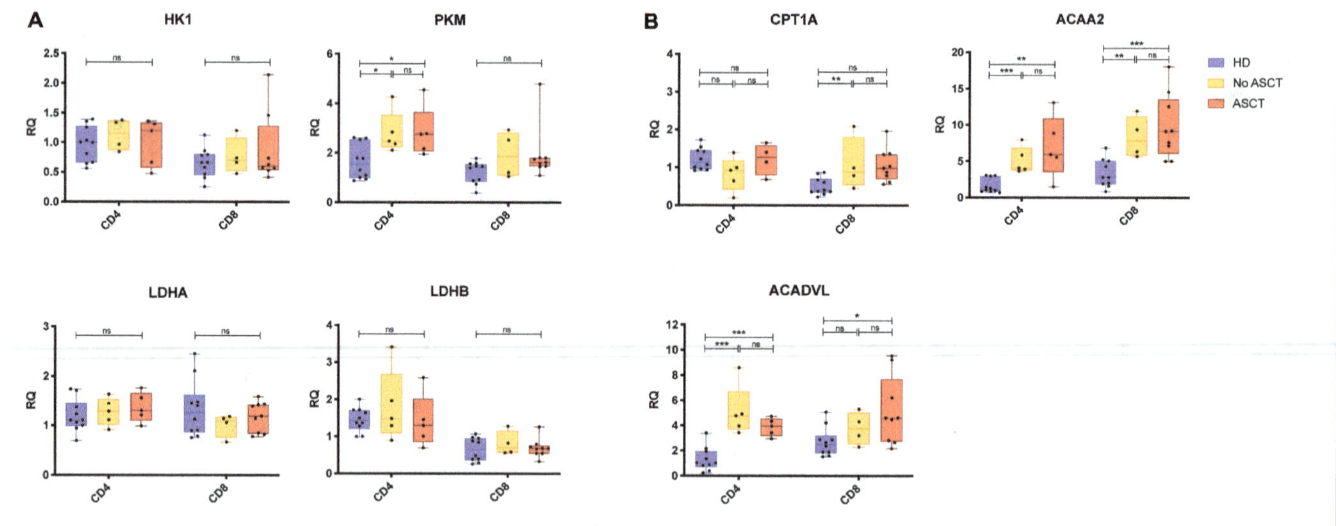

FIGURE 4 | Expression of metabolic genes in CD4+ and CD8+ T cells. Relative transcript expression assessed by qPCR for **(A)** glycolysis-associated genes and **(B)** FAO-associated genes. Study groups: Healthy donor (HD) (n = 12), RRMM No ASCT (n = 5)[1], RRMM ASCT (n = 9)[2]. Statistical significance was determined using the Mann–Whitney test (*$p < 0.05$, **$p < 0.01$, ***$p < 0.001$). [1]Insufficient RNA extracted from one CD8+ sample for analysis. [2]Insufficient RNA extracted from four CD4+ samples for analysis.

both CD4+ and CD8+ T cells from RRMM patients compared with HD (**Figure 5A**); in fact, virtually all T cells had high MTdr expression, unlike HD, where T cells were predominantly MTdr low-intermediate or MTdr negative (**Figure 5B**). This increase in MTdr staining was seen across all T cell subsets in RRMM (**Figure 5C**), but it was most marked in T_N and T_{CM} cells (**Figure 5D**).

Mitochondrial ROS Levels Are Reduced in T Cells in RRMM

CD4+ and CD8+ T cells in RRMM had elevated mitochondrial mass, but these mitochondria may not necessarily be functional. To assess the functionality of mitochondria, we then measured ROS, which are produced during normal mitochondrial respiration, using the CellROX Orange dye. We gated on cells with high mitochondrial mass for internal consistency (**Figure 6A**) and saw that both CD4+ and CD8+ T cells from RRMM patients showed significantly lower ROS levels than HD (**Figure 6B**). This reduction in ROS levels was evident across all T cell populations (**Figure 6C**). In HD, ROS levels were highest in T_{CM} and T_{EM} cells, which would be expected as these cells rely more heavily on mitochondrial respiration to meet their energy demands, but in RRMM, this difference was reduced (**Figure 6D**).

Mitochondrial Membrane Potential (Δψm) Is Increased in CD4+ T_{CM} Cells in RRMM

High mitochondrial mass accompanied by low ROS levels is suggestive of reduced mitochondrial activity. To assess whether mitochondria were still functional, we assessed mitochondrial membrane potential (Δψm) using the tetramethylrhodamine, methyl ester dye (TMRM), which is retained in mitochondria with intact membrane potential. We again gated on cells with high mitochondrial mass for internal consistency and saw that Δψm was significantly higher in the CD4+ T cells from RRMM

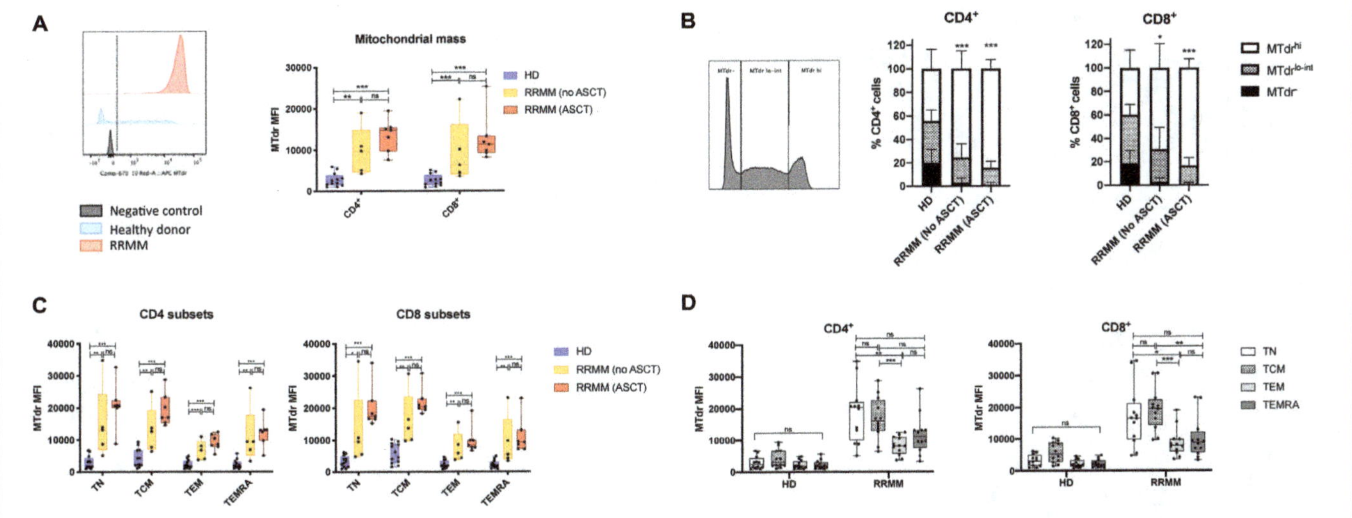

FIGURE 5 | Mitochondrial mass in RRMM. **(A)** Mitochondrial mass measured by geometric mean fluorescence intensity (MFI) of MitoTracker Deep Red (MTdr) in CD4+ and CD8+ T cells from healthy donors and RRMM. Representative histograms (left) and box and whisker plots (right). **(B)** Proportion of CD4/8 T cells with high ($MTdr^{hi}$), low-intermediate ($Mtdr^{lo-int}$), and absent ($MTdr^{-}$) mitochondrial mass by MFI. Representative histogram (left) and stacked bar charts (right). **(C,D)** Box and whisker plots showing mitochondrial mass by MFI in CD4+ and CD8+ T cell subsets from RRMM and HD by **(C)** treatment group or by **(D)** T cell subset (with no ASCT and ASCT combined for RRMM). Study groups as described in **Figure 1**. Statistical significance in all figures was determined using multiple Student's *t* tests with the Holm–Sidak method applied ($^{*}p < 0.05$, $^{**}p < 0.01$, $^{***}p < 0.001$).

patients compared to HD, but there was no significant difference for $CD8^+$ T cells (**Figure 7A**). The RRMM population appeared to be bimodal and, to compare the phenotypic composition of these two subpopulations, we back-gated $TMRM^-$ and $TMRM^+$ events (**Figure 7B**, left). A high proportion of $TMRM^+$ T cells were T_{CM} phenotype, particularly within the $CD4^+$ T cell population (**Figure 7B**, right), suggesting that T_{CM} cells are the most metabolically active subset.

DISCUSSION

Autologous stem cell transplant remains a backbone of MM treatment in medically fit patients, but our findings suggest that ASCT and lymphopenia-inducing therapies in MM have a largely irrecoverable effect on the $CD4^+$ T cell population. We illustrate that these therapies contribute toward a reduction in the CD4:8 ratio (**Figure 1**) and $CD4^+$ T_N cells (**Figure 2**), with a skewing of the T cell population toward a predominance of $CD8^+$ T_{EM} and T_{EMRA} cells, thereby accelerating changes seen with immunosenescence. Prior analysis of these trial populations at baseline additionally identified increased IFNγ production in RRMM, largely from $CD8^+$ T cells (23), which would be consistent with our observation of a predominance of $CD8^+$ T_{EM} and T_{EMRA} cells. The paucity of new thymic emigrants and a heavy reliance on homeostatic proliferation of oligoclonal $CD8^+$ T cells to reconstitute the T cell pool will likely significantly affect an individual's ability to respond to new or recall antigens, whether in the form of vaccination or infection. Analysis of the molecular biomarker $p16^{INK4a}$ (p16) suggested that ASCT induces molecular aging of T cells (37), providing further evidence of the detrimental effect of ASCT.

We acknowledge some limitations in our analysis including the restriction of T cell analysis to the PB compartment [although other studies have pointed to similarities in T cell populations from the PB and BM (23, 38)], the superiority of newer technologies such as mass spectrometry to better identify canonical populations, and the low numbers of samples in the RRMM group.

Nevertheless, our findings are particularly relevant for the utility and production of autologous CAR-T cells in MM. It appears that CAR-T cell production is best achieved with relatively undifferentiated T cells, such as T_N and stem cell memory subsets (39, 40). In mouse models of lymphoma, CAR-T cells derived from T_N and T_{CM} cells were shown to be more efficacious than those from than T_{EM} cells due to superior cytokine production of $CD4^+$ T cells and cytotoxicity of $CD8^+$ T cells (41). Furthermore, the potency of CAR-T cell therapy is dramatically enhanced by generating $CD8^+$ CAR-T cells from T_{CM} cultured with $CD4^+$ T cells. In humans, Garfall et al. (42) found that a higher frequency of $CD8^+CD45RO^-CD27^+$ T cells and a higher CD4:8 ratio at the time of leukapheresis for CAR-T production were the key factors associated with superior clinical outcome. Therefore, a CAR-T product generated from T cells from a heavily pre-treated, immunosenescent individual would be expected to be impaired. A practical approach in the clinic to maximize the effectiveness of a CAR-T cell product in MM patients could be to collect and store T cells prior to ASCT, before the shift in composition of the T cell population, when a higher number of naïve and stem cell memory T cells might be collected.

It was, however, interesting to note that our findings of an increase in the proportion of $CD4^+$ T cells with a T_{CM} phenotype in LEN/DEX-treated RRMM (**Figure 2C**) were also mirrored in the QUIREDEX trial (LEN $\pm$ DEX in high-risk smoldering MM)

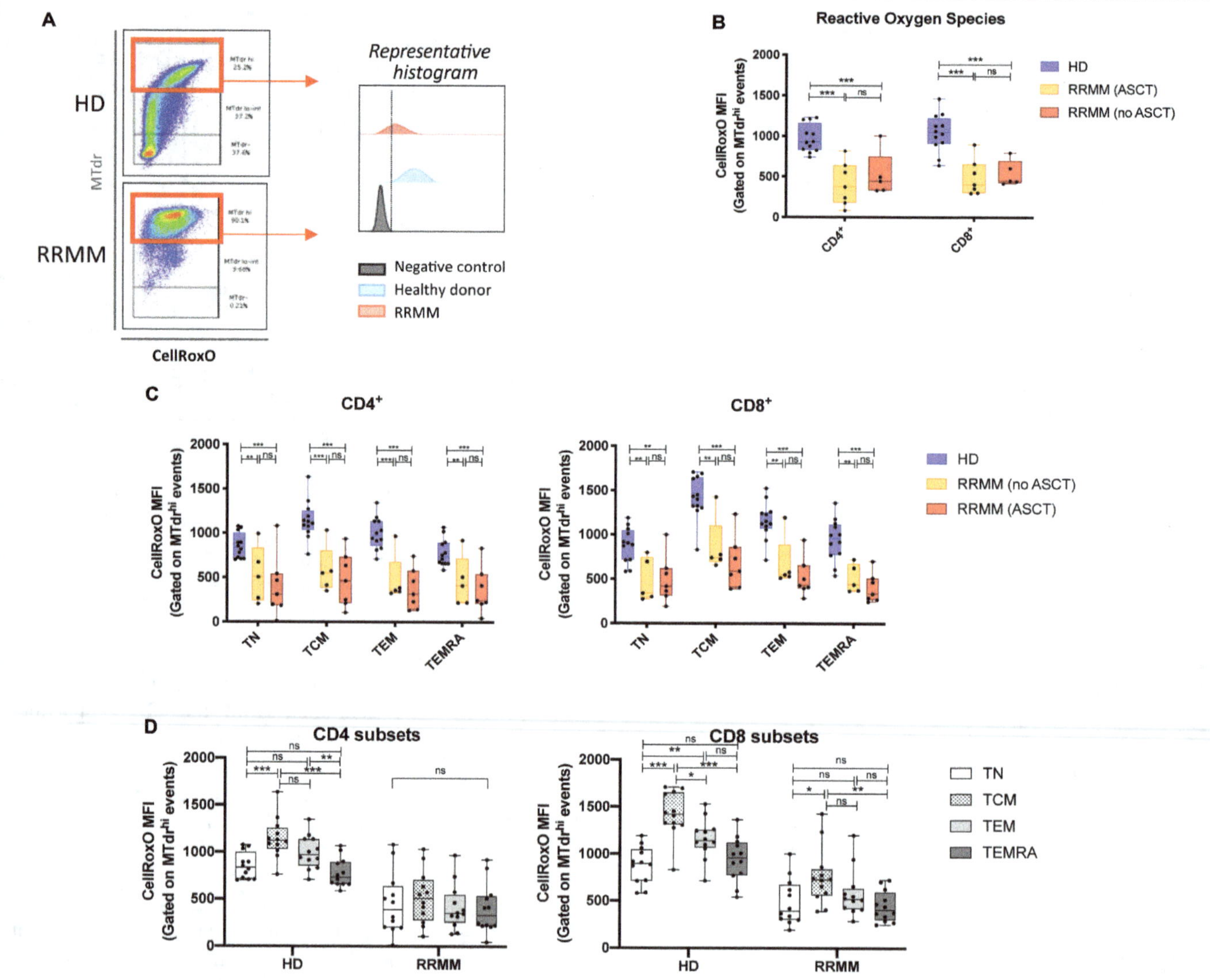

FIGURE 6 | Reactive oxygen species (ROS) levels in RRMM. **(A)** Gating strategy for assessment of ROS in CD4$^+$ and CD8$^+$ T cells with high mitochondrial mass (MTdr hi cells), using geometric mean fluorescence intensity (MFI) of CellRox Orange (CellRoxO). **(B)** Box and whisker plots of CellRoxO MFI in CD4$^+$ and CD8$^+$ T cells from RRMM and HD. **(C)** Box and whisker plots of CellRoxO MFI in CD4$^+$ and CD8$^+$ T cell subsets from RRMM and HD. **(D)** Comparison of CellRoxO MFI in T cell differentiation subsets across RRMM (pooled) and HD. Study groups as described in **Figure 1**. Statistical significance in all figures was determined using multiple Student's *t*-tests with the Holm–Sidak method applied ($^*p < 0.05$, $^{**}p < 0.01$, $^{***}p < 0.001$).

(43). This trial reported a significant increase in the proportion of CD4$^+$ T_{CM} cells by cycle 9 of treatment and, moreover, CD4$^+$ T cells were both functional in terms of cytokine production and proliferative as assessed by expression of activation and proliferation markers. It is not clear, however, whether this change is indicative of re-engagement of the immune system in disease control and/or is related to lenalidomide treatment, and we await the long-term outcome of this trial.

We also show that the frequency of PD1$^+$CD4$^+$ T cells increases post-ASCT and in RRMM, particularly within the CD4$^+$ T_{CM} cell subset (**Figure 3**), which would be expected to impede tumor surveillance and DC vaccination. In previous work, we demonstrated that the frequency of T_{REGS} increases post-ASCT (**Supplementary Figure 5**) and with LEN/DEX in RRMM (44), which could upregulate PD-L1 expression on DCs. However, increased PD-1 expression can also indicate proliferation, as PD-1 is upregulated on initial T cell activation and its expression increases with sustained TCR signaling (45) or chronic antigen stimulation due to infection or tumor. To explore this possibility, further analysis of epitope specificity, TCR repertoire, and telomere length would be of interest. It is possible that a large proportion of these cells are CMV-specific, as oligoclonal expansions can develop in older humans (46), but it is also plausible that this population contains MM-specific T cell clones, the presence of which have been associated with long-term survival (47, 48).

Transcriptional and metabolic analyses of CD4$^+$ and CD8$^+$ T cells in RRMM showed significant increases in FAO transcripts

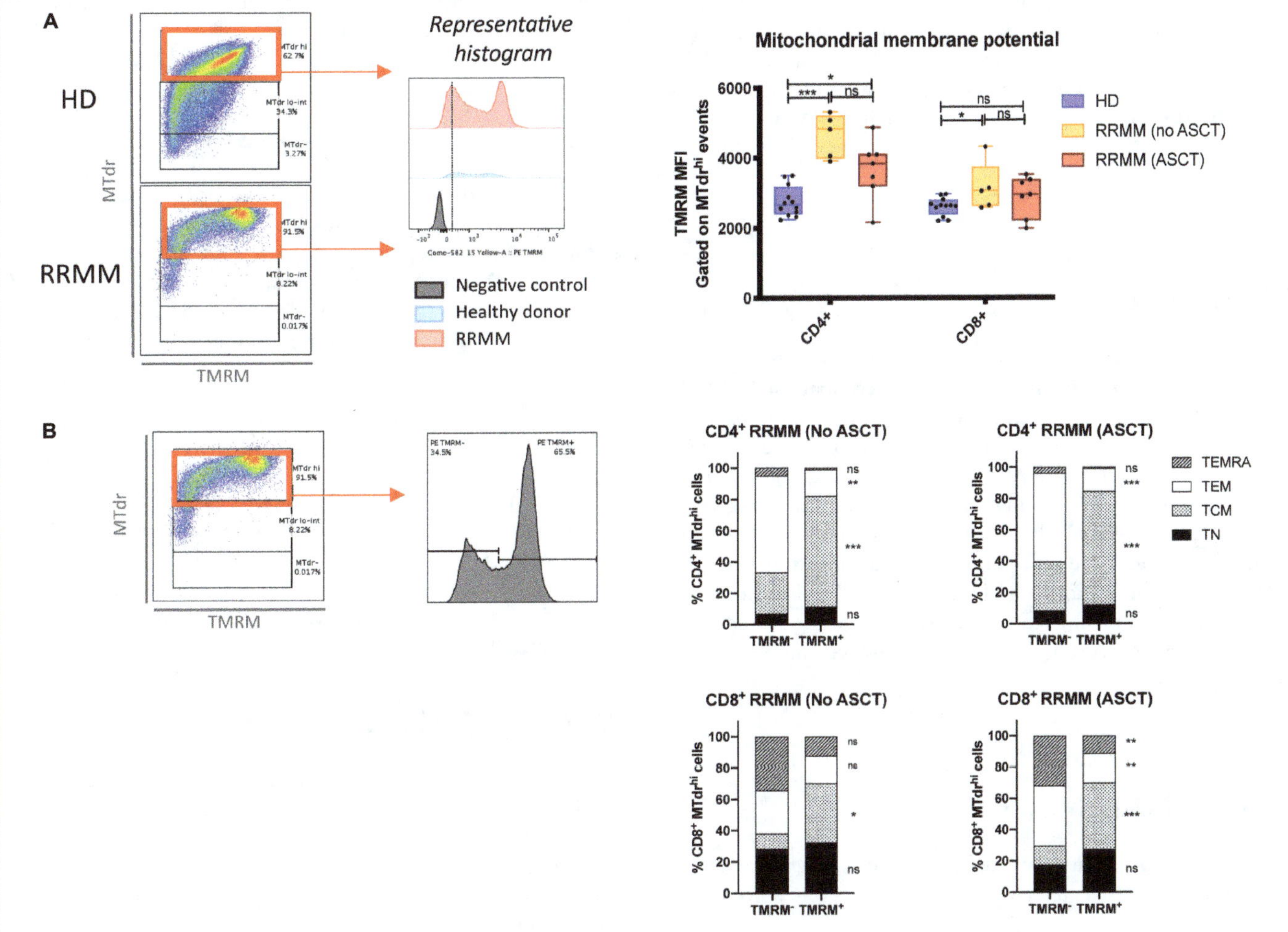

FIGURE 7 | Mitochondrial membrane potential (Δψm) in T cell populations in RRMM. Mitochondrial membrane potential was measured in T cell subsets by geometric mean fluorescence intensity (MFI) of TMRM. **(A)** TMRM MFI in CD4$^+$ and CD8$^+$ T cells from healthy donors and RRMM: (left) Gating strategy and (right) scatter plots. **(B)** CD4$^+$ and CD8$^+$ T cells with high mitochondrial mass (MTdr staining) from RRMM were further subdivided into TMRM$^-$ and TMRM$^+$ events (gating strategy to the left) and backgated into T cell differentiation subsets, as shown in stacked bar charts of the mean frequency (right). Study groups as described in **Figure 1**. Statistical significance was determined using multiple Student's *t*-tests with the Holm–Sidak method applied (*$p < 0.05$, **$p < 0.01$, ***$p < 0.001$).

(**Figure 4**) and increased mitochondrial mass (**Figure 5**). Memory T cells are known to have higher mitochondrial mass and engage FAO for their energy requirements, while T_N cells have low mitochondrial mass and low energy requirements (34). Accordingly, the shift in cell proportions after ACST, with a loss of T_N cells and an increase in $T_{CM/EM}$ cells, is likely to account for some of the increase in FAO transcripts and mitochondrial mass. However, it should be noted that an increase in mitochondrial mass was observed at all T cell differentiation states. This global increase could be driven by lymphopenia-associated IL-15 signaling, as IL-15 is known to promote *CPT1a* expression and FAO engagement and promote mitochondrial biogenesis (49, 50). Mitochondrial mass was highest in T_{CM} cells and, notably, T_N cells. This suggests that the remaining T_N cells are not truly naïve and they may have acquired some memory-associated metabolic characteristics during ASCT, likely from lymphopenia-associated signals.

Given the increased mitochondrial mass in T cells in RRMM, the reduction in ROS levels was unexpected (**Figure 6**). A potential explanation for discordance between mitochondrial mass and ROS production is that the mitochondria that accumulate in RRMM T cells may be less metabolically fit. This is consistent with the relatively low Δψm that was observed in CD8$^+$ T cells with RRMM (**Figure 7A**). This effect may again be driven by lymphopenia-induced IL-15 signaling, as it was recently shown that effector CD8$^+$ T cells transferred into irradiated mice had increased mitochondrial content but lower Δψm compared with those transferred into IL-15-deficient irradiated mice (13). In contrast, RRMM CD4$^+$ T cells exhibited elevated Δψm compared with HD but high Δψm associated with the T_{CM}

subset (**Figure 7B**), highlighting that $CD4^+$ T_{CM} remain a metabolically active subset. Clarification of the metabolic fitness of these cell subsets with further metabolic studies would be beneficial. Unfortunately, this was not feasible in this analysis due to the effects on mitochondria by lengthy cryopreservation of these samples and limited duplicate samples but would be important in future prospective studies.

CONCLUSION

Taken together, our findings show that the composition and metabolic profile of the T cell compartment shifts significantly over time in MM. This is likely a consequence of an interplay between aging, duration of disease, and cumulative treatment, but ASCT clearly has a dominant role. Given the inherent variability in these processes, the use of phenotypic and metabolic biomarkers to immunologically profile a patient at the time of clinical decision making will aid in directing and optimizing therapy for MM. Furthermore, if metabolic remodeling can be attenuated without reducing reconstitution after ASCT, it may better preserve functionality in T cell populations.

ETHICS STATEMENT

The studies involving human participants were reviewed and approved by Peter MacCallum Cancer Centre. The patients/participants provided their written informed consent to participate in this study.

AUTHOR CONTRIBUTIONS

RC designed and performed the laboratory research, analyzed the data, and wrote the manuscript. KQ provided significant assistance with writing. SH, HQ, HP, and DR were principal investigators for the Litvacc and/or RevLite clinical trials. RK and DR assisted with the research design and editing of the manuscript. All authors contributed to the article and approved the submitted version.

FUNDING

This research was funded by the Leukaemia Foundation Australia and supported by the University of Melbourne, the Royal Melbourne Hospital, and the Peter MacCallum Cancer Centre. Bioinformatic analysis of the RNA-Seq data was provided by Jessica Chung at Melbourne Bioinformatics (University of Melbourne).

ACKNOWLEDGMENTS

We acknowledge the assistance of Dr. Sarah Gabriel and Prof. Axel Kallies at the Peter Doherty Institute for Infection and Immunity with the mitochondrial staining experiments. cDNA library preparation and RNA sequencing were performed by the Australian Genome Research Facility (Victorian Comprehensive Cancer Centre, Melbourne).

REFERENCES

1. Rajkumar SV, Dimopoulos MA, Palumbo A, Bladé J, Merlini G, Mateos M-V, et al. International myeloma working group updated criteria for the diagnosis of multiple myeloma. *Lancet Oncol.* (2014) 15:e538–48. doi: 10.1016/S1470-2045(14)70442-5
2. Röllig C, Knop S, Bornhäuser M. Multiple myeloma. *Lancet.* (2015) 385:2197–208.
3. Turesson I, Velez R, Kristinsson SY, Landgren O. Patterns of multiple myeloma during the past 5 decades: stable incidence rates for all age groups in the population but rapidly changing age distribution in the clinic. *Mayo Clin Proc.* (2010) 85:225–30. doi: 10.4065/mcp.2009.0426
4. Harrison SJ, Quach H, Link E, Seymour JF, Ritchie DS, Ruell S, et al. A high rate of durable responses with romidepsin, bortezomib, and dexamethasone in relapsed or refractory multiple myeloma. *Blood.* (2011) 118:6274–83. doi: 10.1182/blood-2011-03-339879
5. Costa LJ, Brill IK, Omel J, Godby K, Kumar SK, Brown EE. Recent trends in multiple myeloma incidence and survival by age, race, and ethnicity in the United States. *Blood Adv.* (2017) 1:282–7. doi: 10.1182/bloodadvances.2016002493
6. Herndler-Brandstetter D, Ishigame H, Flavell RA. How to define biomarkers of human T cell aging and immunocompetence? *Front Immunol.* (2013) 4:136. doi: 10.3389/fimmu.2013.00136
7. Nikolich-Žugich J. Aging of the T cell compartment in mice and humans: from no naive expectations to foggy memories. *J Immunol.* (2014) 193:2622–9. doi: 10.4049/jimmunol.1401174
8. Williams KM, Hakim FT, Gress RE. T cell immune reconstitution following lymphodepletion. *Semin Immunol.* (2007) 19:318–30. doi: 10.1016/j.smim.2007.10.004
9. Douek DC, McFarland RD, Keiser PH, Gage EA, Massey JM, Haynes BF, et al. Changes in thymic function with age and during the treatment of HIV infection. *Nature.* (1998) 396:690–5. doi: 10.1038/25374
10. Mackall CL, Stein D, Fleisher TA, Brown MR, Hakim FT, Bare CV, et al. Prolonged CD4 depletion after sequential autologous peripheral blood progenitor cell infusions in children and young adults. *Blood.* (2000) 96:754–62. doi: 10.1182/blood.v96.2.754
11. Zhang X, Sun S, Hwang I, Tough DF, Sprent J. Potent and selective stimulation of memory-phenotype CD8+ T cells in vivo by IL-15. *Immunity.* (1998) 8:591–9. doi: 10.1016/s1074-7613(00)80564-6
12. Le Saout C, Luckey MA, Villarino AV, Smith M, Hasley RB, Myers TG, et al. IL-7–dependent STAT1 activation limits homeostatic CD4+ T cell expansion. *JCI Insight.* (2017) 2:e96228.
13. Xu A, Bhanumathy KK, Wu J, Ye Z, Freywald A, Leary SC, et al. IL-15 signaling promotes adoptive effector T-cell survival and memory formation in irradiation-induced lymphopenia. *Cell Biosci.* (2016) 6:30.

14. Klarquist J, Chitrakar A, Pennock ND, Kilgore AM, Blain T, Zheng C, et al. Clonal expansion of vaccine-elicited T cells is independent of aerobic glycolysis. *Sci Immunol.* (2018) 3:eaas9822. doi: 10.1126/sciimmunol.aas9822
15. Davenport B, Eberlein J, van der Heide V, Jhun K, Nguyen TT, Victorino F, et al. Aging of antiviral CD8+ memory T cells fosters increased survival, metabolic adaptations, and lymphoid tissue homing. *J Immunol Am Assoc Immunol.* (2019) 202:460–75. doi: 10.4049/jimmunol.1801277
16. Goronzy JJ, Li G, Yang Z, Weyand CM. The janus head of T cell aging – autoimmunity and immunodeficiency. *Front Immunol.* (2013) 4:131. doi: 10.3389/fimmu.2013.00131
17. Henson SM, Lanna A, Riddell NE, Franzese O, Macaulay R, Griffiths SJ, et al. p38 signaling inhibits mTORC1-independent autophagy in senescent human CD8(+) T cells. *J Clin Invest.* (2014) 124:4004–16. doi: 10.1172/jci75051
18. Lanna A, Gomes DCO, Muller-Durovic B, McDonnell T, Escors D, Gilroy DW, et al. A sestrin-dependent Erk-Jnk-p38 MAPK activation complex inhibits immunity during aging. *Nat Immunol.* (2017) 18:354–63. doi: 10.1038/ni.3665
19. Harmer D, Falank C, Reagan MR. Interleukin-6 interweaves the bone marrow microenvironment, bone loss, and multiple myeloma. *Front Endocrinol.* (2019) 9:3397. doi: 10.3389/fendo.2018.00788
20. Joshua DE, Brown RD, Ho PJ, Gibson J. Comprehensive review. *Clini Lymphoma Myeloma.* (2011) 8:283–6.
21. Suen H, Brown R, Yang S, Ho PJ, Gibson J, Joshua D. The failure of immune checkpoint blockade in multiple myeloma with PD-1 inhibitors in a phase 1 study. *Leukemia.* (2015) 29:1621–2. doi: 10.1038/leu.2015.104
22. Cooke RE, Koldej R, Ritchie D. Immunotherapeutics in multiple myeloma: how can translational mouse models help? *J Oncol.* (2019) 2019:18.
23. Cooke RE, Gherardin NA, Harrison SJ, Quach H, Godfrey DI, Prince M, et al. Spontaneous onset and transplant models of the Vk*MYC mouse show immunological sequelae comparable to human multiple myeloma. *J Transl Med.* (2016) 14:259.
24. Gherardin NA. *Unconventional T Cells: from Basic Biology to Multiple Myeloma. Minerva Access.* (2016). Available online at: http://hdl.handle.net/11343/59299
25. Kay NE. Blood levels of immune cells predict survival in myeloma patients: results of an Eastern Cooperative Oncology Group phase 3 trial for newly diagnosed multiple myeloma patients. *Blood.* (2001) 98:23–8. doi: 10.1182/blood.v98.1.23
26. Harrison SJ, Khot AS, Tsin T, Hsu AK, Chen K, Loudovaris M, et al. Low dose lenalidomide and dexamethasone induction followed by autologous transplantation in untreated patients with myeloma is associated with high response rates and preservation of CD8, but not CD4 or NK cellular immunity. *Blood.* (2011) 118:1862. doi: 10.1182/blood.v118.21.1862.1862
27. Hsu AK, Quach H, Tai T, Prince HM, Harrison SJ, Trapani JA, et al. The immunostimulatory effect of lenalidomide on NK-cell function is profoundly inhibited by concurrent dexamethasone therapy. *Blood.* (2011) 117:1605–13. doi: 10.1182/blood-2010-04-278432
28. Hsu AK, Gherardin N, Quach H, Harrison SJ, Prince HM, Ritchie D. CD57+ NK CELLS ARE increased in patients with multiple myeloma and ARE primed effectors for ADCC, but NOT natural cytotoxicty. Neeson P, editor. *Blood.* (2013) 122:1904. doi: 10.1182/blood.v122.21.1904.1904
29. Liu R, Holik AZ, Su S, Jansz N, Chen K, Leong HS, et al. Why weight? Modelling sample and observational level variability improves power in RNA-seq analyses. *Nucleic Acids Res.* (2015) 43:e97. doi: 10.1093/nar/gkv412
30. Chung DJ, Pronschinske KB, Shyer JA, Sharma S, Leung S, Curran SA, et al. T-cell exhaustion in multiple myeloma relapse after autotransplant: optimal timing of immunotherapy. *Cancer Immunol Res.* (2016) 4:61–71 doi: 10.1158/2326-6066.cir-15-0055
31. Hallett WHD, Jing W, Drobyski WR, Johnson BD. Immunosuppressive effects of multiple myeloma are overcome by PD-L1 blockade. *Biol Blood Marrow Transplant.* (2011) 17:1133–45. doi: 10.1016/j.bbmt.2011.03.011
32. Kearl TJ, Jing W, Gershan JA, Johnson BD. Programmed death receptor-1/programmed death receptor ligand-1 blockade after transient lymphodepletion to treat myeloma. *J Immunol.* (2013) 190:5620–8. doi: 10.4049/jimmunol.1202005
33. Tkachev V, Goodell S, Opipari AW, Hao L-Y, Franchi L, Glick GD, et al. Programmed death-1 controls T cell survival by regulating oxidative metabolism. *J Immunol.* (2015) 194:5789–800. doi: 10.4049/jimmunol.1402180
34. Man K, Kallies A. Synchronizing transcriptional control of T cell metabolism and function. *Nat Rev Immunol.* (2015) 15:574–84. doi: 10.1038/nri3874
35. O'Neill LAJ, Kishton RJ, Rathmell J. A guide to immunometabolism for immunologists. *Nat Rev Immunol.* (2016) 16:553–65. doi: 10.1038/nri.2016.70
36. Buck MD, O'Sullivan D, Pearce EL. T cell metabolism drives immunity. *J Exp Med.* (2015) 212:1345–60. doi: 10.1084/jem.20151159
37. Rosko A, Hofmeister C, Benson D, Efebera Y, Huang Y, Gillahan J, et al. Autologous hematopoietic stem cell transplant induces the molecular aging of T-cells in multiple myeloma. *Bone Marrow Transplant.* (2015) 50:1379–81. doi: 10.1038/bmt.2015.143
38. Kourelis TV, Villasboas JC, Jessen E, Dasari S, Dispenzieri A, Jevremovic D, et al. Mass cytometry dissects T cell heterogeneity in the immune tumor microenvironment of common dysproteinemias at diagnosis and after first line therapies. *Blood Cancer J.* (2019) 9:72.
39. Crompton JG, Clever D, Vizcardo R, Rao M, Restifo NP. Reprogramming antitumor immunity. *Trends Immunol.* (2014) 35:178–85. doi: 10.1016/j.it.2014.02.003
40. Sukumar M, Kishton RJ, Restifo NP. Metabolic reprograming of anti-tumor immunity. *Curr Opin Immunol.* (2017) 46:14–22. doi: 10.1016/j.coi.2017.03.011
41. Sommermeyer D, Hudecek M, Kosasih PL, Gogishvili T, Maloney DG, Turtle CJ, et al. Chimeric antigen receptor-modified T cells derived from defined CD8+ and CD4+ subsets confer superior antitumor reactivity in vivo. *Leukemia.* (2015) 30:492–500. doi: 10.1038/leu.2015.247
42. Garfall AL, Dancy EK, Cohen AD, Hwang W-T, Fraietta JA, Davis MM, et al. T-cell phenotypes associated with effective CAR T-cell therapy in postinduction vs relapsed multiple myeloma. *Blood Adv.* (2019) 3:2812–5. doi: 10.1182/bloodadvances.2019000600
43. Paiva B, Mateos M-V, Sanchez-Abarca LI, Puig N, Vidriales M-B, López-Corral L, et al. Immune status of high-risk smoldering multiple myeloma patients and its therapeutic modulation under LenDex: a longitudinal analysis. *Blood.* (2016) 127:1151–62. doi: 10.1182/blood-2015-10-662320
44. Quach H, Ritchie D, Neeson P, Harrison S, Tai T, Tainton K, et al. Regulatory T cells (Treg) are depressed in patients with relapsed/refractory multiple myeloma (MM) and increases towards normal range in responding patients treated with lenalidomide (LEN). *Blood.* (2008) 112:1696–1696. doi: 10.1182/blood.v112.11.1696.1696
45. Chikuma S, Terawaki S, Hayashi T, Nabeshima R, Yoshida T, Shibayama S, et al. PD-1-mediated suppression of IL-2 production induces CD8+ T cell anergy in vivo. *J Immunol.* (2009) 182:6682–9. doi: 10.4049/jimmunol.0900080
46. Tu W, Rao S. Mechanisms underlying T cell immunosenescence: aging and cytomegalovirus infection. *Front Microbiol.* (2016) 7:2111. doi: 10.3389/fmicb.2016.02111
47. Brown RD, Spencer A, Joy Ho P, Kennedy N, Kabani K, Yang S, et al. Prognostically significant cytotoxic T cell clones are stimulated after thalidomide therapy in patients with multiple myeloma. *Leuk Lymphoma.* (2009) 50:1860–4. doi: 10.3109/10428190903216804
48. Bryant C, Suen H, Brown R, Yang S, Favaloro J, Aklilu E, et al. Long-term survival in multiple myeloma is associated with a distinct immunological profile, which includes proliferative cytotoxic T-cell clones and a favourable

Treg/Th17 balance. *Blood Cancer J.* (2013) 3:e148. doi: 10.1038/bcj.2013.34

49. van der Windt GJW, Everts B, Chang C-H, Curtis JD, Freitas TC, Amiel E, et al. Mitochondrial respiratory capacity is a critical regulator of CD8+ T cell memory development. *Immunity.* (2012) 36:68–78. doi: 10.1016/j.immuni.2011.12.007
50. O'Sullivan D, van der Windt GJW, Huang SC-C, Curtis JD, Chang C-H, Buck MD, et al. Memory CD8(+) T cells use cell-intrinsic lipolysis to support the metabolic programming necessary for development. *Immunity.* (2014) 41:75–88. doi: 10.1016/j.immuni.2014.06.005

14

Mutual interaction of basophils and T cells in chronic inflammatory diseases

Marika Sarfati[1], Keiko Wakahara[2], Laurence Chapuy[1] and Guy Delespesse[1]*

[1] Centre de Recherche du Centre Hospitalier de l'Université de Montréal (CRCHUM), Université de Montréal, Montréal, QC, Canada, [2] Department of Respiratory Medicine, Nagoya University Graduate School of Medicine, Nagoya, Japan

Edited by:
Elisabetta Padovan,
University of Basel, Switzerland

Reviewed by:
Raffaele De Palma,
Second University of Naples, Italy
Michaela Fux,
University Hospital Inselspital Bern, Switzerland
Dietmar M. W. Zaiss,
University of Edinburgh, UK

***Correspondence:**
Marika Sarfati,
Immunoregulation Laboratory, Centre de Recherche du Centre Hospitalier de l'Université de Montréal, Tour Viger (R-12/424/204), 900 St-Denis Street East, Montréal, QC H2X0A9, Canada
m.sarfati@umontreal.ca

Basophils are, together with mast cells, typical innate effector cells of allergen-induced IgE-dependent allergic diseases. Both cell types express the high-affinity receptor for IgE (FcεR1), release histamine, inflammatory mediators, and cytokines following FcεR1 cross-linking. Basophils are rare granulocytes in blood, lymphoid, and non-lymphoid tissues, and the difficulties to detect and isolate these cells has hampered the study of their biology and the understanding of their possible role in pathology. Furthermore, the existence of other FcεR1-expressing cells, including professional Ag-presenting dendritic cells, generated some controversy regarding the ability of basophils to express MHC Class II molecules, present Ag and drive naïve T cell differentiation into Th2 cells. The focus of this review is to present the recent advances on the interactions between basophils and peripheral blood and tissue memory Th1, Th2, and Th17 cells, as well as their potential role in IgE-independent non-allergic chronic inflammatory disorders, including human inflammatory bowel diseases. Basophils interactions with the innate players of IgE-dependent allergic inflammation, particularly innate lymphoid cells, will also be considered. The previously unrecognized function for basophils in skewing adaptive immune responses opens novel perspectives for the understanding of their contribution to the pathogenesis of inflammatory diseases.

Keywords: basophils, memory T cells, Th17 cells, Th2 cells, inflammatory bowel diseases

Basophils in Type 2 Immune Responses

Basophils represent <1% of all blood leukocytes. Together with mast cells, they are regarded as typical effector cells of IgE-dependent allergic inflammation (1, 2). Because both types of cells express high levels of the high-affinity receptor for IgE (FcεR1), and rapidly release histamine and inflammatory mediators upon cross-linking of FcεR1 by IgE-allergen complexes, basophils were long considered as redundant granulocytes lacking unique functions (3). Until recently, the investigations of the functional properties of basophils have been hampered by the difficulty of detecting and purifying these rare cells in blood and tissues from mice and humans (4). Despite the development of transgenic mice (IL-4-eGFP, Basoph8) that allow the tracking or transient depletion of basophils *in vivo*, conflicting results were generated regarding the antigen-presenting function of basophils and their ability to trump DCs in the priming of Th2 responses (5–8). However, it was reported that cooperation between highly purified murine basophils and DCs, isolated from blood or lungs, is required to induce *in vitro* Th2 cell differentiation (9, 10). In this context, DCs ensure naïve T cell proliferation and basophils provide IL-4 to drive Th2 polarization. As a consequence, a careful exclusion of trace amounts of MHC class $II^+Fc\varepsilon R1^+$ DCs from basophils preparation is mandatory to draw valid conclusions about any yet unrecognized *in vitro* function of these rare cells, especially in human studies (11).

Despite their low frequency in blood, increased numbers of basophils were detected in the tissues of several IgE-dependent allergic diseases that include allergic rhinitis, atopic dermatitis, and asthma (2, 12). How basophils are attracted to the site of allergen challenge remains to be clarified. Histamine and PGD2, which are produced by mast cells, as well as IL-3 secreted by activated T cells have been proposed to play crucial roles in the recruitment of basophils to tissues, since basophils express histamine receptors, CRTH2 (i.e., PGD2 receptor) and IL-3 receptors (13–15). In tissues, basophils may interact with resident memory T cells, as demonstrated by two-photon microscopy (8). Hence, prolonged contacts between basophils and T cells occurred in the inflamed lungs but not in the mediastinal lymph nodes (LNs) of parasite-infected mice. The same study also revealed that activated T cells induced IL-4 secretion by basophils in affected lungs. Optimal IL-4 production by basophils required a direct cell/cell contact, as well as the presence of IL-3, a cytokine that promotes expansion and survival of basophils. Conversely, *in vitro* interactions between pulmonary basophils and lung $CD4^+$ T cell promoted IL-4-dependent T cell survival and amplified release of Th2 cytokines, without inducing memory T cell expansion (9). In experimental asthma, transfer of lung basophils worsens ongoing Th2 responses by increasing airway inflammation and local IL-4 and IL-13 expression (9). Furthermore, human basophils increase IL-4 expression in effector memory T cells *in vitro*. Notably, responding T cells mainly included $CRTH2^+$ cells, corroborating the *in vivo* and *in vitro* data seen in mice. In addition to Th2 cells that produce IL-4, IL-5, and IL-13, double IL-4- and IL-17-expressing memory $CD4^+$ T cells were detected in severe asthmatic patients and in lungs of mice developing experimental asthma (16). In contrast, human basophils were not reported to promote the generation of Th2/Th17 double positive cells. The basophil enhancing effect on memory Th2 responses was partially contact dependent, but did not involve OX40/OX40L, CTLA4/B7family, and CD2/LFA3 interactions. Because IL-3-stimulated basophils express RANKL and activated Th cells may express RANK (17, 18), we speculate that RANK–RANKL pairs of molecules may represent other potential candidates involved in basophil-T cell interactions.

Cellular aggregates made of basophils and memory $CD4^+$ T cells were detected in the dermis of patients with atopic dermatitis and in a mouse model of TSLP-mediated contact dermatitis, underlying the key role of basophils in T cell-mediated skin allergic disorders (19). However, basophils may regulate type 2 inflammatory responses by interacting with cells other than T cells. Indeed, innate immune cells, such as macrophages, innate lymphoid type 2 (ILC2), and eosinophils, are major contributors of allergic lung and skin inflammatory responses (20, 21). Moreover, keratinocyte-derived TSLP activates basophils that results in local recruitment, activation, and proliferation of ILC2, which is mediated by basophil-derived IL-4 (19). This mechanism initiates experimental atopic dermatitis and appears essential for the development of food allergy induced by the application of food antigen to inflamed skin (22). Furthermore, the interactions of activated basophils with ILC2, fibroblasts, and/or endothelial cells regulate recruitment of eosinophils in experimental models of contact dermatitis and allergic asthma (21, 23).

Taken collectively, these finding indicate that, although basophils do not appear to initiate IgE-dependent allergic disease, the interaction between basophil and memory T cell in inflamed tissues may be bidirectional, thus contributing to the exacerbation of chronic allergic airway inflammation at late stages. In support of this, asthmatic patients are successfully treated by administration of Omalizumab, a monoclonal antibody to IgE that prevents IgE binding to $Fc\varepsilon R1$ and regulates basophil homeostasis (24). It has been suggested that its therapeutic efficacy largely result from its effect on basophils, since these cells have a much shorter life than mast cells. In fact, the improved clinical outcome of allergic patients following Omalizumab therapy was associated with a reduction in circulating basophil numbers (24).

Basophils in IgE-Independent Th Responses

Basophils were historically associated exclusively with IgE-dependent allergic disorders. However, TSLP-activated basophils induce and perpetuate experimental eosinophilic esophagitis (EoE), which may be triggered in the absence of IgE and mast cells (25). Notably, the circulating number of basophils is increased in patients with EoE. Similarly, increased numbers of basophils are observed in blood of patients with chronic inflammatory bowel diseases (IBD) (26). Basophilia is found in both Crohn's disease (CD) and ulcerative colitis (UC), the two main chronic relapsing IBD types that are associated with Th17/Th1 and Th17 or Th2 cells, respectively (27). Strikingly, increased percentages of basophils, but not of mast cells are found in the inflamed relative to the non-inflamed colonic mucosa in both CD and UC patients (26). In contrast, basophils are not detected in the intestinal mucosa of non-IBD individuals. The accumulation of basophils in the inflamed colons of IBD patients suggests that these rare cells contribute to disease pathogenesis by influencing pathogenic T cell responses in tissues.

Indeed, similar to their ability to amplify human memory Th2 responses, basophils promote memory Th17 responses *in vitro* (11). Blood basophils as well as basophils isolated from inflamed colonic mucosa or the mesenteric LNs of IBD patients favor the emergence of memory $IL\text{-}17^+$, $IL\text{-}17^+/IFN\text{-}\gamma^+$ but not $IFN\text{-}\gamma^+$ single positive Th cells (26). Activation of $CD4^+$ T lymphocytes generates functionally distinct antigen-experienced T cells, namely, effector memory $CD62L^{low}CCR7^-$ (T_{EM}) that migrate to peripheral tissues and central memory $CD62L^{high}CCR7^+$ (T_{CM}) T cells, which retain the ability to enter LNs (28). Thus, basophils activated by either IL-3, IL-33, or TSLP increase Th17 and Th17/Th1 responses by IL-2-stimulated T_{EM} in the absence of APC, as well as by TCR-stimulated T_{CM} isolated from blood, which mimic memory T cell activation in mucosa and lymphoid tissues, respectively (11). More specifically, basophils promote cytokine production by autologous T_{EM} cells in a contact-independent manner that involves the ERK1/2-pathway. Basophil-derived histamine partially increases IL-17 expression through H_2 and H_4, but not H_1 receptors.

Interestingly, histamine alone cannot replace basophils in their pro-Th17 activity.

Basophils also enhance IL-22 production by T_{EM} cells but not T_{CM} (11). However, Sharma et al. (29, 30) reported that human basophils lack the ability to drive IL-22 or IL-17 memory $CD4^+$ T cell responses. The reasons for the apparent discrepancies might at least result from the analysis of unfractionated stimulated $CD45RO^+CD25^-$ $CD4^+$ T cells, which mainly comprises T_{CM}, in co-culture with IL-3-activated basophils. Also, the purity of basophils was $94 \pm 5\%$ in the latter studies (29, 30), in contrast to >99% purity in the former studies (11, 26), further highlighting the importance of assessing highly purified basophil preparations.

Lymphoid tissues represent the major site of memory T cells in the body relative to circulating pool (31). It is therefore essential, whenever feasible in humans, to assess the functions of T cells that are found in tissues. Basophils enhance Th17 and Th17/Th1 responses by T_{CM} and T_{EM} CD4 T cells isolated from mLNs of IBD patients (26). Furthermore, a small number of tissue memory T_{EM} express CCR7 in inflamed tissues and $CCR7^+$ T_{EM} cells are prone to exit the tissues and re-circulate (32, 33). Notably, $CCR7^+$ T_{EM} cells are the preferential targets of basophils for enhancing Th17 responses (26). A recent study demonstrates that CCR7 expression controls intestinal Th17 and Th1 balance in a model of TNF-α driven Crohn's-like ileitis (34). The CCR7-deficient mice or mice treated with anti-CCR7 mAb develop an exacerbated ileo-colitis, which is associated with retention of Th effectors in intestinal and extra-intestinal tissues, suggesting that recirculation of $CCR7^+$ T_{EM} contribute to intestinal homeostasis.

Immunoregulatory Activity of Basophils

Although basophils clearly amplify allergic skin and airway inflammation, several studies showed that these rare cells might also exert anti-inflammatory activities in the context of autoimmune disease, contact dermatitis, as well as colitis. In a mouse model of arthritis, IL-4 production by IL-33-activated basophils was found to enhance expression of the inhibitory Fcγ Receptor (FcγRIIb) on inflammatory macrophages and mediates the immunosuppressive response elicited by injection of intravenous immunoglobulin (IVIG) (35). A recent report indicates that upon IL-33 and IgE triggering, human basophils down-modulate monocyte activation *in vitro* (36). Furthermore, basophil-derived IL-4 significantly attenuates the intensity of skin inflammation by mediating the differentiation of inflammatory monocytes into alternatively activated M2 macrophages that are endowed with an immunosuppressive and anti-inflammatory activity (37).

Basophils display immunoregulatory activity by enhancing the suppressive activity of FOXP3-expressing regulatory T cells (Treg) *in vivo* and *in vitro* (38). In a mouse model of contact hypersensitivity, basophils mediate UVB-induced immune suppression by increasing Treg function and this immunosuppressive effect is reduced in amphiregulin (AREG)-deficient mice (39). Indeed, basophils express AREG, an epidermal cell growth factor-like cytokine that enhances Treg function (40). Finally, the *in vivo* role of basophils in pathologies affecting the gastrointestinal tract remains to be clarified. A direct pathogenic role has been proposed for murine basophils in experimental EoE, as well as in allergen-induced colitis in a humanized mice model (25, 41). On the other hand, basophils depletion aggravates colitis induced by adoptive transfer of T cells in lymphopenic mice (42).

Concluding Remarks

Overall, the *in vivo* function of mucosal or lymphoid human basophils warrants further investigations in allergic diseases, CD, and UC. Basophils accumulate in inflamed tissues in IgE-dependent, as well as IgE-independent inflammatory disorders whereby they may directly interact with memory T cells to augment Th2, Th17, and Th17/Th1 effector responses. The accumulation of basophils in tissues indicates that they may contribute to the aggravation and flare up of the disease. Conversely, their increased numbers may as well reflect a negative regulatory feedback mechanism to dampen inflammation. Nonetheless, basophils represent an attractive therapeutic target for patients with chronic inflammatory disorders. This opens therapeutic avenues by targeting basophils and histamine using the clinically safe non-degranulating anti-IgE human monoclonal antibody (Omalizumab) (43) or selective anti-histamine receptor drugs (44).

References

1. Voehringer D. Basophils in allergic immune responses. *Curr Opin Immunol* (2011) **23**(6):789–93. doi:10.1016/j.coi.2011.09.005
2. Siracusa MC, Kim BS, Spergel JM, Artis D. Basophils and allergic inflammation. *J Allergy Clin Immunol* (2013) **132**(4):789–801. doi:10.1016/j.jaci.2013.07.046
3. Merluzzi S, Betto E, Ceccaroni AA, Magris R, Giunta M, Mion F. Mast cells, basophils and B cell connection network. *Mol Immunol* (2015) **63**(1):94–103. doi:10.1016/j.molimm.2014.02.016
4. Duriancik DM, Hoag KA. Mistaken identity: purified basophils likely contaminated with dendritic cells. *Cytometry A* (2014) **85**(7):570–2. doi:10.1002/cyto.a.22476
5. Otsuka A, Kabashima K. Mast cells and basophils in cutaneous immune responses. *Allergy* (2015) **70**(2):131–40. doi:10.1111/all.12526
6. Karasuyama H, Yamanishi Y. Basophils have emerged as a key player in immunity. *Curr Opin Immunol* (2014) **31**:1–7. doi:10.1016/j.coi.2014.07.004
7. Hammad H, Plantinga M, Deswarte K, Pouliot P, Willart MA, Kool M, et al. Inflammatory dendritic cells – not basophils – are necessary and sufficient for induction of Th2 immunity to inhaled house dust mite allergen. *J Exp Med* (2010) **207**(10):2097–111. doi:10.1084/jem.20101563
8. Sullivan BM, Liang HE, Bando JK, Wu D, Cheng LE, McKerrow JK, et al. Genetic analysis of basophil function in vivo. *Nat Immunol* (2011) **12**(6):527–35. doi:10.1038/ni.2036
9. Wakahara K, Van VQ, Baba N, Begin P, Rubio M, Delespesse G, et al. Basophils are recruited to inflamed lungs and exacerbate memory Th2 responses in mice and humans. *Allergy* (2013) **68**(2):180–9. doi:10.1111/all.12072
10. Oh K, Shen T, Le Gros G, Min B. Induction of Th2 type immunity in a mouse system reveals a novel immunoregulatory role of basophils. *Blood* (2007) **109**(7):2921–7. doi:10.182/blood-2006/07.0377739
11. Wakahara K, Baba N, Van VQ, Begin P, Rubio M, Ferraro P, et al. Human basophils interact with memory T cells to augment Th17 responses. *Blood* (2012) **120**(24):4761–71. doi:10.1182/blood-2012-04-424226
12. Borriello F, Granata F, Marone G. Basophils and skin disorders. *J Invest Dermatol* (2014) **134**(5):1202–10. doi:10.1038/jid.2014.16
13. Kanoh M, Maruyama S, Asano Y. *Listeria* infection inhibits IgE production in regional lymph nodes by suppressing chemotaxis of basophils to lymph nodes. *Microbiol Immunol* (2013) **57**(12):842–8. doi:10.1111/1348-0421.12101

14. Royer JF, Schratl P, Carrillo JJ, Jupp R, Barker J, Weyman-Jones C, et al. A novel antagonist of prostaglandin D2 blocks the locomotion of eosinophils and basophils. *Eur J Clin Invest* (2008) **38**(9):663–71. doi:10.1111/j.1365-2362.2008.01989.x
15. Schroeder JT. Basophils: emerging roles in the pathogenesis of allergic disease. *Immunol Rev* (2011) **242**(1):144–60. doi:10.1111/j.1600-065X.2011.01023.x
16. Endo Y, Hirahara K, Yagi R, Tumes DJ, Nakayama T. Pathogenic memory type Th2 cells in allergic inflammation. *Trends Immunol* (2014) **35**(2):69–78. doi:10.1016/j.it.2013.11.003
17. Anderson DM, Maraskovsky E, Billingsley WL, Dougall WC, Tometsko ME, Roux ER, et al. A homologue of the TNF receptor and its ligand enhance T-cell growth and dendritic-cell function. *Nature* (1997) **390**(6656):175–9. doi:10.1038/36593
18. Huber C, Odermatt A, Hagmann B, Dahinden CA, Fux M. In human basophils, IL-3 selectively induces RANKL expression that is modulated by IgER-dependent and IgER-independent stimuli. *Allergy* (2014) **69**(11):1498–505. doi:10.1111/all.12497
19. Kim BS, Wang K, Siracusa MC, Saenz SA, Brestoff JR, Monticelli LA, et al. Basophils promote innate lymphoid cell responses in inflamed skin. *J Immunol* (2014) **193**(7):3717–25. doi:10.4049/jimmunol.1401307
20. Motomura Y, Morita H, Moro K, Nakae S, Artis D, Endo TA, et al. Basophil-derived interleukin-4 controls the function of natural helper cells, a member of ILC2s, in lung inflammation. *Immunity* (2014) **40**(5):758–71. doi:10.1016/j.immuni.2014.04.013
21. Nakashima C, Otsuka A, Kitoh A, Honda T, Egawa G, Nakajima S, et al. Basophils regulate the recruitment of eosinophils in a murine model of irritant contact dermatitis. *J Allergy Clin Immunol* (2014) **134**(1):100–7. doi:10.1016/j.jaci.2014.02.026
22. Muto T, Fukuoka A, Kabashima K, Ziegler SF, Nakanishi K, Matsushita K, et al. The role of basophils and proallergic cytokines, TSLP and IL-33, in cutaneously sensitized food allergy. *Int Immunol* (2014) **26**(10):539–49. doi:10.1093/intimm/dxu058
23. Cheng LE, Sullivan BM, Retana LE, Allen CD, Liang HE, Locksley RM. IgE-activated basophils regulate eosinophil tissue entry by modulating endothelial function. *J Exp Med* (2015) **212**(4):513–24. doi:10.1084/jem.20141671
24. Hill DA, Siracusa MC, Ruymann KR, Tait Wojno ED, Artis D, Spergel JM. Omalizumab therapy is associated with reduced circulating basophil populations in asthmatic children. *Allergy* (2014) **69**(5):674–7. doi:10.1111/all.12375
25. Noti M, Wojno ED, Kim BS, Siracusa MC, Giacomin PR, Nair MG, et al. Thymic stromal lymphopoietin-elicited basophil responses promote eosinophilic esophagitis. *Nat Med* (2013) **19**(8):1005–13. doi:10.1038/nm.3281
26. Chapuy L, Bsat M, Mehta H, Rubio M, Wakahara K, Van VQ, et al. Basophils increase in Crohn disease and ulcerative colitis and favor mesenteric lymph node memory TH17/TH1 response. *J Allergy Clin Immunol* (2014) **134**(4):978.e–81.e. doi:10.1016/j.jaci.2014.05.025
27. Kaser A, Zeissig S, Blumberg RS. Inflammatory bowel disease. *Annu Rev Immunol* (2010) **28**:573–621. doi:10.1146/annurev-immunol-030409-101225
28. Masopust D, Schenkel JM. The integration of T cell migration, differentiation and function. *Nat Rev Immunol* (2013) **13**(5):309–20. doi:10.1038/nri3442
29. Sharma M, Kaveri SV, Bayry J. Human basophils lack the capacity to drive memory CD4(+) T cells toward the IL-22 response. *J Allergy Clin Immunol* (2013) **132**(6):1457–8. doi:10.1016/j.jaci.2013.09.024
30. Sharma M, Stephen-Victor E, Poncet P, Kaveri SV, Bayry J. Basophils are inept at promoting human Th17 responses. *Hum Immunol* (2015) **76**(2–3):176–80. doi:10.1016/j.humimm.2014.12.015
31. Sathaliyawala T, Kubota M, Yudanin N, Turner D, Camp P, Thome JJ, et al. Distribution and compartmentalization of human circulating and tissue-resident memory T cell subsets. *Immunity* (2013) **38**(1):187–97. doi:10.1016/j.immuni.2012.09.020
32. Debes GF, Arnold CN, Young AJ, Krautwald S, Lipp M, Hay JB, et al. Chemokine receptor CCR7 required for T lymphocyte exit from peripheral tissues. *Nat Immunol* (2005) **6**(9):889–94. doi:10.1038/ni1238
33. Bromley SK, Yan S, Tomura M, Kanagawa O, Luster AD. Recirculating memory T cells are a unique subset of CD4+ T cells with a distinct phenotype and migratory pattern. *J Immunol* (2013) **190**(3):970–6. doi:10.4049/jimmunol.1202805
34. McNamee EN, Masterson JC, Veny M, Collins CB, Jedlicka P, Byrne FR, et al. Chemokine receptor CCR7 regulates the intestinal TH1/TH17/Treg balance during Crohn's-like murine ileitis. *J Leukoc Biol* (2015) **97**(6):1011–22. doi:10.1189/jlb.3HI0614-303R
35. Anthony RM, Kobayashi T, Wermeling F, Ravetch JV. Intravenous gammaglobulin suppresses inflammation through a novel T(H)2 pathway. *Nature* (2011) **475**(7354):110–3. doi:10.1038/nature10134
36. Rivellese F, Suurmond J, de Paulis A, Marone G, Huizinga TW, Toes RE. IgE and IL-33-mediated triggering of human basophils inhibits TLR4-induced monocyte activation. *Eur J Immunol* (2014) **44**(10):3045–55. doi:10.1002/eji.201444731
37. Egawa M, Mukai K, Yoshikawa S, Iki M, Mukaida N, Kawano Y, et al. Inflammatory monocytes recruited to allergic skin acquire an anti-inflammatory M2 phenotype via basophil-derived interleukin-4. *Immunity* (2013) **38**(3):570–80. doi:10.1016/j.immuni.2012.11.014
38. Zaiss DM, Gause WC, Osborne LC, Artis D. Emerging functions of amphiregulin in orchestrating immunity, inflammation, and tissue repair. *Immunity* (2015) **42**(2):216–26. doi:10.1016/j.immuni.2015.01.020
39. Meulenbroeks C, van Weelden H, Schwartz C, Voehringer D, Redegeld FA, Rutten VP, et al. Basophil-derived amphiregulin is essential for UVB irradiation-induced immune suppression. *J Invest Dermatol* (2015) **135**(1):222–8. doi:10.1038/jid.2014.329
40. Zaiss DM, van Loosdregt J, Gorlani A, Bekker CP, Grone A, Sibilia M, et al. Amphiregulin enhances regulatory T cell-suppressive function via the epidermal growth factor receptor. *Immunity* (2013) **38**(2):275–84. doi:10.1016/j.immuni.2012.09.023
41. Weigmann B, Schughart N, Wiebe C, Sudowe S, Lehr HA, Jonuleit H, et al. Allergen-induced IgE-dependent gut inflammation in a human PBMC-engrafted murine model of allergy. *J Allergy Clin Immunol* (2012) **129**(4):1126–35. doi:10.1016/j.jaci.2011.11.036
42. Rodriguez Gomez M, Talke Y, Hofmann C, Ketelsen I, Hermann F, Reich B, et al. Basophils control T-cell responses and limit disease activity in experimental murine colitis. *Mucosal Immunol* (2013) **7**(1):188–99. doi:10.1038/mi.2013.38
43. Stokes JR, Casale TB. The use of anti-IgE therapy beyond allergic asthma. *J Allergy Clin Immunol Pract* (2015) **3**(2):162–6. doi:10.1016/j.jaip.2014.10.010
44. Varga C, Horvath K, Berko A, Thurmond RL, Dunford PJ, Whittle BJ. Inhibitory effects of histamine H4 receptor antagonists on experimental colitis in the rat. *Eur J Pharmacol* (2005) **522**(1–3):130–8. doi:10.1016/j.ejphar.2005.08.045

15

Epigenetics of peripheral B-Cell differentiation and the antibody response

Hong Zan* and Paolo Casali*

Department of Microbiology and Immunology, University of Texas School of Medicine, UT Health Science Center, San Antonio, TX, USA

Edited by:
Harry W. Schroeder, University of Alabama at Birmingham, USA

Reviewed by:
Wenxia Song, University of Maryland, USA
Ronald B. Corley, Boston University School of Medicine, USA

****Correspondence:***
Hong Zan
zan@uthscsa.edu;
Paolo Casali
pcasali@uthscsa.edu

Epigenetic modifications, such as histone post-translational modifications, DNA methylation, and alteration of gene expression by non-coding RNAs, including microRNAs (miRNAs) and long non-coding RNAs (lncRNAs), are heritable changes that are independent from the genomic DNA sequence. These regulate gene activities and, therefore, cellular functions. Epigenetic modifications act in concert with transcription factors and play critical roles in B cell development and differentiation, thereby modulating antibody responses to foreign- and self-antigens. Upon antigen encounter by mature B cells in the periphery, alterations of these lymphocytes epigenetic landscape are induced by the same stimuli that drive the antibody response. Such alterations instruct B cells to undergo immunoglobulin (Ig) class switch DNA recombination (CSR) and somatic hypermutation (SHM), as well as differentiation to memory B cells or long-lived plasma cells for the immune memory. Inducible histone modifications, together with DNA methylation and miRNAs modulate the transcriptome, particularly the expression of activation-induced cytidine deaminase, which is essential for CSR and SHM, and factors central to plasma cell differentiation, such as B lymphocyte-induced maturation protein-1. These inducible B cell-intrinsic epigenetic marks guide the maturation of antibody responses. Combinatorial histone modifications also function as histone codes to target CSR and, possibly, SHM machinery to the *Ig* loci by recruiting specific adaptors that can stabilize CSR/SHM factors. In addition, lncRNAs, such as recently reported lncRNA-CSR and an lncRNA generated through transcription of the S region that form G-quadruplex structures, are also important for CSR targeting. Epigenetic dysregulation in B cells, including the aberrant expression of non-coding RNAs and alterations of histone modifications and DNA methylation, can result in aberrant antibody responses to foreign antigens, such as those on microbial pathogens, and generation of pathogenic autoantibodies, IgE in allergic reactions, as well as B cell neoplasia. Epigenetic marks would be attractive targets for new therapeutics for autoimmune and allergic diseases, and B cell malignancies.

Keywords: AID, B cell, Blimp-1, class switch DNA recombination, epigenetics, histone post-translational modification, memory B cell, microRNA, plasma cell differentiation, somatic hypermutation

INTRODUCTION

Epigenetic changes brought about by genetic susceptibility and/or environmental exposure can modulate gene expression and alter cellular functions without altering genomic sequences (1). Epigenetic modifications and factors, such as DNA methylation, histone post-translational modifications and non-coding RNAs, such as microRNAs (miRNAs) and long non-coding RNAs (lncRNAs), comprise the epigenome and interact with genetic programs to regulate immune responses. Immunoglobulin (Ig) class switch DNA recombination (CSR) and somatic hypermutation (SHM) are critical for the production of protective antibodies against microbial pathogens, IgE in allergic responses, as well as pathogenic autoantibodies in autoimmune diseases. CSR recombines S region DNA located upstream of constant heavy-chain (C_H) region exons, thereby encoding new Ig C_H regions that endow antibodies new biological effector functions (2). SHM introduces mostly point mutations in variable regions of Ig heavy and light chains, thereby providing the structural substrate for antigen-mediated selection of B cell mutants with higher affinity B cell receptors (BCRs) (3–5). CSR and SHM occur mainly in germinal center and require activation-induced cytidine deaminase (AID, encoded by *AICDA* in humans and *Aicda* in mice), which is expressed in a differentiation stage-specific fashion in B cells (2–4). Class switched and hypermutated B cells further differentiate into long-lived memory B cells, which can react quickly to a recurrent antigenic challenge, or antibody-secreting plasma cells in a fashion critically dependent on B lymphocyte-induced maturation protein 1 (Blimp-1, encoded by *PRDM1* in humans and *Prdm1* in mice) (6, 7). Epigenetic modifications and factors influence gene expression and modulate critical B cell processes, such as CSR, SHM, and differentiation to memory B cells or plasma cells, thereby informing the antibody response (4, 8–10). Epigenetic dysregulation can result in aberrant antibody responses to exogenous antigens or self-antigens, such as chromatin, histones, and double-strand DNA in lupus.

B cell development and differentiation occur in two sequential stages. The initial, antigen-independent stage occurs in the bone marrow and involves recombination activating gene (RAG)1/RAG2-dependent V-(D)-J DNA rearrangement, which produces clonally unique Ig variable regions that specifically bind antigen. This stage generates mature, immunocompetent B cells that can bind to a unique antigen. The B cells move into the periphery and complete further, antigen-independent maturation into immunocompetent naïve mature B cells. In the periphery lymphoid organs, B cell undergoes the antigen-dependent stage of development or differentiation, upon activation by antigen binding and co-stimulation (5). In this stage, resting naïve mature B cells are induced to undergo cell proliferation, CSR, as well as SHM-mediated antibody affinity maturation, and differentiate into memory B cells, or short- or long-lived antibody-secreting plasma cells (6, 7). Multiple epigenetic changes are associated with each B cell development and differentiation stage. Resting, naïve B cells undergo V_HDJ_H-Cμ transcription, which initiates at the V_H promoter and runs through the intronic Sμ region and Cμ/Cδ exon clusters. This encodes the surface BCR, which comprises *Igμ* and *Igδ* heavy chain genes. These resting B cells display low levels of overall histone acetylation and genome-wide DNA hypermethylation, therefore most regions within the Ig heavy chain (*IgH*) locus are in a closed chromatin state (11), enriched in repressive histone post-translational modifications (e.g., H3K9me3 and H3K27me3) but lacking of activated histone modifications (12, 13). In B cells, epigenetic marks, such as DNA methylation, histone modifications, and miRNAs, are induced by the same stimuli that drive the antibody response, and modulate the transcriptome, especially the expression of AID, which is essential for SHM and CSR, and factors critical for plasma cell differentiation, such as Blimp-1 (4). By functioning as histone codes, combinatorial histone modifications also play a role in the targeting of the CSR and, possibly, SHM machinery to the *Ig* loci through recruiting specific scaffold proteins that stabilize CSR/SHM factors (8). These inducible B cell-intrinsic epigenetic marks control transcription programs that distinguish individual stages of B cell differentiation and underpin the molecular changes that are necessary for antibody response.

In this review, we provide a conceptual framework to understand how epigenetic modifications/factors modulate CSR and SHM, and the generation of plasma cells and memory B cells, with focus on AID-dependent peripheral B cell differentiation into memory B cells and long-lived plasma cells (but not differentiation of naïve B cells to short-lived plasma cells). We also highlight our current understanding of epigenetic modulations of CSR, SHM, and plasma cell differentiation by histone deacetylases (HDACs) inhibitors (HDIs). Finally, we summarize recent discoveries that indicate the importance of B cell epigenetic dysregulation in autoimmunity and B cell neoplasia.

EPIGENETIC REGULATION OF AID INDUCTION

Somatic hypermutation and CSR are initiated by transcription through V(D)J and the donor/acceptor S regions that will undergo recombination, respectively, and are mediated by AID, a 198 amino acid protein, which is structurally and functionally similar to apolipoprotein B RNA-editing cytidine deaminases (APOBEC enzymes) (2, 3). AID shares a conserved catalytic domain with other members of the APOBEC family of cytosine or cytidine deaminases (3). It deaminates deoxycytidines (dCs) into deoxyuracils (dUs) yielding dU:dG mismatches. These mismatches can be repaired by an error-prone DNA repair pathway, which introduce somatic mutations, or processed by uracil DNA glycosylase (Ung), which is recruited to and stabilized on S regions by the scaffold functions of 14-3-3 adaptors, the translesion DNA synthesis (TLS) polymerase Rev1 and replication protein A (RPA), or elements of the mismatch repair (MMR) machinery, such as Msh2 and Msh6, which trigger DNA repair processes leading to introduction of point mutations (SHM) or double-strand DNA breaks (DSBs) (CSR) (2).

As a potent mutator, AID can effectively introduce mutations in not only *Ig* loci but also a variety of non-*Ig* genes, thereby causing genome instability in both B cells and non-B cells, including non-lymphoid cells, and contributing to tumorgenesis (3). Tight regulation of AID expression and function is necessary to maintain genomic stability in both B cells and non-B cells, and to avoid damages, such as chromosomal translocations, resulting from its dysregulation (14–18). This is achieved through fine control of transcription, post-transcription and post-translation regulation, nuclear/cytoplasmic distribution, stability, and activity (3) (**Figure 1**). AID express at a very low level (mostly undetectable) in naïve B cells, it is greatly induced in B cells undergoing SHM/CSR, and repressed in memory B cells and plasma cells to preserve the specificity, affinity, and isotype of antibody and BCR. *Aicda* transcription is under the control of multiple elements, particularly Homeobox protein C4 (HoxC4) (**Figure 1**). HoxC4 is a highly conserved helix-loop-helix homeodomain-containing transcription factor. As we have shown, HoxC4 directly binds to the *Aicda* promoter through an evolutionarily conserved 5′-ATTT-3′ site embedded within a conserved binding site for POU domain-containing transcription factors Oct1 and Oct2 (5′-ATTTGAAT-3′) (19). Sp1/Sp3 and NF-κB also bind the same promoter core and synergize with HoxC4 for *Aicda* induction (19, 20).

Regulation of AID Expression by DNA Modifications and Histone Modifications

The expression of *Aicda* is modulated by changes of *Aicda* epigenetic status. Suppression of *Aicda* expression in naïve B cells is mediated by promoter DNA hypermethylation (21). In naive B cells, in which AID is not expressed, histone H3 acetylation occurs in the *Aicda* gene at low levels comparable to the overall H3 acetylation in the genome and neighboring genes, such as *Mfap5*, which is not

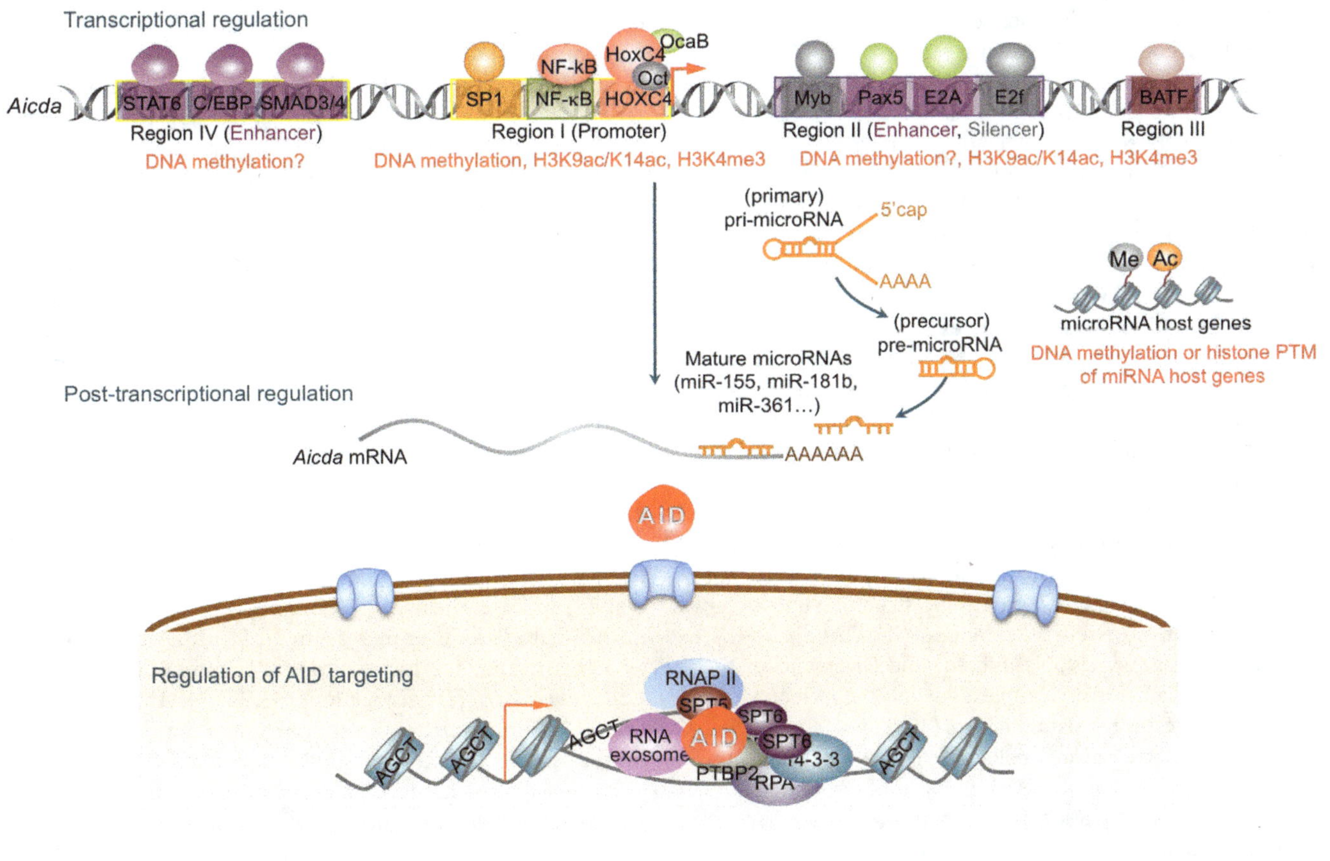

FIGURE 1 | AID is tightly regulated at the transcriptional, post-transcriptional, and post-translational levels. Four distinct DNA regions (regions I–IV) of the AID gene (*Aicda*) locus possess binding sites for multiple transcription factors to regulate *Aicda* expression. Region I functions as promoters containing the binding sites for HoxC4/Oct and NF-κB/Sp1/Sp3, which can be induced by activating the *Aicda* promoter. In resting naive and memory B cells, and non-B cells, silencer elements in region II bind the repressor proteins E2f and c-Myb to counter the activity of the transcriptional activators. Stimulation of B cells with the primary inducing stimuli and cytokines that promote CSR induce activation signals through region IV enhancer in collaboration with the intronic enhancer in region II can overcome the effect of the region II silencer. After transcription, the *Aicda* mRNA can be negatively regulated by miR-155, miR-181b, and miR-361, which specifically bind to the conserved target sites on the 3′ UTR of *Aicda* mRNA. Nuclear AID is either degraded or exported back to the cytoplasm. Only a small proportion of AID molecules are targeted onto DNA at *Ig* or non-*Ig* loci by its co-factors. AID preferentially deaminates single-strand DNA, which emerges from transcription by RNA Pol II and depends on histone modifications in the transcribed locus. AID can be recruited to the open DNA before or during transcription. In CSR, AID recruitment to S regions occurs with interaction of RNA Pol II and AID-interacting factors, such as Spt5, Spt6, PTBP2, RNA exosome, lncRNAs, and 14-3-3 adaptor proteins, which would form a macromolecular complex. AID is enriched and stabilized on the targeted DNA by 14-3-3 adaptor proteins, which access the same S regions as the transcription machinery owing to their open chromatin state. These 14-3-3 adaptors are recruited and/or stabilized through interactions with 5′-AGCT-3′ repeats and possibly by H3K9acS10ph. The RNA exosome also interacts with AID and allows AID to deaminate both the transcribed and the non-transcribed DNA strand in the S regions undergoing transcription. AID deaminate dCs into dUs to yield dU:dG mismatches. Resolution of these lesions can lead to different physiological or pathological outcomes.

significantly expressed in B cells (22). Upon activation of B cells, DNA of the *Aicda* gene is demethylated and the locus becomes enriched in H3K4me3 and H3K9ac/K14ac. B cell activation by LPS plus IL-4, which induces *Aicda* transcription, greatly increases H3 acetylation at the *Aicda* locus, particularly in the *Aicda* regulatory regions (22). These epigenetic modifications, together with induction of nuclear factor NF-κB, homeobox protein HoxC4 and other transcription factors, activate *Aicda* transcription. Transcription elongation depends on the H3K36me3 posttranslational modicification, an intragenic mark of gene activation in the *Aicda* gene body, as suggested by AID down-regulation following depletion of the H3K36me3 methyltransferase Setd2 (3, 23). Post-CSR/SHM down-regulation of *Aicda* transcription probably results from remethylation of the *Aicda* DNA.

Regulation of AID Expression by miRNA

In addition to DNA methylation of the *Aicda* promoter and histone acetylation of the *Aicda* locus, selected miRNAs provide a more important mechanism of modulation of AID expression. miRNAs are small (~21–23 nt), evolutionarily conserved non-coding RNAs derived from much larger primary transcripts encoded by their "host genes." miRNAs bind to complementary sequences within the 3′ untranslated region (3′ UTR) of their target mRNAs and negatively regulate protein expression at the post-transcriptional level. miRNA can recognize its target mRNA through the short (as few as 6–8 nt) "seed sequence" at the 5′ end of the miRNA. miRNA repress gene expression by accelerating mRNA degradation and inhibiting mRNA translation. A given miRNA can potentially target different mRNAs, and a given mRNA can be targeted by multiple miRNAs. The mammalian genome encodes hundreds of miRNAs that collectively impact the expression of about one-third of all genes. miRNAs are transcribed from intergenic genomic DNA by RNA polymerase (Pol) II or Pol III as primary transcripts (pri-miRNAs) that are then cleaved by the nuclear ribonuclease Drosha to generate an about 70 bp long characteristic stem-loop structure, known as a pre-miRNA, and exported to the cytoplasm (24). The pre-miRNA is further processed by cytoplasmic enzyme Dicer into mature miRNA (24), which forms complexes with ribonucleoproteins (RNPs) and expresses regulatory effects (25, 26).

microRNAs control various biological processes by fine-tuning gene expression at the post-transcriptional level. They can modulate a wide range of physiological and pathological processes by regulating cellular function at every aspect, from proliferation and apoptosis to differentiation. miRNAs are present in all human and mouse cells, in which they each modulate the expression of a few to hundreds of target genes. miRNAs likely play important roles in B cell development and peripheral differentiation, as well as T cell stage-specific differentiation and autoimmunity. Naïve B cells, germinal center B cells, memory B cells, and plasma cells show distinct miRNA expression profiles (27, 28). Deletion of Dicer, which is critical for miRNA maturation, in activated B cells resulted in defective generation of germinal center B cells, memory B cells, and plasma cells (29). Indeed, Dicer-deficient B cells showed impaired biogenesis of many miRNAs, including miR-155 and miR-125b, which regulate expression of genes that modulate B cell germinal center reaction and plasma cell differentiation (30, 31). A single miRNA, such as miR-155, can target multiple genes, including *Myd88*, *Pu.1*, and *Aicda*, and regulate sequential stages of B cell differentiation (30, 32–34). By contrast, multiple miRNAs, such as miR-15a and miR-16, can cooperatively repress one critical gene in germinal center B cells, *Bcl2* (27).

miR-155, miR-181b, and miR-361 modulate AID expression by binding to the evolutionarily conserved target sites in the 3′ UTR of *AICDA/Aicda* mRNA, thereby reducing both *AICDA/Aicda* mRNA and AID protein levels (33–37). These miRNAs could suppress AID expression in naïve B cells and in B cells that completed SHM/CSR. miR-155 is the most abundant miRNA that has been shown to silence AID expression. miR-155 is processed from an RNA sequence encoded by miR-155 host gene (*miR155HG*). This was originally identified as a gene transcriptionally activated by promoter insertion at a common retroviral integration site in B-cell lymphomas (*Bic*, B-cell integration cluster). *Bic* RNA is a spliced and polyadenylated but non-protein-coding RNA that accumulates in lymphoma cells (32) and is induced along with AID in B cells activated by CSR-inducing stimuli (33, 34). The sequences of pre-miRNA-155 and mature miR-155 are highly conserved across more than 22 different organisms, including mammals, amphibians, birds, reptiles, sea squirts, and sea lampreys (38).

miR-155 and miR-361 are directly repressed by BCL-6, a transcriptional repressor required for germinal center formation. miR-361 is embedded in the *CHM* gene, which encodes a subunit of a Rab geranylgeranyl transferase and is known for its genetic inactivation in choroideremia (37). BCL-6 display a coordinated activity in sustaining high levels of AID expression in germinal center B cells undergoing CSR and SHM. By direct repressing miR-155 and miR-361, BCL-6 upregulates the expression of the target genes of these miRNAs, including *AICDA* and other elements involved in the maintenance of the germinal center B cell centroblast phenotype (37). The specific effect of miR-155 in the regulation of AID expression was demonstrated by the findings that disruption of the miR-155 binding site in the 3′ UTR of *Aicda* mRNA in B cells led to an increase in *Aicda* mRNA and AID protein by increasing the half-life of *Aicda* mRNA, resulting in increased CSR and *c-Myc/IgH* translocations (33, 34). Nevertheless, the role of miR-155 in regulating B cell function and antibody response is much more than modulating the expression of AID. miR-155 is expressed at a high level in germinal center B cells and plays an important role in germinal center formation and subsequent antibody response following antigen challenge (30, 32, 39). miR-155 deficiency in B cells resulted in reduced extra follicular and germinal center responses, decreased numbers of IgG1^{+} plasma cells and memory B cells, and failed production of high-affinity IgG1 antibodies (30). In B6/*Fas*$^{lpr/lpr}$ mice, deficiency of miR-155 results in a reduced autoantibody production and autoimmunity (40). This is likely stemmed from dysregulation of a variety of genes in multiple immune cells, including derepressed expression of SHIP-1 in B cells, which lead to mitigation of B-cell activation, proliferation and autoantibody production (40).

The 3′ UTR of *Aicda* mRNA contains multiple putative binding sites for miR-181b, which is predominantly expressed in lymphoid cells (10, 41). miR-181b is expressed at the highest levels in resting B cells and is downregulated upon B cell activation by CSR-inducing stimuli (34, 42). Expression of miR-181b in B cells leads to down-regulation of AID at both the transcript and protein levels. It has been suggested that miR-181b and miR-155 have non-overlapping functions in controlling AID expression. miR-181b may inhibit premature AID activity but allows proper AID transcriptional activation at early time points, while miR-155 could narrow AID function at a later stage of activation (34). By controlling AID expression, miR-155 and miR-181b protect resting B cells and non-B cells from AID-mediated mutagenesis. Accordingly, in Burkitt's lymphoma B cells, deficiency of miR-155 expression is associated with high levels of somatic mutations and inter-chromosomal translocations (43).

EPIGENETIC REGULATION OF AID TARGETING IN CSR AND SHM

One fundamental question for B cell biology remains to be answered is how CSR and SHM machineries are targeted to the *Ig* locus. For CSR to take place, the *IgH* genes are subjected to transcriptional activation, RNA splicing, AID-mediated cytidine deamination, as well as DNA cleavage, repair, and recombination. Each of these events is likely associated with, and possibly regulated by specific changes in chromatin structure. Histone modifications in S and V(D)J regions are critical for targeting of the CSR and SHM machinery, respectively (**Table 1**). Chromatin structure that impacts on and likely regulate most aspects of gene expression, also contributes to the regulation of CSR and SHM. In B cells poised to undergo CSR, the *IgH* genes are in an "accessible" chromatin conformation before CSR (44). Upon induction of germ-line transcription, histones H3 and H4 have been shown to be acetylated at the I_H exon promoters and S regions (45, 46).

Epigenetic Targeting of the CSR Machinery

Histone Modifications in CSR Targeting

Histone post-translational modifications are important for targeting of the CSR machinery to the upstream donor and the downstream acceptor S regions that are involved in CSR (**Table 1**). The significant levels of germline Iμ-Sμ-Cμ transcription and activating histone marks, such as H3K4me3, H3K36me3, H2BK5ac, H3K9ac/K14ac, H3K27ac, and H4K8ac, are observed in the donor Sμ region even in resting naïve B cells, suggesting that Sμ is in a constitutively open state and poised for switch recombination (8). CSR induction requires both primary and secondary (CSR-inducing) stimuli. Primary stimuli, such as engagement of B cell CD40 by CD154 expressed on activated T cells, and T-independent dual toll-like receptor (TLR) and BCR engagement, induce B cell activation, proliferation, and differentiation. In conjunction with primary stimuli, secondary stimuli, which comprise cytokines (e.g., IL-4, TGF-β, and IFN-γ), direct class switching to IgG, IgA, or IgE by selecting the acceptor S region, through activation of S region histone modifications and inducing specific germline I_H-S-C_H transcription (46–49). Primary stimuli induce histone-modifying enzymes and trigger chromatin decondensation in downstream S regions by removing repressive H3K9me3 and H3K27me3. These allow histone-modifying enzymes to ride on the RNA Pol II to reach S regions during germline I_H-S-C_H transcription elongation (46, 47, 50–52). Upon RNA Pol II stalling, caused by complex secondary DNA structures, such as cruciform-like structures and R-loop, in S regions (2, 53), histone-modifying enzymes catalyze histone modifications in these regions. DNA transcription together with modified histones opens the chromatin in S regions, thereby allowing for access of CSR factors. The role of histone-modifying enzymes in CSR is further emphasized by the reduced S region histone modifications and CSR in B cells knockdown H3K4 methyltransferase Set1 (48), or H3K9 acetyltransferases Pcaf and Gcn5 (8).

In the donor and acceptor S regions, activating histone modifications, such as H3K9ac and H3K4me3, are enriched at levels much higher than those in the associated I_H promoter and C_H regions (46, 47). These histone marks are read by CSR factors, including 14-3-3 adaptors, which, such as AID and histone-modifying enzymes, are induced by primary CSR stimuli (54). 14-3-3 adaptors directly interact with AID and target it to the upstream and downstream S regions that undergo recombination (2), thereby transducing the epigenetic code. 14-3-3 adaptors specifically bind to the combinatorial histone H3K9acS10ph modification in S regions and 5′-AGCT-3′ (2, 54) repeats. These are characteristic motifs of all *IgH* locus S regions, but not I_H promoters, C_H regions or other genome areas (54). Due to their high affinity for 5′-AGCT-3′ repeats, 14-3-3 can potentially bind all S regions. Nevertheless, these adaptors are recruited only to the S regions that undergo recombination (54). This is due to the open chromatin state of such regions as well as specific binding of 14-3-3 to H3K9acS10ph (8). The specificity of 14-3-3 adaptors for H3K9acS10ph and 5′-AGCT-3′ repeats are evocative of RAG1/RAG2 complex specificity for H3K4me3 and V, D and J gene recombination signal sequences (RSSs) (55).

H3K4 methylation, particularly H3K4me3, plays a critical role in AID-mediated DNA cleavage in S regions during CSR (48). The formation of H3K4me3 at AID target loci is dependent on the histone chaperone complex, facilitates chromatin transcription (FACT), a chromatin-modifying complex during RNA processing (48, 56). We have shown that specific H3K4 methyltransferases and H3K9 acetyltransferases can be induced by TLR or CD40 signaling and catalyze histone H3K4me3 and H3K9ac/K14ac modifications. These are decorated S regions, regardless of whether they are targets of CSR (8). Conversely, the combinatorial histone H3K9acS10ph modification specifically marks the S regions set to recombine and directly recruits 14-3-3 adaptors for AID stabilization (8). 14-3-3 adaptors, which possess no enzymatic activity, function as histone code readers to recruit/stabilize downstream effector molecules, which *per se* cannot read histone codes, consistent with the "histone code hypothesis" (57, 58). Inhibition of the enzymatic activity of Gcn5/Pcaf histone acetyltransferases leads to decreased H3K9acS10ph, 14-3-3 recruitment and AID stabilization in S regions, and CSR.

H3K9me3 is also present, although at a relatively low level, in Sμ but not downstream S regions. In the Sμ region, H3K9me3 recruits the KAP1-HP1γ complex to stabilize AID (13). Accordingly, CSR to IgA can be impaired by deletion of the H3K9 methyltransferase Suv39 (59). Histone modification readers that function as scaffolds, such as 14-3-3 adaptors, translesion DNA synthesis polymerase Rev1 (60) and RPA (61), act as core for the assembly of macromolecular complexes on S region DNA, to stabilize AID and/or Ung for generation of DNA lesions. Histone modifications are also recognized by DNA repair factors, such as p53-binding protein 1 (53BP1), which may functions as a scaffold to recruit/stabilize additional DNA repair factors for CSR. Abrogation of histone methyltransferase MMSET expression impairs H4K20me2 enrichment and 53BP1 recruitment in S regions, and results in reduced CSR (62).

Suppressor of Ty6 (Spt6), a RNA Pol II-interacting histone H3-H4 chaperone, also plays a role in the regulation of H3K4me3 for SHM and CSR (23). Depletion of Spt6 impaired H3K4me3 and AID-mediated DSBs in the S regions in CH12 B cells, which can otherwise be induced to express AID and CSR to IgA (23). In addition, knockdown Spt6 in human Burkitt's lymphoma BL2 cells overexpressing mutant AID (JP8Bdel) that lacks C-terminal 16 aa residues, which are critical for CSR but not to SHM (63), abolished SHM and H3K4me3 in *Ig* V_H region and non-*Ig* AID target genes (23). Thus, activating histone modifications are induced in S regions and create an open chromatin state, which allows for the access of the CSR machinery. Epigenetic specification of CSR targeting entails reading of histone codes by scaffold proteins, which orchestrate the assembly of macromolecular complexes in the sequential DNA lesion and repair stages.

Long Non-Coding RNA and CSR Targeting

Long non-coding RNAs are evolutionarily conserved non-coding RNA molecules that are longer than 200 nt and located within the intergenic loci or regions overlapping antisense transcripts of protein coding genes (64–66). Their expression can be tissue- and cell-type specific. lncRNAs are involved in numerous cellular functions, such as transcriptional regulation, RNA processing, RNA modification and epigenetic silencing. lncRNAs have been recently shown to play an important role in the targeting of the CSR machinery (**Table 1**). They target AID to divergently transcribed loci in B cells (67). In B cells undergoing CSR, the RNA exosome, a cellular

TABLE 1 | Epigenetic marks/factors, and their functions in CSR and SHM.

Target(s)	Epigenetic mark(s)	(Putative) functions	Modulate		Reference
			CSR	SHM	
microRNAs					
Aicda	miR-93 miR-155 miR-181b miR-361	Decrease expression of AID	+	+	(9, 33–37)
lncRNAs					
S regions	Germline I_H-S-C_H transcripts	Increase S region accessibility	+	−	(2)
S regions	Intronic switch RNA	Recruit AID to S region	+	−	(69)
S regions	Antisense S region transcripts	Increase S region accessibility	+	−	(173)
V_HDJ_H	Antisense V_HDJ_H transcripts	Increase V_HDJ_H region accessibility	−	+	(173)
IgH 3′ RR super-enhancer	lncRNA-CSR	Regulate IgH 3′ regulatory region super-enhancer function	+	−	(70)
IgH and other AID target regions	xTSS-RNAs	Recruit AID to ssDNA-forming site	+	+	(67)
DNA METHYLATION					
V(D)J	DNA hypomethylation	Increases V(D)J region accessibility	−	+	(84)
Igh 3′-LCR	DNA hypomethylation	Mediates germline V_HDJ_H and I_H-S-C_H transcription	+	+	(174)
HISTONE MODIFICATIONS					
V(D)J	H3K4me2/3, H3K9ac/K14ac, H4K8ac	Increase V(D)J region accessibility and transcription	−	+	(23, 72, 85)
iEμ	H3K4me3, H3K9ac/K14ac	Activate iEμ and enhance germline VDJ transcription and I_H-S-C_H transcription	+	+	(46, 47)
Igh 3′-LCR	H3K4me1/2 H3K9ac, H3K27ac, H4K8ac, H2BK5ac	Mediate VDJ and germline transcription	+	+	(175) (47)
S region(s)	H3K27me3	Decreases S region(s) accessibility	+	−	(12)
	H3K4me3, H3K9ac/K14ac, H3K27ac, H4K8ac	Increase S region(s) accessibility	+	−	(12, 13, 45–49, 61, 176)
	H3K9me3	Recruits the HP1γ-KAP1 complex and AID to Sμ region	+	−	(13)
	H3K9acS10ph	Recruits 14-3-3 adaptors and AID to S region(s)	+	−	(8)
	H4K20me2	Recruits 53BP1 to S region(s) in the DNA repair stage	+	−	(62)
Aicda	H3K4me3, H3K9ac/K14ac, H3K36me3	Increase transcription of *Aicda*	+	+	(22, 47)

Repressive histone methylation: H3K9me3, H3K27me3.
Activating and recruiting histone modifications include histone acetylation: H3K9ac, H3K14ac, H3K27ac, H4K8ac, H2BK5ac, and H3K9ac; histone methylations: H3K4me2/3, H4K20me2, and H3K36me3; combinatorial histone H3K9acS10ph modification; histone phosphorylation: H2BS14ph; histone ubiquitination: H2AK119ub and H2BK120ub.

RNA-processing/degradation complex is required for optimal CSR (68). The RNA exosome associates with AID, accumulates on S regions in an AID-dependent fashion. Both the cellular RNA exosome complex and a recombinant RNA exosome core complex inform robust transcription-dependent DNA deamination by AID in both strands of transcribed SHM substrates *in vitro*. In B cells, deficiency of *Exosc3* or *Exosc10*, the essential subunits of the RNA exosome complex, impairs CSR and SHM (67, 69). Many novel RNA exosome substrate lncRNAs have been identified by transcriptome analysis of *Exosc3*- or *Exosc10*-deficient B cells. RNA exosome-regulated, antisense-transcribed regions accumulate single-strand DNA structures containing RNA-DNA hybrids and recruit AID in B cell. RNA exosome regulation of lncRNA has been suggested to recruit AID to single-strand DNA-forming sites of antisense and divergent transcription in the B cell genome (67). In addition, a recent study has shown that an lncRNA generated by S region transcription followed by lariat debranching can fold into G-quadruplex structures, which can be directly bound by AID, thereby targeting of AID to S region DNA (70).

Epigenetic Targeting of the SHM Machinery

Activation-induced cytidine deaminase initiates SHM by deaminating cytosine residues in Ig V(D)J genes. It also introduces DNA damages, including point-mutations, in non-*Ig* loci at a lower frequency. How AID is recruited to the target sites is not fully understood. AID has been suggested to target a specific microenvironment rather than a defined set of genes (71). The SHM machinery is targeted to the V(D)J region through unique targeting sequences, transcription, and possibly, DNA demethylation and histone modifications (**Table 1**) (72). Like CSR, SHM requires not only the expression of AID, but also transcription in the target regions. Alterations in chromatin structure at *IgH* may also play an important role in promoting and/or stabilizing AID targeting (73). AID targets a distinct set of hotspots, which are concentrated in genes that are highly transcribed but frequently stalled genes (74). AID associates with RNA Pol II (75). RNA Pol II transcription, as well as several chromatin alterations could facilitate the access of AID to *Ig* loci and give use to single-stranded DNA, a preferential substrate for AID deamination. However, transcription alone is insufficient to recruit AID activity (74). AID targets are predominantly grouped within topological complex, highly transcribed superenhancers and regulatory clusters, which are enriched in chromatin modifications associated with active enhancers (such as H3K27Ac), they are also and marks of active transcription (such as H3K36me3), indicating that these features are universal mediators of AID recruitment (71, 74, 76). In both human and mouse B cells, there is a strong overlap between hypermutated genes and superenhancer domains (71).

The phosphorylated histone H2B (H2BSer14P) correlates tightly with SHM and CSR. In Ig V(D)J and S regions, H2B phosphorylation requires AID and may be mediated by the histone kinase Mst1 (72, 77). It has been suggested that SHM and CSR trigger distinct DNA damage responses and identify a novel histone modification pattern for SHM consisting of H2B (Ser14P) in the absence of γH2AX (72, 77). The non-Ig AID targets share important characteristics with Ig genes, namely, repetitive sequences that can form non-B DNA structures upon efficient transcription, and the accumulation of chromatin H3K4me3 histone marks (78).

The FACT complex may also promote SHM (56). FACT, a histone chaperone-type elongation factor, was originally discovered for its biochemical activity to promote transcription elongation of RNAPII on the nucleosomal DNA template (79). It has been suggested to remove nucleosomal histones and deposit them at the RNAPII of transcription site, and this allows the RNA polymerase to be proceed beyond the nucleosomes (80). FACT is important for inducing H3K4me3, which can be recognized by a protein complex with DNA cleaving activity and accumulates at SHM-targeted genomic regions (48). Furthermore, FACT and histone variant H3.3, a hallmark of replication-independent histone turnover, are enriched at the heavy and light chain V(D)J regions, the light chain Jκ5 region and the Sμ region 5′ flanking sequence (48). The importance of the chromatin histone-exchanging dynamics in SHM target regions, especially Ig genes, is emphasized by high abundant FACT and H3.3 deposition in the most efficient targets of SHM (56, 81). Histone post-translational modifications would also mediate recruitment of DNA repair factors, such as error-prone TLS DNA polymerases, in SHM at the DNA repair stage. H2AK119 ubiquitination (ub) and H2BK120ub are enriched in V_HDJ_H but not C_H regions and colocalize with DNA Pol η, an important TLS polymerase for SHM, in AID nuclear foci (82). Pol η is likely recruited to those loci by H2AK119ub and H2BK120ub, as well as by monoubiquitinated PCNA scaffold, through its ubiquitin-binding domain (83). As mentioned before, AID-dependent histone H2BSer14P mark in the V(D)J region (72) may also contributes to recruitment of DNA repair factors. The role of DNA hypomethylation in SHM has been suggested by the finding that only the hypomethylated allele is hypermutated in B cells carrying two nearly identical pre-rearranged Igκ transgenic alleles, even though transcription of both alleles are comparable (84).

It is possible that DNA demethylation facilitates SHM targeting by promoting histone modifications H3K4me3, H3K9ac/K14ac and H4K8ac, which are enriched in the V(D)J region and associated with an open chromatin state (23, 72, 85). Both H3K4me3 and H4K8ac are involved in SHM. Decreased H3K4me3 in V_HDJ_H regions in human BL2 cells, a Burkitt's lymphoma cell line that can be induced to undergo SHM, upon knockdown of histone chaperone Spt6 is associated with reduced V_HDJ_H mutations (23). In BL2 cells, H4K8ac increases concomitantly with V_HDJ_H mutations upon treatment with HDI trichostatin A (TSA) (85). Persistent H4K8ac in VλJλ region required E2A, whose inactivation result in decreased mutations (72, 86).

Some *cis*-acting regulatory regions, such as *Ig* enhancer and *Ig* enhancer-like sequences, are important for targeting SHM to *Ig* loci (87, 88). In chicken, mouse and human B cells that *Ig* locus enhancers and enhancer-like elements function as core diversification activator (DIVAC) sequences that work together to target SHM (88). In chicken DT40 B cells, short mammalian *Igλ* and *IgH* enhancer fragments can increase mutation rates by more than 20-fold (88). lncRNAs, which are likely to regulate many biological functions, have been recently shown to be link to enhancer activity. lncRNAs are expressed in a lineage-specific fashion and function through RNA–protein, RNA–DNA, or RNA–RNA target interactions. They are induced to modulate innate and adaptive immunity (66). Many regulatory lncRNAs can be categorized as DNA accessibility modulators, and likely play a role in SHM targeting, especially in conjunction with the function of *Ig* enhancers (67). Thus, activating histone modifications, DNA hypomethylation, and possibly lncRNAs increase V(D)J region chromatin accessibility to the SHM machinery, including AID and error-prone DNA repair factors, which can be stabilized by modified histones.

EPIGENETIC REGULATION OF PLASMA CELL DIFFERENTIATION

B cell differentiation is initiated by extracellular stimuli that bind to cellular receptors and trigger a signaling cascade resulting in the induction of transcription factors that reprogram B cells to secrete antibodies. The function of transcription factors is controlled by the accessibility to DNA through epigenetic modifications. Little is known about how the epigenetic mechanisms direct B cell differentiation into antibody-secreting plasma cells (6). Plasma cells are terminally differentiated elements in the B cell lineage that mostly have undergone SHM and CSR. These cells do not proliferate, but secrete large volumes (10^7 molecules/h) of clone-specific antibodies. Plasma cells are derived from either germinal center or memory B cells. Although some memory B cells are IgM$^+$, most memory B cells are class-switched and express mutated V(D)J gene segments. Upon reactivation by specific antigen, memory B cells differentiate into antibody-secreting plasma cells to mediate an anamnestic humoral response (89). Reactivated memory B cells can also reenter into the germinal center reaction and undergo further CSR and/or SHM before differentiating into plasma cells or reverting back to memory B cells (90, 91).

Plasma cells display a transcriptional signature that is distinct from B cells (92). Their changes in gene expression correlated with the acquisition of permissive histone modifications, including H3K4me1 and H3K4me4, which are enriched in active promoters and distal enhancers and play an important role in B cell development (92, 93). Upregulation of Blimp-1, a transcriptional repressor, is central to plasma differentiation (6). Blimp-1 downregulates the expression of *Bcl6*, *Pax5*, and *Spib*, all of which inhibit B cell differentiation into plasma cells by binding to the promoters of these genes (6), and, possibly, deacetylating their promoters. Indeed, *Pax5*, *Spib*, and perhaps *Bcl6* promoters display decreased histone acetylation in plasma cells (94, 95). Furthermore, Blimp-1 can interact with HDACs that remove acetyl groups on a histone (94). In addition, in plasma cells, Blimp-1 down-regulates *c-Myc* expression through a similar epigenetic mechanism (94), thereby maintaining the terminal differentiation state of these cells (6). Finally, Blimp-1 can interact with H3K9 methyltransferase G9a and likely recruits this enzyme to the *Pax5* and *Spib* promoters, thereby increasing H3K9me3 and repressing activation of these promoters (95, 96). Thus, epigenetic induction of Blimp-1 and Blimp-1-mediated epigenetic inhibition of target genes drives plasma cell differentiation, and possibly maintains plasma cell identity. Down-regulation of Pax-5 and Pax-5-driven Bcl-6 lead to derepression of the *Prdm1* promoter from Bcl-6-mediated epigenetic silencing. This is associated with increased histone acetylation in the *Prdm1* promoter, likely resulting from release of Bcl-6-bound HDACs (97, 98). Reduction of Blimp-1 in a plasmacytoid cell line by enforced expression of Bcl-6 resulted in re-expression of B cell markers, including CD19 (98).

Prdm1 mRNA contains a long (>2,000 nt) 3′ UTR, which can be potentially targeted by multiple miRNAs, including miR-9, miR-23b, miR-30, miR-125b, miR-127, and let-7 (10, 27, 28, 31, 99–102). Overexpression of miR-125b in B cells impairs expression of Blimp-1 and inhibits B cell differentiation into plasma cells (31). In addition, miR-125b can downregulate IFN regulatory factor (Irf)-4, which reciprocally regulates Blimp-1 and is required for the generation of plasma cells (27, 31, 103). Furthermore, X-box binding protein (Xbp)-1 that governs late events of plasma cell differentiation can be downregulated by miR-127 (102).

EPIGENETIC REGULATION OF MEMORY B CELL DIFFERENTIATION

B cell memory is a hallmark of adaptive immunity. Memory B cells are antigen-experienced quiescent B cells, which can be generated in response to both T-dependent antigens (usually proteins) and T-independent antigens (usually carbohydrates) (7). B cells quickly react to a second challenge with the same antigen, thereby providing humoral immune protection. While inherit epigenetic information from their active B cell precursors, memory B cells acquire new epigenetic marks, which make these resting B cells poised to quickly respond to experienced antigen. Expression of memory B cell hallmark genes, such as *CD27* (in humans) and *Cd38* (in mice), is likely mediated by histone modifications induced during B cell activation (4). Genes that control B cell identity and function, including *Pax5* and *Spib*, are also expressed in memory B cells, likely reflecting the epigenetic state that originated in naïve B cells and led them to memory B cells differentiation. Post-recombined S–S regions in the *IgH* locus show constitutive (upstream Sμ portion) or induced (downstream Sγ, Sϵ, or Sα portion) histone modifications, which could be transferred to memory B cells and result in comparable epigenetic landscapes in class-switched memory B cells (4). The functional distinction between memory B cells and their naïve counterparts could at least partially result from the epigenetic alterations.

Quiescent and activated B cells display different histone marks (104). In resting cells, histone lysine methylation was reduced as compared to activated cells (105). Enhancer of zeste homolog 2 (Ezh2) catalyzes H3K27me3, which is enriched at transcription start sites of repressed genes, through its SET domain. EZH2 is highly expressed in human germinal center B cells. Inactivation of Ezh2 in mouse germinal center B cells resulted in a profound reduction of germinal center reactions, memory B cell formation, and antibody response (106). Ezh2 protected germinal center B cells against AID mutagenesis and facilitated cell cycle progression. Repression of Blimp-1 and Irf4 expression in germinal center B cells is also necessary to limit plasma cell differentiation (106). In *Ezh2$^{fl/fl}$Cγ1-Cre* mice, the B cell differentiation stage-specific

Ezh2 deficiency resulted in profound impairment of germinal center reactions and memory B cell formation, suggesting that the methyltransferase activity of *Ezh2* is essential for not only germinal center B cell functions but also generation of memory B cells (106). Furthermore, it has been recently shown that histone acetyltransferase monocytic leukemia zinc finger protein (MOZ), which specifically targets H3K9 and plays a role in stem cell self-renewal, regulates B cell memory formation, controlling memory compartment composition (104). This activity of MOZ is B cell-intrinsic and is required for establishing the germinal center gene expression program. B cell stage-specific deletion of MOZ alters fate decisions in both primary and secondary antibody responses. The lack of MOZ affected the functional outcome of antibody responses, with an increase in secondary germinal centers and a corresponding decrease in secondary high-affinity antibody-secreting cell formation (104).

The differentiation of naïve B cells to germinal center B cells and then to plasma cells or memory B cells would also be associated with changes in DNA methylation. Several genes can be silenced by DNA methylation catalyzed by DNA methyltransferases (DNMTs), such as DNMT3a, which is highly expressed in memory B cells (107). In memory B cells, different expression, as compare to naïve B cells, of the immune activation related elements is likely concomitant with distinctive DNA methylation (108). This supports the concept that the memory B cell epigenome is poised to facilitate a more rapid and robust activation response than that of its naive counterparts.

As demonstrated by concomitant miRNA and mRNA profiling, miRNAs play a regulatory role at every stage of the B cell peripheral differentiation process (28). Selected miRNAs, including miR-125b and let-7, negatively regulate *Prdm1* (10, 27, 28, 101). Down-regulation of miR-15a and miR-16, which target *Bcl2*, likely contributes to memory B cell survival (27, 109) and re-expression of Krüppel-like factors (KLFs), which can bind HDACs, mediates memory B cell quiescence (110). miR-223 is enriched in human memory B cells and down-regulates the expression of LMO2, a key transcription factor in B cell differentiation (28). In addition to function as a negative regulator for CSR and SHM by silencing AID, miR-155 also plays an important role in memory B cell responses. miR-155 deficiency greatly reduced memory B cells (111). Several lncRNAs have been shown to be preferentially expressed in human memory B cells, but not in naïve B cells or B1 cells (112), suggesting that lncRNA also play a role in memory B cell differentiation. Thus, DNA methylation, histone modifications and non-coding RNAs, especially miRNAs, control gene expression programs that lead to B cell differentiation into plasma cells and memory B cells, and maintain the identity of these differentiated cells.

EPIGENETIC MODULATION OF AID AND Blimp-1 EXPRESSION, CSR, SHM, AND PLASMA CELL DIFFERENTIATION BY HDAC INHIBITORS

Histone deacetylases are a class of enzymes that remove the acetyl groups from the lysine residues on a histone leading to the formation of a condensed and transcriptionally silenced chromatin. HDIs block this action and can result in histone hyperacetylation, thereby affecting gene expression. HDIs have been shown to alter gene expression by altering chromatin accessibility (113–115). In immune cells, these epigenetic modifiers exert modulatory effects even at moderate concentrations. By using well-characterized short-chain fatty acid (SCFA) HDIs, valproic acid (VPA) (116), and butyrate (117), we have shown that HDIs regulate intrinsic B cell functions that are critical in shaping effective antibody and autoantibody responses. Our findings were further supported by a recent publication showing that HDIs Panobinostat (a novel broad-spectrum HDI) and Vorinostat (suberanilohydroxamic acid or SAHA) significantly impair antibody and autoantibody responses (118). VPA is an FDA-approved drug, widely used as an anticonvulsant and a mood-stabilizer. It selectively inhibits class I HDACs, particularly, HDAC1 and HDAC2, and, less effectively, class IIa HDACs, of the four HDAC classes identified in mammals (116, 119). Butyrate is a major metabolite in the digestive tract, arising from bacterial fermentation of dietary fibers, mainly "resistant" starch (120, 121), and it is widely available as a dietary supplement. Butyrate modulates gene expression by selectively inhibiting HDAC1 and HDAC3, and, less effectively, other members of class I and class IIa HDACs (117). SCFA HDIs have been suggested to display significant selectivity for different HDACs (122). HDAC activity is mostly associated with multiprotein complexes, the role and composition of which are often cell type-specific. HDAC-associated proteins would specify the selectivity of HDI, which display different affinities for different HDAC/co-factor complexes. HDIs with diverse chemical properties target different HDACs and HDAC/co-factor complexes, thereby regulating gene expression in a locus- and cell type-specific fashion (122). In B cells, HDIs would modulate miRNAs selectively, possibly as a result of HDACs existing in unique contexts of HDAC/co-factor complexes, as occurring in these lymphocytes, particularly when in an activated state (10).

Although HDIs may also indirectly modulate antibody responses or diminish autoimmunity by affecting elements other than B cells, such as innate immune cells (123) and T cells (Treg, T_H1, and T_H17 cells), or inhibit proinflammatory cytokines (115, 124–126), HDIs would directly regulate B cell genes that are central to the peripheral differentiation of these lymphocytes and the maturation of antibody and autoantibody responses (**Figure 2**) (10). Silencing of *AICDA/Aicda* and *PRDM1/Prdm1* (and *XBP1/Xbp1*) by HDIs has been found to be intrinsic to B cells and independent of other cellular elements, as shown by our *in vitro* experiments using purified human and mouse B cells, as well as our *in vivo* studies of the T-dependent response to NP-CGG and the T-independent response to NP-LPS. In both *in vivo* and *in vitro*, HDI-mediated down-regulation of *AICDA/Aicda* and *PRDM1/Prdm1* expression was associated with a concomitant increase of the respective B cell targeting miRNAs (miR-155, miR-181b, and miR-361 for *AICDA/Aicda*; miR-23b, miR-30a, and miR-125b for *PRDM1/Prdm1*), in a tight dose-dependent fashion (10). HDI-induced down-regulation of *XBP1/Xbp1* could be secondary to decreased Blimp-1 expression.

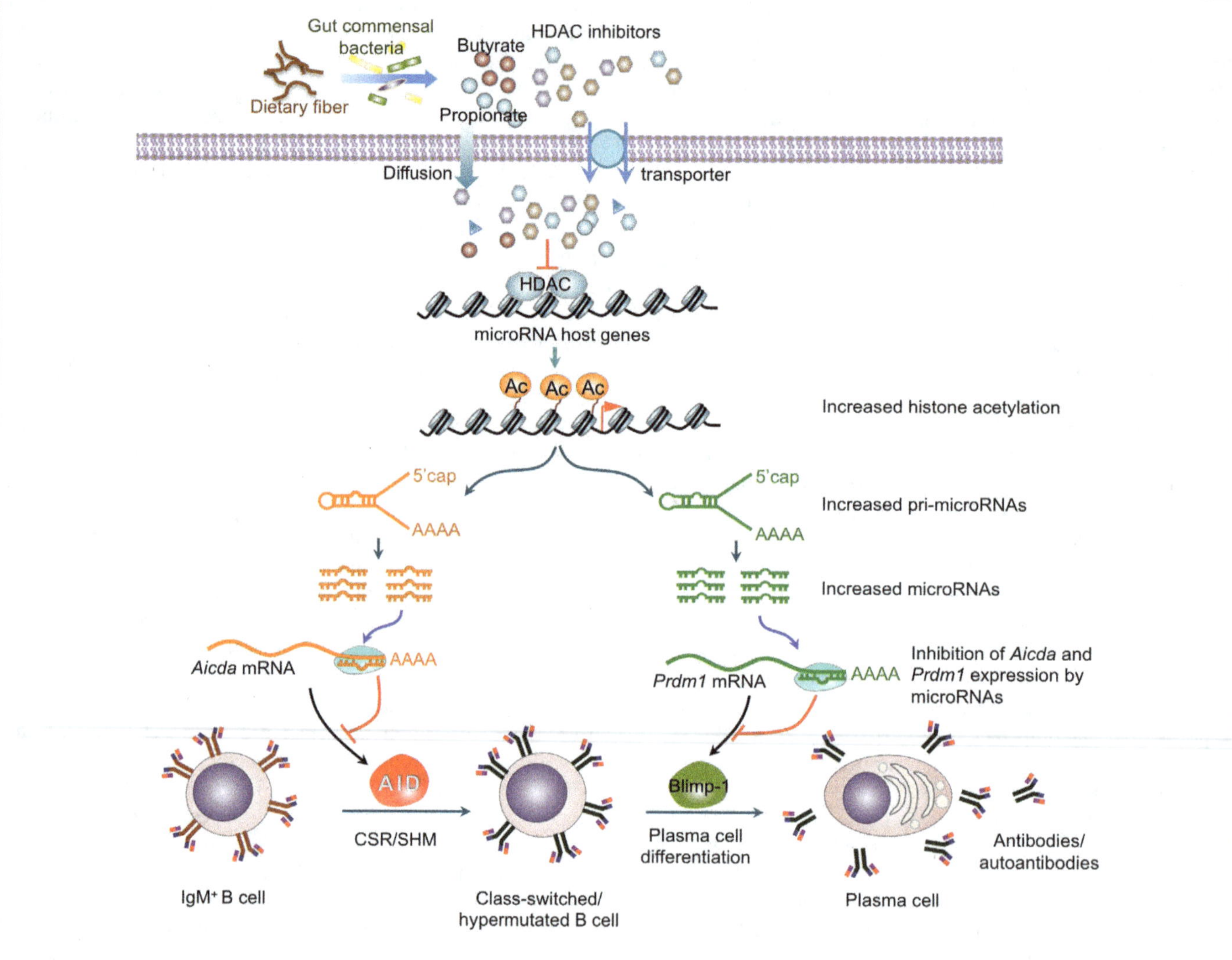

FIGURE 2 | Histone deacetylase inhibitors upregulate selected B cell miRNAs that silence AID and Blimp-1 expression to epigenetically modulate CSR, SHM, plasma cell differentiation and antibody/autoantibody responses. HDAC inhibitors, including short-chain fatty acid butyrate and propionate produced by gut commensal bacteria through fermentation of dietary fiber, epigenetically modify CSR and SHM by upregulating miRNAs, which silence *AICDA/Aicda* mRNA and *PRDM1/Prdm1* mRNA. The upregulation of miRNA expression results from an increase in the histone acetylation of the host genes of these miRNAs. This leads to down-regulation of AID and Blimp-1 expression, and the dampening of CSR, SHM, and plasma cell differentiation.

The selectivity of HDI-mediated silencing of *AICDA/Aicda* and *PRDMI/Prdm1* in B cells that were induced to undergo CSR and plasma cell differentiation was demonstrated by genome-wide mRNA-Seq and further emphasized by the unchanged expression of *Ung*, *Irf4*, *HoxC4*, *Rev1*, and *Bcl6*, as well as the unchanged expression of miR-19a/b, miR-20a, and miR-25, which are not known to regulate *AICDA/Aicda* or *PRDMI/Prdm1* (10, 99). This, however, cannot rule out the possibility that HDI regulated other B cell factors (e.g., NF-κB, Id2/3, or Pax5), which contributed to the reduction of AID or Blimp-1. Nevertheless, relief of the HDI-mediated repression of luciferase activity under the control of *Aicda* and *Prdm1* mRNA 3′ UTRs bearing mutated miR-155, miR-181b, miR-23b, miR-30a, and miR-125b target sites demonstrated that miRNAs are indeed direct effectors of the HDI-mediated repression of such selected genes in B cells (10).

Potential Role for Gut Microbiota-Derived Short-Chain Fatty Acid HDAC Inhibitors in the Modulation of Antibody Response

At ant time, the human body carries 10^{13}–10^{14} microorganisms, a number 10-fold more than the total number of human cells in the body. Human gastrointestinal tract microbiota composed of up to 1,000–1,150 bacterial species, which play an important role in nutritional, metabolic and physiological processes that are crucial for the maintenance of human health. Gut commensal bacteria are critical regulators of health and disease by protecting against pathogen while also maintaining immune tolerance to allergens (127–131). Commensal bacteria may modulate host immunity through metabolite-dependent mechanisms (129, 131). SCFAs, such as acetic acid, propionic acid, and butyric acid, which are generated in the colon by commensal bacteria through digestion of dietary fiber, are among the most abundant of these dietary metabolites. They are important for gut motility and colonocyte development. SCFAs function through binding to host cell surface receptors, such as GPR41, GPR43, and GPR109A, and through their HDI activity (132). It has been suggested that SCFAs produced in the gut could distribute systemically and shape the immunological environment in the respiratory system, thereby influencing the severity of allergic inflammation (132).

Mice fed a low-fiber diet displayed decreased serum levels of SCFAs and increased IgE-mediated allergic inflammation in the lung, while a high-fiber diet increased levels of SCFAs and were protected against allergic airway disease (132). Butyrate and propionate, which are potent HDIs, modulate the function of intestinal macrophages and naive T cells to promote epigenetic changes that regulate the expression of genes responsible for differentiation into regulatory T cells and IL-10-producing T cells (121, 132, 133). Our recent findings that butyrate modulates AID expression and CSR to IgG, IgA, and IgE, as well as plasma cell differentiation through its direct HDI activity on B cells (10), indicates that this SCFA can play an important role in modulating antibody responses of gut lymphoid organs. A diverse microbial population, which would produce an appropriate amount of SCFA HDIs, particularly, butyrate, is required to maintain a baseline immune-regulatory state, including IgG, IgA, and IgE levels. Elevated serum IgE and CSR to IgE in B cells at mucosal sites in the absence of microbial colonization in germ-free mice and in mice with low-diversity gut microbiota (134) further emphasize the important role for gut commensal bacteria-produced butyrate in modulating IgE production. Altered composition and decreased bacterial diversity of gut microbiota would lead to changes in absolute and relative levels of SCFA HDIs and, therefore, changes in systemic IgG, IgA and IgE levels and specificities, which contribute to altered immunity and increased susceptibility to immune-mediated diseases.

B CELL EPIGENETIC DYSREGULATION IN AUTOIMMUNITY AND LYMPHOMAGENESIS

Epigenetic factors also play an important role in the pathogenesis of B cell-related immune disorders, such as autoimmunity, allergic states and B cell malignancies, by integrating the effects of genetic makeup and the environment, two major disease-causing factors. Epigenetic dysregulation would compound genetic susceptibility in the generation of autoantibodies and autoimmunity, as suggested by alterations of histone modifications and DNA methylation in patients with lupus, autoimmunity in mice with miRNA dysregulation (9), and low penetrance (25–45%) of lupus in monozygotic twins (135). The development of allergic diseases has been associated with environmental conditions, such as diet, drugs, toxins, sex hormones, and microbiota, all of which can impact the epigenetic profile (136, 137). Aberrant AID expression that can result from epigenetic dysregulation can lead to autoantibody-mediated autoimmunity, IgE-mediated allergic responses and tumorigenesis (**Figure 3**).

Epigenetic Changes and Autoimmunity

Systemic autoimmune diseases, such as SLE, rheumatoid arthritis, systemic sclerosis, and dermatomyositis, are associated with overall DNA hypomethylation (1, 138, 139). Autoreactive

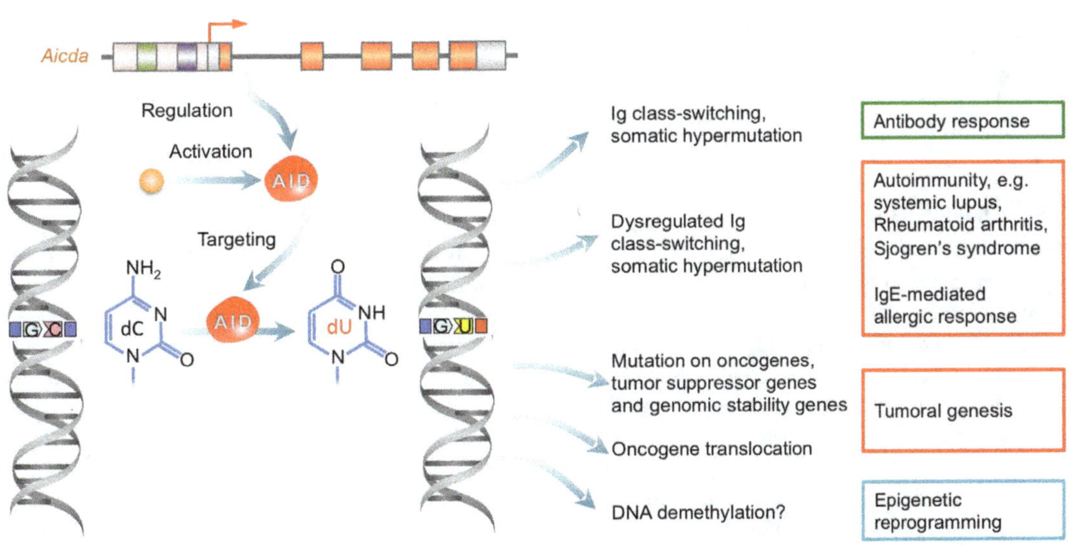

FIGURE 3 | Dysregulation of AID result in autoantibody-mediated autoimmunity, IgE-mediated allergic response and tumoral genesis. AID initiates CSR and SHM by deaminating dCs into dUs yielding dU:dG mismatches, which lead to point-mutations in Ig V(D)J regions and DSBs in S regions. Aberrant AID expression result from epigenetic dysregulation can lead to a dysregulated antibody/autoantibody response and AID-mediated DNA mutagenesis, which can cause autoimmunity, allergic response, or tumoral genesis.

B cells in lupus patients are characterized by lack of ability to induce DNA methylation that extends their survival (140). In mice, prolonged treatment with DNA methylation inhibitors, or adaptive transfer of B cells treated with DNMT inhibitors, resulted in autoantibody production and lupus-like disease (141, 142). The role of DNA methylation in autoimmune diseases is further emphasized by the discordance of SLE in monozygotic twins. B cells isolated from SLE patients displayed profound defects in DNA methylation, as compared to those from healthy monozygotic siblings (135). The decreased DNA methylation in autoreactive B cells likely resulted from reduced DNMT1 and DNMT3b expression; it could also result from active DNA demethylation mediated by AID-mediated cytosine deamination (143). Indeed, AID is upregulated in B cells of lupus patients or lupus-prone mice (3, 9, 144). The contribution of aberrant histone modifications to lupus development has been strongly suggested by the increased histone acetylation and reduced autoantibody production in lupus-prone mice treated with HDIs (1, 10, 145).

Dysregulation of miRNAs has been associated with autoimminty. miRNAs are aberrantly expressed in different cell types and tissues in patients with autoimmune disease. B cell-specific deletion of Dicer, which is critical for miRNA maturation, resulted in a distorted BCR repertoire with increased of autoreactivity, suggesting a role for miRNAs in preventing the generation of self-reactive antibodies (9, 146, 147). In lupus-prone MRL/$Fas^{lpr/lpr}$ mice, miR-150 is downregulated in spleen B cells, as compared to that in MRL/$Fas^{+/+}$ mice (148), possibly as a result of decreased acetylation and transcription of the miR-150 host gene due to defective HDAC activity. Indeed, specific knock-in dominant negative mutant of histone acetyltransferase p300 in B cells resulted in production of class-switched anti-double-stranded DNA autoantibodies and development of lupus-like symptoms (149). Conversely, elevated expression of some miRNAs can also contribute to the development of autoimmunity. In lupus mice, expression miR-21 is upregulated in B cells, silencing of this miRNA ameliorates autoimmune splenomegaly (150). Constitutively expression of miR-17 ~ 92 in transgenic mice results in an increased numbers of germinal center B cells in the spleen and peripheral lymph nodes that may lead to autoimmune response (151).

TABLE 2 | B cell epigenetic dysregulation and lymphomagenesis.

Neoplasm	Epigenetic change	Potential impacts of epigenetic changes	Reference
DLBCL, FL	Loss-of-function mutation of HAT genes *CREBBP* and *EP300*	Reduce P53 and BCL6 acetylation	(177, 178)
HD, NHL	Deregulation of the H3K27 methyltransferase EZH2	Malignant GC B cell transformation	(179)
Multiple myeloma	Overexpression of H3K36 methyltransferase *MMSET/NSD2*	Alter H3K36 and H3K27 methylation, upregulate *c-MYC* expression by reducing *c-MYC* targeting miR-126	(180)
NHL, DLBCL, FL, MLL	Dysregulation of the H3K4 methyltransferase MLL2/MLL3/KMT2D	Modulate cell-type- and stage-specific transcriptional programs by regulating chromatin accessibility at enhancer regulatory sequences	(181)
NHL, DLBCL	Aberrant DNA methylation	Promote aberrant gene expression	(155, 182, 183)
B cell CLL	miR-15a/16-1 depletion	Aberrant expression of cell cycle regulators Ccnd2, Ccnd3, Cdk4, Cdk6 and Chk1, and anti-apoptotic protein BCL2	(171, 184)
NHL, HD, BL	miR-155 deregulation	Enhance/sustain AID mutagenic activity	(37, 185)
DLBCL, BL	Overexpression of the miR-17-92 cluster	Downregulate inhibitors of the PI3K (*Pten*), NF-κB (*A20, Cyld*) and the intrinsic apoptotic (*Bim*) pathways; alter MYC-centered regulatory network	(151, 186, 187)

Epigenetics Changes and Lymphomagenesis

At all stages of cancer development, inappropriate epigenetic marks interact with genetic alterations to promote neoplastic transformation and tumor cell progression (152, 153). The epigenome of B cell lymphomas is characterized by global changes in DNA methylation and histone modification patterns, which varies with chromosomal regions, local gene density, as well as DNA and histone modification status of neighboring genes (**Table 2**) (154, 155). Aberrant DNA hypomethylation of promoters can lead to increased transcription of genes with oncogenic potential, and aberrant DNA hypermethylation can lead to decreased transcription of genes with tumor suppressor function. For example, mantle B cell lymphomas display DNA hypomethylation in promoters of genes that are involved in pathways controlling cell cycle or apoptosis, such as *Cdk5*, and aberrant hypermethylation in the promoter of tumor suppressor genes, such as *Cdkn2b* (156). Hypermethylation is likely associated with increased expression of DNMTs, such as DNMT3b, which is upregulated in diffuse lager B cell lymphomas (157). Accordingly, *Dnmt3b* transgenic mice develop mediastinal B cell lymphomas, which display significantly altered methylation patterns (157). Aberrant hypomethylation could involve AID, which can mediate active DNA demethylation (158) and is upregulated in human B cell non-Hodgkin lymphomas (NHL) (159).

Active DNA demethylation can also be initiated by the 10–11 translocation (Tet) family of proteins Tet1, Tet2, and Tet3, which catalyze the oxidation of 5mC to 5-hydroxymethylcytosine (5hmC), a critical step for ultimate removal of a methyl mark (160, 161). Reduced expression of Tet proteins that lead to decreased 5hmC has been shown to associate with tumor development, suggests an important role of Tet proteins and 5hmC in normal cellular function (162). Tet1 is required for maintaining the normal abundance and distribution of 5hmC, which prevented hypermethylation of DNA in B cells (163). It is important for regulation of the B cell lineage and of genes encoding molecules involved in chromosome maintenance and DNA repair. Tet1 may function as a tumor suppressor of B cell malignancy. Deletion of *Tet1* in mice promotes the development of B cell lymphoma (163).

Altered expression or mutation of the histone-modifying enzymes promotes aberrant gene expression, which is responsible for many tumor changes (164). Aberrant germinal center development is common in many B cell malignancies. EZH2, a histone methyltransferase component of polycomb repression complex (PRC)2 that catalyzes H3K27me3 and promotes tumor growth, is highly expressed in germinal center B cells and is often constitutively activated in germinal center-derive NHLs. EZH2 prevents apoptosis caused by DNA damage, including that generated by AID, facilitated cell cycle progression, and silenced Blimp-1, which can function as tumor suppressor (106). Inhibition of EZH2 in NHL cells induces Blimp-1, which impairs tumor growth. Overexpression of EZH2 is associated with B lymphomagenesis (165). Somatic mutations at Y641 and A677 residues within the catalytic domain of EZH2 have been found in diffuse large B cell lymphoma and follicular lymphoma (166). These mutations promote EZH2 activity and increase H3K27me3 levels in those cells (165). Furthermore, other histone-modifying enzymes, such as histone acetyltransferases CBP and p300, histone methyltransferases MLL2, and histone demethylases UTX and JMJD2C, are frequently mutated in B cell lymphomas (157). Mutations in these enzymes are likely mediated by AID, which is highly expressed in those neoplastic B cells, and result in aberrant patterns of histone modifications and disruption of chromatin structure, ultimately leading to dysregulated gene transcription programs.

Dysregulated miRNA expression also contributes to B lymphomagenesis (28, 167). The miR-17 ~ 92 cluster, which consists of six miRNAs (miR-17, miR-18a, miR-19a, miR-20a, miR-19b-1, and miR-92-1) that target the tumor repressor genes *Bim* and *Pten*, is often increased in human lymphomas (151, 168). Accordingly, ectopic expression of the miR-17 ~ 92 cluster in lymphocytes leads to development of lymphoproliferative disease (151, 168). Conversely, expression of miR-15 and miR-16-1, which target anti-apoptotic oncogene *Bcl-2*, is downregulated in chronic lymphocytic leukemia B cells (169, 170). Knockout miR-15a and miR-16-1 in B cells results in clonal lymphoproliferative disorders (171). B cell lymphomas often express significant amounts of mRNA isoforms with shorter 3′ UTRs, which lack miRNA-binding sites, thereby escaping miRNA-directed silencing (172). For example, a short *Cyclin D1* mRNA isoform that lacks part of the 3′ UTR is expressed in a subset of mantle cell lymphomas (172). These cells have increased expression of Cyclin D1, an important regulator of cell cycle progression, and B cell proliferation. Thus, by allowing selected oncogenes to escape regulation by their modulatory miRNAs, the shortening of 3′ UTRs may provide an important mechanism in B cell neoplastic transformation.

CONCLUDING REMARKS

Epigenetic changes are critical in shaping B cell differentiation functions, such as CSR, SHM, generation of plasma cells as well as memory B cells, for the production of class-switched and high affinity antibodies. In addition, a growing body of evidence implicates the involvement of epigenetic mechanisms in immune programing and development of allergic and autoimmune diseases. Nevertheless, important questions on the nature and role of such epigenetic changes remain to be answered. These include the mechanisms by which histone posttranslational modifications and non-coding RNAs target the CSR and SHM machineries, particularly the selective recruitment of AID, to the *Ig* locus and how the dynamics of these epigenetic modifications orchestrate AID-mediated DNA lesion and DNA repair processes. High-affinity antibodies are generated in germinal centers through SHM and selection of higher affinity B cell submutants for survival and expansion. These B cells will then undergo differentiation to plasma cells or memory B cells. Much needs be understood on the role of epigenetic modifications in the selection of germinal center B cells and in what determines whether a germinal B cell becomes a memory B cell or a plasma cell. These processes would involve unique epigenetic and transcriptional changes. Furthermore, altered DNA methylation, histone methylation and acetylation, and miRNA expression, resulting in immune imbalance, have been shown to be associated with the onset and progression of allergic and autoimmune diseases, as well as B cell lymphomagenesis. Thus, knowledge of the epigenetic profiles associated with B cell development and peripheral differentiation, and molecular mechanisms that cause and result from disease-associated epigenetic patterns in B cells is required to understand the pathophysiology of allergic and autoimmune diseases, as well as B cell malignancies.

ACKNOWLEDGMENTS

We apologize that owing to space limitations only a fraction of the relevant literature was cited in this review article. This work was supported by NIH grants AI 079705 and AI 105813, and the Alliance for Lupus Research Target Identification in Lupus Grant ALR 295955 (to PC) and an Arthritis National Research Foundation grant (to HZ).

REFERENCES

1. Hedrich CM, Tsokos GC. Epigenetic mechanisms in systemic lupus erythematosus and other autoimmune diseases. *Trends Mol Med* (2011) **17**:714–24. doi:10.1016/j.molmed.2011.07.005
2. Xu Z, Zan H, Pone EJ, Mai T, Casali P. Immunoglobulin class-switch DNA recombination: induction, targeting and beyond. *Nat Rev Immunol* (2012) **12**:517–31. doi:10.1038/nri3216
3. Zan H, Casali P. Regulation of *Aicda* expression and AID activity. *Autoimmunity* (2013) **46**:81–99. doi:10.3109/08916934.2012.749244
4. Li G, Zan H, Xu Z, Casali P. Epigenetics of the antibody response. *Trends Immunol* (2013) **34**:460–70. doi:10.1016/j.it.2013.03.006
5. De Silva NS, Klein U. Dynamics of B cells in germinal centres. *Nat Rev Immunol* (2015) **15**:137–48. doi:10.1038/nri3804
6. Nutt SL, Hodgkin PD, Tarlinton DM, Corcoran LM. The generation of antibody-secreting plasma cells. *Nat Rev Immunol* (2015) **15**:160–71. doi:10.1038/nri3795
7. Kurosaki T, Kometani K, Ise W. Memory B cells. *Nat Rev Immunol* (2015) **15**:149–59. doi:10.1038/nri3802
8. Li G, Pone EJ, Lan T, Tran DC, Mai T, Zan H, et al. Combinatorial H3K9acS10ph histone modification in IgH locus S regions targets 14-3-3

adaptors and AID to specify antibody class-switch DNA recombination. *Cell Rep* (2013) **5**:702–14. doi:10.1016/j.celrep.2013.09.031
9. Zan H, Tat C, Casali P. microRNAs in lupus. *Autoimmunity* (2014) **47**:272–85. doi:10.3109/08916934.2014.915955
10. White CA, Pone EJ, Lam T, Tat C, Hayama KL, Li G, et al. Histone deacetylase inhibitors upregulate B cell microRNAs that silence AID and Blimp-1 expression for epigenetic modulation of antibody and autoantibody responses. *J Immunol* (2014) **193**:5933–50. doi:10.4049/jimmunol.1401702
11. Shaknovich R, Cerchietti L, Tsikitas L, Kormaksson M, De S, Figueroa ME, et al. DNA methyltransferase 1 and DNA methylation patterning contribute to germinal center B-cell differentiation. *Blood* (2011) **118**:3559–69. doi:10.1182/blood-2011-06-357996
12. Chowdhury M, Forouhi O, Dayal S, McCloskey N, Gould HJ, Felsenfeld G, et al. Analysis of intergenic transcription and histone modification across the human immunoglobulin heavy-chain locus. *Proc Natl Acad Sci U S A* (2008) **105**:15872–7. doi:10.1073/pnas.0808462105
13. Jeevan-Raj BP, Robert I, Heyer V, Page A, Wang JH, Cammas F, et al. Epigenetic tethering of AID to the donor switch region during immunoglobulin class switch recombination. *J Exp Med* (2011) **208**:1649–60. doi:10.1084/jem.20110118
14. Robbiani DF, Bothmer A, Callen E, Reina-San-Martin B, Dorsett Y, Difilippantonio S, et al. AID is required for the chromosomal breaks in c-myc that lead to c-myc/IgH translocations. *Cell* (2008) **135**:1028–38. doi:10.1016/j.cell.2008.09.062
15. Pasqualucci L, Bhagat G, Jankovic M, Compagno M, Smith P, Muramatsu M, et al. AID is required for germinal center-derived lymphomagenesis. *Nat Genet* (2008) **40**:108–12. doi:10.1038/ng.2007.35
16. Robbiani DF, Bunting S, Feldhahn N, Bothmer A, Camps J, Deroubaix S, et al. AID produces DNA double-strand breaks in non-Ig genes and mature B cell lymphomas with reciprocal chromosome translocations. *Mol Cell* (2009) **36**:631–41. doi:10.1016/j.molcel.2009.11.007
17. Hasham MG, Donghia NM, Coffey E, Maynard J, Snow KJ, Ames J, et al. Widespread genomic breaks generated by activation-induced cytidine deaminase are prevented by homologous recombination. *Nat Immunol* (2010) **11**:820–6. doi:10.1038/ni.1909
18. Chandra V, Bortnick A, Murre C. AID targeting: old mysteries and new challenges. *Trends Immunol* (2015) **36**(9):527–35. doi:10.1016/j.it.2015.07.003
19. Park SR, Zan H, Pal Z, Zhang J, Al-Qahtani A, Pone EJ, et al. HoxC4 binds to the promoter of the cytidine deaminase AID gene to induce AID expression, class-switch DNA recombination and somatic hypermutation. *Nat Immunol* (2009) **10**:540–50. doi:10.1038/ni.1725
20. White CA, Seth Hawkins J, Pone EJ, Yu ES, Al-Qahtani A, Mai T, et al. AID dysregulation in lupus-prone MRL/Fas(lpr/lpr) mice increases class switch DNA recombination and promotes interchromosomal c-Myc/IgH loci translocations: modulation by HoxC4. *Autoimmunity* (2011) **44**:585–98. doi:10.3109/08916934.2011.577128
21. Fujimura S, Matsui T, Kuwahara K, Maeda K, Sakaguchi N. Germinal center B-cell-associated DNA hypomethylation at transcriptional regions of the AID gene. *Mol Immunol* (2008) **45**:1712–9. doi:10.1016/j.molimm.2007.09.023
22. Crouch EE, Li Z, Takizawa M, Fichtner-Feigl S, Gourzi P, Montano C, et al. Regulation of AID expression in the immune response. *J Exp Med* (2007) **204**:1145–56. doi:10.1084/jem.20061952
23. Begum NA, Stanlie A, Nakata M, Akiyama H, Honjo T. The histone chaperone Spt6 is required for activation-induced cytidine deaminase target determination through H3K4me3 regulation. *J Biol Chem* (2012) **287**:32415–29. doi:10.1074/jbc.M112.351569
24. Ha M, Kim VN. Regulation of microRNA biogenesis. *Nat Rev Mol Cell Biol* (2014) **15**:509–24. doi:10.1038/nrm3838
25. Hausser J, Zavolan M. Identification and consequences of miRNA-target interactions-beyond repression of gene expression. *Nat Rev Genet* (2014) **15**:599–612. doi:10.1038/nrg3765
26. Cech TR, Steitz JA. The noncoding RNA revolution-trashing old rules to forge new ones. *Cell* (2014) **157**:77–94. doi:10.1016/j.cell.2014.03.008
27. Malumbres R, Sarosiek KA, Cubedo E, Ruiz JW, Jiang X, Gascoyne RD, et al. Differentiation stage-specific expression of microRNAs in B lymphocytes and diffuse large B-cell lymphomas. *Blood* (2009) **113**:3754–64. doi:10.1182/blood-2008-10-184077
28. Zhang J, Jima DD, Jacobs C, Fischer R, Gottwein E, Huang G, et al. Patterns of microRNA expression characterize stages of human B-cell differentiation. *Blood* (2009) **113**:4586–94. doi:10.1182/blood-2008-09-178186
29. Xu S, Guo K, Zeng Q, Huo J, Lam KP. The RNase III enzyme Dicer is essential for germinal center B-cell formation. *Blood* (2012) **119**:767–76. doi:10.1182/blood-2011-05-355412
30. Thai TH, Calado DP, Casola S, Ansel KM, Xiao C, Xue Y, et al. Regulation of the germinal center response by microRNA-155. *Science* (2007) **316**:604–8. doi:10.1126/science.1141229
31. Gururajan M, Haga CL, Das S, Leu CM, Hodson D, Josson S, et al. microRNA 125b inhibition of B cell differentiation in germinal centers. *Int Immunol* (2010) **22**:583–92. doi:10.1093/intimm/dxq042
32. Vigorito E, Perks KL, Abreu-Goodger C, Bunting S, Xiang Z, Kohlhaas S, et al. microRNA-155 regulates the generation of immunoglobulin class-switched plasma cells. *Immunity* (2007) **27**:847–59. doi:10.1016/j.immuni.2007.10.009
33. Teng G, Hakimpour P, Landgraf P, Rice A, Tuschl T, Casellas R, et al. microRNA-155 is a negative regulator of activation-induced cytidine deaminase. *Immunity* (2008) **28**:621–9. doi:10.1016/j.immuni.2008.03.015
34. Dorsett Y, McBride KM, Jankovic M, Gazumyan A, Thai TH, Robbiani DF, et al. microRNA-155 suppresses activation-induced cytidine deaminase-mediated Myc-Igh translocation. *Immunity* (2008) **28**:630–8. doi:10.1016/j.immuni.2008.04.002
35. de Yebenes VG, Belver L, Pisano DG, Gonzalez S, Villasante A, Croce C, et al. miR-181b negatively regulates activation-induced cytidine deaminase in B cells. *J Exp Med* (2008) **205**:2199–206. doi:10.1084/jem.20080579
36. Borchert GM, Holton NW, Larson ED. Repression of human activation induced cytidine deaminase by miR-93 and miR-155. *BMC Cancer* (2011) **11**:347. doi:10.1186/1471-2407-11-347
37. Basso K, Schneider C, Shen Q, Holmes AB, Setty M, Leslie C, et al. BCL6 positively regulates AID and germinal center gene expression via repression of miR-155. *J Exp Med* (2012) **209**:2455–65. doi:10.1084/jem.20121387
38. Faraoni I, Antonetti FR, Cardone J, Bonmassar E. miR-155 gene: a typical multifunctional microRNA. *Biochim Biophys Acta* (2009) **1792**:497–505. doi:10.1016/j.bbadis.2009.02.013
39. Rodriguez A, Vigorito E, Clare S, Warren MV, Couttet P, Soond DR, et al. Requirement of bic/microRNA-155 for normal immune function. *Science* (2007) **316**:608–11. doi:10.1126/science.1139253
40. Thai TH, Patterson HC, Pham DH, Kis-Toth K, Kaminski DA, Tsokos GC. Deletion of microRNA-155 reduces autoantibody responses and alleviates lupus-like disease in the Fas(lpr) mouse. *Proc Natl Acad Sci U S A* (2013) **110**:20194–9. doi:10.1073/pnas.1317632110
41. Landgraf P, Rusu M, Sheridan R, Sewer A, Iovino N, Aravin A, et al. A mammalian microRNA expression atlas based on small RNA library sequencing. *Cell* (2007) **129**:1401–14. doi:10.1016/j.cell.2007.04.040
42. Stavnezer J. Complex regulation and function of activation-induced cytidine deaminase. *Trends Immunol* (2011) **32**:194–201. doi:10.1016/j.it.2011.03.003
43. Kluiver J, van den Berg A, de Jong D, Blokzijl T, Harms G, Bouwman E, et al. Regulation of pri-microRNA BIC transcription and processing in Burkitt lymphoma. *Oncogene* (2007) **26**:3769–76. doi:10.1038/sj.onc.1210147
44. Fear DJ, McCloskey N, O'Connor B, Felsenfeld G, Gould HJ. Transcription of Ig germline genes in single human B cells and the role of cytokines in isotype determination. *J Immunol* (2004) **173**:4529–38. doi:10.4049/jimmunol.173.7.4529
45. Nambu Y, Sugai M, Gonda H, Lee CG, Katakai T, Agata Y, et al. Transcription-coupled events associating with immunoglobulin switch region chromatin. *Science* (2003) **302**:2137–40. doi:10.1126/science.1092481
46. Wang L, Wuerffel R, Feldman S, Khamlichi AA, Kenter AL. S region sequence, RNA polymerase II, and histone modifications create chromatin accessibility during class switch recombination. *J Exp Med* (2009) **206**:1817–30. doi:10.1084/jem.20081678
47. Daniel JA, Santos MA, Wang Z, Zang C, Schwab KR, Jankovic M, et al. PTIP promotes chromatin changes critical for immunoglobulin class switch recombination. *Science* (2010) **329**:917–23. doi:10.1126/science.1187942
48. Stanlie A, Aida M, Muramatsu M, Honjo T, Begum NA. Histone3 lysine4 trimethylation regulated by the facilitates chromatin transcription complex is critical for DNA cleavage in class switch recombination. *Proc Natl Acad Sci U S A* (2010) **107**:22190–5. doi:10.1073/pnas.1016923108

49. Kuang FL, Luo Z, Scharff MD. H3 trimethyl K9 and H3 acetyl K9 chromatin modifications are associated with class switch recombination. *Proc Natl Acad Sci U S A* (2009) **106**:5288–93. doi:10.1073/pnas.0901368106
50. Rajagopal D, Maul RW, Ghosh A, Chakraborty T, Khamlichi AA, Sen R, et al. Immunoglobulin switch mu sequence causes RNA polymerase II accumulation and reduces dA hypermutation. *J Exp Med* (2009) **206**:1237–44. doi:10.1084/jem.20082514
51. Pavri R, Gazumyan A, Jankovic M, Di Virgilio M, Klein I, Ansarah-Sobrinho C, et al. Activation-induced cytidine deaminase targets DNA at sites of RNA polymerase II stalling by interaction with Spt5. *Cell* (2010) **143**:122–33. doi:10.1016/j.cell.2010.09.017
52. Storck S, Aoufouchi S, Weill JC, Reynaud CA. AID and partners: for better and (not) for worse. *Curr Opin Immunol* (2011) **23**:337–44. doi:10.1016/j.coi.2011.02.002
53. Kenter AL. AID targeting is dependent on RNA polymerase II pausing. *Semin Immunol* (2012) **24**:281–6. doi:10.1016/j.smim.2012.06.001
54. Xu Z, Fulop Z, Wu G, Pone EJ, Zhang J, Mai T, et al. 14-3-3 adaptor proteins recruit AID to 5'-AGCT-3'-rich switch regions for class switch recombination. *Nat Struct Mol Biol* (2010) **17**:1124–35. doi:10.1038/nsmb.1884
55. Schatz DG, Swanson PC. V(D)J recombination: mechanisms of initiation. *Annu Rev Genet* (2011) **45**:167–202. doi:10.1146/annurev-genet-110410-132552
56. Aida M, Hamad N, Stanlie A, Begum NA, Honjo T. Accumulation of the FACT complex, as well as histone H3.3, serves as a target marker for somatic hypermutation. *Proc Natl Acad Sci U S A* (2013) **110**:7784–9. doi:10.1073/pnas.1305859110
57. Wang Z, Zang C, Rosenfeld JA, Schones DE, Barski A, Cuddapah S, et al. Combinatorial patterns of histone acetylations and methylations in the human genome. *Nat Genet* (2008) **40**:897–903. doi:10.1038/ng.154
58. Suganuma T, Workman JL. Signals and combinatorial functions of histone modifications. *Annu Rev Biochem* (2011) **80**:473–99. doi:10.1146/annurev-biochem-061809-175347
59. Bradley SP, Kaminski DA, Peters AH, Jenuwein T, Stavnezer J. The histone methyltransferase Suv39h1 increases class switch recombination specifically to IgA. *J Immunol* (2006) **177**:1179–88. doi:10.4049/jimmunol.177.2.1179
60. Zan H, White CA, Thomas LM, Mai T, Li G, Xu Z, et al. Rev1 recruits ung to switch regions and enhances du glycosylation for immunoglobulin class switch DNA recombination. *Cell Rep* (2012) **2**:1220–32. doi:10.1016/j.celrep.2012.09.029
61. Yamane A, Resch W, Kuo N, Kuchen S, Li Z, Sun HW, et al. Deep-sequencing identification of the genomic targets of the cytidine deaminase AID and its cofactor RPA in B lymphocytes. *Nat Immunol* (2011) **12**:62–9. doi:10.1038/ni.1964
62. Pei H, Wu X, Liu T, Yu K, Jelinek DF, Lou Z. The histone methyltransferase MMSET regulates class switch recombination. *J Immunol* (2013) **190**:756–63. doi:10.4049/jimmunol.1201811
63. Nagaoka H, Ito S, Muramatsu M, Nakata M, Honjo T. DNA cleavage in immunoglobulin somatic hypermutation depends on de novo protein synthesis but not on uracil DNA glycosylase. *Proc Natl Acad Sci U S A* (2005) **102**:2022–7. doi:10.1073/pnas.0409491102
64. Wang KC, Chang HY. Molecular mechanisms of long noncoding RNAs. *Mol Cell* (2011) **43**:904–14. doi:10.1016/j.molcel.2011.08.018
65. Lee JT. Epigenetic regulation by long noncoding RNAs. *Science* (2012) **338**:1435–9. doi:10.1126/science.1231776
66. Satpathy AT, Chang HY. Long noncoding RNA in hematopoiesis and immunity. *Immunity* (2015) **42**:792–804. doi:10.1016/j.immuni.2015.05.004
67. Pefanis E, Wang J, Rothschild G, Lim J, Chao J, Rabadan R, et al. Noncoding RNA transcription targets AID to divergently transcribed loci in B cells. *Nature* (2014) **514**:389–93. doi:10.1038/nature13580
68. Basu U, Meng FL, Keim C, Grinstein V, Pefanis E, Eccleston J, et al. The RNA exosome targets the AID cytidine deaminase to both strands of transcribed duplex DNA substrates. *Cell* (2011) **144**:353–63. doi:10.1016/j.cell.2011.01.001
69. Zheng S, Vuong BQ, Vaidyanathan B, Lin JY, Huang FT, Chaudhuri J. Non-coding RNA Generated following Lariat Debranching Mediates Targeting of AID to DNA. *Cell* (2015) **161**:762–73. doi:10.1016/j.cell.2015.03.020
70. Pefanis E, Wang J, Rothschild G, Lim J, Kazadi D, Sun J, et al. RNA exosome-regulated long non-coding RNA transcription controls super-enhancer activity. *Cell* (2015) **161**:774–89. doi:10.1016/j.cell.2015.04.034
71. Qian J, Wang Q, Dose M, Pruett N, Kieffer-Kwon KR, Resch W, et al. B cell super-enhancers and regulatory clusters recruit AID tumorigenic activity. *Cell* (2014) **159**:1524–37. doi:10.1016/j.cell.2014.11.013
72. Odegard VH, Kim ST, Anderson SM, Shlomchik MJ, Schatz DG. Histone modifications associated with somatic hypermutation. *Immunity* (2005) **23**:101–10. doi:10.1016/j.immuni.2005.05.007
73. Daniel JA, Nussenzweig A. The AID-induced DNA damage response in chromatin. *Mol Cell* (2013) **50**:309–21. doi:10.1016/j.molcel.2013.04.017
74. Wang Q, Oliveira T, Jankovic M, Silva IT, Hakim O, Yao K, et al. Epigenetic targeting of activation-induced cytidine deaminase. *Proc Natl Acad Sci U S A* (2014) **111**:18667–72. doi:10.1073/pnas.1420575111
75. Willmann KL, Milosevic S, Pauklin S, Schmitz KM, Rangam G, Simon MT, et al. A role for the RNA pol II-associated PAF complex in AID-induced immune diversification. *J Exp Med* (2012) **209**:2099–111. doi:10.1084/jem.20112145
76. Meng FL, Du Z, Federation A, Hu J, Wang Q, Kieffer-Kwon KR, et al. Convergent transcription at intragenic super-enhancers targets AID-initiated genomic instability. *Cell* (2014) **159**:1538–48. doi:10.1016/j.cell.2014.11.014
77. Odegard VH, Schatz DG. Targeting of somatic hypermutation. *Nat Rev Immunol* (2006) **6**:573–83. doi:10.1038/nri1896
78. Kato L, Begum NA, Burroughs AM, Doi T, Kawai J, Daub CO, et al. Nonimmunoglobulin target loci of activation-induced cytidine deaminase (AID) share unique features with immunoglobulin genes. *Proc Natl Acad Sci U S A* (2012) **109**:2479–84. doi:10.1073/pnas.1120791109
79. Orphanides G, LeRoy G, Chang CH, Luse DS, Reinberg D. FACT, a factor that facilitates transcript elongation through nucleosomes. *Cell* (1998) **92**:105–16. doi:10.1016/S0092-8674(00)80903-4
80. Belotserkovskaya R, Oh S, Bondarenko VA, Orphanides G, Studitsky VM, Reinberg D. FACT facilitates transcription-dependent nucleosome alteration. *Science* (2003) **301**:1090–3. doi:10.1126/science.1085703
81. Aida M, Honjo T. FACT and H3.3: new markers for the somatic hypermutation. *Cell Cycle* (2013) **12**:2923–4. doi:10.4161/cc.26178
82. Borchert GM, Holton NW, Edwards KA, Vogel LA, Larson ED. Histone H2A and H2B are monoubiquitinated at AID-targeted loci. *PLoS One* (2010) **5**:e11641. doi:10.1371/journal.pone.0011641
83. Kannouche PL, Wing J, Lehmann AR. Interaction of human DNA polymerase eta with monoubiquitinated PCNA: a possible mechanism for the polymerase switch in response to DNA damage. *Mol Cell* (2004) **14**:491–500. doi:10.1016/S1097-2765(04)00259-X
84. Fraenkel S, Mostoslavsky R, Novobrantseva TI, Pelanda R, Chaudhuri J, Esposito G, et al. Allelic 'choice' governs somatic hypermutation in vivo at the immunoglobulin kappa-chain locus. *Nat Immunol* (2007) **8**:715–22. doi:10.1038/ni1476
85. Woo CJ, Martin A, Scharff MD. Induction of somatic hypermutation is associated with modifications in immunoglobulin variable region chromatin. *Immunity* (2003) **19**:479–89. doi:10.1016/S1074-7613(03)00261-9
86. Kitao H, Kimura M, Yamamoto K, Seo H, Namikoshi K, Agata Y, et al. Regulation of histone H4 acetylation by transcription factor E2A in Ig gene conversion. *Int Immunol* (2008) **20**:277–84. doi:10.1093/intimm/dxm140
87. Blagodatski A, Batrak V, Schmidl S, Schoetz U, Caldwell RB, Arakawa H, et al. A cis-acting diversification activator both necessary and sufficient for AID-mediated hypermutation. *PLoS Genet* (2009) **5**:e1000332. doi:10.1371/journal.pgen.1000332
88. Buerstedde JM, Alinikula J, Arakawa H, McDonald JJ, Schatz DG. Targeting of somatic hypermutation by immunoglobulin enhancer and enhancer-like sequences. *PLoS Biol* (2014) **12**:e1001831. doi:10.1371/journal.pbio.1001831
89. McHeyzer-Williams M, Okitsu S, Wang N, McHeyzer-Williams L. Molecular programming of B cell memory. *Nat Rev Immunol* (2012) **12**:24–34. doi:10.1038/nri3128
90. Dogan I, Bertocci B, Vilmont V, Delbos F, Megret J, Storck S, et al. Multiple layers of B cell memory with different effector functions. *Nat Immunol* (2009) **10**:1292–9. doi:10.1038/ni.1814
91. McHeyzer-Williams LJ, Milpied PJ, Okitsu SL, McHeyzer-Williams MG. Class-switched memory B cells remodel BCRs within secondary germinal centers. *Nat Immunol* (2015) **16**:296–305. doi:10.1038/ni.3095
92. Shi W, Liao Y, Willis SN, Taubenheim N, Inouye M, Tarlinton DM, et al. Transcriptional profiling of mouse B cell terminal differentiation defines a

signature for antibody-secreting plasma cells. *Nat Immunol* (2015) **16**:663–73. doi:10.1038/ni.3154
93. Heinz S, Benner C, Spann N, Bertolino E, Lin YC, Laslo P, et al. Simple combinations of lineage-determining transcription factors prime cis-regulatory elements required for macrophage and B cell identities. *Mol Cell* (2010) **38**:576–89. doi:10.1016/j.molcel.2010.05.004
94. Yu J, Angelin-Duclos C, Greenwood J, Liao J, Calame K. Transcriptional repression by blimp-1 (PRDI-BF1) involves recruitment of histone deacetylase. *Mol Cell Biol* (2000) **20**:2592–603. doi:10.1128/MCB.20.7.2592-2603.2000
95. Su ST, Ying HY, Chiu YK, Lin FR, Chen MY, Lin KI. Involvement of histone demethylase LSD1 in Blimp-1-mediated gene repression during plasma cell differentiation. *Mol Cell Biol* (2009) **29**:1421–31. doi:10.1128/MCB.01158-08
96. Gyory I, Wu J, Fejer G, Seto E, Wright KL. PRDI-BF1 recruits the histone H3 methyltransferase G9a in transcriptional silencing. *Nat Immunol* (2004) **5**:299–308. doi:10.1038/ni1046
97. Lemercier C, Brocard MP, Puvion-Dutilleul F, Kao HY, Albagli O, Khochbin S. Class II histone deacetylases are directly recruited by BCL6 transcriptional repressor. *J Biol Chem* (2002) **277**:22045–52. doi:10.1074/jbc.M201736200
98. Fujita N, Jaye DL, Geigerman C, Akyildiz A, Mooney MR, Boss JM, et al. MTA3 and the Mi-2/NuRD complex regulate cell fate during B lymphocyte differentiation. *Cell* (2004) **119**:75–86. doi:10.1016/j.cell.2004.09.014
99. Shen T, Nasrollahi H, Zan H, Casali P. Genome-wide analysis of B cells reveals selective modulation of microRNAs and mRNAs by histone deacetylase inhibitor. *Front Immunol* (2015) **6**:627. doi:10.3389/fimmu.2015.00627
100. West JA, Viswanathan SR, Yabuuchi A, Cunniff K, Takeuchi A, Park IH, et al. A role for Lin28 in primordial germ-cell development and germ-cell malignancy. *Nature* (2009) **460**:909–13. doi:10.1038/nature08210
101. Nie K, Zhang T, Allawi H, Gomez M, Liu Y, Chadburn A, et al. Epigenetic down-regulation of the tumor suppressor gene PRDM1/Blimp-1 in diffuse large B cell lymphomas: a potential role of the microRNA let-7. *Am J Pathol* (2010) **177**:1470–9. doi:10.2353/ajpath.2010.091291
102. Leucci E, Onnis A, Cocco M, De Falco G, Imperatore F, Giuseppina A, et al. B-cell differentiation in EBV-positive Burkitt lymphoma is impaired at posttranscriptional level by miRNA-altered expression. *Int J Cancer* (2010) **126**:1316–26. doi:10.1002/ijc.24655
103. Sciammas R, Shaffer AL, Schatz JH, Zhao H, Staudt LM, Singh H. Graded expression of interferon regulatory factor-4 coordinates isotype switching with plasma cell differentiation. *Immunity* (2006) **25**:225–36. doi:10.1016/j.immuni.2006.07.009
104. Good-Jacobson KL. Regulation of germinal center, B-cell memory, and plasma cell formation by histone modifiers. *Front Immunol* (2014) **5**:596. doi:10.3389/fimmu.2014.00596
105. Baxter J, Sauer S, Peters A, John R, Williams R, Caparros ML, et al. Histone hypomethylation is an indicator of epigenetic plasticity in quiescent lymphocytes. *EMBO J* (2004) **23**:4462–72. doi:10.1038/sj.emboj.7600414
106. Caganova M, Carrisi C, Varano G, Mainoldi F, Zanardi F, Germain PL, et al. Germinal center dysregulation by histone methyltransferase EZH2 promotes lymphomagenesis. *J Clin Invest* (2013) **123**:5009–22. doi:10.1172/JCI70626
107. Luckey CJ, Bhattacharya D, Goldrath AW, Weissman IL, Benoist C, Mathis D. Memory T and memory B cells share a transcriptional program of self-renewal with long-term hematopoietic stem cells. *Proc Natl Acad Sci U S A* (2006) **103**:3304–9. doi:10.1073/pnas.0511137103
108. Lai AY, Mav D, Shah R, Grimm SA, Phadke D, Hatzi K, et al. DNA methylation profiling in human B cells reveals immune regulatory elements and epigenetic plasticity at Alu elements during B-cell activation. *Genome Res* (2013) **23**:2030–41. doi:10.1101/gr.155473.113
109. Klein U, Tu Y, Stolovitzky GA, Keller JL, Haddad J Jr, Miljkovic V, et al. Transcriptional analysis of the B cell germinal center reaction. *Proc Natl Acad Sci U S A* (2003) **100**:2639–44. doi:10.1073/pnas.0437996100
110. Cao Z, Sun X, Icli B, Wara AK, Feinberg MW. Role of Kruppel-like factors in leukocyte development, function, and disease. *Blood* (2010) **116**:4404–14. doi:10.1182/blood-2010-05-285353
111. Calame K. microRNA-155 function in B Cells. *Immunity* (2007) **27**:825–7. doi:10.1016/j.immuni.2007.11.010
112. Ranzani V, Rossetti G, Panzeri I, Arrigoni A, Bonnal RJ, Curti S, et al. The long intergenic noncoding RNA landscape of human lymphocytes highlights the regulation of T cell differentiation by linc-MAF-4. *Nat Immunol* (2015) **16**:318–25. doi:10.1038/ni.3093
113. Gonda H, Sugai M, Nambu Y, Katakai T, Agata Y, Mori KJ, et al. The balance between Pax5 and Id2 activities is the key to AID gene expression. *J Exp Med* (2003) **198**:1427–37. doi:10.1084/jem.20030802
114. Delcuve GP, Khan DH, Davie JR. Roles of histone deacetylases in epigenetic regulation: emerging paradigms from studies with inhibitors. *Clin Epigenetics* (2012) **4**:5. doi:10.1186/1868-7083-4-5
115. Reilly CM, Regna N, Mishra N. HDAC inhibition in lupus models. *Mol Med* (2011) **17**:417–25. doi:10.2119/molmed.2011.00055
116. Gottlicher M, Minucci S, Zhu P, Kramer OH, Schimpf A, Giavara S, et al. Valproic acid defines a novel class of HDAC inhibitors inducing differentiation of transformed cells. *EMBO J* (2001) **20**:6969–78. doi:10.1093/emboj/20.24.6969
117. Davie JR. Inhibition of histone deacetylase activity by butyrate. *J Nutr* (2003) **133**:2485S–93S.
118. Waibel M, Christiansen AJ, Hibbs ML, Shortt J, Jones SA, Simpson I, et al. Manipulation of B-cell responses with histone deacetylase inhibitors. *Nat Commun* (2015) **6**:6838. doi:10.1038/ncomms7838
119. Phiel CJ, Zhang F, Huang EY, Guenther MG, Lazar MA, Klein PS. Histone deacetylase is a direct target of valproic acid, a potent anticonvulsant, mood stabilizer, and teratogen. *J Biol Chem* (2001) **276**:36734–41. doi:10.1074/jbc.M101287200
120. Topping DL, Clifton PM. Short-chain fatty acids and human colonic function: roles of resistant starch and nonstarch polysaccharides. *Physiol Rev* (2001) **81**:1031–64.
121. Furusawa Y, Obata Y, Fukuda S, Endo TA, Nakato G, Takahashi D, et al. Commensal microbe-derived butyrate induces the differentiation of colonic regulatory T cells. *Nature* (2013) **504**:446–50. doi:10.1038/nature12721
122. Bantscheff M, Hopf C, Savitski MM, Dittmann A, Grandi P, Michon AM, et al. Chemoproteomics profiling of HDAC inhibitors reveals selective targeting of HDAC complexes. *Nat Biotechnol* (2011) **29**:255–65. doi:10.1038/nbt.1759
123. Roger T, Lugrin J, Le Roy D, Goy G, Mombelli M, Koessler T, et al. Histone deacetylase inhibitors impair innate immune responses to toll-like receptor agonists and to infection. *Blood* (2011) **117**:1205–17. doi:10.1182/blood-2010-05-284711
124. Dowdell KC, Pesnicak L, Hoffmann V, Steadman K, Remaley AT, Cohen JI, et al. Valproic acid (VPA), a histone deacetylase (HDAC) inhibitor, diminishes lymphoproliferation in the Fas -deficient MRL/lpr(-/-) murine model of autoimmune lymphoproliferative syndrome (ALPS). *Exp Hematol* (2009) **37**:487–94. doi:10.1016/j.exphem.2008.12.002
125. Villagra A, Cheng F, Wang HW, Suarez I, Glozak M, Maurin M, et al. The histone deacetylase HDAC11 regulates the expression of interleukin 10 and immune tolerance. *Nat Immunol* (2009) **10**:92–100. doi:10.1038/ni.1673
126. Akimova T, Beier UH, Liu Y, Wang L, Hancock WW. Histone/protein deacetylases and T-cell immune responses. *Blood* (2012) **119**:2443–51. doi:10.1182/blood-2011-10-292003
127. Hooper LV, Littman DR, Macpherson AJ. Interactions between the microbiota and the immune system. *Science* (2012) **336**:1268–73. doi:10.1126/science.1223490
128. Ivanov II, Honda K. Intestinal commensal microbes as immune modulators. *Cell Host Microbe* (2012) **12**:496–508. doi:10.1016/j.chom.2012.09.009
129. Brestoff JR, Artis D. Commensal bacteria at the interface of host metabolism and the immune system. *Nat Immunol* (2013) **14**:676–84. doi:10.1038/ni.2640
130. Belkaid Y, Hand TW. Role of the microbiota in immunity and inflammation. *Cell* (2014) **157**:121–41. doi:10.1016/j.cell.2014.03.011
131. Thorburn AN, Macia L, Mackay CR. Diet, metabolites, and "western-lifestyle" inflammatory diseases. *Immunity* (2014) **40**:833–42. doi:10.1016/j.immuni.2014.05.014
132. Trompette A, Gollwitzer ES, Yadava K, Sichelstiel AK, Sprenger N, Ngom-Bru C, et al. Gut microbiota metabolism of dietary fiber influences allergic airway disease and hematopoiesis. *Nat Med* (2014) **20**:159–66. doi:10.1038/nm.3444
133. Arpaia N, Campbell C, Fan X, Dikiy S, van der Veeken J, deRoos P, et al. Metabolites produced by commensal bacteria promote peripheral regulatory T-cell generation. *Nature* (2013) **504**:451–5. doi:10.1038/nature12726
134. Cahenzli J, Koller Y, Wyss M, Geuking MB, McCoy KD. Intestinal microbial diversity during early-life colonization shapes long-term IgE levels. *Cell Host Microbe* (2013) **14**:559–70. doi:10.1016/j.chom.2013.10.004
135. Javierre BM, Fernandez AF, Richter J, Al-Shahrour F, Martin-Subero JI, Rodriguez-Ubreva J, et al. Changes in the pattern of DNA methylation

associate with twin discordance in systemic lupus erythematosus. *Genome Res* (2010) **20**:170–9. doi:10.1101/gr.100289.109
136. Kauffmann F, Demenais F. Gene-environment interactions in asthma and allergic diseases: challenges and perspectives. *J Allergy Clin Immunol* (2012) **130**:1229–40. doi:10.1016/j.jaci.2012.10.038
137. Blumenthal MN. Genetic, epigenetic, and environmental factors in asthma and allergy. *Ann Allergy Asthma Immunol* (2012) **108**:69–73. doi:10.1016/j.anai.2011.12.003
138. Ballestar E. Epigenetic alterations in autoimmune rheumatic diseases. *Nat Rev Rheumatol* (2011) **7**:263–71. doi:10.1038/nrrheum.2011.16
139. Portela A, Esteller M. Epigenetic modifications and human disease. *Nat Biotechnol* (2010) **28**:1057–68. doi:10.1038/nbt.1685
140. Garaud S, Le Dantec C, Jousse-Joulin S, Hanrotel-Saliou C, Saraux A, Mageed RA, et al. IL-6 modulates CD5 expression in B cells from patients with lupus by regulating DNA methylation. *J Immunol* (2009) **182**:5623–32. doi:10.4049/jimmunol.0802412
141. Strickland FM, Richardson BC. Epigenetics in human autoimmunity. *Autoimmunity* (2008) **41**:278–86. doi:10.1080/08916930802024616
142. Mazari L, Ouarzane M, Zouali M. Subversion of B lymphocyte tolerance by hydralazine, a potential mechanism for drug-induced lupus. *Proc Natl Acad Sci U S A* (2007) **104**:6317–22. doi:10.1073/pnas.0610434104
143. Wu SC, Zhang Y. Active DNA demethylation: many roads lead to Rome. *Nat Rev Mol Cell Biol* (2010) **11**:607–20. doi:10.1038/nrm2950
144. Zan H, Zhang J, Ardeshna S, Xu Z, Park SR, Casali P. Lupus-prone MRL/*fas*$^{lpr/lpr}$ mice display increased AID expression and extensive DNA lesions, comprising deletions and insertions, in the immunoglobulin locus: concurrent upregulation of somatic hypermutation and class switch DNA recombination. *Autoimmunity* (2009) **42**:89–103. doi:10.1080/08916930802629554
145. Pieterse E, Hofstra J, Berden J, Herrmann M, Dieker J, van der Vlag J. Acetylated histones contribute to the immunostimulatory potential of neutrophil extracellular traps in systemic lupus erythematosus. *Clin Exp Immunol* (2015) **179**:68–74. doi:10.1111/cei.12359
146. Belver L, de Yébenes VG, Ramiro AR. microRNAs prevent the generation of autoreactive antibodies. *Immunity* (2010) **33**:713–22. doi:10.1016/j.immuni.2010.11.010
147. Ceribelli A, Satoh M, Chan EK. microRNAs and autoimmunity. *Curr Opin Immunol* (2012) **24**:686–91. doi:10.1016/j.coi.2012.07.011
148. Dai R, Zhang Y, Khan D, Heid B, Caudell D, Crasta O, et al. Identification of a common lupus disease-associated microRNA expression pattern in three different murine models of lupus. *PLoS One* (2010) **5**:e14302. doi:10.1371/journal.pone.0014302
149. Forster N, Gallinat S, Jablonska J, Weiss S, Elsässer HP, Lutz W. p300 protein acetyltransferase activity suppresses systemic lupus erythematosus-like autoimmune disease in mice. *J Immunol* (2007) **178**:6941–8. doi:10.4049/jimmunol.178.11.6941
150. Garchow BG, Bartulos Encinas O, Leung YT, Tsao PY, Eisenberg RA, Caricchio R, et al. Silencing of microRNA-21 in vivo ameliorates autoimmune splenomegaly in lupus mice. *EMBO Mol Med* (2011) **3**:605–15. doi:10.1002/emmm.201100171
151. Xiao C, Srinivasan L, Calado DP, Patterson HC, Zhang B, Wang J, et al. Lymphoproliferative disease and autoimmunity in mice with increased miR-17-92 expression in lymphocytes. *Nat Immunol* (2008) **9**:405–14. doi:10.1038/ni1575
152. Esteller M. Epigenetics in cancer. *N Engl J Med* (2008) **358**:1148–59. doi:10.1056/NEJMra072067
153. Esteller M. Non-coding RNAs in human disease. *Nat Rev Genet* (2011) **12**:861–74. doi:10.1038/nrg3074
154. Jones PA, Baylin SB. The epigenomics of cancer. *Cell* (2007) **128**:683–92. doi:10.1016/j.cell.2007.01.029
155. De S, Shaknovich R, Riester M, Elemento O, Geng H, Kormaksson M, et al. Aberration in DNA methylation in B-cell lymphomas has a complex origin and increases with disease severity. *PLoS Genet* (2013) **9**:e1003137. doi:10.1371/journal.pgen.1003137
156. Leshchenko VV, Kuo PY, Shaknovich R, Yang DT, Gellen T, Petrich A, et al. Genomewide DNA methylation analysis reveals novel targets for drug development in mantle cell lymphoma. *Blood* (2010) **116**:1025–34. doi:10.1182/blood-2009-12-257485
157. Shaknovich R, Melnick A. Epigenetics and B-cell lymphoma. *Curr Opin Hematol* (2011) **18**:293–9. doi:10.1097/MOH.0b013e32834788cf
158. Fritz EL, Papavasiliou FN. Cytidine deaminases: AIDing DNA demethylation? *Genes Dev* (2010) **24**:2107–14. doi:10.1101/gad.1963010
159. Greeve J, Philipsen A, Krause K, Klapper W, Heidorn K, Castle BE, et al. Expression of activation-induced cytidine deaminase in human B-cell non-Hodgkin lymphomas. *Blood* (2003) **101**:3574–80. doi:10.1182/blood-2002-08-2424
160. Shen L, Song CX, He C, Zhang Y. Mechanism and function of oxidative reversal of DNA and RNA methylation. *Annu Rev Biochem* (2014) **83**:585–614. doi:10.1146/annurev-biochem-060713-035513
161. Schubeler D. Function and information content of DNA methylation. *Nature* (2015) **517**:321–6. doi:10.1038/nature14192
162. Huang Y, Rao A. Connections between TET proteins and aberrant DNA modification in cancer. *Trends Genet* (2014) **30**:464–74. doi:10.1016/j.tig.2014.07.005
163. Cimmino L, Dawlaty MM, Ndiaye-Lobry D, Yap YS, Bakogianni S, Yu Y, et al. TET1 is a tumor suppressor of hematopoietic malignancy. *Nat Immunol* (2015) **16**:653–62. doi:10.1038/ni.3148
164. Rodriguez-Paredes M, Esteller M. Cancer epigenetics reaches mainstream oncology. *Nat Med* (2011) **17**:330–9. doi:10.1038/nm.2305
165. Velichutina I, Shaknovich R, Geng H, Johnson NA, Gascoyne RD, Melnick AM, et al. EZH2-mediated epigenetic silencing in germinal center B cells contributes to proliferation and lymphomagenesis. *Blood* (2010) **116**:5247–55. doi:10.1182/blood-2010-04-280149
166. Yap DB, Chu J, Berg T, Schapira M, Cheng SW, Moradian A, et al. Somatic mutations at EZH2 Y641 act dominantly through a mechanism of selectively altered PRC2 catalytic activity, to increase H3K27 trimethylation. *Blood* (2011) **117**:2451–9. doi:10.1182/blood-2010-11-321208
167. Lu J, Getz G, Miska EA, Alvarez-Saavedra E, Lamb J, Peck D, et al. microRNA expression profiles classify human cancers. *Nature* (2005) **435**:834–8. doi:10.1038/nature03702
168. Baltimore D, Boldin MP, O'Connell RM, Rao DS, Taganov KD. microRNAs: new regulators of immune cell development and function. *Nat Immunol* (2008) **9**:839–45. doi:10.1038/ni.f.209
169. Bonci D, Coppola V, Musumeci M, Addario A, Giuffrida R, Memeo L, et al. The miR-15a-miR-16-1 cluster controls prostate cancer by targeting multiple oncogenic activities. *Nat Med* (2008) **14**:1271–7. doi:10.1038/nm.1880
170. Aqeilan RI, Calin GA, Croce CM. miR-15a and miR-16-1 in cancer: discovery, function and future perspectives. *Cell Death Differ* (2010) **17**:215–20. doi:10.1038/cdd.2009.69
171. Klein U, Lia M, Crespo M, Siegel R, Shen Q, Mo T, et al. The DLEU2/miR-15a/16-1 cluster controls B cell proliferation and its deletion leads to chronic lymphocytic leukemia. *Cancer Cell* (2010) **17**:28–40. doi:10.1016/j.ccr.2009.11.019
172. Rosenwald A, Wright G, Wiestner A, Chan WC, Connors JM, Campo E, et al. The proliferation gene expression signature is a quantitative integrator of oncogenic events that predicts survival in mantle cell lymphoma. *Cancer Cell* (2003) **3**:185–97. doi:10.1016/S1535-6108(03)00028-X
173. Perlot T, Alt FW. Cis-regulatory elements and epigenetic changes control genomic rearrangements of the IgH locus. *Adv Immunol* (2008) **99**:1–32. doi:10.1016/S0065-2776(08)00601-9
174. Giambra V, Volpi S, Emelyanov AV, Pflugh D, Bothwell AL, Norio P, et al. Pax5 and linker histone H1 coordinate DNA methylation and histone modifications in the 3' regulatory region of the immunoglobulin heavy chain locus. *Mol Cell Biol* (2008) **28**:6123–33. doi:10.1128/MCB.00233-08
175. Garrett FE, Emelyanov AV, Sepulveda MA, Flanagan P, Volpi S, Li F, et al. Chromatin architecture near a potential 3' end of the IgH locus involves modular regulation of histone modifications during B-Cell development and *in vivo* occupancy at CTCF sites. *Mol Cell Biol* (2005) **25**:1511–25. doi:10.1128/MCB.25.4.1511-1525.2005
176. Wang L, Whang N, Wuerffel R, Kenter AL. AID-dependent histone acetylation is detected in immunoglobulin S regions. *J Exp Med* (2006) **203**:215–26. doi:10.1084/jem.20051774
177. Pasqualucci L, Dominguez-Sola D, Chiarenza A, Fabbri G, Grunn A, Trifonov V, et al. Inactivating mutations of acetyltransferase genes in B-cell lymphoma. *Nature* (2011) **471**:189–95. doi:10.1038/nature09730
178. Xu Y. DNA damage: a trigger of innate immunity but a requirement for adaptive immune homeostasis. *Nat Rev Immunol* (2006) **6**:261–70. doi:10.1038/nri1804
179. Morin RD, Johnson NA, Severson TM, Mungall AJ, An J, Goya R, et al. Somatic mutations altering EZH2 (Tyr641) in follicular and diffuse large

B-cell lymphomas of germinal-center origin. *Nat Genet* (2010) **42**:181–5. doi:10.1038/ng.518

180. Popovic R, Martinez-Garcia E, Giannopoulou EG, Zhang Q, Zhang Q, Ezponda T, et al. Histone methyltransferase MMSET/NSD2 alters EZH2 binding and reprograms the myeloma epigenome through global and focal changes in H3K36 and H3K27 methylation. *PLoS Genet* (2014) **10**:e1004566. doi:10.1371/journal.pgen.1004566
181. Pasqualucci L. The genetic basis of diffuse large B-cell lymphoma. *Curr Opin Hematol* (2013) **20**:336–44. doi:10.1097/MOH.0b013e3283623d7f
182. Chambwe N, Kormaksson M, Geng H, De S, Michor F, Johnson NA, et al. Variability in DNA methylation defines novel epigenetic subgroups of DLBCL associated with different clinical outcomes. *Blood* (2014) **123**:1699–708. doi:10.1182/blood-2013-07-509885
183. Shaknovich R, Geng H, Johnson NA, Tsikitas L, Cerchietti L, Greally JM, et al. DNA methylation signatures define molecular subtypes of diffuse large B-cell lymphoma. *Blood* (2010) **116**:e81–9. doi:10.1182/blood-2010-05-285320
184. Cimmino A, Calin GA, Fabbri M, Iorio MV, Ferracin M, Shimizu M, et al. miR-15 and miR-16 induce apoptosis by targeting BCL2. *Proc Natl Acad Sci U S A* (2005) **102**:13944–9. doi:10.1073/pnas.0506654102
185. Lawrie CH, Soneji S, Marafioti T, Cooper CD, Palazzo S, Paterson JC, et al. microRNA expression distinguishes between germinal center B cell-like and activated B cell-like subtypes of diffuse large B cell lymphoma. *Int J Cancer* (2007) **121**:1156–61. doi:10.1002/ijc.22800
186. Jin HY, Oda H, Lai M, Skalsky RL, Bethel K, Shepherd J, et al. microRNA-17~92 plays a causative role in lymphomagenesis by coordinating multiple oncogenic pathways. *EMBO J* (2013) **32**:2377–91. doi:10.1038/emboj.2013.178
187. Aguda BD, Kim Y, Piper-Hunter MG, Friedman A, Marsh CB. microRNA regulation of a cancer network: consequences of the feedback loops involving miR-17-92, E2F, and Myc. *Proc Natl Acad Sci U S A* (2008) **105**:19678–83. doi:10.1073/pnas.0811166106

16

Human immunodeficiencies related to defective APC/T cell interaction

Marinos Kallikourdis[1,2]*, Antonella Viola*[3] *and Federica Benvenuti*[4]*

[1] Humanitas University, Rozzano, Italy, [2] Adaptive Immunity Laboratory, Humanitas Clinical and Research Center, Rozzano, Italy, [3] Venetian Institute of Molecular Medicine, Padova, Italy, [4] Cellular Immunology, International Centre for Genetic Engineering and Biotechnology, Trieste, Italy

Edited by:
Elisabetta Padovan,
Basel University Hospital and
University of Basel, Switzerland

Reviewed by:
Benedita Rocha,
Faculté de Médecine Paris
Descartes, France
Loïc Dupré,
Institut National de la Santé et de la
Recherche Médicale, France

***Correspondence:**
Federica Benvenuti,
International Centre for Genetic
Engineering and Biotechnology,
Area di Ricerca, Padriciano 99,
Trieste 34149, Italy
benvenut@icgeb.org

The primary event for initiating adaptive immune responses is the encounter between T lymphocytes and antigen presenting cells (APCs) in the T cell area of secondary lymphoid organs and the formation of highly organized intercellular junctions referred to as immune synapses (IS). *In vivo* live-cell imaging of APC–T cell interactions combined to functional studies unveiled that T cell fate is dictated, in large part, by the stability of the initial contact. Immune cell interaction is equally important during delivery of T cell help to B cells and for the killing of target cells by cytotoxic T cells and NK cells. The critical role of contact dynamics and synapse stability on the immune response is well illustrated by human immune deficiencies in which disease pathogenesis is linked to altered adhesion or defective cross-talk between the synaptic partners. The Wiskott–Aldrich syndrome (WAS) is a severe primary immunodeficiency caused by mutations in the Wiskott–Aldrich syndrome protein (WASp), a scaffold that promotes actin polymerization and links TCR stimulation to T cell activation. Absence or mutations in WASp affects intercellular APC–T cell communications by interfering with multiple mechanisms on both sides of the IS. The warts, hypogammaglobulinemia, infections, and myelokathexis (WHIM) syndrome is caused by mutations in CXCR4, a chemokine receptor that in mutant form leads to impairment of APC–T cell interactions. Present evidences suggest that other recently characterized primary immune deficiencies caused by mutation in genes linked to actin cytoskeletal reorganization, such as WIP and DOCK8, may also depend on altered synapse stability. Here, we will discuss in details the mechanisms of disturbed APC–T cell interactions in WAS and WHIM. Moreover, we will summarize the evidence pointing to a compromised conjugate formation in WIP, DOCK8, and X-linked lymphoproliferative syndrome.

Keywords: immune synapse, immunodeficiencies, actin cytoskeleton, chemokines, T cell activation

Introduction

Cells of the immune system communicate with one another by physical contacts and by soluble signals that may act on the interacting cells or at a distance. The formation of intercellular junctions is essential to bring receptor–ligand couples close enough to trigger downstream signaling and to transmit activatory/inhibitory signals between the two cells. Tight membrane apposition is also a prerequisite to allow focused delivery of soluble factors in a spatially confined fashion, ensuring specificity and effectiveness during killing of targets or polarized secretion of soluble mediators. Immune cell interaction is supported by several interconnected systems that assist the various stages of contact formation from initial scouting to adhesion and stabilization of the junction. The importance of such pathways is underscored by human pathologies caused by mutations in genes controlling these systems.

APC–T Cell Encounter in the T Cell Area of Lymph Nodes

The first challenge for a T cell entering the T cell area of a lymph node is to find its cognate antigen on the surface of a dendritic cell (DC). This process is aided by the strategic distribution of DCs in an extensive network and by chemokine cues that guide motility and positioning in lymph nodes. *In vivo* imaging experiments have shown that lymphocytes entering the T-cell zones move randomly over densely packed networks of DCs and fibroblastic reticular cells (FRCs) (1, 2). This motility is driven by CCR7-binding chemokines. Besides CCL21, other chemokines produced in lymph nodes may coordinate specific encounters between cells. Thus, CCL3 and CCL4 seem to be involved in recruitment of naïve $CD8^+$ T cells, which can upregulate CCR5 expression during inflammation, to sites where they can receive help from $CD4^+$ T cells (3). CXCR3 expression on $CD4^+$T cells is important for the interaction with antigen bearing DCs and for the global intranodal positioning of T cells (4). Moreover, the same chemokine receptor selectively controls repositioning of memory T cells within lymph nodes during a recall response (5).

Interaction of the TCR with cognate antigen results in the activation of phospholipase C-γ and Ca^{2+} influx via calcium release activated channels (CRAC) Orai1/CRACM1 in the plasma membrane (6, 7). Among the other effects, Ca^{2+} influx induces ATP synthesis and release (8) that, in turns, induces P2X4/P2X7-mediated calcium waves in the neighboring lymphocytes and acts as a paracrine signaling molecule that regulates T cell motility during immune responses (9). ATP-induced Ca^{2+} waves induce a "stop" not only in cells that have already found their antigenic partners but also in lymphocytes that may be potentially triggered within the tissue. Several studies have indeed observed that in the lymph node microenvironment there is a significant drop in the velocity of polyclonal T cells during antigenic stimulation of TCR-specific cells (10, 11). The reduced motility of T lymphocytes in a tissue where antigenic recognition is occurring may be strategic for a better scanning of resident DCs and, in this perspective, extracellular ATP may alter the equilibrium between adhesive and chemoattractant forces operating in lymph nodes during T cell priming and thus modify T cell activation. Interestingly, destabilization of T–DCs conjugates *in vivo* by regulatory T cells is, in part, due to high levels of expression of CD39 and CD73, two cell surface ecto-enzymes that hydrolyze extracellular ATP to ADP, AMP and adenosine that, acting through the A2A receptor, prevents activation and proliferation of $CD4^+$ T cells (12, 13).

The Duration of APC–T Cell Contacts and the Consequences for T Cell Activation

The dynamics of cellular contacts and the functional consequences of short and prolonged cellular interactions in terms of T cell activation have been investigated mostly in the context of naïve T cells priming by DCs. *In vitro* studies showed that T cells remain stably attached to DCs in conditions that lead to T cell activation, whereas short intermittent contacts dominate when DCs are immature and unable to induce activation. With the limits of an *in vitro* analysis, these findings provided one of the first correlations between contact duration and function (14). An opposite result, i.e., short contacts may be enough to trigger naïve T cell activation, was obtained when analyzing cells in a collagen 3D matrix, suggesting that the requirements for T cell activation may depend on the context (15). Direct imaging of the immune response in lymph nodes revealed the presence of both sequential, brief, T–DC contacts (kynapses) and long antigen-specific contacts (synapses) (16). Different phases of short- and long-lasting antigen presenting cell (APC)–T contacts alternates during initial priming and longer arrest of T cells on the APC surface predominates in conditions of full T cell activation (17–19). This concept was later refined by studies showing that the affinity of the pMHC for the TCR critically determines contact duration. High-affinity antigens induce a complete T cell stop, whereas low-affinity antigens cause only T cell deceleration (20–22). Interestingly, the presence of bystander cells, such as regulatory T cells, modifies contact dynamics hampering the formation of stable contacts (12, 20). The state of T cell activation is a further critical parameter that determines contact dynamics. Naïve T cells stop and form mostly synapses upon antigen recognition, whereas previously activated T cells can collect activatory signals from kinapses (23). It has also emerged that kinapses may lead to T cell activation when antigen density is high enough to allow integration of signals over multiple serial encounters (24).

Molecular Structure of the Immune Synapse

Ex-vivo analysis of single T cells engaged in contact with APCs has been instrumental to understand the subcellular reorganization occurring in T cells during activation (**Figure 1**). Because of some analogies with the mode of intercellular communication used by neurons, the specialized structure formed between a T cell and an antigen presenting B cell was named as "immune synapse" (25, 26). The immune synapse (IS) was initially described as a central area containing signaling components such as the TCR and PKC-θ kinase (cSMAC), a peripheral ring containing adhesive molecules (pSMAC), and a distal region rich in actin (dSMAC). Subsequent studies using planar bilayer as surrogate APCs allowed the quantitative and dynamic analysis of synapse formation in T cells and to assess the contribution of single receptors (MHC peptide complexes, adhesion, and co-stimulatory molecules) on the reorganization of signaling platforms, cytoskeletal remodeling, and polarized vesicular trafficking (**Figure 1**). These studies revealed that microclusters (MCs) of 10–20 TCRs molecules forms in the dSMAC and are translocated into the cSMAC, where the signaling activity of the TCR extinguishes [(27–30) and reviewed in Ref. (31)]. An essential component to coordinate TCR signaling is the actin cytoskeleton. This is needed to support early events of T cell activation, such as clustering of TCRs in MCs, recruitment of

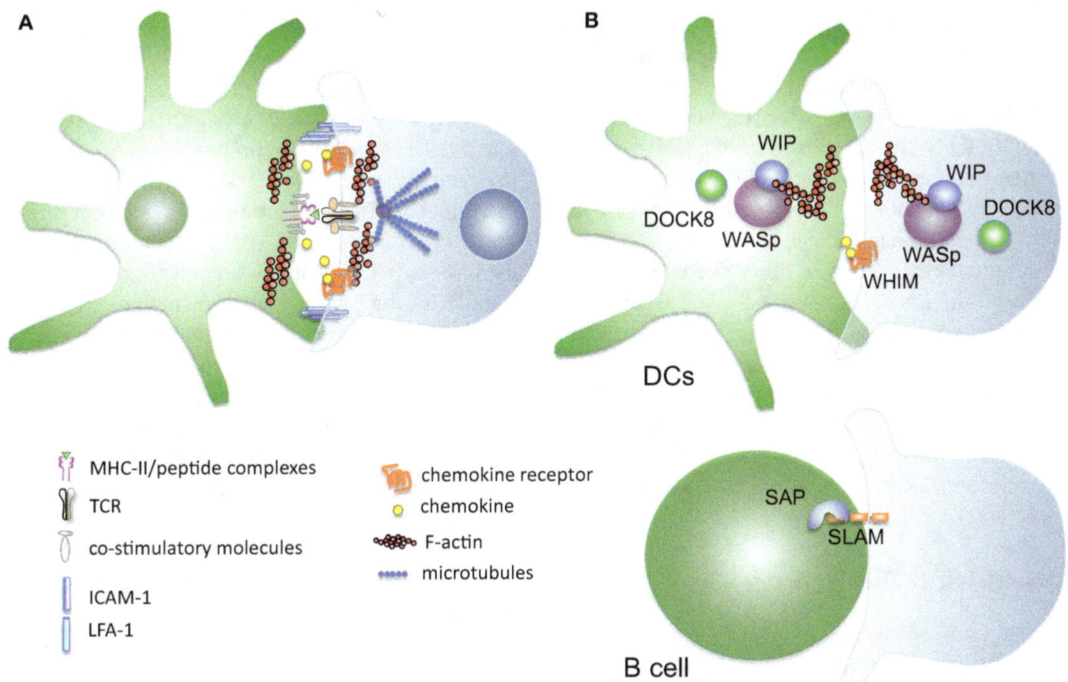

FIGURE 1 | Mutations in proteins controlling synapse stability linked to development of primary immune deficiencies. (A) Schematic representation of the molecules implicated DC–T cells cross-talk during synapse formation. Several interconnected systems, including membrane receptors and cytosolic proteins, contribute to form and stabilize the interaction between the two cell types. **(B)** Disease-causing mutations targeting proteins that control synapse stability. Wiskott–Aldrich syndrome protein WASp, causative of WAS syndrome, is a key node controlling actin polymerization in immune cells. Mutations in WASp have been associated to several defects in synapse formation on both the T-cell and the DC side. Most recently discovered mutations in DOCK8 and WIP cytoskeletal regulators cause immunodeficiency syndromes whose cellular basis include disturbance of the intercellular interactions. SAP, an adaptor for SLAM receptors mutated in XLP syndrome, is affecting selectively the stability of the B–T synapse.

signaling complexes to MC, and later mobility of signaling platforms. In turn, recruited signaling molecules, such as the adaptor LAT, serve as platforms to dock cytoskeletal regulatory proteins, such as Vav and Wiskott–Aldrich syndrome protein (WASp), necessary to sustain T cell activation (30, 32). Most recently, a novel view of the actin cytoskeleton as a global regulator of the cytoplasm poroelasticity and consequently of T cell signaling is emerging (33).

Interconnected to the role of actin cytoskeleton, the integrin LFA-1, acts at several levels in the IS. First of all, lateral movements of LFA-1, ensured by linkage with the underlying actin cytoskeleton, are essential to ensure correct T cell activation (31, 34). Besides its function in supporting synaptic architecture, LFA-1 is also an important co-stimulatory molecule during T cell activation by increasing the sensitivity for antigen by 100-fold. Mechanistically, LFA-1 engagement is known to enhance activation of early TCR signaling molecules and to promote later events of T cell proliferation and cytokine production (35, 36). LFA-1 plays a role also at earlier stages of synapse formation. During scanning in search of matching TCR/pMHC, the initial adhesive interactions between T cells and APC are mediated by LFA-1 and ICAM-1,3 on T cells and APCs, respectively (37). The functional relevance of LFA-1 on contact duration has been addressed by *in vivo* studies that correlated contact duration with acquisition of effector functions. Expression of the LFA-1 ligand ICAM-1 is required to sustain long antigen-specific DC–T contacts, whereas short interactions can still occur in the absence of ICAM-1. Importantly, T cells primed by ICAM-1 deficient DCs undergo early events of activation but fail to differentiate into effective memory CD8 T cells (38, 39). A mirroring finding in CD4 T cells lacking LFA-1 support is the importance of the LFA-1/ICAM-1 adhesion module to achieve optimal T cell priming *in vivo* (38). Interference with positive regulator of integrin activation yielded similar results. For instance, deletion of Talin in T cells leads to unstable contacts with APCs and failure to undergo full T cell activation (40, 41).

Soluble immunotransmitters like chemokines play also an important role in IS stabilization and T cell proliferation (42, 43). When approaching an APC, T cells emit CCR5 (or CXCR4)-enriched protrusions that indent the APC surface; this situation resembles the concentration of chemokine receptors at the leading edge of chemoattractant-stimulated T cells (44). These interactions culminate in the formation of a stable synapse, whereas CCR5 and CXCR4 are stably concentrated. Chemokine release at the immunological synapse and chemokine receptor recruitment into this region result in prolonged T-cell–APC interaction, and facilitate T cell activation by reinforcing T cell–APC pair attraction and delivering co-stimulatory signals (43). Interestingly, chemokine recognition in the context of the immunological synapse induces a $G_{q/11}$-mediated CCR5 signaling, suggesting that chemokine receptor signaling pathways are modified by TCR triggering (43). Notably, coupling of G_q to the chemokine receptors delays their internalization, explaining the accumulation of CCR5 and CXCR4 at the T cell immunological synapse. In this scenario, chemokine receptors prolong the duration of T cell–APC interaction and facilitate T cell activation by increasing LFA-1 affinity (45), reinforcing T cell–APC pair attraction and avoiding pre-mature splitting due to other chemoattractant sources. On the basis of their actions, a dual role for chemokines in T-cell activation has been proposed, while the presence of chemoattractant forces when T cells are searching for the right partner may indeed prevent T cell–APC pairing, production of chemokines by the APCs, and subsequent accumulation and trapping of G_q-coupled chemokine receptors at the IS, may represent a strategy to reinforce T-cell–APC interaction and facilitate T-cell activation (46, 47).

The Wiskott–Aldrich Syndrome

Cytoskeletal remodeling is a highly dynamic process that ensures spatio-temporal coordination of diverse functions, such as mechanical support to the cell cortex, migration, phagocytosis, intercellular interactions, and subcellular distribution of signaling molecules and vesicles flow. Actin dynamics are tightly controlled by several different nucleation-promoting factors in turn activated by multiple complex pathways. Formation of branched actin networks is regulated by the Arp2/3 complex that is induced by the VCA domain contained in the WASp family of actin regulatory proteins. The eight members of the family (N-WASp, WAVE 1–3, WASH, JMY, and WHAM (48)] have different activation modes and control differential functions in various tissues. WASp, the founding member of the family, is expressed exclusively in the hematopoietic lineage and it was first discovered because loss-of-function mutations in its coding gene are associated with the X-linked immunodeficiency Wiskott–Aldrich syndrome (WAS) (49). The disease is characterized by multiple clinical manifestations, including susceptibility to infections, hemorrhages and eczema, and multiple forms of autoimmune disorders (50).

Wiskott–Aldrich syndrome protein mutations impact on disparate cellular functions in different hematopoietic lineages (51, 52). T cells were the first lineage recognized as being heavily affected by WASp mutations. A detailed review on the role of WASp in T cells has been recently published (53). Here, we will recall the main features of WASp deficient T cells and present the emerging defects in WASp null APCs.

Initial studies identified defects in TCR signaling and activation of IL-2 in T cells from WAS patients (54–56). WASp null T cells, similarly to cells of other hematopoietic lineages, also present with alteration of motility (57, 58). Later studies helped to better define how WASp controls selectively multiple sequential events in T cell activation. WASp is recruited to sites of early TCR receptor signaling in multimeric complex together with LAT, SLAP-76, Nck, and the cdc24 GEF Vav (32, 59, 60). At the synaptic interface, binding of activated cdc42, PIP2, and phosphorylation of tyrosine 291 by Src family kinases cooperate to release the auto-inhibited conformation of WASp, exposing the VCA domain and inducing acting nucleating activity [reviewed in Ref. (61)]. Genetic deletion of WASp in T cells causes alterations in the early dynamic events of stabilization of the synapse. Upon TCR triggering cycles of stable symmetric synapse structure alternates to phases of T cell motility when the synaptic structure is lost. WASp is required to reform the synaptic structure after these periodic breaking rather than for the initial synapse formation (62). This is in line with the finding that T cells derived from WASp patients, despite normal conjugate formation, fail to spatially organize signaling in the cSMAC and to polarize the microtubules organizing center (63). Downstream events of T cell activation, such as calcium fluxes, IL-2 production, and T cell proliferation, are also affected by WASp deficiency both in mouse models and in patient's-derived cells (64–68). The exact role of WASp-mediated F-actin dynamics in regulating synaptic structure and downstream signaling is still not fully resolved. A recent study proposes that WASp controls selectively a small fraction of synaptic F-actin required to sustain PLC-γ activation and calcium ion elevation, thereby linking the control of early events to later T cell activation (69). It is also emerging that WASp can have actin-independent activities in T cells, functioning as a transcription factor to regulate transcription of cytokine genes (70). Thus, WASp plays a central role in controlling multiple integrated functions that link TCR signaling to full T cell activation. Moreover, its role varies depending on the T cell subset, reflecting the existence of cell type-specific modes of actin regulation besides common shared mechanism (53).

Regulated cytoskeletal remodeling is needed also to support the function of APCs during synapse formation and maintenance. DCs are active player in synapse formation by virtue of their membrane protrusions that facilitate scanning of the T cell repertoire and interaction with T cells (14, 71, 72). This flypaper membrane activity of DCs is regulated by members of the Rho family of small GTPase and by actin regulatory proteins. Genetic deletion of an upstream regulator of cytoskeletal remodeling, the Rho GTPases Rac, inhibits dendrites extension, resulting in reduced DC–T contact time and inefficient priming (71). In WAS, loss of proper actin cytoskeletal rearrangement hampers the function of DCs at several levels. Defects in adhesion to ICAM-1, polarization and responses to chemokine gradients (73, 74) render DCs unable to properly migrate from site of antigen acquisition in the periphery to lymph nodes. Failure to properly initiate adaptive immunity by WASp deficient DCs arises from defects that go beyond the capacity to properly home to lymph nodes (75). Delivery of the model antigen DEC205-OVA to resident DCs resulted in poor activation of antigen-specific $CD8^+$ T cell in WASp null recipient. Further experiments to dissect the individual contribution of migration, antigen processing and DC–T cell interaction *in vivo* demonstrated that WASp null DCs fail to efficiently prime naïve CD8 T cells even when the migratory defect is compensated (75). Imaging of DC–T cell contacts *in vitro* and by two-photon microscopy *in vivo* indeed showed that WASp null DCs fail to form stable and long-lasting interactions with antigen-specific T cells (75). Interestingly, T cells primed by WASp null DCs can enter the cell cycle but fail to accumulate, similarly to what happens when priming is promoted by Cdc42 knock down DCs, an upstream regulator of WASp (76). A similar defect in the stability of DC–T cell contacts and in the capacity to support formation of an organized synaptic structure was seen also using CD4+ T cells (77). Taken together, these data indicate that defective cytoskeletal organization in WAS DCs affects two key steps during priming, i.e., migration to lymph nodes and formation of stable DC–T cell contacts and T cell activation once in lymph nodes. Thus, not only presentation of antigens that are taken up in the periphery and transported to secondary lymphoid organs but also presentation of blood born antigens by lymph node resident DCs is likely to be compromised in WAS. The impact of DCs to the overall immune deficiency is demonstrated by the fact that rescue of DCs functions upon gene therapy is capable to improve T cell priming (78).

It is also emerging that plasmacytoid DCs and myeloid cells present with defects in innate immunity pathways in WAS (79). The role that an altered cytokine secretion profile may have on synapse stability and signaling at the IS is an intriguing aspect that is currently being investigated by our group.

Wiskott–Aldrich syndrome patient experience recurrent autoimmune manifestations, whose cellular basis are not yet fully understood (80). Functional defects in regulatory T cells are likely to contribute to loss of peripheral tolerance (81–83). DC–T cell interactions are critical for the establishment of peripheral T tolerance besides initiation of adaptive immunity (17, 84). It is interesting to speculate that besides cell intrinsic Tregs abnormalities, defective interaction with APC may contribute to loss of peripheral tolerance in WAS.

Other Actin-Related Immune Deficiencies

Recently, a new cytoskeletal-related immunodeficiency caused by mutation in the WASp interacting protein WIP has been identified (85). WIP controls WASp activity in at least three different ways: regulating its stability, controlling its activation by Cdc42, and bringing WASp to sites of active polymerization (86). Indeed, a stop codon mutation in the WIP sequence that silenced protein expression resulted in almost undetectable WASp level, and clinical features similar to WAS (85). At the cellular level, WIP was shown to control podosomes assembly and cell migration in DCs (87, 88). In addition, WIP binds to actin and controls cytoskeletal integrity independently of WASp. The WASp-independent actin regulation exerted by WIP is essential for T cell homing to infected tissue (89). A further interesting function that has been attributed to WIP, independently of its binding to WASp, is the control of lytic granule secretion in NK cells. The failure in cytolytic activity of WIP null NK cells is due to lack of transport and polarization of granules at the IS (90). The role of WIP in controlling IS formation in T cells and DCs has not yet been addressed. However, it is likely that priming will not be efficient because of defects on both sides of the IS, thus explaining the poor immune responses (91).

A further example of immunodeficiency arising form cytoskeletal abnormalities that affect synapse formation is DOCK8 deficiency. DOCK8 is a GTP-exchange factor for Rho and Rac GTPases that controls conversion of extracellular signals into activation of actin regulatory proteins. Mutations in DOCK8 were found to be the genetic basis of a combined immunodeficiency characterized by increased susceptibility to skin viral infections, hyper IgE syndrome, T cell lymphopenia, and impaired antibody response (92). At the cellular level, DOCK8 was shown to be required for the accumulation of the integrin ICAM-1 at the B cell synapse and its mutation compromise synaptic architecture and B cell functions (93). Marginal zone B cells are highly reduced in DOCK8, similarly to what has been observed in WAS (94). DOCK8 mutant T cells were also shown to have defective LFA-1 polarization in synapse, resulting in decreased T cell proliferation and survival (95). The DC compartment is also affected in a way reminiscent of defects observed in WAS, such as defective homing to lymph nodes and reduced T cell priming activity (96). Although the direct role of DOCK8 in controlling the stability of the DC-T synapse has not been addressed, it is reasonable to predict that alterations in contact duration may contribute to disease pathology.

The WHIM Syndrome

As discussed above, chemokines and their receptors have a dual role in localization of T cells and APCs within secondary lymphoid organs, as well as in enhancing the strength of the T–APC interaction. Intriguingly, the relevance of the chemokine–chemokine receptor axis in promoting stable synapses has been further emphasized by recent studies on the rare immune deficiency warts, hypogammaglobulinemia, infections, and myelokathexis (WHIM). A chemokine-mediated regulation of the duration of T–APC interactions was shown to contribute to the cellular basis of T cell-dependent response defects in this disease (47). The WHIM syndrome is an inherited immunodeficiency that features a wide range of symptoms, including recurring infections, human papillomavirus (HPV)-induced warts, reduced long-term immunoglobulin G (IgG) titers, myelokathexis, and leukopenia (97–100). The syndrome is associated with dominant mutations in the chemokine receptor CXCR4 that lead to truncation of its carboxy-terminal domain. This leads to a defect in the ability of the receptor to internalize after binding its cognate ligand, CXCL12. As a consequence, immune cells bearing the WHIM-mutant receptor display increased signaling and enhanced migration after stimulation by chemokine (98, 101–103). Historically, this enhanced functionality of the mutant CXCR4 has provided a mechanistic explanation for the abnormal retention of neutrophils in the bone marrow (myelokathexis), as demonstrated by experiments in a human-to-mouse *in vivo* xenograft model and in a zebrafish model (101, 104). Yet, symptoms of WHIM syndrome patients, such as the inability to successfully mount responses to a recurring pathogen and the decreased capacity to produce hypermutated IgG signify that antigen-specific memory responses, antibody class-switching and affinity maturation are defective in these individuals (99). The finding that CXCR4, along with other chemokines, is utilized in the organization of lymphoid organ follicles enabled the speculation that possible aberrations in lymphoid organ architecture could be the cause of the above adaptive immunity defects in WHIM (99). Reports of disrupted lymph node spatial organization in a recent mouse knock-in model of WHIM support this hypothesis (105). Nonetheless, the generation of antigen-specific memory, Ig class switching and affinity maturation do depend on the formation of successful T cell–APC interactions via immunological synapses (106). Recent work has identified that T cells from WHIM patients, or indeed healthy donor T cells transfected with the dominant, WHIM-mutant CXCR4, form less stable conjugates with superantigen-pulsed B cells. Importantly, this only occurs in the presence of competing migratory ("go") signals from exogenous CXCL12, which appear to affect the mutant but not the wild-type receptor. A very similar impairment of T–APC immunological synapse stability occurs between antigen-specific WHIM-mutant T cells and antigen-loaded DCs in *ex vivo* lymph node slice cultures derived from a retrogenic model of WHIM, imaged via 2-photon microscopy (47). While both wild-type and WHIM-mutant CXCR4 are recruited to the immunological synapse, exogenous CXCL12, which is present in lymph nodes (107), is able to "distract" only the hyperfunctional WHIM-mutant CXCR4 away from the synapse. Indeed, wild-type CXCR4 is unable to impair immunological synapse formation (108) and has no effect on T cell activation (109, 110). Intriguingly, however, the hyperfunctional WHIM-mutant CXCR4 appears to exceed a threshold that favors motility over formation of stable immunological synapses, resulting in aberrant T cell activation (47). Further molecular studies will tell us more about the regulation of T–APC interactions. Nonetheless, the finding that many of the WHIM defects are reversible using a pharmacological inhibitor of CXCR4 is an interesting demonstration of how chemokines and their receptors, in specific circumstances, have the ability to affect T cell function.

Synaptic Defects in Patients with X-Linked Lymphoproliferative Disease

X-linked lymphoproliferative disease (XLP) is caused by loss-of-function mutations in signaling lymphocyte activation molecule-associated protein (SAP), an adaptor linking SLAM family receptors to downstream signaling. The protein is primarily expressed in T cells, NK cells, and B cells. XLP patients are subjected to severe Epstein–Barr viral infections and develop lymphomas and lymphoproliferative disorders (111). At the cellular level, the disease is characterized by a defect in germinal center formation and consequently poor humoral response, abnormalities in NKT cell development, NK cell cytotoxicity, and cytokine production (112). In the context of this review, it is interesting to discuss the evidences pointing to disturbed B–T cell interaction to explain poor germinal center formation. Upon initial activation of T cells by DCs in lymph nodes, the second circuit of immune cell interaction includes motile but prolonged interactions between activated B cells and T cells at the border between the follicle and the T cell zone, followed by translocation of T cells in the germinal center to sustain the germinal center reaction. Follicular helper T cells, specialized in this process, express high levels of SAP and SLAM (113). *In vivo* imaging of B–T interactions during T cell-dependent B cell-activation revealed that SAP-deficient T cells are intrinsically unable to form stable contact with B cells. Interestingly, this defect is selective for B–T cell interaction, as DC–T cell interactions proceed normally. These data show that SAP-associated family members controls, selectively, adhesive mechanism required to stabilize T cell–B cell conjugates required to deliver to B cells the signals supporting full B cell proliferation (112, 114). Further insight into the role of SAP and SLAM receptor in assembling B–T synapse comes from the finding that the SLAM receptor Ly108 is a potent negative regulator of T–B cell adhesion, counteracted by SAP, that act by recruiting the phosphatase SHP-1 at the synapse (115).

SAP functions also in controlling adhesion during cytolysis. SAP-deficient cytotoxic T lymphocytes fail to assemble a proper synaptic structure during conjugation to target cells, with altered polarization of perforin granules and lipid raft at the contact site (116, 117). In line with this observation, SAP-deficient NKT cells fail to polarize the microtubule-organizing center toward the target cell, resulting in reduced killing ability (118).

Conclusion

A class of primary immunodeficiency is caused by pathogenic mutations in genes controlling immune cell trafficking and cellular interactions dynamics (**Figure 1**). The cellular basis of these diseases has been increasingly investigated helping to improve patients management. Moreover, analysis of these naturally arising mutant cells revealed important insights into basic functioning of the immune system. As a prominent example, WASp mutant cells have been instrumental in understanding actin-mediated signal transduction during TCR triggering and to unveil the importance of an intact actin cytoskeleton in APCs. Characterization of mutant T cells in less common immunodeficiency like WHIM, WIP, DOCK8, and SAP is still at early stages and it will help to dissect subtle details of immune cell interaction regulation. Further analysis is needed to understand the reciprocal contribution of alterations on both sides of the IS to gain an integrated view of the parameters that control, in normal and pathological conditions, the transfer of information between APC and T cells during priming of adaptive immune responses.

Acknowledgments

The authors wish to thank Telethon GGP06267 and GGP10231 on WAS syndrome to FB and Telethon GGP07134 and GGP10170 on the WHIM syndrome to AV, FIRB (RBFR10HP97, to MK).

References

1. Miller MJ, Wei SH, Cahalan MD, Parker I. Autonomous T cell trafficking examined in vivo with intravital two-photon microscopy. *Proc Natl Acad Sci U S A* (2003) **100**:2604–9. doi:10.1073/pnas.2628040100
2. Bajenoff M, Egen JG, Koo LY, Laugier JP, Brau F, Glaichenhaus N, et al. Stromal cell networks regulate lymphocyte entry, migration, and territoriality in lymph nodes. *Immunity* (2006) **25**:989–1001. doi:10.1016/j.immuni.2006.10.011
3. Castellino F, Huang AY, Altan-Bonnet G, Stoll S, Scheinecker C, Germain RN. Chemokines enhance immunity by guiding naive CD8+ T cells to sites of CD4+ T cell-dendritic cell interaction. *Nature* (2006) **440**:890–5. doi:10.1038/nature04651
4. Groom JR, Richmond J, Murooka TT, Sorensen EW, Sung JH, Bankert K, et al. CXCR3 chemokine receptor-ligand interactions in the lymph node

optimize CD4+ T helper 1 cell differentiation. *Immunity* (2012) **37**:1091–103. doi:10.1016/j.immuni.2012.08.016

5. Sung JH, Zhang H, Moseman EA, Alvarez D, Iannacone M, Henrickson SE, et al. Chemokine guidance of central memory T cells is critical for antiviral recall responses in lymph nodes. *Cell* (2012) **150**:1249–63. doi:10.1016/j.cell.2012.08.015
6. Feske S, Gwack Y, Prakriya M, Srikanth S, Puppel SH, Tanasa B, et al. A mutation in Orai1 causes immune deficiency by abrogating CRAC channel function. *Nature* (2006) **441**:179–85. doi:10.1038/nature04702
7. Prakriya M, Feske S, Gwack Y, Srikanth S, Rao A, Hogan PG. Orai1 is an essential pore subunit of the CRAC channel. *Nature* (2006) **443**:230–3. doi:10.1038/nature05122
8. Schenk U, Westendorf AM, Radaelli E, Casati A, Ferro M, Fumagalli M, et al. Purinergic control of T cell activation by ATP released through pannexin-1 hemichannels. *Sci Signal* (2008) **1**:ra6. doi:10.1126/scisignal.1160583
9. Wang CM, Ploia C, Anselmi F, Sarukhan A, Viola A. Adenosine triphosphate acts as a paracrine signaling molecule to reduce the motility of T cells. *EMBO J* (2014) **33**:1354–64. doi:10.15252/embj.201386666
10. McKee AS, Burchill MA, Munks MW, Jin L, Kappler JW, Friedman RS, et al. Host DNA released in response to aluminum adjuvant enhances MHC class II-mediated antigen presentation and prolongs CD4 T-cell interactions with dendritic cells. *Proc Natl Acad Sci U S A* (2013) **110**:E1122–31. doi:10.1073/pnas.1300392110
11. Salgado-Pabon W, Celli S, Arena ET, Nothelfer K, Roux P, Sellge G, et al. *Shigella* impairs T lymphocyte dynamics in vivo. *Proc Natl Acad Sci U S A* (2013) **110**:4458–63. doi:10.1073/pnas.1300981110
12. Tadokoro CE, Shakhar G, Shen S, Ding Y, Lino AC, Maraver A, et al. Regulatory T cells inhibit stable contacts between CD4+ T cells and dendritic cells in vivo. *J Exp Med* (2006) **203**:505–11. doi:10.1084/jem.20050783
13. Tang Q, Adams JY, Tooley AJ, Bi M, Fife BT, Serra P, et al. Visualizing regulatory T cell control of autoimmune responses in nonobese diabetic mice. *Nat Immunol* (2006) **7**:83–92. doi:10.1038/ni1289
14. Benvenuti F, Lagaudriere-Gesbert C, Grandjean I, Jancic C, Hivroz C, Trautmann A, et al. Dendritic cell maturation controls adhesion, synapse formation, and the duration of the interactions with naive T lymphocytes. *J Immunol* (2004) **172**:292–301. doi:10.4049/jimmunol.172.1.292
15. Gunzer M, Schafer A, Borgmann S, Grabbe S, Zanker KS, Brocker EB, et al. Antigen presentation in extracellular matrix: interactions of T cells with dendritic cells are dynamic, short lived, and sequential. *Immunity* (2000) **13**:323–32. doi:10.1016/S1074-7613(00)00032-7
16. Dustin ML. T-cell activation through immunological synapses and kinapses. *Immunol Rev* (2008) **221**:77–89. doi:10.1111/j.1600-065X.2008.00589.x
17. Hugues S, Fetler L, Bonifaz L, Helft J, Amblard F, Amigorena S. Distinct T cell dynamics in lymph nodes during the induction of tolerance and immunity. *Nat Immunol* (2004) **5**:1235–42. doi:10.1038/ni1134
18. Mempel TR, Henrickson SE, Von Andrian UH. T-cell priming by dendritic cells in lymph nodes occurs in three distinct phases. *Nature* (2004) **427**:154–9. doi:10.1038/nature02238
19. Celli S, Lemaitre F, Bousso P. Real-time manipulation of T cell-dendritic cell interactions in vivo reveals the importance of prolonged contacts for CD4+ T cell activation. *Immunity* (2007) **27**:625–34. doi:10.1016/j.immuni.2007.08.018
20. Pace L, Tempez A, Arnold-Schrauf C, Lemaitre F, Bousso P, Fetler L, et al. Regulatory T cells increase the avidity of primary CD8+ T cell responses and promote memory. *Science* (2012) **338**:532–6. doi:10.1126/science.1227049
21. Moreau HD, Lemaitre F, Terriac E, Azar G, Piel M, Lennon-Dumenil AM, et al. Dynamic in situ cytometry uncovers T cell receptor signaling during immunological synapses and kinapses in vivo. *Immunity* (2012) **37**:351–63. doi:10.1016/j.immuni.2012.05.014
22. Skokos D, Shakhar G, Varma R, Waite JC, Cameron TO, Lindquist RL, et al. Peptide-MHC potency governs dynamic interactions between T cells and dendritic cells in lymph nodes. *Nat Immunol* (2007) **8**:835–44. doi:10.1038/ni1490
23. Azar GA, Lemaitre F, Robey EA, Bousso P. Subcellular dynamics of T cell immunological synapses and kinapses in lymph nodes. *Proc Natl Acad Sci U S A* (2010) **107**:3675–80. doi:10.1073/pnas.0905901107
24. Marangoni F, Murooka TT, Manzo T, Kim EY, Carrizosa E, Elpek NM, et al. The transcription factor NFAT exhibits signal memory during serial T cell interactions with antigen-presenting cells. *Immunity* (2013) **38**:237–49. doi:10.1016/j.immuni.2012.09.012
25. Dustin ML, Olszowy MW, Holdorf AD, Li J, Bromley S, Desai N, et al. A novel adaptor protein orchestrates receptor patterning and cytoskeletal polarity in T-cell contacts. *Cell* (1998) **94**:667–77. doi:10.1016/S0092-8674(00)81608-6
26. Monks CR, Freiberg BA, Kupfer H, Sciaky N, Kupfer A. Three-dimensional segregation of supramolecular activation clusters in T cells. *Nature* (1998) **395**:82–6. doi:10.1038/25764
27. Varma R, Campi G, Yokosuka T, Saito T, Dustin ML. T cell receptor-proximal signals are sustained in peripheral microclusters and terminated in the central supramolecular activation cluster. *Immunity* (2006) **25**:117–27. doi:10.1016/j.immuni.2006.04.010
28. Vardhana S, Choudhuri K, Varma R, Dustin ML. Essential role of ubiquitin and TSG101 protein in formation and function of the central supramolecular activation cluster. *Immunity* (2010) **32**:531–40. doi:10.1016/j.immuni.2010.04.005
29. Campi G, Varma R, Dustin ML. Actin and agonist MHC-peptide complex-dependent T cell receptor microclusters as scaffolds for signaling. *J Exp Med* (2005) **202**:1031–6. doi:10.1084/jem.20051182
30. Yokosuka T, Sakata-Sogawa K, Kobayashi W, Hiroshima M, Hashimoto-Tane A, Tokunaga M, et al. Newly generated T cell receptor microclusters initiate and sustain T cell activation by recruitment of Zap70 and SLP-76. *Nat Immunol* (2005) **6**:1253–62. doi:10.1038/ni1272
31. Fooksman DR, Vardhana S, Vasiliver-Shamis G, Liese J, Blair DA, Waite J, et al. Functional anatomy of T cell activation and synapse formation. *Annu Rev Immunol* (2010) **28**:79–105. doi:10.1146/annurev-immunol-030409-101308
32. Barda-Saad M, Braiman A, Titerence R, Bunnell SC, Barr VA, Samelson LE. Dynamic molecular interactions linking the T cell antigen receptor to the actin cytoskeleton. *Nat Immunol* (2005) **6**:80–9. doi:10.1038/ni1143
33. Beemiller P, Krummel MF. Regulation of T-cell receptor signaling by the actin cytoskeleton and poroelastic cytoplasm. *Immunol Rev* (2013) **256**:148–59. doi:10.1111/imr.12120
34. Springer TA, Dustin ML. Integrin inside-out signaling and the immunological synapse. *Curr Opin Cell Biol* (2012) **24**:107–15. doi:10.1016/j.ceb.2011.10.004
35. Li D, Molldrem JJ, Ma Q. LFA-1 regulates CD8+ T cell activation via T cell receptor-mediated and LFA-1-mediated Erk1/2 signal pathways. *J Biol Chem* (2009) **284**:21001–10. doi:10.1074/jbc.M109.002865
36. Perez OD, Mitchell D, Jager GC, South S, Murriel C, McBride J, et al. Leukocyte functional antigen 1 lowers T cell activation thresholds and signaling through cytohesin-1 and Jun-activating binding protein 1. *Nat Immunol* (2003) **4**:1083–92. doi:10.1038/ni984
37. de la Fuente H, Mittelbrunn M, Sanchez-Martin L, Vicente-Manzanares M, Lamana A, Pardi R, et al. Synaptic clusters of MHC class II molecules induced on DCs by adhesion molecule-mediated initial T-cell scanning. *Mol Biol Cell* (2005) **16**:3314–22. doi:10.1091/mbc.E05-01-0005
38. Kandula S, Abraham C. LFA-1 on CD4+ T cells is required for optimal antigen-dependent activation in vivo. *J Immunol* (2004) **173**:4443–51. doi:10.4049/jimmunol.173.7.4443
39. Scholer A, Hugues S, Boissonnas A, Fetler L, Amigorena S. Intercellular adhesion molecule-1-dependent stable interactions between T cells and dendritic cells determine CD8+ T cell memory. *Immunity* (2008) **28**:258–70. doi:10.1016/j.immuni.2007.12.016
40. Wernimont SA, Wiemer AJ, Bennin DA, Monkley SJ, Ludwig T, Critchley DR, et al. Contact-dependent T cell activation and T cell stopping require talin1. *J Immunol* (2011) **187**:6256–67. doi:10.4049/jimmunol.1102028
41. Ilani T, Vasiliver-Shamis G, Vardhana S, Bretscher A, Dustin ML. T cell antigen receptor signaling and immunological synapse stability require myosin IIA. *Nat Immunol* (2009) **10**:531–9. doi:10.1038/ni.1723
42. Karpus WJ, Lukacs NW, Kennedy KJ, Smith WS, Hurst SD, Barrett TA. Differential CC chemokine-induced enhancement of T helper cell cytokine production. *J Immunol* (1997) **158**:4129–36.
43. Molon B, Gri G, Bettella M, Gomez-Mouton C, Lanzavecchia A, Martinez AC, et al. T cell costimulation by chemokine receptors. *Nat Immunol* (2005) **6**:465–71. doi:10.1038/ni1191
44. Gomez-Mouton C, Lacalle RA, Mira E, Jimenez-Baranda S, Barber DF, Carrera AC, et al. Dynamic redistribution of raft domains as an organizing platform for signaling during cell chemotaxis. *J Cell Biol* (2004) **164**:759–68. doi:10.1083/jcb.200309101

45. Shamri R, Grabovsky V, Gauguet JM, Feigelson S, Manevich E, Kolanus W, et al. Lymphocyte arrest requires instantaneous induction of an extended LFA-1 conformation mediated by endothelium-bound chemokines. *Nat Immunol* (2005) **6**:497–506. doi:10.1038/ni1194
46. Viola A, Contento RL, Molon B. T cells and their partners: The chemokine dating agency. *Trends Immunol* (2006) **27**:421–7. doi:10.1016/j.it.2006.07.004
47. Kallikourdis M, Trovato AE, Anselmi F, Sarukhan A, Roselli G, Tassone L, et al. The CXCR4 mutations in WHIM syndrome impair the stability of the T-cell immunologic synapse. *Blood* (2013) **122**:666–73. doi:10.1182/blood-2012-10-461830
48. Matalon O, Reicher B, Barda-Saad M. Wiskott-Aldrich syndrome protein – dynamic regulation of actin homeostasis: from activation through function and signal termination in T lymphocytes. *Immunol Rev* (2013) **256**:10–29. doi:10.1111/imr.12112
49. Derry JM, Ochs HD, Francke U. Isolation of a novel gene mutated in Wiskott-Aldrich syndrome. *Cell* (1994) **79**:922. following,
50. Albert MH, Notarangelo LD, Ochs HD. Clinical spectrum, pathophysiology and treatment of the Wiskott-Aldrich syndrome. *Curr Opin Hematol* (2011) **18**:42–8. doi:10.1097/MOH.0b013e32834114bc
51. Bosticardo M, Marangoni F, Aiuti A, Villa A, Grazia Roncarolo M. Recent advances in understanding the pathophysiology of Wiskott-Aldrich syndrome. *Blood* (2009) **113**:6288–95. doi:10.1182/blood-2008-12-115253
52. Moulding DA, Record J, Malinova D, Thrasher AJ. Actin cytoskeletal defects in immunodeficiency. *Immunol Rev* (2013) **256**:282–99. doi:10.1111/imr.12114
53. Cotta-de-Almeida V, Dupre L, Guipouy D, Vasconcelos Z. Signal integration during T Lymphocyte activation and function: lessons from the Wiskott-Aldrich syndrome. *Front Immunol* (2015) **6**:47. doi:10.3389/fimmu.2015.00047
54. Zhang J, Shehabeldin A, da Cruz LA, Butler J, Somani AK, McGavin M, et al. Antigen receptor-induced activation and cytoskeletal rearrangement are impaired in Wiskott-Aldrich syndrome protein-deficient lymphocytes. *J Exp Med* (1999) **190**:1329–42. doi:10.1084/jem.190.9.1329
55. Snapper SB, Rosen FS. The Wiskott-Aldrich syndrome protein (WASP): roles in signaling and cytoskeletal organization. *Annu Rev Immunol* (1999) **17**:905–29. doi:10.1146/annurev.immunol.17.1.905
56. Gallego MD, Santamaria M, Pena J, Molina IJ. Defective actin reorganization and polymerization of Wiskott-Aldrich T cells in response to CD3-mediated stimulation. *Blood* (1997) **90**:3089–97.
57. Snapper SB, Meelu P, Nguyen D, Stockton BM, Bozza P, Alt FW, et al. leads to global defects of directed leukocyte migration in vitro and in vivo. *J Leukoc Biol* (2005) **77**:993–8. doi:10.1189/jlb.0804444
58. Lafouresse F, Cotta-de-Almeida V, Malet-Engra G, Galy A, Valitutti S, Dupre L. Wiskott-Aldrich syndrome protein controls antigen-presenting cell-driven CD4+ T-cell motility by regulating adhesion to intercellular adhesion molecule-1. *Immunology* (2012) **137**:183–96. doi:10.1111/j.1365-2567.2012.03620.x
59. Zeng R, Cannon JL, Abraham RT, Way M, Billadeau DD, Bubeck-Wardenberg J, et al. SLP-76 coordinates Nck-dependent Wiskott-Aldrich syndrome protein recruitment with Vav-1/Cdc42-dependent Wiskott-Aldrich syndrome protein activation at the T cell-APC contact site. *J Immunol* (2003) **171**:1360–8. doi:10.4049/jimmunol.171.3.1360
60. Burkhardt JK, Carrizosa E, Shaffer MH. The actin cytoskeleton in T cell activation. *Annu Rev Immunol* (2008) **26**:233–59. doi:10.1146/annurev.immunol.26.021607.090347
61. Thrasher AJ, Burns SO. WASP: a key immunological multitasker. *Nat Rev Immunol* (2010) **10**:182–92. doi:10.1038/nri2724
62. Sims TN, Soos TJ, Xenias HS, Dubin-Thaler B, Hofman JM, Waite JC, et al. Opposing effects of PKCtheta and WASP on symmetry breaking and relocation of the immunological synapse. *Cell* (2007) **129**:773–85. doi:10.1016/j.cell.2007.03.037
63. Calvez R, Lafouresse F, De Meester J, Galy A, Valitutti S, Dupre L. The Wiskott-Aldrich syndrome protein permits assembly of a focused immunological synapse enabling sustained T-cell receptor signaling. *Haematologica* (2011) **96**:1415–23. doi:10.3324/haematol.2011.040204
64. Snapper SB, Rosen FS, Mizoguchi E, Cohen P, Khan W, Liu CH, et al. Wiskott-Aldrich syndrome protein-deficient mice reveal a role for WASP in T but not B cell activation. *Immunity* (1998) **9**:81–91. doi:10.1016/S1074-7613(00)80590-7
65. Cianferoni A, Massaad M, Feske S, de la Fuente MA, Gallego L, Ramesh N, et al. Defective nuclear translocation of nuclear factor of activated T cells and extracellular signal-regulated kinase underlies deficient IL-2 gene expression in Wiskott-Aldrich syndrome. *J Allergy Clin Immunol* (2005) **116**:1364–71. doi:10.1016/j.jaci.2005.09.006
66. Dupre L, Aiuti A, Trifari S, Martino S, Saracco P, Bordignon C, et al. Wiskott-Aldrich syndrome protein regulates lipid raft dynamics during immunological synapse formation. *Immunity* (2002) **17**:157–66. doi:10.1016/S1074-7613(02)00360-6
67. Trifari S, Sitia G, Aiuti A, Scaramuzza S, Marangoni F, Guidotti LG, et al. Defective Th1 cytokine gene transcription in CD4+ and CD8+ T cells from Wiskott-Aldrich syndrome patients. *J Immunol* (2006) **177**:7451–61. doi:10.4049/jimmunol.177.10.7451
68. Cannon JL, Burkhardt JK. Differential roles for Wiskott-Aldrich syndrome protein in immune synapse formation and IL-2 production. *J Immunol* (2004) **173**:1658–62. doi:10.4049/jimmunol.173.3.1658
69. Kumari S, Depoil D, Martinelli R, Judokusumo E, Carmona G, Gertler FB, et al. Actin foci facilitate activation of the phospholipase C-gamma in primary T lymphocytes via the WASP pathway. *eLife* (2015) **4**:e04953. doi:10.7554/eLife.04953
70. Taylor MD, Sadhukhan S, Kottangada P, Ramgopal A, Sarkar K, D'Silva S, et al. Nuclear role of WASp in the pathogenesis of dysregulated TH1 immunity in human Wiskott-Aldrich syndrome. *Sci Transl Med* (2010) **2**:37ra44. doi:10.1126/scitranslmed.3000813
71. Benvenuti F, Hugues S, Walmsley M, Ruf S, Fetler L, Popoff M, et al. Requirement of Rac1 and Rac2 expression by mature dendritic cells for T cell priming. *Science* (2004) **305**:1150–3. doi:10.1126/science.1099159
72. Miller MJ, Hejazi AS, Wei SH, Cahalan MD, Parker I. T cell repertoire scanning is promoted by dynamic dendritic cell behavior and random T cell motility in the lymph node. *Proc Natl Acad Sci U S A* (2004) **101**:998–1003. doi:10.1073/pnas.0306407101
73. de Noronha S, Hardy S, Sinclair J, Blundell MP, Strid J, Schulz O, et al. Impaired dendritic-cell homing in vivo in the absence of Wiskott-Aldrich syndrome protein. *Blood* (2005) **105**:1590–7. doi:10.1182/blood-2004-06-2332
74. Burns S, Hardy SJ, Buddle J, Yong KL, Jones GE, Thrasher AJ. Maturation of DC is associated with changes in motile characteristics and adherence. *Cell Motil Cytoskeleton* (2004) **57**:118–32. doi:10.1002/cm.10163
75. Pulecio J, Tagliani E, Scholer A, Prete F, Fetler L, Burrone OR, et al. Expression of Wiskott-Aldrich syndrome protein in dendritic cells regulates synapse formation and activation of naive CD8+ T cells. *J Immunol* (2008) **181**:1135–42. doi:10.4049/jimmunol.181.2.1135
76. Pulecio J, Petrovic J, Prete F, Chiaruttini G, Lennon-Dumenil AM, Desdouets C, et al. Cdc42-mediated MTOC polarization in dendritic cells controls targeted delivery of cytokines at the immune synapse. *J Exp Med* (2010) **207**:2719–32. doi:10.1084/jem.20100007
77. Bouma G, Mendoza-Naranjo A, Blundell MP, de Falco E, Parsley KL, Burns SO, et al. Cytoskeletal remodeling mediated by WASp in dendritic cells is necessary for normal immune synapse formation and T-cell priming. *Blood* (2011) **118**:2492–501. doi:10.1182/blood-2011-03-340265
78. Catucci M, Prete F, Bosticardo M, Castiello MC, Draghici E, Locci M, et al. Dendritic cell functional improvement in a preclinical model of lentiviral-mediated gene therapy for Wiskott-Aldrich syndrome. *Gene Ther* (2012) **19**:1150–8. doi:10.1038/gt.2011.202
79. Prete F, Catucci M, Labrada M, Gobessi S, Castiello MC, Bonomi E, et al. Wiskott-Aldrich syndrome protein-mediated actin dynamics control type-I interferon production in plasmacytoid dendritic cells. *J Exp Med* (2013) **210**:355–74. doi:10.1084/jem.20120363
80. Catucci M, Castiello MC, Pala F, Bosticardo M, Villa A. Autoimmunity in Wiskott-Aldrich syndrome: an unsolved enigma. *Front Immunol* (2012) **3**:209. doi:10.3389/fimmu.2012.00209
81. Humblet-Baron S, Sather B, Anover S, Becker-Herman S, Kasprowicz DJ, Khim S, et al. Wiskott-Aldrich syndrome protein is required for regulatory T cell homeostasis. *J Clin Invest* (2007) **117**:407–18. doi:10.1172/JCI29539
82. Maillard MH, Cotta-de-Almeida V, Takeshima F, Nguyen DD, Michetti P, Nagler C, et al. The Wiskott-Aldrich syndrome protein is required for the function of CD4(+)CD25(+)Foxp3(+) regulatory T cells. *J Exp Med* (2007) **204**:381–91. doi:10.1084/jem.20061338
83. Marangoni F, Trifari S, Scaramuzza S, Panaroni C, Martino S, Notarangelo LD, et al. WASP regulates suppressor activity of human and murine CD4(+)

CD25(+)FOXP3(+) natural regulatory T cells. *J Exp Med* (2007) **204**:369–80. doi:10.1084/jem.20061334

84. Steinman RM, Hawiger D, Liu K, Bonifaz L, Bonnyay D, Mahnke K, et al. Dendritic cell function in vivo during the steady state: a role in peripheral tolerance. *Ann N Y Acad Sci* (2003) **987**:15–25. doi:10.1111/j.1749-6632.2003.tb06029.x
85. Lanzi G, Moratto D, Vairo D, Masneri S, Delmonte O, Paganini T, et al. A novel primary human immunodeficiency due to deficiency in the WASP-interacting protein WIP. *J Exp Med* (2012) **209**:29–34. doi:10.1084/jem.20110896
86. de la Fuente MA, Sasahara Y, Calamito M, Anton IM, Elkhal A, Gallego MD, et al. WIP is a chaperone for Wiskott-Aldrich syndrome protein (WASP). *Proc Natl Acad Sci U S A* (2007) **104**:926–31. doi:10.1073/pnas.0610275104
87. Chou HC, Anton IM, Holt MR, Curcio C, Lanzardo S, Worth A, et al. WIP regulates the stability and localization of WASP to podosomes in migrating dendritic cells. *Curr Biol* (2006) **16**:2337–44. doi:10.1016/j.cub.2006.10.037
88. Banon-Rodriguez I, Monypenny J, Ragazzini C, Franco A, Calle Y, Jones GE, et al. The cortactin-binding domain of WIP is essential for podosome formation and extracellular matrix degradation by murine dendritic cells. *Eur J Cell Biol* (2011) **90**:213–23. doi:10.1016/j.ejcb.2010.09.001
89. Massaad MJ, Oyoshi MK, Kane J, Koduru S, Alcaide P, Nakamura F, et al. Binding of WIP to actin is essential for T cell actin cytoskeleton integrity and tissue homing. *Mol Cell Biol* (2014) **34**:4343–54. doi:10.1128/MCB.00533-14
90. Krzewski K, Chen X, Strominger JL. WIP is essential for lytic granule polarization and NK cell cytotoxicity. *Proc Natl Acad Sci U S A* (2008) **105**:2568–73. doi:10.1073/pnas.0711593105
91. Fried S, Matalon O, Noy E, Barda-Saad M. WIP: more than a WASp-interacting protein. *J Leukoc Biol* (2014) **96**:713–27. doi:10.1189/jlb.2RU0314-162R
92. Zhang Q, Davis JC, Lamborn IT, Freeman AF, Jing H, Favreau AJ, et al. Combined immunodeficiency associated with DOCK8 mutations. *N Engl J Med* (2009) **361**:2046–55. doi:10.1056/NEJMoa0905506
93. Randall KL, Lambe T, Johnson AL, Treanor B, Kucharska E, Domaschenz H, et al. Dock8 mutations cripple B cell immunological synapses, germinal centers and long-lived antibody production. *Nat Immunol* (2009) **10**:1283–91. doi:10.1038/ni.1820
94. Westerberg LS, de la Fuente MA, Wermeling F, Ochs HD, Karlsson MC, Snapper SB, et al. WASP confers selective advantage for specific hematopoietic cell populations and serves a unique role in marginal zone B-cell homeostasis and function. *Blood* (2008) **112**:4139–47. doi:10.1182/blood-2008-02-140715
95. Randall KL, Chan SS, Ma CS, Fung I, Mei Y, Yabas M, et al. DOCK8 deficiency impairs CD8 T cell survival and function in humans and mice. *J Exp Med* (2011) **208**:2305–20. doi:10.1084/jem.20110345
96. Harada Y, Tanaka Y, Terasawa M, Pieczyk M, Habiro K, Katakai T, et al. DOCK8 is a Cdc42 activator critical for interstitial dendritic cell migration during immune responses. *Blood* (2012) **119**:4451–61. doi:10.1182/blood-2012-01-407098
97. Zuelzer W. "MYELOKATHEXIS" – a new form of chronic granulocytopenia. Report of a case. *N Engl J Med* (1964) **270**:699–704.
98. Hernandez P, Gorlin R, Lukens J, Taniuchi S, Bohinjec J, Francois F, et al. Mutations in the chemokine receptor gene CXCR4 are associated with WHIM syndrome, a combined immunodeficiency disease. *Nat Genet* (2003) **34**:70–4. doi:10.1038/ng1149
99. Mc Guire P, Cunningham-Rundles C, Ochs H, Diaz G. Oligoclonality, impaired class switch and B-cell memory responses in WHIM syndrome. *Clin Immunol* (2010) **135**:412–21. doi:10.1016/j.clim.2010.02.006
100. McDermott D, Liu Q, Ulrick J, Kwatemaa N, Anaya-O'Brien S, Penzak S, et al. The CXCR4 antagonist plerixafor corrects panleukopenia in patients with WHIM syndrome. *Blood* (2011) **118**:4957–62. doi:10.1182/blood-2011-07-368084
101. Kawai T, Choi U, Cardwell L, DeRavin S, Naumann N, Whiting-Theobald N, et al. WHIM syndrome myelokathexis reproduced in the NOD/SCID mouse xenotransplant model engrafted with healthy human stem cells transduced with C-terminus-truncated CXCR4. *Blood* (2007) **109**:78–84. doi:10.1182/blood-2006-05-025296
102. Kawai T, Choi U, Whiting-Theobald N, Linton G, Brenner S, Sechler J, et al. Enhanced function with decreased internalization of carboxy-terminus truncated CXCR4 responsible for WHIM syndrome. *Exp Hematol* (2005) **33**:460–8. doi:10.1016/j.exphem.2005.01.001
103. Balabanian K, Lagane B, Pablos J, Laurent L, Planchenault T, Verola O, et al. WHIM syndromes with different genetic anomalies are accounted for by impaired CXCR4 desensitization to CXCL12. *Blood* (2005) **105**:2449–57. doi:10.1182/blood-2004-06-2289
104. Walters K, Green J, Surfus J, Yoo S, Huttenlocher A. Live imaging of neutrophil motility in a zebrafish model of WHIM syndrome. *Blood* (2010) **116**:2803–11. doi:10.1182/blood-2010-03-276972
105. Balabanian K, Brotin E, Biajoux V, Bouchet-Delbos L, Lainey E, Fenneteau O, et al. Proper desensitization of CXCR4 is required for lymphocyte development and peripheral compartmentalization in mice. *Blood* (2012) **119**:5722–30. doi:10.1182/blood-2012-01-403378
106. Notarangelo L, Lanzi G, Peron S, Durandy A. Defects of class-switch recombination. *J Allergy Clin Immunol* (2006) **117**:855–64. doi:10.1016/j.jaci.2006.01.043
107. Allen C, Ansel K, Low C, Lesley R, Tamamura H, Fujii N, et al. Germinal center dark and light zone organization is mediated by CXCR4 and CXCR5. *Nat Immunol* (2004) **5**:943–52. doi:10.1038/ni1100
108. Bromley S, Peterson D, Gunn M, Dustin M. Cutting edge: hierarchy of chemokine receptor and TCR signals regulating T cell migration and proliferation. *J Immunol* (2000) **165**:15–9. doi:10.4049/jimmunol.165.1.15
109. Asperti-Boursin F, Real E, Bismuth G, Trautmann A, Donnadieu E. CCR7 ligands control basal T cell motility within lymph node slices in a phosphoinositide 3-kinase-independent manner. *J Exp Med* (2007) **204**:1167–79. doi:10.1084/jem.20062079
110. Okada T, Cyster J. CC chemokine receptor 7 contributes to Gi-dependent T cell motility in the lymph node. *J Immunol* (2007) **178**:2973–8. doi:10.4049/jimmunol.178.5.2973
111. Morra M, Howie D, Grande MS, Sayos J, Wang N, Wu C, et al. X-linked lymphoproliferative disease: a progressive immunodeficiency. *Annu Rev Immunol* (2001) **19**:657–82. doi:10.1146/annurev.immunol.19.1.657
112. Schwartzberg PL, Mueller KL, Qi H, Cannons JL. SLAM receptors and SAP influence lymphocyte interactions, development and function. *Nat Rev Immunol* (2009) **9**:39–46. doi:10.1038/nri2456
113. Yusuf I, Kageyama R, Monticelli L, Johnston RJ, Ditoro D, Hansen K, et al. Germinal center T follicular helper cell IL-4 production is dependent on signaling lymphocytic activation molecule receptor (CD150). *J Immunol* (2010) **185**:190–202. doi:10.4049/jimmunol.0903505
114. Qi H, Cannons JL, Klauschen F, Schwartzberg PL, Germain RN. SAP-controlled T-B cell interactions underlie germinal centre formation. *Nature* (2008) **455**:764–9. doi:10.1038/nature07345
115. Kageyama R, Cannons JL, Zhao F, Yusuf I, Lao C, Locci M, et al. The receptor Ly108 functions as a SAP adaptor-dependent on-off switch for T cell help to B cells and NKT cell development. *Immunity* (2012) **36**:986–1002. doi:10.1016/j.immuni.2012.05.016
116. Dupre L, Andolfi G, Tangye SG, Clementi R, Locatelli F, Arico M, et al. SAP controls the cytolytic activity of CD8+ T cells against EBV-infected cells. *Blood* (2005) **105**:4383–9. doi:10.1182/blood-2004-08-3269
117. Zhao F, Cannons JL, Dutta M, Griffiths GM, Schwartzberg PL. Positive and negative signaling through SLAM receptors regulate synapse organization and thresholds of cytolysis. *Immunity* (2012) **36**:1003–16. doi:10.1016/j.immuni.2012.05.017
118. Das R, Bassiri H, Guan P, Wiener S, Banerjee PP, Zhong MC, et al. The adaptor molecule SAP plays essential roles during invariant NKT cell cytotoxicity and lytic synapse formation. *Blood* (2013) **121**:3386–95. doi:10.1182/blood-2012-11-468868

17

Non-human primate regulatory T Cells and their assessment as cellular therapeutics in preclinical transplantation models

Angus W. Thomson[1,2], Kazuki Sasaki[1] and Mohamed B. Ezzelarab[1]*

[1] Department of Surgery, Thomas E. Starzl Transplantation Institute, University of Pittsburgh School of Medicine, Pittsburgh, PA, United States, [2] Department of Immunology, University of Pittsburgh School of Medicine, Pittsburgh, PA, United States

Edited by:
Ling Lu,
Nanjing Medical University, China

Reviewed by:
Zengli Guo,
University of North Carolina at Chapel Hill, United States
Isabel Ishizuka,
Genentech Inc., United States

***Correspondence:**
Angus W. Thomson
thomsonaw@upmc.edu

Non-human primates (NHP) are an important resource for addressing key issues regarding the immunobiology of regulatory T cells (Treg), their *in vivo* manipulation and the translation of adoptive Treg therapy to clinical application. In addition to their phenotypic and functional characterization, particularly in cynomolgus and rhesus macaques, NHP Treg have been isolated and expanded successfully *ex vivo*. Their numbers can be enhanced *in vivo* by administration of IL-2 and other cytokines. Both polyclonal and donor antigen (Ag) alloreactive NHP Treg have been expanded *ex vivo* and their potential to improve long-term outcomes in organ transplantation assessed following their adoptive transfer in combination with various cytoreductive, immunosuppressive and "Treg permissive" agents. In addition, important insights have been gained into the *in vivo* fate/biodistribution, functional stability, replicative capacity and longevity of adoptively-transferred Treg in monkeys. We discuss current knowledge of NHP Treg immunobiology, methods for their *in vivo* expansion and functional validation, and results obtained testing their safety and efficacy in organ and pancreatic islet transplantation models. We compare and contrast results obtained in NHP and mice and also consider prospects for future, clinically relevant studies in NHP aimed at improved understanding of Treg biology, and innovative approaches to promote and evaluate their therapeutic potential.

Keywords: regulatory T cells, non-human primates, transplantation, cell therapy, immunobiology

INTRODUCTION

NHP are a valuable resource for translational research on innovative therapies with potential for clinical application. These include strategies to promote transplant tolerance without the toxicities and morbidities associated with immunosuppressive (IS) drugs that fail to induce clinical tolerance (Knechtle et al., 2019). Mouse models of tolerance induction are inadequate predictors of tolerance in both NHP and humans (Sachs, 2003). This reflects the fact that unlike the latter species, specific pathogen-free (spf) laboratory mice do not acquire heterologous immunity, i.e., virus-induced T

Abbreviations: Ab, antibody; Ag, antigen; (a)APC, (artificial) antigen-presenting cell; ATG, anti-thymocyte globulin; Co-SB, co-stimulation blockade; Cy, cyclophosphamide; darTreg, donor antigen alloreactive regulatory T cells; IS, immunosuppression/immunosuppressive; NHP, non-human primate; PBMC, peripheral blood mononuclear cells; spf, specific pathogen free; Teff, T effector cell(s); TGFβ, transforming growth factor β; Tmem, memory T cell(s); Treg, regulatory T cell(s).

cell memory that constitutes a powerful barrier to tolerance induction (Adams et al., 2003). In addition, whereas MHC class II Ags that are key to induction of alloimmunity are absent from rodent vascular endothelium, they are expressed constitutively by these cells in large animals (Choo et al., 1997; Houser et al., 2004). Due to (i) similarities between NHP and human immune systems, (ii) cross-reactivity between drug targets in these species, (iii) the outbred nature of NHP, (iv) their natural exposure to environmental pathogens, and (v) their longevity compared with mice, NHP are important models for studying mechanisms underlying immune regulation and tolerance (Fitch et al., 2019). NHP also allow evaluation of the scalability and safety of innovative therapeutic strategies (e.g., monitoring and management of adverse events, such as potential infusion reactions and infectious complications) and associated techniques, e.g., leukapheresis in conjunction with cell therapy, that are not practiced in rodents.

NHP Treg phenotype and function resemble those of human Treg (Anderson et al., 2008; Haanstra et al., 2008). As in humans, testing of their efficacy is dependent on their isolation, massive expansion and product validation. The ability to assess the *in vivo* stability and migration of adoptively-transferred Treg is also an important translational aspect of studies of these cells in NHP and crucial for their assessment as cellular therapeutics.

ISOLATION, PURIFICATION, *EX VIVO* EXPANSION AND VALIDATION OF NHP TREG

Details of methods developed for isolation and purification of NHP Tregs from blood or tissues, and for expansion and testing of polyclonal, polyspecific or donor Ag-alloreactive (dar) NHP Treg are summarized in **Table 1**. Thus, *ex vivo* expansion of cynomolgus or rhesus Treg after immunomagnetic bead or/and flow sorting has been well-described in response to either polyclonal stimuli (Gansuvd et al., 2007; Anderson et al., 2008), allogeneic PBMC (Porter et al., 2007) or dendritic cells (DCs) (Moreau et al., 2008), artificial (a)APCs (Weiner et al., 2015; Zhang et al., 2015) or CD40L-stimulated allogeneic B cells (sBc) (Ezzelarab et al., 2020; Alonso-Guallart et al., 2021). Most recent attention has focused on expansion of alloreactive Tregs using various protocols. Thus, Alonso-Guallart et al. (2021) expanded highly suppressive cynomolgus polyspecific Tregs using a combination of CD40L−engineered B cells from 3 to 4 animals representative of diverse MHCs. The expanded Tregs expressed high levels of Foxp3 and Helios, a high incidence of Treg-specific demethylated region demethylation, and markedly suppressed naïve T cell responses *in vitro*. Importantly, these Tregs also expanded after cryopreservation, an important benefit allowing protocol flexibility. Specificity assays confirmed they were suppressive following activation by any APCs whose MHC expression was shared by the CD40L−sBc used during their expansion, proving that they were polyspecific (Alonso-Guallart et al., 2021). Recently, Ezzelarab et al. (2020) also used CD40L−sBc of donor origin to expand cynomolgus darTregs that were adoptively-transferred to transplant recipients.

Weiner et al. (2015) flow-sorted $CD4^{+}CD25^{hi}$ cells from baboon PBMC, followed by expansion with IL-2, anti-CD3 Ab, aAPCs (transfected with human CD58, CD32, and CD80), and rapamycin, with weekly restimulation. Expanded Treg were cryopreserved for 2 months, after which they were thawed and cultured for 48 h with the same stimulating agents. The purified Treg were expanded > 10,000-fold and exhibited excellent suppressive function. Cryopreservation reduced the cells' suppressive function without changing their phenotype, but increasing levels of reactivation post-thawing improved cell viability and function, with a shift toward greater Treg purity. Thus, both the phenotype and function of the Tregs were preserved or even enhanced by increasing levels of restimulation post-thawing, reinforcing the concept of banking expanded recipient Tregs.

MIGRATORY PROPERTIES

Treg migratory ability is considered key to their *in vivo* homing to lymphoid tissues and sites of inflammation considered critical locations of their immunosuppressive function. While Treg markers are expressed in either accepted or rejected NHP kidney allografts (Haanstra et al., 2007), Treg recruitment to the interstitium of the graft has been implicated in metastable kidney transplant tolerance in rhesus macaques (Torrealba et al., 2004). Numerous studies, including those in transplanted animals (Chen and Bromberg, 2006; Lamarche and Levings, 2018; Mempel and Marangoni, 2019) have shown that the expression of specific chemokine receptors, integrins and selectins is required for Treg activity *in vivo* (Qin et al., 2008; Zhang et al., 2009) and that maximal graft protection occurs when Tregs migrate to both the transplant and the draining lymphoid tissue. Thus, optimization of procedures for generation of highly suppressive NHP Treg needs to include evaluation of the expression of a range of chemokine receptors compatible with their *in vivo* migration to both the allograft and lymphoid tissues. Zhang et al. (2015) reported that *ex vivo*-expanded polyclonal cynomolgus Treg expressed high levels of CXCR3/low levels of CD62L and CCR7, consistent with their potential accumulation at sites of inflammation.

IN VIVO MOBILIZATION AND DEPLETION

The influence of cytokine and other biological agent administration on Treg in NHP has been investigated (**Table 2**). Thus, specific hematopoietic growth factors have been evaluated for their ability to selectively increase Treg *in vivo*, with potential to enhance their therapeutic efficacy, whereas Treg-selective depleting agents enable assessment of the dependency of tolerance-promoting protocols on these cells.

IL-2

Inoculation of low dose IL-2 (10^5–5×10^6 IU/m^2) expands $CD4^{+}Foxp3^{+}$ Tregs preferentially due to the cells' expression of the high affinity IL-2 receptor alpha chain (CD25)

TABLE 1 | Timeline of reports of Treg isolation, expansion and suppressive activity in NHP species.

Species	Treg selection (purity)	Cell yield	Expansion method	Expansion rate	Suppressive activity	Reference(s)
Rhesus macaque	T cells from spleen	200 × 10^6 cells per recipient (splenectomized)	Donor splenocytes + anti-CD80/CD86; 13 days	2–4-fold	*In vivo* infusion 13 days post allogeneic kidney transplant; donor-specific inhibition of rejection	Bashuda et al., 2005
Rhesus	MACS (90%) or FACS (98%) $CD4^+$ $CD25^+$	Not indicated	Anti-CD3/CD28 beads + IL-2; 4 weeks	300–2,000-fold	Up to 1:8^a ratio, suppression of autologous PBMC proliferation	Gansuvd et al., 2007
Rhesus	Anti-CD8 and anti-CD20 Dynabeads, or $CD4^+$ MACS, followed by anti-CD25 MACS (82%)	10% of $CD3^+CD4^+$ T cells	Fresh cells used; no expansion	n/a	Proliferation of Teff in response anti-CD3 or irradiated PBMC decreased at 1:1^a ratio, however variation between animals	Haanstra et al., 2008
Rhesus	FACS $CD4^+CD25^{hi}$ or $CD4^+CD25^+CD127^-$	10^5 cells/mL blood	Anti-CD3/CD28 beads + IL-2; 4 weeks	Up to 450-fold	CFSE-MLR, up to 1:100^a ratio; suppression of alloreactive response by responder-specific or third-party Treg	Anderson et al., 2008
Rhesus	MACS $CD4^+CD127^{-/lo}$	7% of $CD4^+$/1.3% of total PBMC; 3.7 × 10^4 cells/ml blood	Immature $Mo\text{-}DC^+$ $IL\text{-}2^+$ IL-15; 14 days, or 10 days followed by 2 days without DC	No expansion	Suppression up to 1:40^a ratio; donor-specific	Zahorchak et al., 2009
Rhesus	FACS $CD4^+$ CD25- $CD127^-$/lo cells (> 80%)	>or = 10^6	Stimulation with anti-CD3 and anti-CD28 microbeads (1 cell: 2 beads) + IL-2 (2,000 U/ml) ± rapamycin (1,000 nM); re-stimulation at 7 and 14 days; harvested on day 21	210–760-fold	Strong suppression of $CD4^+$ and $CD8^+$ T cell proliferation in CFSE-MLR	Singh K. et al., 2012
Cynomolgus macaque	FACS $CD4^+$ $CD25^+CD127^-$ (> 98%)	0.4% of PBMC	Allo DC (BM-DC/Mo-DC) + IL-2; 7 days	12–25-fold	CFSE-MLR, $PBMC^+$ anti-$CD3/CD28^+$ Treg: 30% inhibition at 1:3^a ratio. Treg suppressive function stimulated by BM-DC > Mo-DC	Moreau et al., 2008
Cynomolgus (MS model)	MACS $CD4^+$ $CD25^+$ (>90%)	6.4% of T cells	Fresh cells used; no expansion	n/a	Proliferation to anti-CD3/CD28 or CD3/CD46 stimulation impaired during active MS	Ma et al., 2009
Cynomolgus	FACS $CD4^+CD25^{hi}CD127^-$ from PBMC	5% total $CD4^+$ cells	NHP-specific anti-CD2/3/28 microbeads (cell: bead ratio 1:2), rhu IL-2 (1,000 U/ml) and rhu TGF-b; 5 ng/mL); 20 day culture	>80-fold	Strong suppressive effect at ratios up to 1:4 (Treg:Teff) on $CD4^+$ and $CD8^+$ T cell proliferation	Dons et al., 2013
Cynomolgus	FACS $CD4^+CD25^+CD127^-$ (>95%)	4.7 (2–6.9)% of blood $CD4^+$ cells	Artificial (a)APCs (L32) loaded with anti-CD3 (1:1 ratio) for 7–8 days with IL-2 + rapamycin; restimulation with aAPCs on days 7 and 14 without rapamycin; harvested on day 21	1,000-fold	Potent suppression of anti-CD3/CD28-indiced CD4 and CD8 T cell proliferation	Guo et al., 2015; Zhang et al., 2015
Cynomolgus	FACS $CD4^+CD25^{hi}CD127^{lo}$	0.5–1% of total PBMC	Donor Ag alloreactive Tregs stimulated with donor CD40L-activated B cells + IL-2; harvest on day 9 and co-culture with aAPCs (L32 cells) + IL-2 for 2 subsequent rounds of 7 days	10,000-fold	Strong suppression (>polyclonal Tregs) of autologous T cell proliferation in MLR in response to donor APCs.	Ezzelarab et al., 2020
Cynomolgus	FACS CD4 + $CD8^-CD25^{hi}CD127^-$	Top 1% $CD25^+$ cells in the $CD4^+$ $CD8^-CD127^-$ gate	Polyspecific Tregs expanded with a panel of CD40L-stimulated B cells (CD40L–sBc)	10,000-fold after 28 days (4 rounds)	Expanded Tregs suppressive after activation by any APCs whose MHC was shared by CD40L–sBc used during expansion	Alonso-Guallart et al., 2021

(Continued)

TABLE 1 | Continued

Species	Treg selection (purity)	Cell yield	Expansion method	Expansion rate	Suppressive activity	Reference(s)
Baboon	MACSFACS sorting (> 95%) $CD4^+CD25^{hi}$	1.7% spleen, 3.1% lymph node, 1.9% blood T cells; 10×10^4 cells/ml blood	Pig $PBMC^+$ IL-2; 3–4 week + 7–10 days without PBMC	≤ 2,000-fold, depending on IL-2 concentration	1:1[a], strong xenogeneic suppression, donor-specific: 4–10 x less efficient to third-party	Porter et al., 2007
Baboon	$CD4^+CD25^{hi}$FACS-sorted from PBMC (> 95% purity)	1–2% of $CD4^+$ cells	Stimulation with irradiated pig PBMC or anti-CD3/CD28 in cultures supplemented with IL-2 and rapamycin for 4 weeks	200-fold	Suppression of autologous anti-pig T effector cell and B cell proliferation	Singh A. K. et al., 2012
Baboon	FACS $CD4^+CD25^{hi}$ (top 1% of $CD25^+$ cells) from PBMC	10^5 Treg isolated from 20 ml blood	Culture for 26 days with IL-2, anti-CD3 Ab, aAPCs (transfected with human CD58, CD32, and CD80) and rapamycin, with weekly restimulation	>10,000-fold	Excellent suppressive function,. preserved or even enhanced by increasing amounts of restimulation after thawing	Weiner et al., 2015
Baboon	$CD4^+$ T cells	n/a	Stimulation with tolerogenic, baboon Mo-derived DCs loaded with porcine-specific *in vitro*-transcribed RNA in cocultures supplemented with IL-2 and rapamycin for 10 days	Fivefold within 10 days	Highly suppressive effects on porcine-specific T effector cell proliferation; reduced IFNg/enhanced IL-10/TGFb production	Li et al., 2018

(a)APC, (artificial) antigen-presenting cell; BM-DC, bone-marrow derived dendritic cells; CD40L-sBc, CD40 ligand-stimulated B cells; CFSE-MLR, carboxyfluorescein succinimidyl ester-mixed leukocyte reaction; FACS, fluorescence-activated cell sorting; LN, lymph node; MACS, magnetic-activated cell sorting; Mo-derived DC, monocyte-derived dendritic cells; MS, multiple sclerosis; TGFb, transforming growth factor b.

(Zorn et al., 2006; Sakaguchi et al., 2008; Liao et al., 2013). Aoyama et al. (2012) reported that administration of low-dose IL-2 (1 million international units/m^2 BSA/day) significantly expanded peripheral blood $CD4^+$ and $CD8^+$Tregs in normal cynomolgus macaques, with restricted expansion of non-Tregs. The expanded Tregs were principally $CD45RA^-$ $Foxp3^{hi}$ activated Tregs, with strong immunosuppressive activity *in vitro*.

Exposure of Treg to high IL-2 concentrations during their expansion can render the cells sensitive to "cytokine withdrawal–induced death" (Larsen et al., 2017) following their adoptive transfer. This phenomenon could potentially be alleviated by systemic IL-2 administration. Thus, Furlan et al. (2020) found that, in non-transplanted monkeys, adding low dose IL-2 (1 million units/m^2/day) to rapamycin *in vivo* (target trough level: 5–15 ng/ml) promoted a logarithmic increase in the half-life/persistence of adoptively-transferred, autologous NHP Treg, in effect doubling the number of stable circulating Treg compared with Treg infusion in combination with rapamycin alone.

Yamada et al. (2015) examined the influence of systemic IL-2 on T cell alloreactivity and the maintenance of tolerance to MHC mis-matched kidney allografts induced in cynomolgus macaques via mixed hematopoietic cell chimerism. When given low doses of IL-2 ($0.6–3 \times 10^6$ IU/m^2), animals that had accepted their grafts for 1–10 years in the absence of IS rejected acutely, with reactivation/expansion of alloreactive effector memory T cells. After stopping IL-2 administration, graft rejection was reversed and normal renal function restored.

Hematopoietic Growth Factors

Kean et al. (2011) found that a small molecule antagonist of CXCR4- and CXCL12-mediated chemotaxis (AMD3100; Plerixafor) mobilized circulating lymphocytes in rhesus macaques, with significant increases in Tregs. $CD4^+CD25^{hi}CD127^{lo}FoxP3^+$ Tregs were mobilized efficiently, with increases as great as fourfold in leukapheresis products when compared with G-CSF administration alone. Overall, the results indicated that AMD3100 could mobilize a T cell repertoire that might provide protection against GVHD, and thus be of potential benefit in allogeneic hematopoietic stem cell transplantation. Also, in rhesus macaques, Sasaki et al. (2020) observed that combining GM-CSF and G-CSF administration increased the incidence of Treg in both blood and leukapheresis products. In these studies, the mobilized Treg exhibited a similar range of transcription factors, surface markers and chemokine receptors to Treg in normal monkey peripheral blood Treg. Moreover, when the mobilized Treg were expanded *ex vivo*, they displayed similar capacity to inhibit autologous $CD4^+$ and $CD8^+$ T cell proliferation.

Depletion of Treg

Intravenous injection of cynomolgus monkeys with two doses of an IL-2-diphtheria toxin fusion protein (denileukin diftitox; 8 or 18 μg/kg) resulted in a rapid, but short- duration reduction in circulating resting Tregs ($CD4^+CD45RA^+Foxp3^+$) accompanied by a transient elevation in activated Tregs ($CD4^+CD45RA^-Foxp3^{hi}$), followed by their partial depletion (50–60%) (Yamada et al., 2012a). Wang et al. (2016)

TABLE 2 | Agents used to selectively enhance or deplete Tregs in NHP species.

Agent	Species	Dosage	Reported effect	References
Enhancing agents				
IL-2	Cynomolgus macaque	10^6 IU/m^2/day	Increased peripheral blood CD4 and CD8 Tregs (mainly CD45RA$^-$ Foxp3^{hi})	Aoyama et al., 2012
IL-2	Rhesus macaque	10^6 U/m^2/day in combination with adoptively-transferred autologous Treg and rapamycin	Doubling of peripheral blood Treg compared with Treg infusion and rapamycin alone; stable expression of Treg gene transcripts	Furlan et al., 2020
IL-2	Cynomolgus macaque	0.6–3 × 10^6 IU/m^2	Acute cellular rejection of tolerated renal allografts 1–10 years post-transplant; reactivation and expansion of alloreactive T effector memory cells	Yamada et al., 2015
AMD3100 (Plerixafor),-antagonist of CXCR4 and CXCL12-mediated chemotaxis	Rhesus macaque	1 mg/kg (single dose)	CD4$^+$/CD25^{hi}CD127^{lo}FoxP3$^+$ Tregs mobilized efficiently using AMD3100-containing regimens; up to fourfold enrichment in leukapheresis products compared with use of G-CSF alone	Kean et al., 2011
GM-CSF and G-CSF	Rhesus macaque	GM-CSF (Leukine; 10 μg/kg/day); G-CSF (Neupogen; 10 μg/kg/day)	Significant elevation of Treg in peripheral blood and leukapheresis products	Sasaki et al., 2020
Depleting agents				
IL-2-diphtheria toxin fusion protein	Cynomolgus macaque	Two doses (8 or 18 μg/kg)	Rapid, but short-lived decrease in peripheral blood resting Tregs (CD4$^+$CD45RA$^+$Foxp3$^+$) with a transient increase in activated Tregs (CD4$^+$CD45RA$^-$Foxp3^{hi}), followed by their depletion by50–60%	Yamada et al., 2012b
Anti-human CCR4 immunotoxin	Cynomolgus macaque	25 mg/kg twice a day for four consecutive days, 6 h apart	78–89% CCR4$^+$Foxp3$^+$ Treg reduction in peripheral blood for approx 10 days; 89–96% CCR4$^+$Foxp3$^+$ Treg depletion in lymph nodes	Wang et al., 2016

G(M)-CSF, granulocyte (macrophage)-stimulating factor.

demonstrated that an anti-human CCR4 immunotoxin bound and depleted cynomolgus CCR4$^+$ cells *in vitro*. In addition, they showed that the immunotoxin bound to the CCR4$^+$Foxp3$^+$ monkey Tregs *in vitro*. *In vivo* studies carried out in two naive cynomolgus revealed 78–89% CCR4$^+$Foxp3$^+$ Treg depletion in the peripheral blood that lasted about 10 days. In lymph nodes (LN), 89–96% CCR4$^+$Foxp3$^+$ Tregs were depleted. However, no effect was observed on other immune cell populations, including other CD4$^+$ cells, CD8$^+$ T cells, B cells and NK cells.

INFLUENCE OF IS REGIMENS ON TREG IN ALLOGRAFT RECIPIENTS

The existence of Treg in NHP kidney allografts during their rejection has been considered integral to the rejection response (Haanstra et al., 2007). On the other hand, specific induction of Tregs by donor Ags and intragraft enrichment of Tregs may be key to long-lasting tolerance in NHP induced by transient mixed chimerism (Hotta et al., 2016; Matsunami et al., 2019). Co-stimulation blockade (Co-SB) of the CD28 pathway is deleterious to Treg function, due likely to the importance of the complimentary CTLA4-CD80/86 pathway in Treg development and homeostasis. Thus, administration of CTLA4-Ig (Abatacept) decreases circulating Tregs in MHC-mismatched rhesus renal transplant recipients (Anderson et al., 2019). However, Poirier et al. (2015) found that a novel antagonistic pegylated anti-CD28 Fab' Ab fragment (FR104), together with low dose tacrolimus or rapamycin in a steroid-free treatment regimen, prevented acute allograft rejection and alloAb development, with accumulation of Helios$^-$ Tregs in the blood and graft. Blocking CD28 using a monovalent, non-activating single chain anti-CD28 Fv fragment linked to alpha-1 anti-trypsin (sc28AT) synergized with CNI in cynomolgus kidney and heart transplantation, increasing absolute numbers of peripheral Tregs (Zhang et al., 2018). Kim et al. (2017) found that a novel anti-human CD40L (CD154) domain Ab (dAb) that prolonged rhesus renal allograft survival without thromboembolism, and that synergized with conventional IS to more markedly control graft rejection, increased CD4$^+$CD25$^+$Foxp3$^+$ Treg frequency.

Ezzelarab et al. (2013, 2018) reported that infusion of donor-derived DCreg 1 week before transplant prolonged rhesus renal allograft survival in combination with CD28 Co-SB and rapamycin and promoted maintenance of donor-reactive CD4$^+$CTLA4^{hi} Tregs.

TREG THERAPEUTIC PROTOCOLS IN TRANSPLANT RECIPIENTS

Successful development of a therapeutic protocol based on adoptive transfer of Treg must address: (i) Treg efficacy and the number of cells required to achieve a therapeutic effect; (ii) stability of the suppressive phenotype; (iii) the Treg migratory pattern that assures their optimal regulatory function; (iv) the Ag specificity required for safe/effective control of rejection; (v) the impact of lymphocyte depletion/concomitant IS therapy on Treg function and durable control of rejection; (vi) conditions permissive to regulation of memory T cell responses. Several NHP studies (**Table 3**) have assessed feasibility, safety and therapeutic efficacy of adoptively-transferred, autologous Treg in transplant recipients. In a direct comparison of the persistence of transferred autologous vs. allogeneic Treg in peripheral blood of immunosuppressed, but not transplanted cynomolgus, we found that autologous Tregs survived much longer than the former (Zhang et al., 2015), a property suggesting more durable potential efficacy of autologous Tregs.

Renal Transplantation

The earliest work (Bashuda et al., 2005) was conducted in rhesus macaques given MHC-mismatched renal allografts. Thus, autologous spleen-derived "suppressive T cells" (approx 10^7/kg) that were rendered anergic by co-culture with donor alloAg together with anti-CD80/CD86 mAbs were infused

TABLE 3 | Assessment of adoptive Treg therapy in NHP transplant recipients.

Type of graft (species)	IS therapy/conditioning	Type of Tregs (number/infusions)	Result	References
Kidney (rhesus) $n = 6$	Cyclosporine and post-transplant cyclophosphamide	Autologous splenocyte-derived "suppressive T cells" (approx 10^7/kg) rendered anergic following co-culture with donor alloAg and anti-CD80/86 mAbs ($10^2 \pm 67 \times 10^6$ total on day 13 post-transplant)	Donor-specific tolerance in 50% of graft recipients	Bashuda et al., 2005
Kidney (cynomolgus) $n = 4$	ATG and low dose rapamycin	Expanded, donor Ag-specific, host splenocyte–derived $CD4^+CD25^+$Treg (14 daily infusions; 10^7 per day)	Graft MST prolonged from 22 to 48.5 days	Ma et al., 2011
Kidney (cynomolgus) ($n = 5$)	Non-myeloablative conditioning and MHC-mismatched BMT. Renal transplantation (from the same BMT donor) conducted 4 months after BMT, with no IS	Expanded polyclonal autologous Treg ($15–53 \times 10^6$/infusion) during the 1st week post-transplant (days 0, 2, 5, 7) and day + 50 (total dose: $88–96 \times 10^6$/kg)	Two of 5 evaluable recipients of Treg + BMT displayed T cell chimerism up to 335 days post-BMT. In one long-term surviving animal, the delayed kidney graft survived > 294 days without IS, however, non-Treg BMT recipients rejected their delayed kidney grafts within 3–4 weeks	Duran-Struuck et al., 2017
Heart (cynomolgus) $n = 5$	ATG, tacrolimus, anti-IL-6R mAb and tapered rapamycin maintenance IS therapy	Expanded polyclonal Tregs (single or multiple doses (up to a maximum cumulative cell dose of 1.87 billion cells during the early post-transplant period (up to 1 month post-transplant)	Inferior graft function with multiple infusions; elevated incidences of T effector memory cells, increased IFNγ production by host $CD8^+$ T cells, enhanced levels of proinflammatory cytokines and anti-donor alloAb	Ezzelarab et al., 2016
Heart (cynomolgus) $n = 5$	ATG, tacrolimus and anti-IL-6R with tacrolimus conversion to rapamycin at 2 weeks (early cell infusion within 3 weeks post-transplant); ATG and tacrolimus with tacrolimus conversion to rapamycin at 2.5 weeks (delayed cell infusion, 6–8 weeks post-transplant)	Expanded donor Ag alloreactive Tregs; $20.5–120 \times 10^6$/kg for each of 2–4 infusions	No prolongation of graft survival; loss of regulatory signature and proliferative/survival capacity by transferred Tregs	Ezzelarab et al., 2020
Pig pancreatic islets (xeno; rhesus) $n = 3$	ATG, CVF, anti-CD154 mAb, and rapamycin	Intraportal infusion (x1 or x2) of expanded $CD4^+CD25^{hi}CD127^{lo}$ autologous Tregs ($1.87–62.0 \times 10^6$) following ATG depletion	Treg infusion associated with more stable and durable normoglycemia	Shin et al., 2015
Pig pancreatic islets (xeno; rhesus) $n = 2$	ATG, CVF, anti-CD154 mAb and rapamycin	As above (ref 65)	Engrafted pig islets rejected by activated T cells following withdrawal of maintenance IS	Shin et al., 2016
Pig skin graft (xeno; baboon) $n = 4$	Splenectomy, TBI, ATG, TI, rapamycin, CVF, GalKO/huCD46/huCD47 transgenic donor pig HSCs, anti-CD40LAb, methylprednisolone	25×10^6/kg (8 infusions)	Prolonged donor skin graft acceptance	Stern et al., 2017

ATG, anti-thymocyte globulin; BMT, bone marrow transplantation; CVF, cobra venom factor; Gal KO, α1,3-galactosyltransferase gene-knockout; HSCs, hematopoietic stem cells; hu, human; IS, immunosuppression; MST, mean/median graft survival time; TBI, total body irradiation; TI, thymic irradiation.

once, 13 days post-transplant to splenectomized hosts that receiving brief cyclosporine and cyclophosphamide (Cy) treatment. Grafts survived long-term and donor-specific tolerance was achieved in 50% of recipients (n = 6), but not in controls, confirming the potential of a Treg therapy in NHP organ transplantation. These findings provided the basis for a clinical trial in living donor liver transplantation, in which splenic T cells rendered anergic to donor and administered 13 days post-transplant after Cy, induced operational tolerance in 7/10 recipients (Todo et al., 2016). However, infusion of similarly generated Tregs 12 days post-transplant into living donor kidney transplant patients resulted in high rates of rejection upon subsequent IS drug withdrawal (Koyama et al., 2020).

Ma et al. (2011) reported that *ex vivo*-expanded autologous Treg prolonged renal transplant survival in ATG-treated cynomolgus monkeys. In this study, a much greater number of infusions (fourteen) of expanded, donor alloAg-specific, spleen–derived $CD4^+CD25^+$Treg were infused (10^7 per day). The infusions started at the time of transplantation (i.e., 1 day following a 3-day course of ATG) and were administered together with low-dose rapamycin for 14 days. Thus, kidney graft survival was prolonged significantly, but unlike in the aforementioned study, no grafts survived indefinitely.

Duran-Struuck et al. (2017) reported that recipient Treg co-transfer could enhance bone marrow (BM) engraftment/hematopoietic cell chimerism and prevent cynomolgus kidney allograft rejection. Eight monkeys were subjected to non-myeloablative conditioning and MHC-mismatched BM transplantation (BMT), either with or without infusion of Treg. Transplantation (from the same BM donor) was undertaken 4 months post-BMT, in the absence of IS to evaluate robust, donor-specific tolerance. Five animals received *ex vivo*-expanded polyclonal autologous Treg during the first week post-transplant (days 0, 2, 5, 7) and also on day 50. Transient mixed chimerism, without significant T cell chimerism, was observed in those monkeys given BMT but no Treg (n = 3). By contrast, the 2 of 5 monkeys given Treg + BMT that could be evaluated showed multilineage (including T cell) chimerism up to 335 days after BMT. It was notable that, in the monkey that survived long-term, >90% of donor T cells were found to be new thymic emigrants. In this monkey, the delayed (to 4 months) renal transplant was accepted for >294 days without IS therapy, whereas non-Treg BMT recipients rejected their delayed kidney grafts within 3–4 weeks. Early reactivation of cytomegalovirus (CMV) and anti-viral treatment was linked with early failure of chimerism, irrespective of Treg administration. Overall, these observations reveal that, without early CMV reactivation (and consequent BM-toxic anti-viral therapy), administration of host Treg can promote both prolonged multilineage chimerism and robust donor tolerance.

Heart Transplantation

Addressing the hypothesis that markedly reduced T cell numbers in graft recipients would favor the therapeutic efficacy of adoptively-transferred Tregs, Ezzelarab et al. (2016) infused *ex vivo*-expanded, polyclonal Treg into ATG-treated, MHC-mismatched cynomolgus monkey heart transplant recipients before the homeostatic recovery of effector T cells. Tacrolimus, anti-IL-6R mAb and tapered rapamycin maintenance treatment was also administered. Infusion of Treg in either single or multiple doses during the early post-transplant period (up to a month post-transplant) during which time host T cells were markedly depleted, resulted in poorer heart graft function compared with non-Treg-infused controls. This was accompanied by an increased incidence of circulating effector memory T cells, elevated IFNγ production by $CD8^+$ T cells, and enhanced levels of circulating proinflammatory cytokines and anti-donor alloAb. These observations suggest that Treg infusion early post-transplant period following lymphodepletion should be avoided in human clinical trials. Thus, despite marked but transient increases in circulating Treg relative to effector T cells and the use of so-called "Treg-friendly" agents, environmental conditions and host immune effector mechanisms that prevail under these conditions may negate the potential therapeutic efficacy of the infused transferred Treg.

In a more recent study (Ezzelarab et al., 2020), cynomolgus monkey autologous darTreg were expanded from flow-sorted, circulating Treg using activated donor B lymphocytes and infused after transplant into MHC-mismatched heart graft recipients. While the darTreg selectively suppressed proliferative responses of autologous T cells to donor alloAgs *in vitro*, their adoptive transfer post-transplant failed to prolong graft survival. Early (within 2 weeks post-transplant; under ATG, tacrolimus and anti-IL-6R) or delayed (6–8 weeks post-transplant; under rapamycin) darTreg infusion resulted in a rapid reduction in transferred cells in the circulation. After early or delayed infusion, dye-labeled darTreg could be observed in lymphoid and non-lymphoid tissues and in the heart graft at low percentages (<4% $CD4^+$ T cells). Notably, the infused darTreg displayed reduced expression of Foxp3, CTLA4, Helios, the proliferative marker Ki67, and anti-apoptotic Bcl2, compared with pre-infusion darTreg and endogenous Treg.

Comparison of Doses of darTreg Tested in NHP and Human Allograft Recipients

Doses of darTreg tested in cynomolgus heart allograft recipients following lymphodepletion with ATG (Ezzelarab and Thomson, 2020) were similar to or greater than doses of autologous T cells rendered anergic to donor Ag and infused post-transplant to Cy-treated, renal-allografted monkeys (Bashuda et al., 2005) and that induced donor-specific tolerance. However, they also resemble the single doses of similarly generated Tregs (14–36 × 10^6/kg) infused 12 days post-transplant to living donor kidney transplant patients, including those given Cy, that, by contrast, exhibited high rates of rejection upon subsequent IS drug withdrawal (Koyama et al., 2020). In other clinical studies of darTeg in living donor kidney transplantation, lower doses of darTreg have been targeted (i.e., 2 × 10^3–2 × 10^6/kg or 0.5–10 × 10^6/kg, respectively) in small numbers of patients at separate centers in the ONE Study (Sawitzki et al., 2020) in which overall safety of cell therapy and similar 1-year graft survival compared to a reference standard of care group have been reported. In human living donor liver transplantation, doses of 23.3–14.4 $\times$ 10^6 T cells rendered anergic to donor and administered 13 days post-transplant after Cy induced operational tolerance in 7/10 recipients (Todo et al., 2016). A total of 300–500 $\times$ 10^6 darTreg have been targeted in a liver transplantation IS drug withdrawal study at UCSF (NCT02474199).

TRACKING/MONITORING OF POLYCLONAL OR DARTREGS IN NORMAL NHP OR ORGAN ALLOGRAFT RECIPIENTS

The *in vivo* persistence and migration of adoptively-transferred polyclonal Tregs to secondary lymphoid tissues documented in rodents have been confirmed by NHP studies that have determined the survival, migration, and function of exogenous Tregs. Detection of autologous or allogeneic Tregs infused into normal macaques has been accomplished by direct dye-labeling and subsequent tracking of the Tregs in blood, LNs and spleen at various times after their infusion (Singh et al., 2014; Zhang et al., 2015). Pharmacokinetic analysis of dye-labeled autologous Tregs has revealed an initial rapid period of elimination from the blood between day 0 and 3 post-infusion, after which the transferred Tregs persist at low levels for up to 3 weeks (Zhang et al., 2015). Staining for the cell proliferation marker Ki67 further demonstrates that label dilution as a result of cell proliferation does not contribute to the apparent disappearance of transferred Tregs from blood. Labeled autologous Tregs have been detected in LNs on day 1–2 post-infusion, however analysis on day 6 failed to demonstrate sustained persistence of infused Tregs in secondary lymphoid organs (Zhang et al., 2015).

Concurrent IS therapy markedly increases the survival of adoptively-transferred autologous Tregs in the peripheral blood and LNs. Labeled autologous Tregs persist longer in monkeys given rapamycin and in greater numbers compared to non-immunosuppressed conditions at least 50 days post-infusion (Furlan et al., 2020). Low dose IL-2 together with rapamycin further prolongs the half-life of adoptively-transferred Tregs in NHPs, with detection of labeled cells in the periphery up to 84 days after infusion. These findings highlight a wide variability in the survival of infused Tregs under different conditions, including the use and type of IS, in addition to cell production methods, including cryopreservation.

XENOTRANSPLANTATION

Treg in xenotransplantation has been reviewed (Ezzelarab, 2018). Baboon Treg expanded in response to irradiated pig PBMC for potential use in pig-to-baboon xenotransplantation (Porter et al., 2007) proved strongly suppressive *in vitro* and donor-specific suppression was achieved. Huang et al. (2017) found that baboon autologous Tregs expanded by stimulation with pig PBMC could prevent porcine islet xenograft rejection in NOD-SCID IL-2r$\gamma^{-/-}$ mice reconstituted with baboon PBMC. Prolonged xenograft survival to >100 days correlated with Treg engraftment and intragraft CD39 and Foxp3 gene expression. Shin et al. (2016) transplanted two diabetic rhesus with pancreatic islets isolated from wild-type miniature pigs with IS comprising ATG, cobra venom factor, anti-CD154 mAb and sirolimus. Expanded $CD4^+CD25^{hi}CD127^{lo}$ autologous Tregs were infused during the peri-transplant period, however following withdrawal of maintenance IS, engrafted pig islets were rejected, indicating failure of tolerance induction by the autologous Tregs in this model.

CONCLUSION AND FUTURE STUDIES

NHP have the inherent advantage over rodent or humanized/primatized mouse models of closely resembling the human condition. Endogenous Treg in NHP can be increased or selectively depleted *in vivo*, and both polyclonal and darTreg have been expanded successfully *ex vivo*. In NHP kidney, heart and pancreatic islet transplantation, single or multiple infusions of autologous Treg have yielded results ranging from indefinite, IS-free graft survival to exacerbation of acute rejection, depending on the experimental model and IS regimen. In addition to valuable safety and graft outcome data that help guide clinical trial design, important insights have been gained into the biodistribution, stability and longevity of the transferred cells, and their influence on anti-donor immunity. These findings have drawn attention to the biological and logistical challenges encountered when transitioning testing of Treg therapeutic efficacy in inbred, spf mouse models, usually at very high/unphysiological Treg/effector cell ratios, to more clinically relevant NHP species. Exciting, newly evolving approaches to generation of stable, Ag-specific Tregs (Ferreira et al., 2019; Raffin et al., 2020), include gene editing of bulk T cells (Honaker et al., 2020) and production of CAR Tregs engineered to promote their Ag specificity and homing (MacDonald et al., 2016; Dawson et al., 2019; Hoeppli et al., 2019; Mohseni et al., 2020). Although there are no published reports of these developments as yet in NHP models, testing of such advances in NHP organ transplantation is keenly anticipated.

AUTHOR CONTRIBUTIONS

AT, KS, and ME participated in planning of the manuscript, literature searches, and in the writing of the mini-review. All authors contributed to the article and approved the submitted version.

FUNDING

This work was supported by the National Institutes of Health Non-human Primate Cooperative Study Group Grant U19 AI131453.

REFERENCES

Adams, A. B., Pearson, T. C., and Larsen, C. P. (2003). Heterologous immunity: an overlooked barrier to tolerance. *Immunol. Rev.* 196, 147–160. doi: 10.1046/j.1600-065x.2003.00082.x

Alonso-Guallart, P., Llore, N., Lopes, E., Kofman, S. B., Ho, S. H., Stern, J., et al. (2021). CD40L-stimulated B cells for ex-vivo expansion of polyspecific non-human primate regulatory T cells for translational studies. *Clin. Exp. Immunol.* 203, 480–492. doi: 10.1111/cei.13537

Anderson, A., Martens, C. L., Hendrix, R., Stempora, L. L., Miller, W. P., Hamby, K., et al. (2008). Expanded nonhuman primate Tregs exhibit a unique gene expression signature and potently downregulate alloimmune responses. *Am. J. Transplant.* 8, 2252–2264. doi: 10.1111/j.1600-6143.2008.02376.x

Anderson, D. J., Lo, D. J., Leopardi, F., Song, M., Strobert, E. A., Jenkins, J. B., et al. (2019). Corticosteroids and methotrexate as adjuvants to costimulation blockade in non-human primate renal transplantation. *Clin. Transplant.* 33:e13568.

Aoyama, A., Klarin, D., Yamada, Y., Boskovic, S., Nadazdin, O., Kawai, K., et al. (2012). Low-dose IL-2 for in vivo expansion of CD4+ and CD8+ regulatory T cells in nonhuman primates. *Am. J. Transplant.* 12, 2532–2537. doi: 10.1111/j.1600-6143.2012.04133.x

Bashuda, H., Kimikawa, M., Seino, K., Kato, Y., Ono, F., Shimizu, A., et al. (2005). Renal allograft rejection is prevented by adoptive transfer of anergic T cells in nonhuman primates. *J. Clin. Invest.* 115, 1896–1902. doi: 10.1172/jci23743

Chen, D., and Bromberg, J. S. (2006). T regulatory cells and migration. *Am. J. Transplant.* 6, 1518–1523. doi: 10.1111/j.1600-6143.2006.01372.x

Choo, J. K., Seebach, J. D., Nickeleit, V., Shimizu, A., Lei, H., Sachs, D. H., et al. (1997). Species differences in the expression of major histocompatibility complex class II antigens on coronary artery endothelium: implications for cell-mediated xenoreactivity. *Transplantation* 64, 1315–1322. doi: 10.1097/00007890-199711150-00014

Dawson, N. A., Lamarche, C., Hoeppli, R. E., Bergqvist, P., Fung, V. C., McIver, E., et al. (2019). Systematic testing and specificity mapping of alloantigen-specific chimeric antigen receptors in regulatory T cells. *JCI Insight* 4:e123672.

Dons, E. M., Raimondi, G., Zhang, H., Zahorchak, A. F., Bhama, J. K., Lu, L., et al. (2013). Ex vivo-expanded cynomolgus macaque regulatory T cells are resistant to alemtuzumab-mediated cytotoxicity. *Am. J. Transplant.* 13, 2169–2178. doi: 10.1111/ajt.12248

Duran-Struuck, R., Sondermeijer, H. P., Buhler, L., Alonso-Guallart, P., Zitsman, J., Kato, Y., et al. (2017). Effect of ex vivo-expanded recipient regulatory T cells on hematopoietic chimerism and kidney allograft tolerance across MHC barriers in Cynomolgus Macaques. *Transplantation* 101, 274–283. doi: 10.1097/tp.0000000000001559

Ezzelarab, M. B. (2018). Regulatory T cells from allo- to xenotransplantation: opportunities and challenges. *Xenotransplantation* 25:e12415. doi: 10.1111/xen.12415

Ezzelarab, M. B., and Thomson, A. W. (2020). Plasmacytoid dendritic cells and the spontaneous acceptance of kidney allografts. *Transplantation* 104, 15–16. doi: 10.1097/tp.0000000000002868

Ezzelarab, M. B., Lu, L., Shufesky, W. F., Morelli, A. E., and Thomson, A. W. (2018). Donor-derived regulatory dendritic cell infusion maintains donor-reactive CD4(+)CTLA4(hi) T cells in non-human primate renal allograft recipients treated with CD28 co-stimulation blockade. *Front. Immunol.* 9:250.

Ezzelarab, M. B., Zahorchak, A. F., Lu, L., Morelli, A. E., Chalasani, G., Demetris, A. J., et al. (2013). Regulatory dendritic cell infusion prolongs kidney allograft survival in nonhuman primates. *Am. J. Transplant.* 13, 1989–2005. doi: 10.1111/ajt.12310

Ezzelarab, M. B., Zhang, H., Guo, H., Lu, L., Zahorchak, A. F., Wiseman, R. W., et al. (2016). Regulatory T cell infusion can enhance memory T cell and alloantibody responses in lymphodepleted nonhuman primate heart allograft recipients. *Am. J. Transplant.* 16, 1999–2015. doi: 10.1111/ajt.13685

Ezzelarab, M. E., Zhang, H., Sasaki, K., Lu, L., Zahorchak, A. F., Van der Windt, D., et al. (2020). Ex vivo expanded donor alloreactive regulatory T cells lose immunoregulatory, proliferation and anti-apoptotic markers after infusion into ATG-lymphodepleted, nonhuman primate heart allograft recipients. *Transplantation* doi: 10.1097/TP.0000000000003617 Online ahead of print.

Ferreira, L. M. R., Muller, Y. D., Bluestone, J. A., and Tang, Q. (2019). Next-generation regulatory T cell therapy. *Nat. Rev. Drug Discov.* 18, 749–769. doi: 10.1038/s41573-019-0041-4

Fitch, Z., Schmitz, R., Kwun, J., Hering, B., Madsen, J., and Knechtle, S. J. (2019). Transplant research in nonhuman primates to evaluate clinically relevant immune strategies in organ transplantation. *Transplant. Rev.* 33, 115–129. doi: 10.1016/j.trre.2019.03.002

Furlan, S. N., Singh, K., Lopez, C., Tkachev, V., Hunt, D. J., Hibbard, J., et al. (2020). IL-2 enhances ex vivo-expanded regulatory T-cell persistence after adoptive transfer. *Blood Adv.* 4, 1594–1605. doi: 10.1182/bloodadvances.2019001248

Gansuvd, B., Asiedu, C. K., Goodwin, J., Jargal, U., Deckard, L. A., Andrades, P., et al. (2007). Expansion of CD4+CD25+ suppressive regulatory T cells from rhesus macaque peripheral blood by FN18/antihuman CD28-coated Dynal beads. *Hum. Immunol.* 68, 478–490. doi: 10.1016/j.humimm.2007.02.011

Guo, H., Zhang, H., Lu, L., Ezzelarab, M. B., and Thomson, A. W. (2015). Generation, cryopreservation, function and in vivo persistence of ex vivo expanded cynomolgus monkey regulatory T cells. *Cell. Immunol.* 295, 19–28. doi: 10.1016/j.cellimm.2015.02.006

Haanstra, K. G., van der Maas, M. J., t Hart, B. A., and Jonker, M. (2008). Characterization of naturally occurring CD4+CD25+ regulatory T cells in rhesus monkeys. *Transplantation* 85, 1185–1192. doi: 10.1097/tp.0b013e31816b15b9

Haanstra, K. G., Wubben, J. A., Korevaar, S. S., Kondova, I., Baan, C. C., and Jonker, M. (2007). Expression patterns of regulatory T-cell markers in accepted and rejected nonhuman primate kidney allografts. *Am. J. Transplant.* 7, 2236–2246. doi: 10.1111/j.1600-6143.2007.01917.x

Hoeppli, R. E., MacDonald, K. N., Leclair, P., Fung, V. C. W., Mojibian, M., Gillies, J., et al. (2019). Tailoring the homing capacity of human Tregs for directed migration to sites of Th1-inflammation or intestinal regions. *Am. J. Transplant.* 19, 62–76. doi: 10.1111/ajt.14936

Honaker, Y., Hubbard, N., Xiang, Y., Fisher, L., Hagin, D., Sommer, K., et al. (2020). Gene editing to induce FOXP3 expression in human CD4(+) T cells leads to a stable regulatory phenotype and function. *Sci. Transl. Med.* 12:eaay6422. doi: 10.1126/scitranslmed.aay6422

Hotta, K., Aoyama, A., Oura, T., Yamada, Y., Tonsho, M., Huh, K. H., et al. (2016). Induced regulatory T cells in allograft tolerance via transient mixed chimerism. *JCI Insight* 1:e86419.

Houser, S. L., Benjamin, L. C., Wain, J. C., Madsen, J. C., and Allan, J. S. (2004). Constitutive expression of major histocompatibility complex class II antigens in pulmonary epithelium and endothelium varies among different species. *Transplantation* 77, 605–607. doi: 10.1097/01.tp.0000114285.63313.e7

Huang, D., Wang, Y., Hawthorne, W. J., Hu, M., Hawkes, J., Burns, H., et al. (2017). Ex vivo-expanded baboon CD39 + regulatory T cells prevent rejection of porcine islet xenografts in NOD-SCID IL-2r$\gamma^{-/-}$ mice reconstituted with baboon peripheral blood mononuclear cells. *Xenotransplantation* 24:e12344. doi: 10.1111/xen.12344

Kean, L. S., Sen, S., Onabajo, O., Singh, K., Robertson, J., Stempora, L., et al. (2011). Significant mobilization of both conventional and regulatory T cells with AMD3100. *Blood* 118, 6580–6590. doi: 10.1182/blood-2011-06-359331

Kim, S. C., Wakwe, W., Higginbotham, L. B., Mathews, D. V., Breeden, C. P., Stephenson, A. C., et al. (2017). Fc-Silent Anti-CD154 domain antibody effectively prevents nonhuman primate renal allograft rejection. *Am. J. Transplant.* 17, 1182–1192. doi: 10.1111/ajt.14197

Knechtle, S. J., Shaw, J. M., Hering, B. J., Kraemer, K., and Madsen, J. C. (2019). Translational impact of NIH-funded nonhuman primate research in transplantation. *Sci. Transl. Med.* 11:aau0143.

Koyama, I., Bashuda, H., Uchida, K., Seino, K. I., Habu, S., Nakajima, I., et al. (2020). A clinical trial with adoptive transfer of ex vivo-induced, donor-specific immune-regulatory cells in kidney transplantation-a second report. *Transplantation* 104, 2415–2423. doi: 10.1097/tp.0000000000003149

Lamarche, C., and Levings, M. K. (2018). Guiding regulatory T cells to the allograft. *Curr. Opin. Organ. Transplant.* 23, 106–113. doi: 10.1097/mot.0000000000000483

Larsen, S. E., Voss, K., Laing, E. D., and Snow, A. L. (2017). Differential cytokine withdrawal-induced death sensitivity of effector T cells derived from distinct human CD8(+) memory subsets. *Cell Death Discov.* 3:17031.

Li, M., Eckl, J., Abicht, J.-M., Mayr, T., Reichart, B., Schendel, D. J., et al. (2018). Induction of porcine-specific regulatory T cells with high specificity and expression of IL-10 and TGF-$^{\beta}$1 using baboon-derived tolerogenic dendritic cells. *Xenotransplantation* 25:e12355. doi: 10.1111/xen.12355

Liao, W., Lin, J. X., and Leonard, W. J. (2013). Interleukin-2 at the crossroads of effector responses, tolerance, and immunotherapy. *Immunity* 38, 13–25. doi: 10.1016/j.immuni.2013.01.004

Ma, A., Qi, S., Song, L., Hu, Y., Dun, H., Massicotte, E., et al. (2011). Adoptive transfer of CD4+CD25+ regulatory cells combined with low-dose sirolimus and anti-thymocyte globulin delays acute rejection of renal allografts in Cynomolgus monkeys. *Int. Immunopharmacol.* 11, 618–629. doi: 10.1016/j.intimp.2010.11.001

Ma, A., Xiong, Z., Hu, Y., Qi, S., Song, L., Dun, H., et al. (2009). Dysfunction of IL-10-producing type 1 regulatory T cells and CD4(+)CD25(+) regulatory T cells in a mimic model of human multiple sclerosis in Cynomolgus monkeys. *Int. Immunopharmacol.* 9, 599–608. doi: 10.1016/j.intimp.2009.01.034

MacDonald, K. G., Hoeppli, R. E., Huang, Q., Gillies, J., Luciani, D. S., Orban, P. C., et al. (2016). Alloantigen-specific regulatory T cells generated with a chimeric antigen receptor. *J. Clin. Invest.* 126, 1413–1424. doi: 10.1172/jci82771

Matsunami, M., Rosales, I. A., Adam, B. A., Oura, T., Mengel, M., Smith, R. N., et al. (2019). Long-term kinetics of intragraft gene signatures in renal allograft tolerance induced by transient mixed chimerism. *Transplantation* 103:e334. doi: 10.1097/tp.0000000000002911

Mempel, T. R., and Marangoni, F. (2019). Guidance factors orchestrating regulatory T cell positioning in tissues during development, homeostasis, and response. *Immunol. Rev.* 289, 129–141. doi: 10.1111/imr.12761

Mohseni, Y. R., Tung, S. L., Dudreuilh, C., Lechler, R. I., Fruhwirth, G. O., and Lombardi, G. (2020). The future of regulatory T cell therapy: promises and challenges of implementing CAR technology. *Front. Immunol.* 11:1608.

Moreau, A., Chiffoleau, E., Beriou, G., Deschamps, J. Y., Heslan, M., Ashton-Chess, J., et al. (2008). Superiority of bone marrow-derived dendritic cells over monocyte-derived ones for the expansion of regulatory T cells in the macaque. *Transplantation* 85, 1351–1356. doi: 10.1097/tp.0b013e31816f22d6

Poirier, N., Dilek, N., Mary, C., Ville, S., Coulon, F., Branchereau, J., et al. (2015). FR104, an antagonist anti-CD28 monovalent fab' antibody, prevents alloimmunization and allows calcineurin inhibitor minimization in nonhuman primate renal allograft. *Am. J. Transplant.* 15, 88–100. doi: 10.1111/ajt.12964

Porter, C. M., Horvath-Arcidiacono, J. A., Singh, A. K., Horvath, K. A., Bloom, E. T., and Mohiuddin, M. M. (2007). Characterization and expansion of baboon CD4+CD25+ Treg cells for potential use in a non-human primate xenotransplantation model. *Xenotransplantation* 14, 298–308. doi: 10.1111/j.1399-3089.2007.00416.x

Qin, S., Sui, Y., Soloff, A. C., Junecko, B. A., Kirschner, D. E., Murphey-Corb, M. A., et al. (2008). Chemokine and cytokine mediated loss of regulatory T cells in lymph nodes during pathogenic simian immunodeficiency virus infection. *J. Immunol.* 180, 5530–5536. doi: 10.4049/jimmunol.180.8.5530

Raffin, C., Vo, L. T., and Bluestone, J. A. (2020). Treg cell-based therapies: challenges and perspectives. *Nat. Rev. Immunol.* 20, 158–172. doi: 10.1038/s41577-019-0232-6

Sachs, D. H. (2003). Tolerance: of mice and men. *J. Clin. Invest.* 111, 1819–1821. doi: 10.1172/jci18926

Sakaguchi, S., Yamaguchi, T., Nomura, T., and Ono, M. (2008). Regulatory T cells and immune tolerance. *Cell* 133, 775–787. doi: 10.1016/j.cell.2008.05.009

Sasaki, K., Wang, Y. C., Lu, L., Hughes, J., Vujevich, V., Thomson, A. W., et al. (2020). Combined GM-CSF and G-CSF administration mobilizes CD4(+) CD25(hi) Foxp3(hi) Treg in leukapheresis products of rhesus monkeys. *Am. J. Transplant.* 20, 1691–1702. doi: 10.1111/ajt.15761

Sawitzki, B., Harden, P. N., Reinke, P., Moreau, A., Hutchinson, J. A., Game, D. S., et al. (2020). Regulatory cell therapy in kidney transplantation (The ONE Study): a harmonised design and analysis of seven non-randomised, single-arm, phase 1/2A trials. *Lancet* 395, 1627–1639.

Shin, J. S., Kim, J. M., Kim, J. S., Min, B. H., Kim, Y. H., Kim, H. J., et al. (2015). Long-term control of diabetes in immunosuppressed nonhuman primates (NHP) by the transplantation of adult porcine islets. *Am. J. Transplant.* 15, 2837–2850. doi: 10.1111/ajt.13345

Shin, J. S., Min, B. H., Kim, J. M., Kim, J. S., Yoon, I. H., Kim, H. J., et al. (2016). Failure of transplantation tolerance induction by autologous regulatory T cells in the pig-to-non-human primate islet xenotransplantation model. *Xenotransplantation* 23, 300–309. doi: 10.1111/xen.12246

Singh, A. K., Seavey, C. N., Horvath, K. A., and Mohiuddin, M. M. (2012). Ex-vivo expanded baboon CD4+ CD25 Hi Treg cells suppress baboon anti-pig T and B cell immune response. *Xenotransplantation* 19, 102–111. doi: 10.1111/j.1399-3089.2012.00697.x

Singh, K., Kozyr, N., Stempora, L., Kirk, A. D., Larsen, C. P., Blazar, B. R., et al. (2012). Regulatory T cells exhibit decreased proliferation but enhanced suppression after pulsing with sirolimus. *Am. J. Transplant.* 12, 1441–1457. doi: 10.1111/j.1600-6143.2011.03963.x

Singh, K., Stempora, L., Harvey, R. D., Kirk, A. D., Larsen, C. P., Blazar, B. R., et al. (2014). Superiority of rapamycin over tacrolimus in preserving nonhuman primate Treg half-life and phenotype after adoptive transfer. *Am. J. Transplant.* 14, 2691–2703. doi: 10.1111/ajt.12934

Stern, J., Kofman, S. B., Alonso-Guallart, P., Berglund, E., Danton, M., Weiner, J., et al. (2017). Autologous expanded Tregs and Porcine hematopoietic cells to prolong xenogeneic pig skin graft acceptance in baboons. *Am. J. Transplant.* 17, 522–528.

Todo, S., Yamashita, K., Goto, R., Zaitsu, M., Nagatsu, A., Oura, T., et al. (2016). A pilot study of operational tolerance with a regulatory T-cell-based cell therapy in living donor liver transplantation. *Hepatology* 64, 632–643. doi: 10.1002/hep.28459

Torrealba, J. R., Katayama, M., Fechner, J. H., Jankowska-Gan, E., Kusaka, S., Xu, Q., et al. (2004). Metastable tolerance to rhesus monkey renal transplants is correlated with allograft TGF-beta 1+CD4+ T regulatory cell infiltrates. *J. Immunol.* 172, 5753–5764. doi: 10.4049/jimmunol.172.9.5753

Wang, Z., Pratts, S. G., Zhang, H., Spencer, P. J., Yu, R., Tonsho, M., et al. (2016). Treg depletion in non-human primates using a novel diphtheria toxin-based anti-human CCR4 immunotoxin. *Mol. Oncol.* 10, 553–565. doi: 10.1016/j.molonc.2015.11.008

Weiner, J., Duran-Struuck, R., Zitsman, J., Buhler, L., Sondermeijer, H., McMurchy, A. N., et al. (2015). Restimulation after Cryopreservation and thawing preserves the phenotype and function of expanded baboon regulatory T cells. *Transplant. Direct* 1, 1–7. doi: 10.1097/txd.0000000000000511

Yamada, Y., Aoyama, A., Tocco, G., Boskovic, S., Nadazdin, O., Alessandrini, A., et al. (2012a). Differential effects of denileukin diftitox IL-2 immunotoxin on NK and regulatory T cells in nonhuman primates. *J. Immunol.* 188, 6063–6070. doi: 10.4049/jimmunol.1200656

Yamada, Y., Boskovic, S., Aoyama, A., Murakami, T., Putheti, P., Smith, R. N., et al. (2012b). Overcoming memory T-cell responses for induction of delayed tolerance in nonhuman primates. *Am. J. Transplant.* 12, 330–340. doi: 10.1111/j.1600-6143.2011.03795.x

Yamada, Y., Nadazdin, O., Boskovic, S., Lee, S., Zorn, E., Smith, R. N., et al. (2015). Repeated injections of IL-2 break renal allograft tolerance induced via mixed hematopoietic Chimerism in monkeys. *Am. J. Transplant.* 15, 3055–3066. doi: 10.1111/ajt.13382

Zahorchak, A. F., Raimondi, G., and Thomson, A. W. (2009). Rhesus monkey immature monocyte-derived dendritic cells generate alloantigen-specific regulatory T cells from circulating CD4+CD127-/lo T cells. *Transplantation* 88, 1057–1064. doi: 10.1097/tp.0b013e3181ba6b1f

Zhang, H., Guo, H., Lu, L., Zahorchak, A. F., Wiseman, R. W., Raimondi, G., et al. (2015). Sequential monitoring and stability of ex vivo-expanded autologous and nonautologous regulatory T cells following infusion in nonhuman primates. *Am. J. Transplant.* 15, 1253–1266. doi: 10.1111/ajt.13113

Zhang, N., Schroppel, B., Lal, G., Jakubzick, C., Mao, X., Chen, D., et al. (2009). Regulatory T cells sequentially migrate from inflamed tissues to draining lymph nodes to suppress the alloimmune response. *Immunity* 30, 458–469. doi: 10.1016/j.immuni.2008.12.022

Zhang, T., Azimzadeh, A. M., Sun, W., O'Neill, N. A., Sievert, E., Bergbower, E., et al. (2018). Selective CD28 inhibition modulates alloimmunity and cardiac allograft vasculopathy in Anti-CD154-treated monkeys. *Transplantation* 102, e90–e100.

Zorn, E., Nelson, E. A., Mohseni, M., Porcheray, F., Kim, H., Litsa, D., et al. (2006). IL-2 regulates FOXP3 expression in human CD4+CD25+ regulatory T cells through a STAT-dependent mechanism and induces the expansion of these cells in vivo. *Blood* 108, 1571–1579. doi: 10.1182/blood-2006-02-004747

18

Modulation of APC function and anti-tumor immunity by anti-cancer drugs

Kea Martin[1†], Jens Schreiner[1†] and Alfred Zippelius[1,2]*

[1] Department of Biomedicine, University Hospital Basel, University of Basel, Basel, Switzerland, [2] Department of Medical Oncology, University Hospital Basel, Basel, Switzerland

Edited by:
Stefan F. Martin,
University of Freiburg, Germany

Reviewed by:
María Marcela Barrio,
Fundación Cáncer FUCA, Argentina
Gabi Niedermann,
University of Freiburg, Germany

***Correspondence:**
Alfred Zippelius,
Department of Medical Oncology,
University Hospital Basel,
Petersgraben 4, Basel CH-4031,
Switzerland
alfred.zippelius@usb.ch

[†]Kea Martin and Jens Schreiner have contributed equally to this work.

Professional antigen-presenting cells (APCs), such as dendritic cells (DCs), are central to the initiation and regulation of anti-cancer immunity. However, in the immunosuppressive environment within a tumor APCs may antagonize anti-tumor immunity by inducing regulatory T cells (Tregs) or anergy of effector T cells due to lack of efficient costimulation. Hence, in an optimal setting, anti-cancer drugs have the power to reduce tumor size and thereby may induce the release of tumor antigens and, at the same time, modulate APC function toward efficient priming of antigen-specific effector T cells. Selected cytotoxic agents may revert APC dysfunction either by directly maturing DCs or through induction of immunogenic tumor cell death. Furthermore, specific cytotoxic agents may support adaptive immunity by selectively depleting regulatory subsets, such as Tregs or myeloid-derived suppressor cells. Perspectively, this will allow developing effective combination strategies with novel immunotherapies to exert complementary pressure on tumors via direct toxicity as well as immune activation. We, here, review our current knowledge on the capacity of anti-cancer drugs to modulate APC functions to promote durable anti-cancer immune responses.

Keywords: chemotherapy, dendritic cells, anti-tumor immunity, antigen-presenting cell, tumor-induced T cell dysfunction, immunogenic cell death

DCs are Central to the Initiation and Regulation of Anti-Cancer Immunity

Both the induction of endogenous anti-tumor immune responses and the successful implementation of immunotherapy protocols rely on adequate activation of adaptive immunity by antigen-presenting cells (APCs). Although innate and adaptive immune cells act in concert to fight cancer cells, T cells play a superior role in inducing and maintaining sustained anti-tumor immune responses (1–4). Professional APCs include B-cells, macrophages, dendritic cells (DCs), and skin-resident Langerhans cells. Among these, DCs are by far the most potent activators of adaptive immunity owing to their unique capacity to induce primary T cell responses (5, 6).

To initiate T cell responses in the tumor setting, DCs must first recognize tumor cells as "abnormal" cells. Tumor cells differ from normal cells due to expression of altered-self or neo-antigens that arise as a consequence of genetic instability and high mutation rates in transformed cells (7, 8). Efficient activation of naïve and central memory T cells requires at least three signals delivered by APCs (9, 10). Along with the uptake of tumor-associated antigens and presentation in the context of MHC molecules, professional APCs are further required to provide lymphocyte costimulation, such as through expression of the B7 molecules (CD80 and CD86) or CD40. Expression of T cell-directing cytokines and additional costimulatory surface receptors by DCs subsequently provides the impulse for appropriate

CD4+ T helper cell polarization (11). Importantly, DC maturation is regulated by the type, duration, and timing of danger/stress signals, such as pathogen-associated molecular patterns (PAMPs) or damage-associated molecular patterns (DAMPs), both of which trigger DC-intrinsic pattern-recognition receptors (12–14). Consequently, these signals determine the quality and quantity of costimulation provided by DCs and thus have the power to define the outcome of T cell immunity.

Tumor cells may undergo cell death due to hypoxia and nutrient deprivation (15) resulting in the release of host-derived DAMPs as an indicator of a dying or "stressed" cell. Thus, on theoretical grounds, tumors may provide the basic elements needed for the initiation of successful anti-tumor immune responses. However, it is well established that the immune-suppressive microenvironment of progressive tumors may severely interfere with both APC and T cell activation, thereby limiting the induction of endogenous anti-tumor immunity and the success of immunotherapies. Importantly, numerous tumor-mediated mechanisms may induce DC dysfunction, leading to immature or semi-mature DCs that are incapable of providing the necessary activation signals (16, 17). Consequently, under these circumstances, antigen presentation will typically provoke T cell tolerance including T cell anergy, peripheral T cell clonal deletion, or the induction of regulatory T cells (Tregs) (18–21).

In light of the recent success of novel immunotherapy approaches, future therapeutic efforts will ultimately focus on the development of effective combination strategies that exert complementary pressure on tumors via immune activation and additional direct toxicity. Of note, accumulating evidence reveals unrecognized immune-modulatory features of chemo- and radiotherapy (22, 23). In addition to reducing the primary tumor burden and thereby, at least in part, reverting the immunosuppressive microenvironment, specific compound classes can also induce DC maturation, enhance antigen cross-presentation, selectively eliminate immunosuppressive cells, or induce immunogenic cell death (ICD) (24, 25). These mechanisms may provide the basis for initiation of anti-tumor immunity and therefore support the successful implementation of T cell-mediated immunotherapy protocols, such as blockade of inhibitory receptors. Consequently, chemo-immunotherapy protocols are being evaluated in numerous clinical studies with promising therapeutic activity (26).

A major drawback of cytotoxic anti-cancer agents is their possible interference with T cell activation and clonal expansion (27, 28). A precise definition of the immune-modulating properties of cytotoxic therapies is, therefore, crucial for optimizing chemo-immunotherapy regimens. Here, we review the current knowledge on the capacity of anti-cancer drugs to modulate the phenotype and function of APCs, and in particular, the impact of these agents on T cell effector functions.

Modulation of APC Function by Anti-Cancer Chemotherapeutics

Direct DC Maturation by Cytotoxic Anti-Cancer Agents

A lack of T cell effector function is mostly caused by inefficient expression of costimulatory molecules on tumor-associated DCs or by dysregulation of DC maturation pathways (29). Therefore, understanding how cytotoxic agents influence DC maturation is vital for designing effective chemo-immunotherapy protocols. An improved DC phenotype associated with T cell activation *in vitro* was reported after treatment of immature DCs with the topoisomerase I inhibitor topotecan. In contrast, treatment of lipopolysaccharide-matured DCs with topotecan resulted in decreased allogeneic T cell responses accompanied with a shift toward T_H2 responses and increased IL-10 in co-cultures (30). Therefore, topoisomerase inhibitors might down-modulate responses of previously activated tumor-resident DCs, suggesting limited suitability for T cell immunotherapy combinations. Studies on other topoisomerase I inhibitors report conflicting results on DC maturation (31, 32). Also, using a DC-based reporter system, nine of 12 investigated compounds were identified as DC stimulatory (33). The effects of topoisomerase inhibitors on the induction of anti-tumor immunity as well as T cell activation and expansion *in vivo*, therefore, require further investigations.

Liu and colleagues revealed mechanistic insights into the molecular events associated with chemotherapy-induced DC maturation (32). Expression of the cell cycle regulator $p21^{waf1/cip1}$ in human DCs was associated with a favorable DC phenotype and was shown to be upregulated by cytotoxic agents. $p21^{waf1/cip1}$ expression correlated with enhanced expression of CD83 and CD86 in response to the anti-malaria agent artesunate and several anti-cancer compounds including camptothecin, lenalidomide, and docetaxel (32). When considering the "two-signal model" in innate immune activation (34), it seems plausible that p21, which generally indicates intrinsic cell stress, is activated in response to cytotoxicity. This "cell stress" or "abnormal condition" in the innate cell itself may deliver the necessary secondary signal for complete activation of innate immune cells and therefore result in enhanced DC maturation.

Along the same line, microtubule-destabilizing agents (MDAs), such as the *Vinca*-alkaloids, dolastatins, or maytansines, can directly affect DC maturation. Early studies indicated that microtubule disruption by colchicine, vinblastine, and vincristine induced marked expression of IL-1 in monocytes (35). Interestingly, rupture of the actin filaments by cytochalasins could not recapitulate this effect. Broad immune-stimulatory effects on murine DCs upon colchicine or vinblastine treatment, including expression of further pro-inflammatory cytokines and enhanced cross-presentation, have subsequently been confirmed by Takashima and colleagues (33, 36, 37). In extension of those data, we were able to demonstrate that two further families of MDAs, the dolastatins and maytansines, potently induced DC maturation. Importantly, DC pre-treatment with these agents induced profound T cell immunity, while treatment of tumor-bearing mice synergized with blockade of CTLA-4 and PD-1. Mechanistically, tumor rejection could be explained by enhanced infiltration of lymphocytes into the tumors and a shift toward an increased effector T cell to Treg ratio (38–40). Experiments to elucidate DC signaling pathways induced by MDAs are currently ongoing.

In stark contrast, we did not detect significant changes in DC phenotype or cytokine expression upon exposure to microtubule-stabilizing agents (MSA), such as the taxane-family of compounds (38).

Various studies have reported modulation of DC phenotype upon exposure to low, non-cytotoxic, concentrations of paclitaxel and other chemotherapeutics (41–44). However, these studies mostly evaluated DC function and phenotypic maturation in the context of paclitaxel pre-treated tumor cells or in combination with lipopolysaccharide treatment. Direct effects of paclitaxel and other MSAs on DCs were generally very moderate and thus are largely consistent with our data. The stimulatory effects of paclitaxel on tumor-associated macrophages, which subsequently may lead to activation of intra-tumoral immune cells, such as DCs, NK cells, and cytotoxic T lymphocytes, are comprehensively reviewed elsewhere (45).

Antibody-drug conjugates (ADCs) are emerging as powerful treatment strategies with outstanding target specificity and high therapeutic activity in cancer patients. The immune-modulatory capacities of dolastatins and maytansines are of particular clinical interest as their synthetic analogs, i.e., monomethyl auristatin E (MMAE) and DM1, are used as cytotoxic payloads of ADCs (46). Importantly, in tumor-bearing mice, DC activation upon treatment with such ADCs is equally potent as observed after administration of the respective free compound. Upon internalization, the cytotoxic payload is released into the tumor cell cytoplasm but may also diffuse into the surrounding microenvironment (47). Notably, the latter may induce maturation of tumor-resident DCs. We detected increased CD8 and CD4 T cell infiltrates, activation of APCs and T cells as well as reduced Treg frequencies in patients treated with the MMAE-carrying ADC Brentuximab Vedotin (BV) (39). Furthermore, induction of long-lasting tumor-specific T cells was detected in relapsed lymphoma patients responding to BV (with or without donor lymphocyte infusions) post-allogeneic HSCT (48, 49).

DC Stimulation via Immunogenic Cell Death

Apoptotic cell death was historically considered to be non-immunogenic. However, some types of cell death have been demonstrated to induce an immune response against antigens released from dying cells, commonly referred to as immunogenic cell death (ICD). Immunogenic signals released by dying tumor cells can induce antigen uptake as well as antigen processing and presentation by the APC. Although cytotoxic anti-cancer therapies generally induce apoptosis, ICD is only induced in treatment with some of these agents, particularly, anthracyclines (50), oxaliplatin (51), and cyclophosphamide (52) as well as for irradiation (50). ICD is characterized by the induction of endoplasmic reticulum (ER) stress and autophagy, which is in distinction to non-immunogenic apoptosis (53, 54). Hallmarks of ICD include the pre-apoptotic exposure of calreticulin (CRT) on the cell surface, the secretion of adenosine triphophosphate (ATP), and the post-apoptotic release of the chromatin-binding protein high-mobility group box 1 (HMGB1) (50, 55, 56). Importantly, the suppression of each of these signals abolishes the immunogenicity of cell death, demonstrating the non-redundancy of each of these pathways (50, 55, 56).

Cytotoxic agents that trigger ICD are also efficient inducers of CRT cell-surface exposure. CRT is under normal circumstances located at the membrane of the ER. Following the induction of an ER stress response, CRT translocates to the cell surface where it serves as an established "eat me signal" for apoptotic cells (50, 54). This occurs well before the induction of apoptotic changes, such as the surface exposure of phosphatidylserine. Binding of CRT to CD91 on phagocytes induces phagocytosis and macropinocytosis leading to the efficient clearance of these cells (57). CRT is also detectable on the surface of viable cells; however, the expression of the surface molecule CD47 and its binding to SIRP-α on phagocytes efficiently inhibits the uptake of viable cells (57). The induction of CRT surface expression on tumor cells by cytotoxic agents efficiently mediates their uptake by DCs (50). Importantly, CRT-CD91 interaction leads to signaling through NF-κB in DCs and to the release of inflammatory cytokines, in particular TNF, IL-6, IL-1β, and IL-12. This cytokine milieu induced by CRT exposure leads to Th17 priming in an immunosuppressive, TGF-β containing, microenvironment (58).

Adenosine triphophosphate release by dying tumor cells manifests the second hallmark of ICD and is one of the most prominent "find-me" signals for myeloid cells. Upon treatment with selected cytotoxic agents, tumor cells secrete ATP in an autophagy-dependent fashion (53, 59). ATP induces recruitment of myeloid cells into the tumor upon its binding to P2Y2 receptors (55). In the second step, ATP facilitates myeloid cells to differentiate into inflammatory DCs. Furthermore, ATP activates P2RX7 receptors on DCs, which activates the NLRP3 inflammasome leading to IL-1β release. Of note, IL-1β then is required for the priming of $CD8^+$ T cells (60). Importantly, priming of T cells appears to occur predominantly in the tumor microenvironment as no significant abrogation in T cell priming is maintained in a mouse model upon surgical removal of draining lymph nodes (55).

High-mobility group box 1 is a chromatin-binding factor found within the nucleus that can be released by injured cells as they undergo primary or secondary necrosis and thereby induces inflammation (61). Treatment of tumor cells by ICD-inducing cytotoxic compounds leads to a post-apoptotic release of HMGB1, which is recognized by TLR4 on DCs. TLR4 controls the tumor antigen processing and is, therefore, indispensable for efficient cross-presentation of tumor cell antigens by DCs (56). In the absence of TLR4 stimulation, phagosomes fuse with lysosomes, which results in degradation of dying cells in the lysosomal compartment, and consequently inefficient antigen presentation (56, 62). In esophageal squamous cell carcinoma, levels of HMGB1 within the tumor microenvironment were significantly upregulated upon preoperative chemoradiotherapy and patients with a high HMGB1 levels showed a better overall survival compared to those with weak HMGB1 expression (63). These findings underline the clinical relevance of HMGB1 expression. However, the inter-patient variability of HMGB1 expression remains poorly understood. HMGB1 can also bind the T cell immunoglobulin- and mucin-domain containing molecule (Tim-3) that is preferentially expressed on tumor-infiltrating DCs (64). Galectin-9 independent ligation of Tim-3 with HMGB1 leads to a negative regulation of nucleic acid-mediated innate immune responses. It is, therefore, reasonable to hypothesize that the balance between a positive signal through TLR4 ligation and a negative signal through Tim-3 ligation might regulate the ICD induced activation of tumor-resident DCs.

While the described mechanisms leading to ICD are able to induce efficient antigen presentation and cytokine secretion, costimulatory molecules might not be upregulated in most of these ICD-inducing chemotherapeutic regiments (50, 55, 56), leaving a gap for more efficient selection of chemotherapeutics or the additional administration of adjuvants.

Cytotoxic Agents Targeting Tumor-Resident Immunosuppressive Cells

Regulatory T cells interfere with anti-tumor immune responses by several mechanisms [reviewed in Ref. (65)]. For example, Tregs may inhibit DC maturation via CTLA-4/CD80/CD86 interaction and induce expression of the immunosuppressive enzyme indoleamine-2,3-dioxygenase (IDO) (66, 67). Several cytotoxic agents are able to target Tregs and thereby promote adaptive anti-tumor immunity. One of the first drugs reported to interfere with Tregs was cyclophosphamide. At low doses, cyclophosphamide depletes Tregs and inhibits their effector functions and homeostatic proliferation, as demonstrated in mouse models and patients (68–71). Consequently, low-dose cyclophosphamide treatment promotes tumor-specific immune responses when combined with different vaccination strategies, including DC-derived exosomes (DEX) (72) and oncolytic adenovirus (73). Yet, the mechanisms underlying this synergy need to be further elucidated. However, it is reasonable, that in the absence of Tregs, CD4$^+$ T cells might activate tumor-resident DCs through CD40L–CD40 interaction, which then can efficiently present tumor antigen and promote T cell activation (74, 75). Additional chemotherapeutic agents targeting Tregs include paclitaxel, which selectively induces apoptosis of Tregs by upregulation of the cell death receptor Fas (76), and low-dose temozolomide, which reduces Treg numbers through poorly understood molecular mechanisms (77, 78).

Myeloid-derived suppressor cells (MDSCs) are a heterogeneous population of immature myeloid cells located in the tumor microenvironment and lymphatic organs. These cells can inhibit innate and adaptive immune responses [reviewed in Ref. (79)]. Several chemotherapeutic drugs can promote anti-tumor immunity by either inducing apoptosis of MDSCs or inducing their differentiation into mature myeloid cells with features of DCs or macrophages. 5-Fluorouracil (5-FU) and gemcitabine substantially reduce the numbers of MDSCs by induction of apoptosis (80, 81). In addition, both 5-FU and gemcitabine induce activation of NLRP3 in dying MDSCs following release of cathepsin B from lysosomes. Active NLRP3 triggers secretion of IL-1β, which may induce IL-17 production by T cells, resulting in priming of Th17 cells, neoangiogenesis, and promotion of tumor growth (82). As 5-FU and gemcitabine, however, do not induce ICD, the measured IL-1β concentrations appear to be low compared to the IL-1β secretion triggered by ICD-inducing chemotherapeutics (80). Importantly, at low concentrations, IL-1β does not support the priming of CD8$^+$ T cells and the detrimental effects of IL-1β prevail. Therefore, the therapeutic potential of 5-FU and gemcitabine treatment could be enhanced by co-administration of IL-1β inhibitors. Importantly, 5-FU-induced depletion of MDSCs acts synergistically with Treg depletion induced by low-dose cyclophosphamide treatment, enhancing T cell functions and anti-tumor responses (80). A similar selective depletion of MDSCs and subsequent enhancement of T cell immunity was seen during treatment with doxorubicin or 5-azacytidine (83, 84).

In contrast, non-toxic, low doses of paclitaxel stimulate the differentiation of MDSCs into functional DCs expressing MHCII and costimulatory molecules (85, 86). These functional DCs have lost their suppressive capacity and contribute to the induction of T cell responses. Similarly, docetaxel treatment polarizes MDSCs toward an M1 phenotype with loss of suppressive effects, higher levels of MHCII and CD80 expression, and a shift from IL-10 to IL-12 secretion (87).

Concluding Remarks

The cytotoxic agents that have been used for several decades for anti-cancer therapy were originally selected for their ability to kill tumor cells. Some, but not all, of these reagents are now known to stimulate anti-tumor immunity, which contributes to their therapeutic effect. A detailed characterization of the immune-stimulatory effects of currently used chemotherapeutic agents should guide the way for rational combinations with immunotherapeutic approaches, which should stimulate anti-tumor immune responses in a synergistic fashion. Cytotoxic agents that directly induce DC maturation or ICD are ideal candidates for combining with inhibitors of immune checkpoints such as PD-1 or CTLA-4, which may result in a long-lasting population of effector memory CD8$^+$ T cells (38, 39). In addition, the selective depletion of immune-inhibitory subsets, such as Tregs and MDSCs induced by chemotherapeutic agents, may complement active vaccination strategies and/or checkpoint blockade, by strengthening effector T cell populations (72, 73). The findings discussed here provide the basis for the further development of rational immunotherapeutic protocols in the near future.

Acknowledgments

This work was supported by the Wilhelm Sander-Stiftung für Krebsforschung, a SAKK/Amgen Research Grant, the Swiss National Science Foundation, the Krebsliga beider Basel, the Sassella-Stiftung, the Huggenberger-Bischoff Stiftung zur Krebsforschung, and the Freiwillige Akademische Gesellschaft Basel.

References

1. Shankaran V, Ikeda H, Bruce AT, White JM, Swanson PE, Old LJ, et al. IFNgamma and lymphocytes prevent primary tumour development and shape tumour immunogenicity. *Nature* (2001) **410**(6832):1107–11. doi:10.1038/35074122
2. Galon J, Pages F, Marincola FM, Thurin M, Trinchieri G, Fox BA, et al. The immune score as a new possible approach for the classification of cancer. *J Transl Med* (2012) **10**:1. doi:10.1186/1479-5876-10-1
3. Waitz R, Solomon SB, Petre EN, Trumble AE, Fasso M, Norton L, et al. Potent induction of tumor immunity by combining tumor cryoablation with anti-CTLA-4 therapy. *Cancer Res* (2012) **72**(2):430–9. doi:10.1158/0008-5472.CAN-11-1782
4. Sato E, Olson SH, Ahn J, Bundy B, Nishikawa H, Qian F, et al. Intraepithelial CD8+ tumor-infiltrating lymphocytes and a high CD8+/regulatory T cell ratio are associated with favorable prognosis in ovarian cancer. *Proc Natl Acad Sci U S A* (2005) **102**(51):18538–43. doi:10.1073/pnas.0509182102
5. Banchereau J, Briere F, Caux C, Davoust J, Lebecque S, Liu YJ, et al. Immunobiology of dendritic cells. *Annu Rev Immunol* (2000) **18**:767–811. doi:10.1146/annurev.immunol.18.1.767
6. Banchereau J, Steinman RM. Dendritic cells and the control of immunity. *Nature* (1998) **392**(6673):245–52. doi:10.1038/32588

7. Chen YT, Scanlan MJ, Sahin U, Tureci O, Gure AO, Tsang S, et al. A testicular antigen aberrantly expressed in human cancers detected by autologous antibody screening. *Proc Natl Acad Sci U S A* (1997) **94**(5):1914–8. doi:10.1073/pnas.94.5.1914
8. Linnemann C, van Buuren MM, Bies L, Verdegaal EM, Schotte R, Calis JJ, et al. High-throughput epitope discovery reveals frequent recognition of neo-antigens by CD4+ T cells in human melanoma. *Nat Med* (2015) **21**(1):81–5. doi:10.1038/nm.3773
9. Boesteanu AC, Katsikis PD. Memory T cells need CD28 costimulation to remember. *Semin Immunol* (2009) **21**(2):69–77. doi:10.1016/j.smim.2009.02.005
10. Bernard A, Lamy And L, Alberti I. The two-signal model of T cell activation after 30 years. *Transplantation* (2002) **73**(1 Suppl):S31–5. doi:10.1097/00007890-200201151-00011
11. Kaiko GE, Horvat JC, Beagley KW, Hansbro PM. Immunological decision-making: how does the immune system decide to mount a helper T cell response? *Immunology* (2008) **123**(3):326–38. doi:10.1111/j.1365-2567.2007.02719.x
12. Matzinger P. Tolerance, danger, and the extended family. *Annu Rev Immunol* (1994) **12**:991–1045. doi:10.1146/annurev.iy.12.040194.005015
13. Matzinger P. The danger model: a renewed sense of self. *Science* (2002) **296**(5566):301–5. doi:10.1126/science.1071059
14. Seya T, Shime H, Ebihara T, Oshiumi H, Matsumoto M. Pattern recognition receptors of innate immunity and their application to tumor immunotherapy. *Cancer Sci* (2010) **101**(2):313–20. doi:10.1111/j.1349-7006.2009.01442.x
15. Zeh HJ III, Lotze MT. Addicted to death: invasive cancer and the immune response to unscheduled cell death. *J Immunother* (2005) **28**(1):1–9. doi:10.1097/00002371-200501000-00001
16. Gabrilovich D. Mechanisms and functional significance of tumour-induced dendritic-cell defects. *Nat Rev Immunol* (2004) **4**(12):941–52. doi:10.1038/nri1498
17. Hargadon KM. Tumor-altered dendritic cell function: implications for anti-tumor immunity. *Front Immunol* (2013) **4**:192. doi:10.3389/fimmu.2013.00192
18. Lutz MB, Kurts C. Induction of peripheral CD4+ T cell tolerance and CD8+ T cell cross-tolerance by dendritic cells. *Eur J Immunol* (2009) **39**(9):2325–30. doi:10.1002/eji.200939548
19. Gimmi CD, Freeman GJ, Gribben JG, Gray G, Nadler LM. Human T cell clonal anergy is induced by antigen presentation in the absence of B7 costimulation. *Proc Natl Acad Sci U S A* (1993) **90**(14):6586–90. doi:10.1073/pnas.90.14.6586
20. Hoyne GF. Mechanisms that regulate peripheral immune responses to control organ-specific autoimmunity. *Clin Dev Immunol* (2011) **2011**:294968. doi:10.1155/2011/294968
21. Redmond WL, Marincek BC, Sherman LA. Distinct requirements for deletion versus anergy during CD8 T cell peripheral tolerance in vivo. *J Immunol* (2005) **174**(4):2046–53. doi:10.4049/jimmunol.174.4.2046
22. Lake RA, Robinson BW. Immunotherapy and chemotherapy – a practical partnership. *Nat Rev Cancer* (2005) **5**(5):397–405. doi:10.1038/nrc1613
23. Menard C, Martin F, Apetoh L, Bouyer F, Ghiringhelli F. Cancer chemotherapy: not only a direct cytotoxic effect, but also an adjuvant for antitumor immunity. *Cancer Immunol Immunother* (2008) **57**(11):1579–87. doi:10.1007/s00262-008-0505-6
24. Zitvogel L, Apetoh L, Ghiringhelli F, Kroemer G. Immunological aspects of cancer chemotherapy. *Nat Rev Immunol* (2008) **8**(1):59–73. doi:10.1038/nri2216
25. Bracci L, Schiavoni G, Sistigu A, Belardelli F. Immune-based mechanisms of cytotoxic chemotherapy: implications for the design of novel and rationale-based combined treatments against cancer. *Cell Death Differ* (2014) **21**(1):15–25. doi:10.1038/cdd.2013.67
26. Vanneman M, Dranoff G. Combining immunotherapy and targeted therapies in cancer treatment. *Nat Rev Cancer* (2012) **12**(4):237–51. doi:10.1038/nrc3237
27. Litterman AJ, Zellmer DM, Grinnen KL, Hunt MA, Dudek AZ, Salazar AM, et al. Profound impairment of adaptive immune responses by alkylating chemotherapy. *J Immunol* (2013) **190**(12):6259–68. doi:10.4049/jimmunol.1203539
28. Kang DH, Weaver MT, Park NJ, Smith B, McArdle T, Carpenter J. Significant impairment in immune recovery after cancer treatment. *Nurs Res* (2009) **58**(2):105–14. doi:10.1097/NNR.0b013e31818fcecd
29. Melief CJ. Cancer immunotherapy by dendritic cells. *Immunity* (2008) **29**(3):372–83. doi:10.1016/j.immuni.2008.08.004
30. Trojandt S, Knies D, Pektor S, Ritz S, Mailander V, Grabbe S, et al. The chemotherapeutic agent topotecan differentially modulates the phenotype and function of dendritic cells. *Cancer Immunol Immunother* (2013) **62**(8):1315–26. doi:10.1007/s00262-013-1431-9
31. Hu J, Kinn J, Zirakzadeh AA, Sherif A, Norstedt G, Wikstrom AC, et al. The effects of chemotherapeutic drugs on human monocyte-derived dendritic cell differentiation and antigen presentation. *Clin Exp Immunol* (2013) **172**(3):490–9. doi:10.1111/cei.12060
32. Liu WM, Scott KA, Thompson M, Dalgleish AG. Dendritic cell phenotype can be improved by certain chemotherapies and is associated with alterations to p21(waf1/cip1.). *Cancer Immunol Immunother* (2013) **62**(10):1553–61. doi:10.1007/s00262-013-1456-0
33. Tanaka H, Matsushima H, Mizumoto N, Takashima A. Classification of chemotherapeutic agents based on their differential in vitro effects on dendritic cells. *Cancer Res* (2009) **69**(17):6978–86. doi:10.1158/0008-5472.CAN-09-1101
34. Fontana MF, Vance RE. Two signal models in innate immunity. *Immunol Rev* (2011) **243**(1):26–39. doi:10.1111/j.1600-065X.2011.01037.x
35. Ferrua B, Manie S, Doglio A, Shaw A, Sonthonnax S, Limouse M, et al. Stimulation of human interleukin 1 production and specific mRNA expression by microtubule-disrupting drugs. *Cell Immunol* (1990) **131**(2):391–7. doi:10.1016/0008-8749(90)90263-Q
36. Mizumoto N, Tanaka H, Matsushima H, Vishwanath M, Takashima A. Colchicine promotes antigen cross-presentation by murine dendritic cells. *J Invest Dermatol* (2007) **127**(6):1543–6. doi:10.1038/sj.jid.5700699
37. Tanaka H, Matsushima H, Nishibu A, Clausen BE, Takashima A. Dual therapeutic efficacy of vinblastine as a unique chemotherapeutic agent capable of inducing dendritic cell maturation. *Cancer Res* (2009) **69**(17):6987–94. doi:10.1158/0008-5472.CAN-09-1106
38. Martin K, Muller P, Schreiner J, Prince SS, Lardinois D, Heinzelmann-Schwarz VA, et al. The microtubule-depolymerizing agent ansamitocin P3 programs dendritic cells toward enhanced anti-tumor immunity. *Cancer Immunol Immunother* (2014) **63**(9):925–38. doi:10.1007/s00262-014-1565-4
39. Muller P, Martin K, Theurich S, Schreiner J, Savic S, Terszowski G, et al. Microtubule-depolymerizing agents used in antibody-drug conjugates induce antitumor immunity by stimulation of dendritic cells. *Cancer Immunol Res* (2014) **2**(8):741–55. doi:10.1158/2326-6066.CIR-13-0198
40. Muller P, Martin K, Theurich S, von Bergwelt-Baildon M, Zippelius A. Cancer chemotherapy agents target intratumoral dendritic cells to potentiate antitumor immunity. *Oncoimmunology* (2014) **3**(8):e954460. doi:10.4161/21624011.2014.954460
41. Shurin GV, Tourkova IL, Kaneno R, Shurin MR. Chemotherapeutic agents in noncytotoxic concentrations increase antigen presentation by dendritic cells via an IL-12-dependent mechanism. *J Immunol* (2009) **183**(1):137–44. doi:10.4049/jimmunol.0900734
42. Kaneno R, Shurin GV, Tourkova IL, Shurin MR. Chemomodulation of human dendritic cell function by antineoplastic agents in low noncytotoxic concentrations. *J Transl Med* (2009) **7**:58. doi:10.1186/1479-5876-7-58
43. Pfannenstiel LW, Lam SS, Emens LA, Jaffee EM, Armstrong TD. Paclitaxel enhances early dendritic cell maturation and function through TLR4 signaling in mice. *Cell Immunol* (2010) **263**(1):79–87. doi:10.1016/j.cellimm.2010.03.001
44. Marin-Esteban V, Charron D, Gelin C, Mooney N. Chemotherapeutic agents targeting the tubulin cytoskeleton modify LPS-induced cytokine secretion by dendritic cells and increase antigen presentation. *J Immunother* (2010) **33**(4):364–70. doi:10.1097/CJI.0b013e3181cd1094
45. Javeed A, Ashraf M, Riaz A, Ghafoor A, Afzal S, Mukhtar MM. Paclitaxel and immune system. *Eur J Pharm Sci* (2009) **38**(4):283–90. doi:10.1016/j.ejps.2009.08.009
46. Mullard A. Maturing antibody-drug conjugate pipeline hits 30. *Nat Rev Drug Discov* (2013) **12**(5):329–32. doi:10.1038/nrd4009
47. Kovtun YV, Goldmacher VS. Cell killing by antibody-drug conjugates. *Cancer Lett* (2007) **255**(2):232–40. doi:10.1016/j.canlet.2007.04.010
48. Theurich S, Malcher J, Wennhold K, Shimabukuro-Vornhagen A, Chemnitz J, Holtick U, et al. Brentuximab vedotin combined with donor lymphocyte infusions for early relapse of Hodgkin lymphoma after allogeneic stem-cell transplantation induces tumor-specific immunity and sustained clinical remission. *J Clin Oncol* (2013) **31**(5):e59–63. doi:10.1200/JCO.2012.43.6832

49. Theurich S, Wennhold K, Wedemeyer I, Rothe A, Hubel K, Shimabukuro-Vornhagen A, et al. CD30-targeted therapy with brentuximab vedotin and DLI in a patient with T cell posttransplantation lymphoma: induction of clinical remission and cellular immunity. *Transplantation* (2013) **96**(3):e16–8. doi:10.1097/TP.0b013e31829a9258
50. Obeid M, Tesniere A, Ghiringhelli F, Fimia GM, Apetoh L, Perfettini JL, et al. Calreticulin exposure dictates the immunogenicity of cancer cell death. *Nat Med* (2007) **13**(1):54–61. doi:10.1038/nm1523
51. Tesniere A, Schlemmer F, Boige V, Kepp O, Martins I, Ghiringhelli F, et al. Immunogenic death of colon cancer cells treated with oxaliplatin. *Oncogene* (2010) **29**(4):482–91. doi:10.1038/onc.2009.356
52. Schiavoni G, Sistigu A, Valentini M, Mattei F, Sestili P, Spadaro F, et al. Cyclophosphamide synergizes with type I interferons through systemic dendritic cell reactivation and induction of immunogenic tumor apoptosis. *Cancer Res* (2011) **71**(3):768–78. doi:10.1158/0008-5472.CAN-10-2788
53. Michaud M, Martins I, Sukkurwala AQ, Adjemian S, Ma Y, Pellegatti P, et al. Autophagy-dependent anticancer immune responses induced by chemotherapeutic agents in mice. *Science* (2011) **334**(6062):1573–7. doi:10.1126/science.1208347
54. Panaretakis T, Kepp O, Brockmeier U, Tesniere A, Bjorklund AC, Chapman DC, et al. Mechanisms of pre-apoptotic calreticulin exposure in immunogenic cell death. *EMBO J* (2009) **28**(5):578–90. doi:10.1038/emboj.2009.1
55. Ma Y, Adjemian S, Mattarollo SR, Yamazaki T, Aymeric L, Yang H, et al. Anticancer chemotherapy-induced intratumoral recruitment and differentiation of antigen-presenting cells. *Immunity* (2013) **38**(4):729–41. doi:10.1016/j.immuni.2013.03.003
56. Apetoh L, Ghiringhelli F, Tesniere A, Obeid M, Ortiz C, Criollo A, et al. Toll-like receptor 4-dependent contribution of the immune system to anticancer chemotherapy and radiotherapy. *Nat Med* (2007) **13**(9):1050–9. doi:10.1038/nm1622
57. Gardai SJ, McPhillips KA, Frasch SC, Janssen WJ, Starefeldt A, Murphy-Ullrich JE, et al. Cell-surface calreticulin initiates clearance of viable or apoptotic cells through trans-activation of LRP on the phagocyte. *Cell* (2005) **123**(2):321–34. doi:10.1016/j.cell.2005.08.032
58. Pawaria S, Binder RJ. CD91-dependent programming of T-helper cell responses following heat shock protein immunization. *Nat Commun* (2011) **2**:521. doi:10.1038/ncomms1524
59. Martins I, Wang Y, Michaud M, Ma Y, Sukkurwala AQ, Shen S, et al. Molecular mechanisms of ATP secretion during immunogenic cell death. *Cell Death Differ* (2014) **21**(1):79–91. doi:10.1038/cdd.2013.75
60. Ghiringhelli F, Apetoh L, Tesniere A, Aymeric L, Ma Y, Ortiz C, et al. Activation of the NLRP3 inflammasome in dendritic cells induces IL-1beta-dependent adaptive immunity against tumors. *Nat Med* (2009) **15**(10):1170–8. doi:10.1038/nm.2028
61. Scaffidi P, Misteli T, Bianchi ME. Release of chromatin protein HMGB1 by necrotic cells triggers inflammation. *Nature* (2002) **418**(6894):191–5. doi:10.1038/nature00858
62. Shiratsuchi A, Watanabe I, Takeuchi O, Akira S, Nakanishi Y. Inhibitory effect of Toll-like receptor 4 on fusion between phagosomes and endosomes/lysosomes in macrophages. *J Immunol* (2004) **172**(4):2039–47. doi:10.4049/jimmunol.172.4.2039
63. Suzuki Y, Mimura K, Yoshimoto Y, Watanabe M, Ohkubo Y, Izawa S, et al. Immunogenic tumor cell death induced by chemoradiotherapy in patients with esophageal squamous cell carcinoma. *Cancer Res* (2012) **72**(16):3967–76. doi:10.1158/0008-5472.CAN-12-0851
64. Chiba S, Baghdadi M, Akiba H, Yoshiyama H, Kinoshita I, Dosaka-Akita H, et al. Tumor-infiltrating DCs suppress nucleic acid-mediated innate immune responses through interactions between the receptor TIM-3 and the alarmin HMGB1. *Nat Immunol* (2012) **13**(9):832–42. doi:10.1038/ni.2376
65. Vignali DA, Collison LW, Workman CJ. How regulatory T cells work. *Nat Rev Immunol* (2008) **8**(7):523–32. doi:10.1038/nri2343
66. Onishi Y, Fehervari Z, Yamaguchi T, Sakaguchi S. Foxp3+ natural regulatory T cells preferentially form aggregates on dendritic cells in vitro and actively inhibit their maturation. *Proc Natl Acad Sci U S A* (2008) **105**(29):10113–8. doi:10.1073/pnas.0711106105
67. Grohmann U, Orabona C, Fallarino F, Vacca C, Calcinaro F, Falorni A, et al. CTLA-4-Ig regulates tryptophan catabolism in vivo. *Nat Immunol* (2002) **3**(11):1097–101. doi:10.1038/ni846
68. Ghiringhelli F, Menard C, Terme M, Flament C, Taieb J, Chaput N, et al. CD4+CD25+ regulatory T cells inhibit natural killer cell functions in a transforming growth factor-beta-dependent manner. *J Exp Med* (2005) **202**(8):1075–85. doi:10.1084/jem.20051511
69. Lutsiak ME, Semnani RT, De Pascalis R, Kashmiri SV, Schlom J, Sabzevari H. Inhibition of CD4(+)25+ T regulatory cell function implicated in enhanced immune response by low-dose cyclophosphamide. *Blood* (2005) **105**(7):2862–8. doi:10.1182/blood-2004-06-2410
70. Ghiringhelli F, Menard C, Puig PE, Ladoire S, Roux S, Martin F, et al. Metronomic cyclophosphamide regimen selectively depletes CD4+CD25+ regulatory T cells and restores T and NK effector functions in end stage cancer patients. *Cancer Immunol Immunother* (2007) **56**(5):641–8. doi:10.1007/s00262-006-0225-8
71. Ge Y, Domschke C, Stoiber N, Schott S, Heil J, Rom J, et al. Metronomic cyclophosphamide treatment in metastasized breast cancer patients: immunological effects and clinical outcome. *Cancer Immunol Immunother* (2012) **61**(3):353–62. doi:10.1007/s00262-011-1106-3
72. Taieb J, Chaput N, Schartz N, Roux S, Novault S, Menard C, et al. Chemoimmunotherapy of tumors: cyclophosphamide synergizes with exosome based vaccines. *J Immunol* (2006) **176**(5):2722–9. doi:10.4049/jimmunol.176.5.2722
73. Cerullo V, Diaconu I, Kangasniemi L, Rajecki M, Escutenaire S, Koski A, et al. Immunological effects of low-dose cyclophosphamide in cancer patients treated with oncolytic adenovirus. *Mol Ther* (2011) **19**(9):1737–46. doi:10.1038/mt.2011.113
74. Schoenberger SP, Toes RE, van der Voort EI, Offringa R, Melief CJ. T cell help for cytotoxic T lymphocytes is mediated by CD40-CD40L interactions. *Nature* (1998) **393**(6684):480–3. doi:10.1038/31002
75. Ridge JP, Di Rosa F, Matzinger P. A conditioned dendritic cell can be a temporal bridge between a CD4+ T-helper and a T-killer cell. *Nature* (1998) **393**(6684):474–8. doi:10.1038/30989
76. Zhang L, Dermawan K, Jin M, Liu R, Zheng H, Xu L, et al. Differential impairment of regulatory T cells rather than effector T cells by paclitaxel-based chemotherapy. *Clin Immunol* (2008) **129**(2):219–29. doi:10.1016/j.clim.2008.07.013
77. Ridolfi L, Petrini M, Granato AM, Gentilcore G, Simeone E, Ascierto PA, et al. Low-dose temozolomide before dendritic-cell vaccination reduces (specifically) CD4+CD25++Foxp3+ regulatory T cells in advanced melanoma patients. *J Transl Med* (2013) **11**:135. doi:10.1186/1479-5876-11-135
78. Banissi C, Ghiringhelli F, Chen L, Carpentier AF. Treg depletion with a low-dose metronomic temozolomide regimen in a rat glioma model. *Cancer Immunol Immunother* (2009) **58**(10):1627–34. doi:10.1007/s00262-009-0671-1
79. Gabrilovich DI, Nagaraj S. Myeloid-derived suppressor cells as regulators of the immune system. *Nat Rev Immunol* (2009) **9**(3):162–74. doi:10.1038/nri2506
80. Vincent J, Mignot G, Chalmin F, Ladoire S, Bruchard M, Chevriaux A, et al. 5-Fluorouracil selectively kills tumor-associated myeloid-derived suppressor cells resulting in enhanced T cell-dependent antitumor immunity. *Cancer Res* (2010) **70**(8):3052–61. doi:10.1158/0008-5472.CAN-09-3690
81. Suzuki E, Kapoor V, Jassar AS, Kaiser LR, Albelda SM. Gemcitabine selectively eliminates splenic Gr-1+/CD11b+ myeloid suppressor cells in tumor-bearing animals and enhances antitumor immune activity. *Clin Cancer Res* (2005) **11**(18):6713–21. doi:10.1158/1078-0432.CCR-05-0883
82. Bruchard M, Mignot G, Derangere V, Chalmin F, Chevriaux A, Vegran F, et al. Chemotherapy-triggered cathepsin B release in myeloid-derived suppressor cells activates the Nlrp3 inflammasome and promotes tumor growth. *Nat Med* (2013) **19**(1):57–64. doi:10.1038/nm.2999
83. Alizadeh D, Trad M, Hanke NT, Larmonier CB, Janikashvili N, Bonnotte B, et al. Doxorubicin eliminates myeloid-derived suppressor cells and enhances the efficacy of adoptive T cell transfer in breast cancer. *Cancer Res* (2014) **74**(1):104–18. doi:10.1158/0008-5472.CAN-13-1545
84. Mikyskova R, Indrova M, Vlkova V, Bieblova J, Simova J, Parackova Z, et al. DNA demethylating agent 5-azacytidine inhibits myeloid-derived suppressor cells induced by tumor growth and cyclophosphamide treatment. *J Leukoc Biol* (2014) **95**(5):743–53. doi:10.1189/jlb.0813435
85. Michels T, Shurin GV, Naiditch H, Sevko A, Umansky V, Shurin MR. Paclitaxel promotes differentiation of myeloid-derived suppressor cells into dendritic

cells in vitro in a TLR4-independent manner. *J Immunotoxicol* (2012) **9**(3):292–300. doi:10.3109/1547691X.2011.642418
86. Sevko A, Michels T, Vrohlings M, Umansky L, Beckhove P, Kato M, et al. Antitumor effect of paclitaxel is mediated by inhibition of myeloid-derived suppressor cells and chronic inflammation in the spontaneous melanoma model. *J Immunol* (2013) **190**(5):2464–71. doi:10.4049/jimmunol.1202781
87. Kodumudi KN, Woan K, Gilvary DL, Sahakian E, Wei S, Djeu JY. A novel chemoimmunomodulating property of docetaxel: suppression of myeloid-derived suppressor cells in tumor bearers. *Clin Cancer Res* (2010) **16**(18):4583–94. doi:10.1158/1078-0432.CCR-10-0733

19

Functional specialization of skin dendritic cell subsets in regulating T cell responses

Björn E. Clausen[1] and Patrizia Stoitzner[2]**

[1] Institute for Molecular Medicine, University Medical Center of the Johannes Gutenberg-University Mainz, Mainz, Germany,
[2] Department of Dermatology and Venereology, Division of Experimental Dermatology, Medical University of Innsbruck, Innsbruck, Austria

Edited by:
Stefan F. Martin,
University of Freiburg, Germany

Reviewed by:
Miriam Wittmann,
University of Leeds, UK
Susan Kovats,
Oklahoma Medical Research Foundation, USA

***Correspondence:**
Björn E. Clausen
bclausen@uni-mainz.de;
Patrizia Stoitzner
patrizia.stoitzner@i-med.ac.at

Dendritic cells (DC) are a heterogeneous family of professional antigen-presenting cells classically recognized as most potent inducers of adaptive immune responses. In this respect, Langerhans cells have long been considered to be prototypic immunogenic DC in the skin. More recently this view has considerably changed. The generation of *in vivo* cell ablation and lineage tracing models revealed the complexity of the skin DC network and, in particular, established the existence of a number of phenotypically distinct Langerin$^+$ and negative DC populations in the dermis. Moreover, by now we appreciate that DC also exert important regulatory functions and are required for the maintenance of tolerance toward harmless foreign and self-antigens. This review summarizes our current understanding of the skin-resident DC system in the mouse and discusses emerging concepts on the functional specialization of the different skin DC subsets in regulating T cell responses. Special consideration is given to antigen cross-presentation as well as immune reactions toward contact sensitizers, cutaneous pathogens, and tumors. These studies form the basis for the manipulation of the human counterparts of the murine DC subsets to promote immunity or tolerance for the treatment of human disease.

Keywords: contact hypersensitivity, cross-presentation, dendritic cells, immunotherapy, infectious skin disease, Langerhans cells, Langerin, skin cancer

INTRODUCTION

The skin is the second largest barrier organ to the outside world besides the intestine. As such it is not only exposed to physical stress but also to a wide variety of environmental antigens, including chemicals, commensal bacteria, and pathogens. Hence, the skin immune system must be prepared to detect and discriminate between these diverse antigens and subsequently induce appropriate tolerogenic or protective immune responses. To this aim, the skin contains a heterogeneous population of dendritic cells (DC, from Greek *dendron* "tree") that represent key regulators of both innate and adaptive immune responses. While skin DC play a critical role in guarding the host against invading pathogens and at the same time limiting collateral tissue damage, they are also associated with the breakdown of peripheral tolerance leading to chronic immune-mediated inflammatory diseases such as allergic contact dermatitis and psoriasis. As essential mediators of cutaneous immune reactions and homeostasis, considerable work has been focused to unravel the origins, phenotypic, and functional differences of the cells of the skin DC network (1–3).

Anatomically, the skin can be divided into an outer epidermis and the underlying dermis, which are separated by a basement membrane. The cell-free basement membrane acts as a mechanical barrier, however, its primary function is to anchor the epithelium (epidermis) to the loose connective tissue (dermis) underneath. The epidermis represents a stratified epithelial layer composed of keratinocytes that generate the water-impermeable *stratum corneum*. The dermis is a cell-poor layer consisting of fibroblasts that produce the extracellular matrix containing proteoglycans and entwined collagen and elastic fibers. Together they enable the skin to resist stretching and tearing forces. In addition to forming the primary physical barrier, keratinocytes also actively contribute to the immunological barrier of the skin. They are equipped with most toll-like receptors (TLR), except TLR7 and TLR8 (4–6). Following TLR triggering and NOD-like receptor (NLR)-mediated inflammasome activation, keratinocytes secrete antimicrobial peptides and many proinflammatory cytokines as well as chemokines for the recruitment of neutrophils. Thereby keratinocytes participate in adaptive immune activation, via inducing DC mobilization and migration to skin-draining lymph nodes (LN), and innate immune modulation (7).

DC can be subdivided into conventional DC and plasmacytoid DC (pDC). Healthy skin contains no or very few pDC (8, 9); they only enter inflamed skin to promote wound healing through type-I interferons (9) or mediate the proinflammatory reaction that develops after TLR7 stimulation, for example, during psoriasis (10). An excellent overview of pDC biology and plasticity has recently been published elsewhere and these cells are not further discussed here (11).

In the steady state, the conventional DC residing in the skin are not inactive. Rather as immature cells, they constantly probe their environment for invading pathogens and continuously sample self- and environmental antigens (**Figure 1**). To this aim, epidermal Langerhans cells (LC) exhibit a unique behavior characterized by rhythmic extension and retraction of their dendrites through intercellular spaces between keratinocytes, which is amplified during inflammation (12). In fact, LC can extend dendrites through tight junctions to survey the skin surface and elicit humoral immunity to antigens that have not yet violated the epidermal barrier, providing preemptive immunity against potentially pathogenic skin microbes (13).

A small fraction of LC and dermal DC undergoes spontaneous maturation through a mechanism that is not yet understood (14). This *homeostatic* or *phenotypic maturation* involves the upregulation of chemokine receptor CCR7, which enables DC migration to the skin-draining LN (15), and in the case of LC downregulation of E-cadherin to detach themselves from the surrounding keratinocytes (16). Moreover, disruption of E-cadherin binding may actively promote a tolerogenic LC phenotype via the release and nuclear localization of β-catenin (17, 18). During their migration to the T cell areas of local LN, the cells upregulate surface expression of MHC/peptide complexes for recognition of and interaction with antigen-specific naïve T cells (**Figure 1**) (19–22). Upon encounter with potentially autoreactive T cells that have escaped central tolerance or with T cells recognizing peptides derived from innocuous foreign antigens, these DC induce T cell anergy or deletional T cell tolerance (*tolerizing function*) (23–26). In addition, the frequent T cell–DC contacts during T cell scanning of DC in lymphoid organs, i.e., in the absence of cognate antigen, induce a basal activation level in T cells required for rapid responsiveness to subsequent encounters with foreign antigen during inflammation (27).

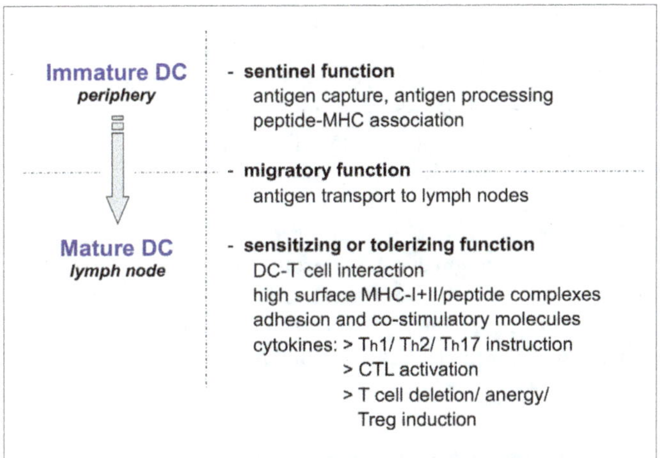

FIGURE 1 | The Langerhans cell paradigm: Ralph Steinman's scheme of key dendritic cell functions. DC, including epidermal LC, exist in two phenotypically and functionally distinct states: as immature cells highly specialized in antigen uptake and processing and as mature cells committed to antigen presentation that activate or tolerize naïve T cells. The two functional programs are connected by DC migration from peripheral tissues to draining LN, which is essential for naïve T cells to encounter their cognate antigen.

Pathogen invasion together with proinflammatory signals drive the full *functional maturation* of skin DC. Beyond the homeostatic differentiation program, the cells now also upregulate the expression of costimulatory molecules and, in particular, proinflammatory cytokines. Together these promote clonal expansion of naïve antigen-specific T cells and instruct the T cells to acquire appropriate effector functions specifically tailored to eliminate the invading pathogen (*sensitizing function*) (**Figure 1**) (19).

In this review, we describe our current understanding of the composition of the skin DC network and summarize the transcription and growth factor requirements for the development of the different skin DC populations. We then discuss the functional specialization of skin DC subsets in the context of allergic and infectious skin disease models, as well as their cross-presentation capacity and their role in skin cancer. Finally, we focus on how this knowledge may be applied to harness skin DC for therapeutic purposes and, to this aim, conclude with a comparison of mouse and human skin DC subsets.

THE SKIN-RESIDENT DENDRITIC CELL NETWORK

After the discovery of DC by Ralph Steinman and Zanvil Cohn in 1973 (28), it was only in 1985 that epidermal LC (**Figure 2**), first described by Paul Langerhans as "*Nerven der menschlichen Haut*" more than a century before (29), were unequivocally placed into the DC family (30, 31). One of the most important findings of these early studies on LC was that DC exist in two phenotypically and functionally distinct states: as immature cells that are highly phagocytic and specialized to take up and process antigen, and as mature cells dedicated to identify and stimulate rare antigen-specific naïve T cells in secondary lymphoid organs (**Figure 1**). This observation is directly linked to another unique function of DC, namely, their migration via afferent lymphatics into the T cell areas of secondary lymphoid organs (19). In fact, in early mixed lymphocyte reaction (MLR) experiments DC turned out to be about 100-fold more efficient at inducing naive T cell proliferation than macrophages (32–34), which also do not travel from peripheral tissues to local LN (35). Owing to their easy accessibility and a large body of *in vitro* work, which almost inevitably triggers LC functional maturation, much of what we know today about the role of DC as most potent inducers of T cell immune responses stems from studying LC biology. Hence, for a long time LC were considered prototypic immunogenic DC for which Wilson and Villadangos later coined the term "*LC paradigm*" (36) and dermal DC were largely overlooked.

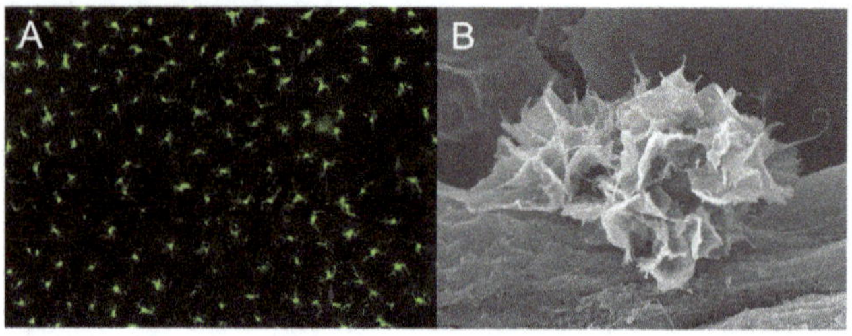

FIGURE 2 | Langerhans cells: sentinels of the skin. **(A)** LC network visualized in an epidermal sheet of mouse ear skin with MHC-II antibody staining (green fluorescence) (37). Photograph by courtesy of Julia Ober-Blöbaum and Björn Clausen. **(B)** Scanning electron microscopy of a LC sitting on a keratinocyte (38). Photograph by courtesy of Kristian Pfaller and Patrizia Stoitzner.

This picture began to change dramatically with the identification of Langerin (CD207), a novel C-type lectin specific to LC (39–41) and the generation of anti-Langerin monoclonal antibodies (42, 43). Although originally described as a LC-specific marker, in combination with constitutive and inducible Langerin$^+$ cell depletion models and a Langerin-EGFP knock-in allele (44–46), this led to the discovery of a small Langerin$^+$ dermal DC subset that is ontogenetically and phenotypically distinct of epidermal LC (47–49). Largely owing to the comprehensive analysis of the Malissen lab to disentangle the complexity of the skin DC network, we can currently distinguish five distinct DC subsets in healthy mouse skin (**Figure 3**) (50, 51). All of these DC populations express CD11c and MHC class II (MHC-II). (*i*) LC in the epidermis as well as in the dermis – en route to skin-draining LN – can be identified as Langerin$^+$CD11b$^+$EpCam$^+$Sirpα^+ cells, and distinguished from CD11b$^+$Sirpα^+ dermal DC by their absence of Langerin and EpCam staining. (*ii*) CD11b$^+$ DC are the most abundant subset and comprise about 65% of all dermal DC (51). (*iii* and *iv*) Langerin$^+$CD11b^{neg} dermal DC, on the other hand, are unambiguously recognized by expression of the chemokine receptor XCR1, lack EpCam and Sirp1α, and can be further divided into a CD103$^+$ and negative subset. Expression of XCR1 is shared by all CD11b^{neg} non-lymphoid and CD8α^+

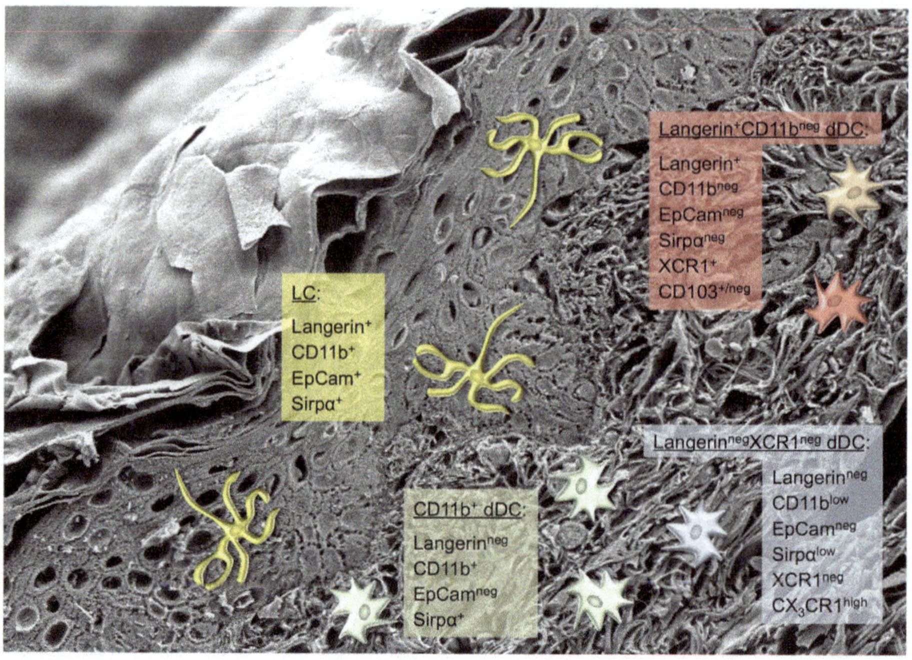

FIGURE 3 | Skin dendritic cell subsets in mice. Scanning electron microscopy picture of a skin section depicting several layers of keratinocytes and the collagen meshwork of the dermis (38). Photograph by courtesy of Kristian Pfaller and Patrizia Stoitzner. Phenotypically distinct murine skin-resident DC subsets are depicted, including the most commonly used markers for their identification. The color code matches the human counterparts shown in **Figure 4**.

lymphoid tissue DC, respectively, but only XCR1$^+$CD11b^{neg} DC in the dermis co-express Langerin (52, 53). Of note, in the skin surface expression of CD24 correlates with that of Langerin and can be used for the purification of viable LC and Langerin$^+$ dermal DC by flow cytometry. (*v*) Finally, the dermis harbors a minor population of Langerin^{neg}XCR1^{neg} double-negative DC that express low levels of CD11b and Sirpα, and are uniquely CX$_3$CR1^{high} (51). These five conventional skin DC populations can be separated from dermal macrophages and monocyte-derived DC by the use of CD64 (35). In particular during inflammation, large numbers of monocytes infiltrate the skin where they differentiate into CD11b$^+$Ly6C$^+$CD64$^+$ monocyte-derived DC that have very low or lack CD11c expression. These recently identified cells play a role mainly in activating skin-resident T cells and disappear after resolution of the inflammation (35). The functional specialization of LC and the different dermal DC populations that are present in mouse skin will be discussed below.

ORIGIN, TRANSCRIPTION FACTOR, AND SURVIVAL FACTOR REQUIREMENTS OF SKIN DENDRITIC CELL POPULATIONS

LC are radio-resistant cells that reside in the supra-basal layer of the epidermis, closely attached to the surrounding keratinocytes via E-cadherin containing adherens junctions. In the steady state, LC exhibit a low rate of proliferation that – unlike dermal DC – is sufficient to maintain the cells locally throughout life as has been demonstrated by parabiosis experiments in mice (54) and could also be observed in human skin of hand transplant patients (55). Only in response to inflammatory changes leading to an increased loss from the epidermis are LC replaced by blood-borne progenitors. These precursors were recruited in a CCR2-dependent way and identified to represent Ly6C^{high} monocytes that enter inflamed skin and differentiate into LC in the epidermis (56, 57). Whether these monocyte-derived LC are functionally similar and equally capable to maintain themselves *in situ* remains elusive. Recent experiments indicate that the initial wave of monocyte-derived LC reconstitution after UV radiation and contact sensitizer exposure generates only short-term LC that are transient and replaced by a second wave of steady-state precursor-derived long-term LC (58, 59). On the other hand, all dermal DC populations in healthy skin are radiosensitive, have a short lifespan, and are continuously replaced by a circulating pool of bone marrow-derived DC precursors (60).

In contrast to dermal DC that originate from DC-restricted progenitors [reviewed in Ref. (2, 60)], during ontogeny LC arise first from yolk sac-derived primitive myeloid precursors around embryonic day 18 that are largely replaced by fetal liver-derived monocytes during late embryogenesis (61). These LC precursors then acquire a DC morphology and phenotype, including CD11c and MHC-II expression immediately after birth (62), whereas Langerin expression becomes apparent only 2–3 days after birth and reaches adult levels of intensity only by 3 weeks of age (63). Moreover, between postnatal days 2 and 7 the LC undergo a massive proliferative burst (62), before reaching a typical density of about 700–1,000 LC/mm^2 in the epidermis of adult mice (37) (**Figure 2**). Intriguingly, LC share this embryonic ancestry from myeloid precursors and the capacity of self-maintenance throughout life without any input from the bone marrow with brain microglia. While macrophage colony-stimulating factor 1 (M-CSF or CSF-1) is essential for the development of most tissue macrophages and partly for CD11b$^+$ dermal DC (64), CSF-1R-deficient mice in addition lack both LC and microglia. Their development requires the presence of the alternative CSF-1R ligand IL-34 that is constitutively produced by keratinocytes and neurons (65, 66). Based on this unique life cycle and the shared pedigree with certain tissue macrophages, LC have recently been grouped into the same lineage as macrophages (67, 68). Although ontogenetically LC and macrophages are closely related cells, in stark contrast to the sessile tissue macrophages LC migrate to LN where they prime naïve T cells to induce regulatory or effector responses. Since migration and naïve T cell priming represent cardinal features characterizing conventional DC (**Figure 1**), we strongly favor to keep LC in the DC family. Reciprocally, from a semantic point of view it has to be stressed that the term "macrophage" (from Greek *makrós* "large, big" and *phagein* "eat" = "big eaters") describes a function for which DC are certainly not specialized as has been worked out so beautifully by Ralph Steinman (69–71).

Another cytokine that has been known for a long time to be essential for LC differentiation is transforming growth factor-β1 (TGF-β1) (72). Although TGF-β1 is produced by both LC and keratinocytes, LC promote their own development through an autocrine loop of TGF-β1 secretion and signaling (73). In addition, TGF-β1 is required to maintain the network of immature LC in the epidermis (74, 75). In line with the critical role of TGF-β1 for LC development, mice lacking the TGF-β1-induced transcription factor inhibitor of DNA binding 2 (Id2), or the transcription factor Runx3 that mediates DC responses to TGF-β1 both also lack LC (76–78). Moreover, Id2$^{-/-}$ mice have dramatically reduced numbers of lymphoid organ CD8$^+$ and non-lymphoid tissue CD103$^+$ DC (64).

The cytokine Flt3L is a key mediator of DC commitment during hematopoiesis (79) and injection of Flt3L into mice dramatically increased DC numbers in various tissues (80). Beyond its role in DC differentiation, Flt3L regulates the homeostatic proliferation of DC to maintain peripheral DC numbers in the steady state (81). With respect to skin DC subsets, LC are not affected by the absence of Flt3 or its ligand, whereas dermal DC were reduced in Flt3$^{-/-}$ and Flt3L$^{-/-}$ mice (64, 82). Granulocyte/macrophage colony-stimulating factor (GM-CSF or CSF-2) is essential for DC differentiation (83), and mice lacking either CSF-2 or its receptor display a reduction of LC and CD103$^+$ dermal DC (84, 85). In the absence of macrophage colony-stimulating factor (M-CSF or CSF-1), LC numbers were halved (86), and mice that lack the M-CSF receptor (CSF-1R) have no LC and reduced CD11b$^+$ dermal DC, while CD103$^+$ dermal DC develop normally (56, 64).

Moreover, a number of interferon regulatory factors (IRF) and other transcription factors have been implicated in the development of different DC subsets, albeit with incomplete available information concerning their effects on LC and dermal DC. IRF2-deficient mice exhibit reduced numbers of splenic $CD4^+$ DC and epidermal LC, while dermal DC subsets have not been assessed (87); $IRF4^{-/-}$ mice harbor reduced numbers of splenic $CD4^+$ DC and of migratory LN DC due to a defect in dermal DC migration, which leads to an accumulation of $CD103^+$ and $CD11b^+$ dermal DC in the skin (88–90); and $IRF8^{-/-}$ mice lack splenic $CD8^+$ DC and non-lymphoid tissue $CD103^+$ DC, including $CD103^+$ dermal DC, whereas LC are unaffected (64, 76, 91–93). In addition, IRF8 also contributes to DC function: IRF8 controls $CD8^+$ DC maturation and IL-12 production (94), antigen uptake and MHC-II presentation (95), the migration of LC and dermal DC to local LN (96), and the tolerogenic function of DC by inducing the expression of indoleamine 2,3-dioxygenase (IDO) (97). Although the basic leucine zipper transcription factor ATF-like 3 (Batf3) is expressed in all conventional DC, including $CD11b^+$ DC, $Batf3^{-/-}$ mice reveal a selective deficiency of $CD8^+$ and $CD103^+$ DC, however, the penetrance of the $CD8^+$ DC defect seems to depend on the inbred background (91, 98). The transcription factor Zbtb46 represents a negative regulator of DC activation and Zbtb46-deficient mice display no alterations in DC numbers (99, 100). Nevertheless, in Zbtb46-DTR bone marrow chimeras LC and all dermal DC subsets are depleted by the injection of diphtheria toxin (82). The deletion of the late endosomal adaptor molecule p14 (LAMTOR2) caused a gradual loss of LC from newborn mice due to increased apoptosis and a defect in homeostatic LC proliferation. This effect is partly mediated by the downregulation of TGF-β receptor II on LC (59, 101). The phenotypes of different cytokine-, growth factor-, and transcription factor-deficient mice lacking distinct DC subsets are summarized in **Table 1**.

In conclusion, the various skin DC subsets vary in their dependency on different transcription and growth factors, which allows the manipulation of particular subsets to investigate their functional properties. Our current knowledge on the specific roles of cutaneous DC subsets in allergic and infectious skin diseases as well as in skin cancer will be discussed in the following sections.

FUNCTIONAL REDUNDANCY OF SKIN DENDRITIC CELLS IN CONTACT HYPERSENSITIVITY

Contact hypersensitivity (CHS) responses to topically applied haptens in mice represent a relevant model for allergic contact dermatitis. Following percutaneous penetration, the hapten covalently binds to host proteins thereby generating a neo-antigen that is eventually recognized by the immune system (102, 103). The emergence of CHS critically depends on the activation of hapten-specific naïve T cells in skin-draining LN during hapten sensitization, which then proliferate and differentiate into effector T cells that mediate a transient ear swelling reaction at the time of hapten challenge. In agreement with the LC paradigm, although haptens can passively drain to LN via afferent lymphatics, the induction of a productive T cell response hinges on the transport of haptenized antigens by migratory skin DC to the T cell areas of the nodes. Therefore, when the first *in vivo* LC ablation mouse models were introduced, it came as a surprise that CHS was similar (46) or reduced, but not absent (44), after inducible depletion of LC in the skin prior to hapten sensitization (**Table 2**). These findings suggested that LC were not essential to induce the ear swelling reaction and that dermal DC contributed to T cell activation in CHS. Moreover, LC had no role in regulating the effector T cell response as was demonstrated by comparable ear swelling following diphtheria toxin treatment after sensitization but prior to hapten challenge (46, 104).

When the $Langerin^+$ dermal DC subset was discovered in 2007 (47–49), it became clear that these initial experiments had been performed in the absence of both $Langerin^+$ skin DC

TABLE 1 | Phenotypes of transcription factor and growth factor/receptor knockout mice lacking specific skin-resident dendritic cell subsets[a].

Transcription/growth factor/receptor knockout	Lymphoid tissue DC		Skin/non-lymphoid tissue DC			Reference
	$CD8^+$ DC	$CD8^{neg}$ DC	LC	$CD103^+$ DC	$CD11b^+$ DC	
Batf3	–	↔	↔	–	↔	(91, 92, 98)
CSF-1 (M-CSF)	↔	↔	↓	n.d.	n.d.	(86)
Csf-1R	↔	↔	–	↔	↓	(56, 64–66)
CSF-2 (GM-CSF)	↔	↔	↓	↓	↔	(83–85)
Csf-2R	↔	↔	↔	↓	↔	(84, 85)
IL-34	↔	↔	–	↔	↔	(65, 66)
Flt3	↓	↓	↔	↓	↓	(64, 79, 81, 82)
Id2	–	↔	–	–	↔	(64, 76, 78)
IRF2	↑	↓	↓	n.d.	n.d.	(87)
IRF4	↑	↓	↔	↑	↑	(76, 88–90, 93)
IRF8	–	↔	↔	–	↔	(64, 76, 91–93, 98)
LAMTOR	↔	↔	–	↓	n.d.	(59)
Runx3	↑	↓	–	n.d.	n.d.	(77)
TGF-β1	↔	↔	–	↔	↔	(72–75)
Zbtb46[b]	↔	↔	↓	↓	↓	(82, 99, 100)

[a]– indicates an absent cell population, ↓ indicates a reduction, ↔ no change, and ↑ an increase in cell number.
[b]Includes data from diphtheria toxin-treated Zbtb46-DTR bone marrow chimeras.
n.d. = not determined.

TABLE 2 | Contact hypersensitivity reactions in mice with specific defects in skin dendritic cell subsets[a].

Mouse strain	Epidermal LC	Langerin^{+}CD103^{+} dermal DC	Langerin^{neg}CD11b^{+}dermal DC	CHS	Reference
DT inducible cell depletion systems					
Langerin-DTR (DT days −1 to −3)	–	–	↔	↓ or ↔ (dependent on hapten conc.)	(44, 46, 47, 104, 105)
Langerin-DTR (DT days −7 to −13)	–	↓ (30%)	↔	↓ or ↔ (dependent on hapten conc.)	(47, 105)
Langerin-DTR BM → WT chimeras	↔	–	↔	↔	(106)
hLangerin-DTR	–	↔	↔	↑	(107)
Constitutive cell deficiency					
hLangerin-DTA	–	↔	↔	↑	(45)
LC/DC-specific TGF-βR1$^{-/-}$	–	↔	↔	↓	(75, 108)
LC/DC-specific p14$^{-/-}$	–	↔	↔	↓	(59)
Batf3$^{-/-}$	↔	–	↔	↔	(91)

[a]– indicates an absent cell population, ↓ indicates a reduction and ↔ means no change in cell number, functionality or CHS intensity, and ↑ indicates an increase in the CHS reaction.

populations and not in the selective absence of epidermal LC as one had assumed [because all Langerin^{+} DC in the dermis were considered to be LC en route to local LN (46)]. However, in agreement with their continuous replenishment from blood-borne precursors, it turned out that following injection of diphtheria toxin the dermal Langerin^{+} DC recovered much faster, i.e., within 7–10 days, while the long-lived self-maintaining LC stayed away for a prolonged period of time, i.e., at least 2–4 weeks (44, 47, 105). Using timed diphtheria toxin treatments, this enabled researchers to induce CHS when both Langerin^{+} skin DC (administration of diphtheria toxin 1–3 days prior to hapten sensitization) or only LC (diphtheria toxin treatment 7–13 days before sensitization) were lacking. Alternatively, Langerin-DTR into wild-type bone marrow chimeras permitted the selective depletion of only Langerin^{+} dermal DC before the induction of CHS (106). From this comprehensive analysis by a number of different laboratories, it became clear that the intensity of the CHS reaction is directly correlated with the efficiency of T cell priming, as was suggested by inefficient antigen transport to draining LN in the absence of Langerin^{+} skin DC (104). Consequently, and in agreement with early dose–response studies (109), LC are required for efficient induction of CHS responses, in particular, at low hapten doses, while at higher hapten concentrations sufficient amounts of antigen can be picked up by dermal DC – both Langerin^{+} and negative – for effective elicitation of CHS in the absence of LC (37, 47, 105, 106, 110, 111). Taken together, there is overwhelming evidence indicating functional redundancy of the different skin DC subsets in CHS (**Table 2**).

In contrast to these inducible Langerin-DTR knock-in mouse models, which harbor physiologic numbers of LC and Langerin^{+} dermal DC until the injection of diphtheria toxin, human (h) Langerin-DTA BAC transgenic mice that constitutively lack LC throughout life mounted enhanced ear swelling responses (45). Although this observation suggested that LC may exert a down-regulatory function in CHS, the great amount of data discussed above rather support compensatory roles of the different skin DC populations during the sensitization and elicitation of CHS (37, 47, 105, 106, 110, 111). Apart from these reports, it is difficult to conceive how negative regulatory properties of LC could develop or be maintained in the highly inflammatory setting of a CHS sensitizing reaction (112). However, the reason for the discrepancy between the inducible and the constitutive LC ablation models remains elusive. On the one hand, hLangerin-DTA mice may develop increased CHS as a result of some unknown failing peripheral tolerance mechanism in the lifelong absence of LC and therefore may respond differently during hapten sensitization and/or may possess altered T cell properties (37, 111, 113). On the other hand, the Langerin^{+} dermal DC that return after the toxin treatment in Langerin-DTR mice may differ from the cells that originally developed during ontogeny (58), and which are left untouched in hLangerin-DTA mice, presumably due to differences in the transcriptional regulation of the mouse and human *langerin* promotors. Both of these hypothetical explanations seem unlikely, however, because all transgenic mouse strains that constitutively lack LC (or Langerin^{+} dermal DC) as a result of varying genetic defects, i.e., independently of the diphtheria toxin/DTR system, and that have been tested in CHS mount similar or attenuated ear swelling reactions than LC-competent controls (**Table 2**) (75, 91, 101, 108). Instead, hLangerin-DTA mice may develop aggravated CHS due to changes in the homeostasis of dermal DC populations, i.e., an increased number of CD103^{+} dermal DC (92), or due to unknown DNA sequences that have been introduced with the human *langerin*-containing BAC. Although speculative as well, the latter may be implied, because to date hLangerin-DTR mice generated with the same BAC construct are the only other mouse model that mount enhanced CHS responses, i.e., after acute diphtheria toxin-mediated ablation of LC (107).

In conclusion, while LC clearly have regulatory potential that may have evolved to prevent inappropriate immune activation to keratinocyte-derived antigens or by commensal skin microbiota (see below), the vast majority of the available evidence indicates that LC promote the induction of CHS reactions, but are only essential at low hapten concentrations, and that dermal DC also contribute to CHS.

FUNCTIONAL SPECIALIZATION OF CUTANEOUS DENDRITIC CELLS IN INFECTIOUS SKIN DISEASE AND HOMEOSTASIS TO COMMENSAL MICROBIOTA

One of the first observations questioning the LC paradigm was the finding that during cutaneous herpes simplex virus-1 (HSV-1) infections not epidermal LC, but instead CD8α^{+} LN-resident DC were responsible for T cell priming and induction of the anti-HSV-1 response (114). Notably, LC were still required to process and transport HSV-derived antigens to the LN, where they transferred their antigenic cargo to the CD8α^{+} LN DC for cross-presentation to naïve T cells (115). Another study using an HSV-2 infection model of the vagina also revealed that epithelial LC did not present viral antigens to LN T cells (116). In this case, submucosal CD8α^{neg} migratory DC carried the viral peptides to the LN and induced the protective T helper (Th) type-1 response to HSV-2. A key question concerning these HSV infection models remains why LC played no direct role in antigen presentation and T cell activation. Was it merely because they were infected and killed by the cytopathic herpes viruses (117, 118); essentially leaving no other option for the apoptotic LC than being taken up and cross-presented to CD8^{+} T cells by LN-resident DC (119).

This hypothesis is supported in an apoptosis-inducing vaccinia virus infection model, in which cytotoxic T cell activation was similarly taken over by CD8α^{+} LN-resident DC, i.e., after uptake and cross-presentation of apoptotic skin-derived DC. On the other hand, in a cutaneous lentiviral infection model where LC/DC stay alive, migratory skin DC are perfectly capable to present antigen to T cells in the draining LN (120). Eventually, this concept was also confirmed for the HSV model, at least for Langerin^{+}CD103^{+} dermal DC (121). In contrast to the primary infection via superficial skin scarification, during reactivation of the virus from its natural reservoir in the cutaneous nerves, HSV antigen presentation to CD8^{+} T cells occurred by both Langerin^{+}CD103^{+} skin DC and CD8α^{+} LN DC. LC still played a minor role in direct antigen presentation, most likely due to higher sensitivity to this cytolytic virus than dermal DC. Although this concept that antigen-carrying skin DC, in particular LC, are taken up for cross-presentation by CD8α^{+} LN-resident DC cannot be generalized (119), it was later found that Langerin^{+}CD103^{+} dermal DC cross-present keratinocyte-derived antigens irrespective of the presence of epidermal LC (see below) (51). A comprehensive overview of the role of DC in primary HSV infections beyond these basic principles has been published recently (122).

LC were originally also considered to be critical for the induction of protective immunity in another infectious skin disease, namely cutaneous leishmaniasis, because they were shown to transport the parasites from the site of infection to skin-draining LN (123). This view was challenged when it was reported – at about the same time that the seminal HSV infection studies were published (114, 116) – that Langerin^{neg}CD8α^{neg} presumably dermal DC, but not LC, act as principal antigen-presenting cells (APC) in experimental *Leishmania major* infection (124). Resistance to *L. major* infection and healing of the skin lesions both in mice and men critically depends on the efficient induction of a Th1/T cytotoxic (Tc) type-1 response (125, 126). Langerin-DTR mice in combination with timed diphtheria toxin treatments (see above) revealed that activation of *L. major*-specific CD8^{+} T cells is significantly reduced during the early phase of the immune response following depletion of Langerin^{+} DC, without affecting the CD4^{+} T cell response and clearance of the infection (127). This demonstrated that Langerin^{neg} dermal DC were indeed essential for effective priming of CD4^{+} Th1 cells, whereas Langerin^{+} dermal DC were involved in early priming of CD8^{+} Tc1 cells.

Moreover, formation of CD4^{+} follicular helper (T_{FH})/B cell conjugates is crucial for B cell differentiation and class switch recombination to generate high-affinity antibodies for host protection following infection with *L. major* parasites (128). Recently, LC were shown to promote germinal center formation and thus antibody affinity maturation in response to *Leishmania*-derived cutaneous antigens (129), although these experiments used non-physiologic high doses of parasites that might blur early events during infection. In a model of physiologic low-dose infection with *L. major* infectious-stage promastigotes (1,000 parasites), mice depleted of all Langerin^{+} DC developed smaller ear lesions, decreased parasite loads and a reduced number of CD4^{+}Foxp3^{+} Treg cells, which was accompanied by increased production of interferon γ (IFNγ) (130). Of note, despite repeated administration of diphtheria toxin over a prolonged period of time (20 weeks) Langerin^{+} DC were efficiently depleted from the skin, confirming the absence of anti-diphtheria toxin neutralizing antibody formation as had previously been demonstrated (113, 131). Intriguingly, selective depletion of LC at the time of low-dose *L. major* inoculation demonstrated that the absence of LC, and not Langerin^{+} dermal DC, was responsible for the reduced Treg cell immigration and the enhanced Th1 response, resulting in attenuated disease (130). Hence, LC act as negative regulators of the anti-*Leishmania* response in mice. This may be important to prevent complete eradication of the parasites from the host, which leads to the loss of T cell memory and susceptibility to reinfection (132, 133).

Candida albicans is a dimorphic fungus accountable for chronic cutaneous and systemic infections in immune-compromised hosts. On the *stratum corneum* of the skin, commensal *C. albicans* grows as budding yeast, while pathogenic *C. albicans* in the dermis and internal organs exists predominantly in its filamentous form, i.e., as pseudo-hyphae (134). This yeast-to-hyphae transition during epidermal invasion is required for both virulence and the generation of protective Th17 responses to cutaneous *C. albicans* (134, 135). On the other hand, systemic fungal immunity is achieved by innate immune mechanisms regulated by IL-17-mediated licensing of NK cells to promote the fungicidal activity of neutrophils (136).

Taking advantage of a superficial skin infection model that does not bypass the epidermis in combination with LC-deficient hLangerin-DTA mice, it was demonstrated that LC are essential for the induction of antigen-specific Th17, but not cytotoxic T lymphocyte (CTL) responses (137). Somewhat inconsistent, despite reduced IL-17 and similar IFNγ responses in the absence of LC, hLangerin-DTA mice mounted significantly increased DTH reactions after epicutaneous *C. albicans* infection, similar to the unique phenotype of these transgenic mice in CHS [(45) and as discussed above]. However, using human Langerin-specific antibodies for targeted antigen delivery to LC in hLangerin-DTR mice (not treated with diphtheria toxin), LC were also found to be sufficient for inducing Th17 cell differentiation.

By contrast, Langerin$^+$ dermal DC promoted antigen-specific Th1 and efficiently cross-presented fungal antigens to activate CTL responses. At the same time, Langerin$^+$ dermal DC suppressed the ability of LC to drive the generation of Th17 cells (137). A follow-up study indicated that infection with *C. albicans* yeast but not pseudo-hyphae was capable of inducing Th17 responses through a mechanism that required Dectin-1 ligation on LC and, as a consequence, LC-derived IL-6 (138). In the dermis, absent Dectin-1 engagement by *C. albicans* pseudo-hyphae prevents Th17 induction by CD11b$^+$ dermal DC. Moreover, Th17 cells were found to provide protection against secondary cutaneous infection whereas Th1 cells were protective against systemic reinfection (138). Together these elegant studies established that distinct and opposing Th cell responses are determined by a combination of differences in *C. albicans* morphology and functional specialization of skin-resident DC subsets.

Beyond the functional specialization of skin DC subsets to deal with particular pathogens, there is accumulating evidence that the interactions between the resident skin microbiota and DC autonomously shape tissue homeostasis and local immunity (139). Skin tissue of mice housed under specific pathogen-free (SPF) conditions harbors Foxp3$^+$ Treg as well as $\alpha\beta^+$ and $\gamma\delta^+$ T cells with the potential to produce IFNγ and/or IL-17A, respectively. Microbial products from skin commensals tightly regulate this balance between Treg and effector T cells as was indicated by the increase in Treg and the reduction in IFNγ and IL-17A producing T cells in germfree mice lacking microbial products from their skin (139). Consequently, protective immunity against *L. major* is severely impaired in germfree mice, as is disease-associated pathology. Intriguingly, colonization with the single skin commensal *Staphylococcus epidermidis* was sufficient to rescue cutaneous IL-17A production in germfree mice, which was dependent on IL-1 signaling in the skin. Monoassociation of germfree mice with *S. epidermidis* at the time of infection also restored immunity to *L. major* as well as pathology with increased necrosis (139). These results suggest that defects in T cell function in the steady state or during inflammation can result from an impaired IL-1-mediated dialog with skin commensals.

Moreover, colonization of the skin of SPF mice that contained a diverse microbiota with *S. epidermidis* led to an accumulation of IL-17A$^+$ CD8$^+$ T cells in the epidermis that enhanced innate barrier immunity by upregulation of antimicrobial peptides and limited skin invasion of the pathogen *C. albicans*. In agreement with the unique role of CD103$^+$ dermal DC in antigen cross-presentation (see below), these Tc17 cells failed to develop in Batf3$^{-/-}$ and IRF8$^{-/-}$ (see **Table 1**), while the IL-17A secreting CD8$^+$ T cells developed normally in constitutively LC-deficient hLangerin-DTA mice (92). Furthermore, CD11b$^+$ dermal DC were required to promote the induction and/or maintenance of Tc17 cells through their capacity to produce IL-1 in response to *S. epidermidis* colonization of the skin. In conclusion, these findings reveal that the skin immune system is highly dynamic and can be readily reshaped by the coordinated action of the different skin DC subsets upon encounter of defined commensals (92).

Hence, in agreement with the extended *LC paradigm* (**Figure 1**), LC exhibit a great degree of functional plasticity and become tolerogenic or immunogenic depending on the nature of the invading pathogen they encounter in the skin.

CROSS-PRESENTATION BY SKIN DENDRITIC CELLS: QUESTION FINALLY ANSWERED?

For developing immunotherapeutic approaches against cancer, one prerequisite is to understand how the various skin DC subsets induce CTL responses. There has been a long-standing debate on the ability of LC to cross-present exogenous antigen to CD8$^+$ T cells (37). The start of this debate was the report that LC are dispensable for the induction of cytotoxic T cell responses against skin infection with herpes virus (see above) (114), which was later confirmed for vaccinia virus (140). Subsequent work clarified that cytopathic viruses induce apoptosis in LC rendering them sole transporters of antigen. As a consequence these cells are no longer capable of directly inducing T cell responses, however, LN-resident DC and other skin DC subsets, such as Langerin$^+$ dermal DC, can step in and cross-present antigen to CD8$^+$ T cells (115, 141, 142).

The debate was further fueled by studies on cross-presentation of self-antigen. For this approach, transgenic mice overexpressing ovalbumin protein in an inducible or constitutive way under control of the keratinocyte-specific K5- or K14-promoter in the skin were employed (143–145). Now it was possible to examine cross-presentation of self-antigen by the various skin DC subsets in the steady state and inflammation. Early studies demonstrated that Langerin$^+$ cells can cross-present ovalbumin to antigen-specific CD8$^+$ T cells (26, 146, 147). This cross-presentation ability was not necessarily restricted to Langerin$^+$ dermal DC, since LC purified from trypsinized epidermis and migratory LC from epidermal explants also efficiently cross-presented ovalbumin to CD8$^+$ T cells *in vitro* (144, 148). Chimeric mice in which antigen cross-presentation was restricted to LC proved that LC are able to cross-present self-antigen also *in vivo*. Interestingly, cross-presentation by Langerin$^+$ skin DC led to tolerance induction through deletion of antigen-specific CD8$^+$ T cells (26). After the discovery of Langerin$^+$ dermal DC, it came as a big surprise, when studies using K5-ovalbumin transgenic mice established that Langerin$^+$ dermal DC are the sole cross-presenters of keratinocyte-derived antigen (51, 121). The localization of Langerin$^+$ dermal DC adjacent to hair follicles where K5$^+$ keratinocytes are present explained how this DC subset gains access to an epidermal antigen (49, 149). Moreover, in human skin keratinocyte-derived keratin bodies were found in the dermis (150). The discrepancy to the earlier studies, proving that LC can cross-present antigen, may be due to the low migratory capacity of LC in the steady state, which ensures that the LC network stays intact until inflammation causes accelerated emigration of LC to LN (21, 43, 151). Indeed, the turnover of LC in the skin is much lower than that of dermal DC as demonstrated by BrdU incorporation assays (51).

The migration of all skin DC populations increases dramatically in an inflammatory setting, though with different kinetics, so that dermal DC arrive in LN much earlier than LC (46, 152). Hence, it would be interesting to investigate the cross-presentation of skin-derived antigen in an inflammatory setting at different time points after the onset of inflammation. Aside from this, most of the studies performed to date used transgenic mice overexpressing the model antigen ovalbumin in keratinocytes. Because of the high-affinity T cell receptor binding and very strong responsiveness of ovalbumin-specific $CD8^+$ T cells, these findings might not reflect what happens in real life (37). Thus, these studies need to be confirmed in a more physiological setting investigating the cross-presentation of genuine self-antigens in the skin.

For the development of immunotherapeutic strategies exploiting skin DC, exogenous antigen needs to be delivered through the skin (see below). Studies on skin immunization added more issues to the controversy whether LC can cross-present exogenous antigen. First of all, LC can induce CTL when they are loaded with soluble ovalbumin *in vitro* and co-cultured with $CD8^+$ T cells (148). Most importantly, topical application of ovalbumin onto the skin by either epicutaneous immunization (153) or by dissolving micro-needles (154) confirmed that $Langerin^+$ DC are involved in cross-priming of $CD8^+$ T cells and that LC are superior to $Langerin^+$ dermal DC, in particular, when the antigen is encapsulated in nanoparticles (154). In line with this, antibody-mediated targeting of the model antigen ovalbumin to $Langerin^+$ cells by intradermal injection proved that both, LC and $Langerin^+$ dermal DC, can cross-present antigen to $CD8^+$ T cells *in vivo* (155).

Finally, to answer the question asked above, yes, both LC and $Langerin^+$ dermal DC in the skin can cross-present exogenous antigen to $CD8^+$ T cells *in vitro* and *in vivo*. We would like to emphasize that cross-presentation and cross-priming must not be equated. There is the very likely possibility that the various skin DC subsets induce different functional outcomes in $CD8^+$ T cell differentiation as exemplified in a recent report. Despite initial $CD8^+$ T cell proliferation induced by LC and $Langerin^+$ dermal DC after loading them *in situ* with protein antigen (proving cross-presentation), LC did not cross-prime T cells but rather induced cross-tolerance. By contrast, $Langerin^+$ dermal DC promoted cytotoxicity, indicating that they indeed cross-primed the T cells (155). Thus, we need to better understand the differential contributions of the various skin DC subsets in $CD8^+$ T cell activation leading to either CTL differentiation or tolerance induction. This knowledge is indispensable for the future development of DC-based immunotherapy of cancer.

SKIN DENDRITIC CELLS IN CANCER

Novel immunotherapeutic strategies to vaccinate through the skin are a promising area of research for the future development of anti-cancer therapies. The rationale behind this approach comes from reports on the involvement of DC in tumor immunity and their outstanding potential in promoting T cell responses. The presence of DC has been reported in many different tumors, however, their specific role in tumor immunity is still incompletely understood (156, 157). Aside from this, tumors also strongly impair DC function and actively prevent efficient immunosurveillance by DC (158). With respect to cutaneous cancer, such as squamous cell carcinoma (SCC), basal cell carcinoma (BCC), and melanoma, several reports indicate that the numbers and function of skin DC are affected by tumor growth.

So far few studies attempted to analyze the specific role of skin DC present in cutaneous tumors. Non-melanoma skin cancer, such as SCC and BCC, are tumors of basal keratinocytes, making it very likely that LC are the first APC getting in contact with transformed cells. Two studies used patient samples from SCC to investigate LC and DC in regard to numbers, phenotype, and T cell stimulatory capacity. In the first study, the numbers of LC in the SCC tumor lesions were decreased as compared to healthy epidermis. Less myeloid cells, including dermal DC, were found around tumor nests than in normal skin. Tumor-associated myeloid DC were poor stimulators of allogeneic T cells despite displaying an activated phenotype (159, 160). The second study demonstrated that tumor-infiltrating LC are more activated and induced higher $CD4^+$ and $CD8^+$ allogeneic T cell proliferation as well as IFNγ production than LC from adjacent healthy skin (161). Thus, LC and myeloid DC found in human SCC samples display an activated phenotype, but only LC induce allogeneic T cell responses. Although suggestive, these studies do not allow any conclusion on the functional ability of these DC subsets to promote tumor immunity to non-melanoma skin cancer since tumor-specific T cell responses were not investigated. However, unhindered tumor growth despite the activation of LC/DC indicates that the immunosuppressive milieu in SCC tumors, which contains high concentrations of TGF-β1 counteracts successful tumor immunity (159).

Another study used a murine model of chemically induced SCC to investigate the role of LC during tumor development (162). Chemical carcinogenesis was induced by application of the carcinogen 7,12-dimethylbenz(a)anthracene (DMBA) that causes Hras mutations, followed by the tumor-promoting agent 12-O-tetra-decanoyl-phorbol-13-acetate (TPA) leading to development of papilloma and subsequent SCC. The observation that hLangerin-DTA mice, lacking LC throughout their lifetime, are completely protected from tumor development is somehow surprising, but may be related to the intrinsically enhanced elicitation of adaptive immune responses, i.e., in CHS and DTH reactions, in this as opposed to other LC-deficient mouse models (see above). However, the authors propose the interesting concept that LC mediate the metabolic conversion of DMBA to its mutagenic metabolite that in turn leads to DNA damage and carcinogenesis. They further suggest that compared to keratinocytes LC express higher levels of CYP1B1, an enzyme of the cytochrome P-450 family responsible for the mutagenic metabolism of DMBA (162). How the metabolite is transferred from LC to keratinocytes to exert its DNA-damaging function was not investigated. Moreover, these data are difficult to reconcile with the fact that keratinocytes themselves express all required enzymes for DMBA metabolism (163, 164). In a follow-up paper, the authors demonstrated that LC exert pro-carcinogenic effects also independently of the enzyme CYP1B1 (165), possibly by aryl hydrocarbon receptor-mediated transcription of other CYP enzymes that trigger DNA damage (166).

In addition, LC played an important role in the progression of tumors by affecting the hyperproliferation of keratinocytes in the DMBA-induced SCC model (165) as well as in UVB-induced SCC (167), likely by augmenting IL-22 production by keratinocytes. Notably, this direct carcinogenic role of LC may be amplified by LC-driven immunosuppression, which is the induction of antigen-specific Treg cells upon UV radiation exposure (166, 168). It will be interesting to compare the growth of chemically and UVB-induced SCC in the hLangerin-DTA mouse model (165, 167) to one of the inducible Langerin-DTR knock-in mice (44, 46), since the constitutive absence of LC in hLangerin-DTA mice may have a distinct effect on the development of the skin immune system (see above). Intriguingly, a recent report revealed an unaltered expression profile of cytochrome P-450 enzymes in the absence of LC and Langerin^{+} dermal DC upon DMBA application in Langerin-DTR mice (169).

Similar as in SCC and BCC, the role of the different skin DC in the immunosurveillance of melanoma is incompletely understood. Over 20 years ago first reports described decreased numbers of LC above invasive human melanoma (170, 171). In line with these findings, the presence of transplantable tumors lowered the number and impaired the migration of LC from murine skin (172). The types and relative proportions of tumor-infiltrating DC in melanoma have not been determined so far, such that information on the functional potential of distinct skin DC subsets to control melanoma is lacking. For instance, in melanoma the accumulation of mature DC of unknown origin in draining LN metastases was associated with the expansion of antigen-specific cytotoxic T cells (173). A recent effort to identify the various myeloid cell types within a transplantable murine melanoma model demonstrated that the CD103^{+} DC subset, which most likely includes Langerin^{+} dermal DC, was superior over CD11b^{+}CD103^{neg} DC in cross-presenting tumor antigens (174). Future studies using multi-color flow cytometry including a comprehensive panel of markers to discriminate individual DC subsets (**Figures 3** and **4**) will be required to obtain a detailed picture on the involvement of distinct skin DC in tumor immunity (175). This knowledge will form the basis for the design of novel and for the improvement of existing immunotherapies harnessing the potential of skin DC for the immunotherapy of cancer.

HARNESSING SKIN DENDRITIC CELLS AS TARGETS FOR IMMUNOTHERAPY OF CANCER

From the time of the experiments of William Coley in the early 1900s immunotherapy of cancer was in the minds of immunologists (176), though it played a rather marginal role. Next to T cells, cytokines and antibodies, DC became promising targets for immunotherapy of cancer owing to the pioneering work by the late Ralph Steinman, who received the 2011 Nobel Prize in Physiology or Medicine for "his discovery of the DC and its role in adaptive immunity" (177). His ultimate goal was to harness the outstanding immunogenic properties of DC for immunotherapy and thereby "taking dendritic cells into medicine" (178). Since the first report of treatment of a B cell lymphoma with antigen-pulsed DC from blood (179), many clinical and basic research centers have been working to improve the efficacy of DC-based strategies to treat cancer patients. The first adoptive DC therapy for cancer (Provenge™, a tumor antigen-pulsed cell suspension containing DC) was approved by the FDA in 2010, and this constituted a milestone in the development of cellular therapies. A parallel development in cancer immunotherapy occurred over the past few years when the so-called "checkpoint inhibitors" were introduced into clinical practice. These antibodies against CTLA-4, PD-1, or PD-L1 (and presumably other inhibitory mediators in the future) switch off down-regulatory signaling pathways in T cells. They are therefore able to powerfully unleash anti-cancer immunity that exists in patients but is obviously insufficient or suppressed by various mechanisms (180). Clinical responses in patients are impressive, but so are side effects (autoimmunity), particularly with the anti-CTLA-4 antibodies. Still, these clinical observations have earned this therapeutic approach the title of "Breakthrough of the Year" in 2013 by *Science* (181).

In spite of these encouraging developments targeting T cells, the potential of DC-based therapies remains high for several reasons. (*i*) Only a variable part of patients treated by checkpoint blockade responds to the treatment (180, 182, 183). (*ii*) Even though undesired autoimmunity can be clinically managed, it would be advantageous to avoid or minimize it from the beginning. (*iii*) Most importantly, checkpoint blockade can only boost those cancer-specific T cells that are already preexisting in the patient. By contrast, DC therapy would be able to generate *de novo* immune responses (182, 183). Such responses would be desired against neo-antigens ("private mutations") in patients' tumors (182, 184). DC-induced T cell responses against such mutated tumor antigens would additionally lack autoimmune danger.

The *ex vivo* generation of DC for therapy is laborious, nevertheless, therapy with tumor antigen-pulsed autologous DC proved to be safe and effective, though not curative, in patients with solid tumors (185). The continuing importance of DC therapy is highlighted by recent publications, indicating persuasive ways of improving DC vaccines. For instance, DC were loaded with peptides derived from neo-antigens identified from the patient's own tumor material, instead of the commonly used peptides from overexpressed self-antigens. This strategy augments T cell responses by broadening the antigenic diversity of the anti-tumor response in the absence of autoimmunity (186). Another approach is the conditioning of the injection site with a potent recall antigen, such as tetanus toxoid, TLR ligands, or cytokines. The pretreatment of the skin site with antigen or danger signals improved the migration of adoptively transferred DC and boosted T cell responses in tumor-bearing mice (187–189). Moreover, the co-administration of tumor-binding allogeneic antibodies enhanced the internalization of tumor antigens by DC and dramatically increased therapy outcome in murine tumor models (190). Furthermore, the choice of DC subset could enhance the efficacy of DC therapy as has been demonstrated for LC-like cells generated from CD34^{+} precursor cells that were able to overcome tolerance to differentiation antigens commonly overexpressed in cancer patients and used for vaccination (191).

Yet another imaginative approach that has been pioneered many years ago in Ralph Steinman's laboratory (192, 193) is the use of antibody-mediated antigen targeting constructs to specifically deliver antigenic peptides or proteins to DC *in situ*. The basic idea is to target the antigen of interest to endocytic receptors specific for DC (subsets) resident in the skin or lymphatic organs to enable them to efficiently incorporate antigen for presentation to T cells. This approach would be much less laborious than the *ex vivo* generation of DC from patients' monocytes and their subsequent loading with tumor antigens. Intriguingly, antigen delivered without adjuvant can induce tolerance, whereas concomitant administration of TLR ligands and agonistic anti-CD40 antibody causes strong induction of $CD4^+$ and $CD8^+$ T cell responses (192, 194). In addition, this approach allows delivering antigen into the various skin DC subsets by aiming at different lectin receptors (195, 196). The most interesting candidate receptors for these *in vivo* antigen targeting approaches are C-type lectins, which are expressed by skin DC, e.g., DEC-205, Langerin, and Dectin-1 (197–199). Specific delivery of the model antigen ovalbumin into $Langerin^+$ cells proved that both LC and $Langerin^+$ dermal DC can cross-present antigen to $CD8^+$ T cells, however, only the dermal DC promoted the development of cytotoxicity while LC induced tolerance (155). Targeting antigens to $DEC\text{-}205^+$ DC led to tumor control or even eradication in murine tumor models, albeit the relative roles of skin DC and LN-resident DC were not investigated in these studies (194, 200, 201). The chemokine receptor XCR1, which is preferentially expressed on $Langerin^+$ dermal DC (52, 53) (**Figure 3**), is another promising target due to the fact that this DC subset excels in inducing cytotoxicity in $CD8^+$ T cells (155). Immunization with the chemokine XCL1 conjugated to ovalbumin protein intravenously or through skin pre-treated with a laser to form pores led to $CD4^+$ and $CD8^+$ T cell activation and inhibited the growth of transplanted tumors in mice (202, 203). First clinical trials have been initiated and so far demonstrated induction of some humoral and cellular immunity by targeting the tumor antigen NY-ESO-1 conjugated to DEC-205 antibody into DC of patients with various solid tumors (204). These data demonstrate the proof-of-concept of the targeting approach in human cancer, but they also call for intense further study to substantially improve this strategy.

Immunization strategies through the skin are very attractive for their easiness of use and, ultimately, the possibility of self-medication in case of topical treatment. Several approaches have been developed such as epicutaneous immunization, micro-needles, laserporation, or powder injection (205). The epicutaneous approach allows to topically apply antigens in protein and peptide form onto the skin (206). The disruption of the skin barrier and the addition of an adjuvant proved to be essential to elicit powerful cytotoxic T cell responses that inhibit tumor growth (153, 207, 208). The involvement of $Langerin^+$ skin DC in $CD8^+$ T cell responses was confirmed in experiments with Langerin-DTR mice in a tumor setting. In line with findings in the CHS model (see above), the antigen dose of ovalbumin protein determined which skin DC subset presented the tumor antigen. The inhibition of tumor growth by epicutaneous immunization with low-dose antigen was completely abrogated in the Langerin-DTR mice depleted for $Langerin^+$ DC, whereas application of a higher dose of antigen still partly inhibited tumor growth even in the absence of $Langerin^+$ DC (153). This supports the notion of the high plasticity of skin DC subsets. The epicutaneous immunization approach has already been clinically tested and proved to be promising for the treatment of cancer and infection (209, 210).

Another very elegant approach is the application of dissolving micro-needles that allow delivery of antigens right into the tissue where skin DC are located. This strategy has been successfully used to vaccinate against influenza (211) and to treat tumors, at least in murine models (154). The latter study demonstrated that LC can be superior to dermal DC in cross-presentation of antigen delivered with micro-needles into the skin. Interestingly, the nature of the antigen determined which skin DC subset induced $CD8^+$ T cell proliferation, in that encapsulated antigen was preferentially cross-presented by LC whereas soluble antigen required $Langerin^+$ dermal DC for $CD8^+$ T cell activation. The $CD4^+$ T cell response was promoted by all skin DC subsets, however, LC dominated the induction of Th1 and Th17 responses (154).

For the future, it will be worthwhile to investigate the potential of the various cutaneous DC subsets in skin immunization and translate the findings from murine tumor models to the patient situation. Undoubtedly, skin DC are critically involved in surveying the skin in order to prevent tumor growth and clearly fulfill an immunogenic role during vaccination against cancer. Yet their precise roles are still unclear and need to be clarified before we will arrive at urgently needed more effective DC-based treatment options for cancer.

HUMAN SKIN DENDRITIC CELL SUBSETS

The human and murine skin DC network seems to be highly conserved between the two species. While this justifies *in vivo* experiments in mice to gain mechanistic insight into the functional specialization of cutaneous DC subsets in regulating immunity and tolerance, we need to identify the human counterparts of the murine DC subtypes in order to translate this knowledge to treating patients. In the recent years, human skin DC subsets were better defined and found to be homologous to murine DC (**Figure 4**) (212–214). In humans, the epidermis contains LC expressing Langerin and high levels of CD1a, whereas in the dermis three subsets of dermal DC can be distinguished (37, 215). The largest population is represented by the $CD1c^+CD1a^+$ dermal DC, which correspond to the murine $CD11b^+$ dermal DC (216, 217). The smallest subset of DC in human dermis is characterized by high expression of CD141 and XCR1 and is homologous to the murine $Langerin^+CD103^+$ dermal DC, which also express XCR1 (214, 218). Very recently evidence for yet another small subset of (weakly) $Langerin^+CD1c^+$ dermal DC was presented, highlighting that similar to mice Langerin expression may not be strictly confined to LC in human skin (219). The $CD14^+$ dermal DC are monocyte-derived cells that are transcriptionally aligned rather to monocytes/macrophages than to DC (216). A corresponding tissue-resident DC subset with the phenotype $CD11b^+Ly6C^-CD64^{lo\text{-}hi}$ has been described in murine dermis (35).

In regard to functional aspects, both human LC and $CD1c^+$ dermal DC can polarize Th1 and Th2 responses (220), depending

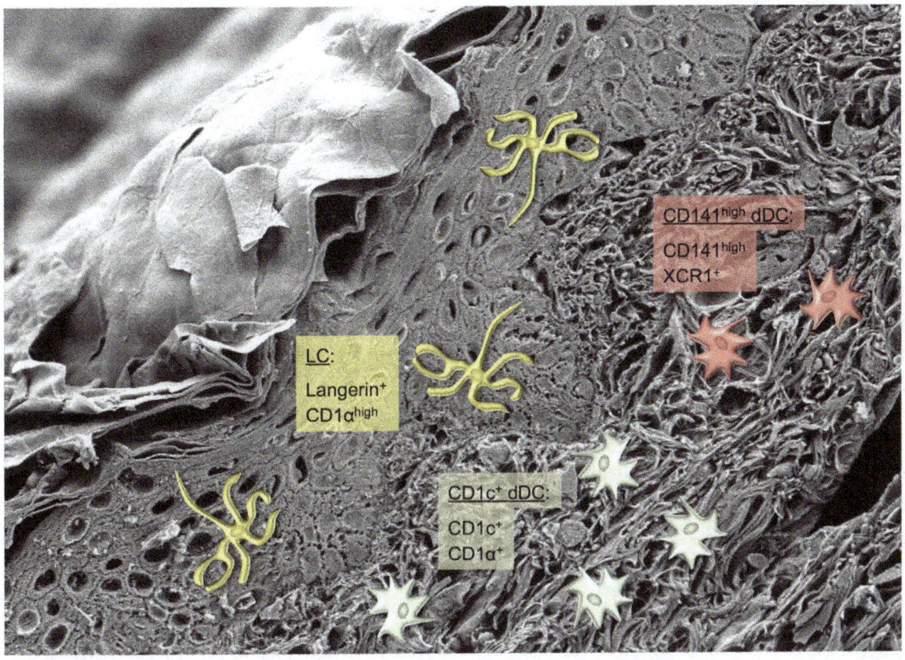

FIGURE 4 | Dendritic cell subsets in human skin. Scanning electron microscopy picture of a section through the skin depicting several layers of keratinocytes and the collagen meshwork of the dermis (38). Photograph by courtesy of Kristian Pfaller and Patrizia Stoitzner. Phenotypically distinct human skin-resident DC subsets are described by their most prominent markers. The color code represents the murine counterparts shown in **Figure 3**.

on the cytokine milieu in the skin (221), and cross-present exogenous antigen to CD8^{+} T cells (215). However, the recently discovered CD141^{hi} dermal DC excel in cross-priming of CD8^{+} T cells comparable to murine Langerin^{+} dermal DC (214). There still exists some controversy in the field on the suitability of XCR1 and CD141 as markers for cross-presenting DC since both molecules can also be expressed by some CD1a^{+} and CD14^{+} dermal DC (218, 222, 223). Importantly, the methods used for the preparation of skin DC differ strongly between the many studies published. Notably, DC isolated from skin tissue by enzymatic digestion or derived from skin explant culture after emigration from the tissue ("crawl-outs") represent immature and mature DC, respectively. This has major influence on their phenotype/function and the presence/absence of cell surface markers. One example is CD141, which is differently expressed on freshly isolated dermal DC and migratory dermal DC. While CD141 is upregulated on CD14^{+} dermal DC upon emigration from skin explants as compared to DC enzymatically isolated from skin, its expression on CD141^{high} CD14^{neg} dermal DC remains unaltered upon migration (214, 223). Humoral immunity is mainly modulated by CD14^{+} dermal DC since they can activate the differentiation of T_{FH} cells (220). Moreover, CD14^{+} dermal DC support memory T cell activation, most likely *in situ* in the skin, but they are poor stimulators of naïve T cells (216). During inflammation, several inflammatory DC subsets, e.g., inflammatory dendritic epidermal cells (IDEC), 6-sulfoLacNAc^{+} (slan) DC, and TNF-α/iNOS-producing (Tip) DC, are recruited to the skin and have a strong impact on the course of inflammatory skin diseases such as psoriasis and atopic dermatitis (215, 224, 225).

Despite the high degree of homology between mouse and human skin DC, functional disparities do exist. Some examples are listed here: (*i*) For instance, with the help of IL-15 released into the immunological synapse, human LC cross-prime cytotoxic CD8^{+} T cell responses (226, 227). As a consequence human LC are able to break tolerance to self-antigens and stimulate cytotoxic T cell responses (191). So far hardly any information on the production of IL-15 by murine skin DC is available. (*ii*) CD70, a molecule involved in DC–T cell interaction and important for activation of CD8^{+} T cells and IFNγ production (228), is highly expressed by human LC (229, 230), whereas murine LC show very low levels of CD70 even after stimulation (155). These functional disparities between murine and human LC are supported by recently published gene transcription profiles of human skin DC subsets, indicating that human LC are more closely related to murine Langerin^{+} dermal DC than to murine LC (222). (*iii*) Another example for functional differences stems from the fact that murine LC, despite initial cross-presentation and induction of CD8^{+} T cell proliferation (148), fail to stimulate cytotoxicity in CD8^{+} T cells and instead induce cross-tolerance (155). Notably, the TLR ligands used in the latter study specifically activate Langerin^{+} dermal DC (231), thus we need to evaluate the potential of LC in cross-priming with TLR ligands suitable for their activation. The knowledge on functional properties of the various murine and human skin DC subsets is of eminent importance when we envisage novel immunotherapeutic approaches that need first to be tested in preclinical murine studies before they can be translated into the clinics.

CONCLUSION

The skin, as one of the barrier tissues to the environment, harbors particular challenges to the resident DC network. While the cells continuously probe their surroundings for invading pathogens, DC have to discriminate harmless from dangerous microbes, prevent inappropriate immune reactions against self-antigens, and limit collateral tissue damage once inflammation occurs during protective immune responses. The original concept that immature DC confer tolerance and mature DC initiate immunity (232) turned out to be too simplistic and was further developed to give way to the hypothesis of functional specialization of particular DC subsets (233), including distinct pathway(s) of tolerogenic DC maturation (14, 17, 18). Through major advancements in multi-color flow cytometry, next-generation transcriptomics and proteomics, and the generation of novel cell type-specific gene targeting, cell labeling, and cell ablation mouse models, we can now dissect an increasing number of phenotypically distinct DC subsets in the skin (as well as other barrier tissues) and are beginning to unravel their functional heterogeneity (1, 3, 37). From these exciting *in vivo* experiments, it is becoming increasingly clear that specific DC subsets indeed exert specialized functions, but that this "*division of labor*" is not intrinsically defined by or fixed within one type of DC and rather determined by the signals the DC receive from their micro-environment (234). For example, LC induce Treg during *L. major* and Th17 cells upon *C. albicans* infection (130, 137), Th2 cells under the influence of pro-allergic TSLP (221) and strong Th1 responses when conditioned by a tumor environment (161). Thus, despite their context-dependent specialization, overall DC subsets display an amazing functional plasticity ("*multitasking*"). The future challenge lies in better understanding (*i*) the unique contribution of the different DC subsets to particular chronic inflammatory diseases and (*ii*) the context-dependent signals that control the function of individual DC subsets in a given disease state. This knowledge will be vital to harness (skin) DC subsets for the treatment of human diseases ranging from allergy and autoimmunity to chronic infections and cancer.

ACKNOWLEDGMENTS

The authors would like to thank the former and present members of their laboratories for their manifold contributions to the work discussed in this review, Drs. Niki Romani and Julia Ober-Blöbaum for many helpful discussions and critical reading of this manuscript, and Drs. Ari Waisman and Niki Romani for their continuous support. The work in our laboratories has been supported by grants from the Netherlands Organization for Scientific Research (NWO, VIDI 617-76-365), the German Research Foundation (DFG)-NWO bilateral cooperation program (DN 93-525), and the Forschungszentrum für Immuntherapie (FZI) of the University Medical Center Mainz to BEC, as well as grants from the Austrian Science Fund (FWF-21487-B13, FWF-27001-B13, FWF-W11001-B15) to PS.

REFERENCES

1. Malissen B, Tamoutounour S, Henri S. The origins and functions of dendritic cells and macrophages in the skin. *Nat Rev Immunol* (2014) **14**(6):417–28. doi:10.1038/nri3683
2. Merad M, Sathe P, Helft J, Miller J, Mortha A. The dendritic cell lineage: ontogeny and function of dendritic cells and their subsets in the steady state and the inflamed setting. *Annu Rev Immunol* (2013) **31**:563–604. doi:10.1146/annurev-immunol-020711-074950
3. Scott CL, Henri S, Guilliams M. Mononuclear phagocytes of the intestine, the skin, and the lung. *Immunol Rev* (2014) **262**(1):9–24. doi:10.1111/imr.12220
4. Iram N, Mildner M, Prior M, Petzelbauer P, Fiala C, Hacker S, et al. Age-related changes in expression and function of toll-like receptors in human skin. *Development* (2012) **139**(22):4210–9. doi:10.1242/dev.083477
5. Lebre MC, van der Aar AM, van Baarsen L, van Capel TM, Schuitemaker JH, Kapsenberg ML, et al. Human keratinocytes express functional toll-like receptor 3, 4, 5, and 9. *J Invest Dermatol* (2007) **127**(2):331–41. doi:10.1038/sj.jid.5700530
6. Miller LS, Modlin RL. Toll-like receptors in the skin. *Semin Immunopathol* (2007) **29**(1):15–26. doi:10.1007/s00281-007-0061-8
7. Tan S, Roediger B, Weninger W. The role of chemokines in cutaneous immunosurveillance. *Immunol Cell Biol* (2015) **93**(4):337–46. doi:10.1038/icb.2015.16
8. Ebner S, Ehammer Z, Holzmann S, Schwingshackl P, Forstner M, Stoitzner P, et al. Expression of c-type lectin receptors by subsets of dendritic cells in human skin. *Int Immunol* (2004) **16**(6):877–87. doi:10.1093/intimm/dxh088
9. Gregorio J, Meller S, Conrad C, Di Nardo A, Homey B, Lauerma A, et al. Plasmacytoid dendritic cells sense skin injury and promote wound healing through type I interferons. *J Exp Med* (2010) **207**(13):2921–30. doi:10.1084/jem.20101102
10. Nestle FO, Kaplan DH, Barker J. Psoriasis. *N Engl J Med* (2009) **361**(5):496–509. doi:10.1056/NEJMra0804595
11. Reizis B, Bunin A, Ghosh HS, Lewis KL, Sisirak V. Plasmacytoid dendritic cells: recent progress and open questions. *Annu Rev Immunol* (2011) **29**:163–83. doi:10.1146/annurev-immunol-031210-101345
12. Nishibu A, Ward BR, Jester JV, Ploegh HL, Boes M, Takashima A. Behavioral responses of epidermal langerhans cells in situ to local pathological stimuli. *J Invest Dermatol* (2006) **126**(4):787–96. doi:10.1038/sj.jid.5700107
13. Ouchi T, Kubo A, Yokouchi M, Adachi T, Kobayashi T, Kitashima DY, et al. Langerhans cell antigen capture through tight junctions confers preemptive immunity in experimental staphylococcal scalded skin syndrome. *J Exp Med* (2011) **208**(13):2607–13. doi:10.1084/jem.20111718
14. Dalod M, Chelbi R, Malissen B, Lawrence T. Dendritic cell maturation: functional specialization through signaling specificity and transcriptional programming. *EMBO J* (2014) **33**(10):1104–16. doi:10.1002/embj.201488027
15. Ohl L, Mohaupt M, Czeloth N, Hintzen G, Kiafard Z, Zwirner J, et al. CCR7 governs skin dendritic cell migration under inflammatory and steady-state conditions. *Immunity* (2004) **21**(2):279–88. doi:10.1016/j.immuni.2004.06.014
16. Tang A, Amagai M, Granger LG, Stanley JR, Udey MC. Adhesion of epidermal langerhans cells to keratinocytes mediated by e-cadherin. *Nature* (1993) **361**(6407):82–5. doi:10.1038/361082a0
17. Jiang A, Bloom O, Ono S, Cui W, Unternaehrer J, Jiang S, et al. Disruption of e-cadherin-mediated adhesion induces a functionally distinct pathway of dendritic cell maturation. *Immunity* (2007) **27**(4):610–24. doi:10.1016/j.immuni.2007.08.015
18. Mellman I, Clausen BE. Immunology. Beta-catenin balances immunity. *Science* (2010) **329**(5993):767–9. doi:10.1126/science.1194185
19. Banchereau J, Steinman RM. Dendritic cells and the control of immunity. *Nature* (1998) **392**(6673):245–52. doi:10.1038/32588
20. Hemmi H, Yoshino M, Yamazaki H, Naito M, Iyoda T, Omatsu Y, et al. Skin antigens in the steady state are trafficked to regional lymph nodes by transforming growth factor-beta1-dependent cells. *Int Immunol* (2001) **13**(5):695–704. doi:10.1093/intimm/13.5.695
21. Weinlich G, Heine M, Stössel H, Zanella M, Stoitzner P, Ortner U, et al. Entry into afferent lymphatics and maturation in situ of migrating

murine cutaneous dendritic cells. *J Invest Dermatol* (1998) **110**(4):441–8. doi:10.1046/j.1523-1747.1998.00161.x

22. Wilson NS, Young LJ, Kupresanin F, Naik SH, Vremec D, Heath WR, et al. Normal proportion and expression of maturation markers in migratory dendritic cells in the absence of germs or toll-like receptor signaling. *Immunol Cell Biol* (2008) **86**(2):200–5. doi:10.1038/sj.icb.7100125
23. Probst HC, Lagnel J, Kollias G, van den Broek M. Inducible transgenic mice reveal resting dendritic cells as potent inducers of CD8+ T cell tolerance. *Immunity* (2003) **18**(5):713–20. doi:10.1016/S1074-7613(03)00120-1
24. Spörri R, Reis e Sousa C. Inflammatory mediators are insufficient for full dendritic cell activation and promote expansion of CD4+ T cell populations lacking helper function. *Nat Immunol* (2005) **6**(2):163–70. doi:10.1038/ni1162
25. Steinman RM, Hawiger D, Nussenzweig MC. Tolerogenic dendritic cells. *Annu Rev Immunol* (2003) **21**:685–711. doi:10.1146/annurev.immunol.21.120601.141040
26. Waithman J, Allan RS, Kosaka H, Azukizawa H, Shortman K, Lutz MB, et al. Skin-derived dendritic cells can mediate deletional tolerance of class i-restricted self-reactive T cells. *J Immunol* (2007) **179**(7):4535–41. doi:10.4049/jimmunol.179.7.4535
27. Hochweller K, Wabnitz GH, Samstag Y, Suffner J, Hämmerling GJ, Garbi N. Dendritic cells control T cell tonic signaling required for responsiveness to foreign antigen. *Proc Natl Acad Sci U S A* (2010) **107**(13):5931–6. doi:10.1073/pnas.0911877107
28. Steinman RM, Cohn ZA. Identification of a novel cell type in peripheral lymphoid organs of mice. I. Morphology, quantitation, tissue distribution. *J Exp Med* (1973) **137**(5):1142–62. doi:10.1084/jem.137.5.1142
29. Langerhans P. Über die nerven der menschlichen haut. *Virchows Arch* (1868) **44**(2):325–37. doi:10.1007/BF01959006
30. Schuler G, Steinman RM. Murine epidermal langerhans cells mature into potent immunostimulatory dendritic cells in vitro. *J Exp Med* (1985) **161**(3):526–46. doi:10.1084/jem.161.3.526
31. Schuler G, Romani N, Steinman RM. A comparison of murine epidermal langerhans cells with spleen dendritic cells. *J Invest Dermatol* (1985) **85**(1 Suppl):99s–106s. doi:10.1111/1523-1747.ep12275566
32. Nussenzweig MC, Steinman RM. Contribution of dendritic cells to stimulation of the murine syngeneic mixed leukocyte reaction. *J Exp Med* (1980) **151**(5):1196–212. doi:10.1084/jem.151.5.1196
33. Steinman RM, Witmer MD. Lymphoid dendritic cells are potent stimulators of the primary mixed leukocyte reaction in mice. *Proc Natl Acad Sci U S A* (1978) **75**(10):5132–6. doi:10.1073/pnas.75.10.5132
34. Steinman RM, Gutchinov B, Witmer MD, Nussenzweig MC. Dendritic cells are the principal stimulators of the primary mixed leukocyte reaction in mice. *J Exp Med* (1983) **157**(2):613–27. doi:10.1084/jem.157.2.613
35. Tamoutounour S, Guilliams M, Montanana Sanchis F, Liu H, Terhorst D, Malosse C, et al. Origins and functional specialization of macrophages and of conventional and monocyte-derived dendritic cells in mouse skin. *Immunity* (2013) **39**(5):925–38. doi:10.1016/j.immuni.2013.10.004
36. Wilson NS, Villadangos JA. Lymphoid organ dendritic cells: beyond the langerhans cells paradigm. *Immunol Cell Biol* (2004) **82**(1):91–8. doi:10.1111/j.1440-1711.2004.01216.x
37. Romani N, Clausen BE, Stoitzner P. Langerhans cells and more: langerin-expressing dendritic cell subsets in the skin. *Immunol Rev* (2010) **234**(1):120–41. doi:10.1111/j.0105-2896.2009.00886.x
38. Stoitzner P, Pfaller K, Stössel H, Romani N. A close-up view of migrating langerhans cells in the skin. *J Invest Dermatol* (2002) **118**(1):117–25. doi:10.1046/j.0022-202x.2001.01631.x
39. Takahara K, Omatsu Y, Yashima Y, Maeda Y, Tanaka S, Iyoda T, et al. Identification and expression of mouse langerin (CD207) in dendritic cells. *Int Immunol* (2002) **14**(5):433–44. doi:10.1093/intimm/14.5.433
40. Valladeau J, Ravel O, Dezutter-Dambuyant C, Moore K, Kleijmeer M, Liu Y, et al. Langerin, a novel c-type lectin specific to langerhans cells, is an endocytic receptor that induces the formation of birbeck granules. *Immunity* (2000) **12**(1):71–81. doi:10.1016/S1074-7613(00)80160-0
41. Valladeau J, Clair-Moninot V, Dezutter-Dambuyant C, Pin JJ, Kissenpfennig A, Mattéi MG, et al. Identification of mouse langerin/CD207 in langerhans cells and some dendritic cells of lymphoid tissues. *J Immunol* (2002) **168**(2):782–92. doi:10.4049/jimmunol.168.2.782
42. Cheong C, Idoyaga J, Do Y, Pack M, Park SH, Lee H, et al. Production of monoclonal antibodies that recognize the extracellular domain of mouse langerin/CD207. *J Immunol Methods* (2007) **324**(1–2):48–62. doi:10.1016/j.jim.2007.05.001
43. Stoitzner P, Holzmann S, McLellan AD, Ivarsson L, Stössel H, Kapp M, et al. Visualization and characterization of migratory langerhans cells in murine skin and lymph nodes by antibodies against langerin/CD207. *J Invest Dermatol* (2003) **120**(2):266–74. doi:10.1046/j.1523-1747.2003.12042.x
44. Bennett CL, van Rijn E, Jung S, Inaba K, Steinman RM, Kapsenberg ML, et al. Inducible ablation of mouse langerhans cells diminishes but fails to abrogate contact hypersensitivity. *J Cell Biol* (2005) **169**(4):569–76. doi:10.1083/jcb.200501071
45. Kaplan DH, Jenison MC, Saeland S, Shlomchik WD, Shlomchik MJ. Epidermal langerhans cell-deficient mice develop enhanced contact hypersensitivity. *Immunity* (2005) **23**(6):611–20. doi:10.1016/j.immuni.2005.10.008
46. Kissenpfennig A, Henri S, Dubois B, Laplace-Builhé C, Perrin P, Romani N, et al. Dynamics and function of langerhans cells in vivo: dermal dendritic cells colonize lymph node areas distinct from slower migrating langerhans cells. *Immunity* (2005) **22**(5):643–54. doi:10.1016/j.immuni.2005.04.004
47. Bursch LS, Wang L, Igyarto B, Kissenpfennig A, Malissen B, Kaplan DH, et al. Identification of a novel population of langerin+ dendritic cells. *J Exp Med* (2007) **204**(13):3147–56. doi:10.1084/jem.20071966
48. Ginhoux F, Collin MP, Bogunovic M, Abel M, Leboeuf M, Helft J, et al. Blood-derived dermal langerin+ dendritic cells survey the skin in the steady state. *J Exp Med* (2007) **204**(13):3133–46. doi:10.1084/jem.20071733
49. Poulin LF, Henri S, de Bovis B, Devilard E, Kissenpfennig A, Malissen B. The dermis contains langerin+ dendritic cells that develop and function independently of epidermal langerhans cells. *J Exp Med* (2007) **204**(13):3119–31. doi:10.1084/jem.20071724
50. Henri S, Guilliams M, Poulin LF, Tamoutounour S, Ardouin L, Dalod M, et al. Disentangling the complexity of the skin dendritic cell network. *Immunol Cell Biol* (2010) **88**(4):366–75. doi:10.1038/icb.2010.34
51. Henri S, Poulin LF, Tamoutounour S, Ardouin L, Guilliams M, de Bovis B, et al. CD207+ CD103+ dermal dendritic cells cross-present keratinocyte-derived antigens irrespective of the presence of langerhans cells. *J Exp Med* (2010) **207**(1):189–206. doi:10.1084/jem.20091964
52. Bachem A, Hartung E, Güttler S, Mora A, Zhou X, Hegemann A, et al. Expression of XCR1 characterizes the batf3-dependent lineage of dendritic cells capable of antigen cross-presentation. *Front Immunol* (2012) **3**:214. doi:10.3389/fimmu.2012.00214
53. Crozat K, Tamoutounour S, Vu Manh TP, Fossum E, Luche H, Ardouin L, et al. Cutting edge: expression of XCR1 defines mouse lymphoid-tissue resident and migratory dendritic cells of the cd8α+ type. *J Immunol* (2011) **187**(9):4411–5. doi:10.4049/jimmunol.1101717
54. Merad M, Manz MG, Karsunky H, Wagers A, Peters W, Charo I, et al. Langerhans cells renew in the skin throughout life under steady-state conditions. *Nat Immunol* (2002) **3**(12):1135–41. doi:10.1038/ni852
55. Kanitakis J, Morelon E, Petruzzo P, Badet L, Dubernard JM. Self-renewal capacity of human epidermal langerhans cells: observations made on a composite tissue allograft. *Exp Dermatol* (2011) **20**(2):145–6. doi:10.1111/j.1600-0625.2010.01146.x
56. Ginhoux F, Tacke F, Angeli V, Bogunovic M, Loubeau M, Dai XM, et al. Langerhans cells arise from monocytes in vivo. *Nat Immunol* (2006) **7**(3):265–73. doi:10.1038/ni1307
57. Nagao K, Kobayashi T, Moro K, Ohyama M, Adachi T, Kitashima DY, et al. Stress-induced production of chemokines by hair follicles regulates the trafficking of dendritic cells in skin. *Nat Immunol* (2012) **13**(8):744–52. doi:10.1038/ni.2353
58. Seré K, Baek JH, Ober-Blöbaum J, Müller-Newen G, Tacke F, Yokota Y, et al. Two distinct types of langerhans cells populate the skin during steady state and inflammation. *Immunity* (2012) **37**(5):905–16. doi:10.1016/j.immuni.2012.07.019
59. Sparber F, Scheffler JM, Amberg N, Tripp CH, Heib V, Hermann M, et al. The late endosomal adaptor molecule p14 (LAMTOR2) represents a novel regulator of langerhans cell homeostasis. *Blood* (2014) **123**(2):217–27. doi:10.1182/blood-2013-08-518555

60. Geissmann F, Manz MG, Jung S, Sieweke MH, Merad M, Ley K. Development of monocytes, macrophages, and dendritic cells. *Science* (2010) **327**(5966):656–61. doi:10.1126/science.1178331
61. Hoeffel G, Wang Y, Greter M, See P, Teo P, Malleret B, et al. Adult langerhans cells derive predominantly from embryonic fetal liver monocytes with a minor contribution of yolk sac-derived macrophages. *J Exp Med* (2012) **209**(6):1167–81. doi:10.1084/jem.20120340
62. Chorro L, Sarde A, Li M, Woollard KJ, Chambon P, Malissen B, et al. Langerhans cell (LC) proliferation mediates neonatal development, homeostasis, and inflammation-associated expansion of the epidermal LC network. *J Exp Med* (2009) **206**(13):3089–100. doi:10.1084/jem.20091586
63. Tripp CH, Chang-Rodriguez S, Stoitzner P, Holzmann S, Stössel H, Douillard P, et al. Ontogeny of langerin/CD207 expression in the epidermis of mice. *J Invest Dermatol* (2004) **122**(3):670–2. doi:10.1111/j.0022-202X.2004.22337.x
64. Ginhoux F, Liu K, Helft J, Bogunovic M, Greter M, Hashimoto D, et al. The origin and development of nonlymphoid tissue CD103+ dcs. *J Exp Med* (2009) **206**(13):3115–30. doi:10.1084/jem.20091756
65. Greter M, Lelios I, Pelczar P, Hoeffel G, Price J, Leboeuf M, et al. Stroma-derived interleukin-34 controls the development and maintenance of langerhans cells and the maintenance of microglia. *Immunity* (2012) **37**(6):1050–60. doi:10.1016/j.immuni.2012.11.001
66. Wang Y, Szretter KJ, Vermi W, Gilfillan S, Rossini C, Cella M, et al. IL-34 is a tissue-restricted ligand of CSF1R required for the development of langerhans cells and microglia. *Nat Immunol* (2012) **13**(8):753–60. doi:10.1038/ni.2360
67. Guilliams M, Ginhoux F, Jakubzick C, Naik SH, Onai N, Schraml BU, et al. Dendritic cells, monocytes and macrophages: a unified nomenclature based on ontogeny. *Nat Rev Immunol* (2014) **14**(8):571–8. doi:10.1038/nri3712
68. Satpathy AT, Wu X, Albring JC, Murphy KM. Re(de)fining the dendritic cell lineage. *Nat Immunol* (2012) **13**(12):1145–54. doi:10.1038/ni.2467
69. Mellman I, Steinman RM. Dendritic cells: specialized and regulated antigen processing machines. *Cell* (2001) **106**(3):255–8. doi:10.1016/S0092-8674(01)00449-4
70. Steinman RM, Cohn ZA. Identification of a novel cell type in peripheral lymphoid organs of mice. II. Functional properties in vitro. *J Exp Med* (1974) **139**(2):380–97. doi:10.1084/jem.139.6.1431
71. Witmer-Pack MD, Crowley MT, Inaba K, Steinman RM. Macrophages, but not dendritic cells, accumulate colloidal carbon following administration in situ. *J Cell Sci* (1993) **105**(Pt 4):965–73.
72. Borkowski TA, Letterio JJ, Farr AG, Udey MC. A role for endogenous transforming growth factor beta 1 in langerhans cell biology: the skin of transforming growth factor beta 1 null mice is devoid of epidermal langerhans cells. *J Exp Med* (1996) **184**(6):2417–22. doi:10.1084/jem.184.6.2417
73. Kaplan DH, Li MO, Jenison MC, Shlomchik WD, Flavell RA, Shlomchik MJ. Autocrine/paracrine tgfbeta1 is required for the development of epidermal langerhans cells. *J Exp Med* (2007) **204**(11):2545–52. doi:10.1084/jem.20071401
74. Bobr A, Igyarto BZ, Haley KM, Li MO, Flavell RA, Kaplan DH. Autocrine/paracrine tgf-β1 inhibits langerhans cell migration. *Proc Natl Acad Sci U S A* (2012) **109**(26):10492–7. doi:10.1073/pnas.1119178109
75. Kel JM, Girard-Madoux MJ, Reizis B, Clausen BE. TGF-beta is required to maintain the pool of immature langerhans cells in the epidermis. *J Immunol* (2010) **185**(6):3248–55. doi:10.4049/jimmunol.1000981
76. Chopin M, Seillet C, Chevrier S, Wu L, Wang H, Morse HC, et al. Langerhans cells are generated by two distinct PU.1-dependent transcriptional networks. *J Exp Med* (2013) **210**(13):2967–80. doi:10.1084/jem.20130930
77. Fainaru O, Woolf E, Lotem J, Yarmus M, Brenner O, Goldenberg D, et al. Runx3 regulates mouse tgf-beta-mediated dendritic cell function and its absence results in airway inflammation. *EMBO J* (2004) **23**(4):969–79. doi:10.1038/sj.emboj.7600085
78. Hacker C, Kirsch RD, Ju XS, Hieronymus T, Gust TC, Kuhl C, et al. Transcriptional profiling identifies id2 function in dendritic cell development. *Nat Immunol* (2003) **4**(4):380–6. doi:10.1038/ni903
79. Liu K, Victora GD, Schwickert TA, Guermonprez P, Meredith MM, Yao K, et al. In vivo analysis of dendritic cell development and homeostasis. *Science* (2009) **324**(5925):392–7. doi:10.1126/science.1170540
80. Maraskovsky E, Brasel K, Teepe M, Roux ER, Lyman SD, Shortman K, et al. Dramatic increase in the numbers of functionally mature dendritic cells in flt3 ligand-treated mice: multiple dendritic cell subpopulations identified. *J Exp Med* (1996) **184**(5):1953–62. doi:10.1084/jem.184.5.1953
81. Waskow C, Liu K, Darrasse-Jèze G, Guermonprez P, Ginhoux F, Merad M, et al. The receptor tyrosine kinase flt3 is required for dendritic cell development in peripheral lymphoid tissues. *Nat Immunol* (2008) **9**(6):676–83. doi:10.1038/ni.1615
82. Mollah SA, Dobrin JS, Feder RE, Tse SW, Matos IG, Cheong C, et al. Flt3L dependence helps define an uncharacterized subset of murine cutaneous dendritic cells. *J Invest Dermatol* (2014) **134**(5):1265–75. doi:10.1038/jid.2013.515
83. Vremec D, Lieschke GJ, Dunn AR, Robb L, Metcalf D, Shortman K. The influence of granulocyte/macrophage colony-stimulating factor on dendritic cell levels in mouse lymphoid organs. *Eur J Immunol* (1997) **27**(1):40–4. doi:10.1002/eji.1830270107
84. Greter M, Helft J, Chow A, Hashimoto D, Mortha A, Agudo-Cantero J, et al. GM-CSF controls nonlymphoid tissue dendritic cell homeostasis but is dispensable for the differentiation of inflammatory dendritic cells. *Immunity* (2012) **36**(6):1031–46. doi:10.1016/j.immuni.2012.03.027
85. Kingston D, Schmid MA, Onai N, Obata-Onai A, Baumjohann D, Manz MG. The concerted action of GM-CSF and flt3-ligand on in vivo dendritic cell homeostasis. *Blood* (2009) **114**(4):835–43. doi:10.1182/blood-2009-02-206318
86. Witmer-Pack MD, Hughes DA, Schuler G, Lawson L, McWilliam A, Inaba K, et al. Identification of macrophages and dendritic cells in the osteopetrotic (op/op) mouse. *J Cell Sci* (1993) **104**(Pt 4):1021–9.
87. Ichikawa E, Hida S, Omatsu Y, Shimoyama S, Takahara K, Miyagawa S, et al. Defective development of splenic and epidermal CD4+ dendritic cells in mice deficient for IFN regulatory factor-2. *Proc Natl Acad Sci U S A* (2004) **101**(11):3909–14. doi:10.1073/pnas.0400610101
88. Akbari M, Honma K, Kimura D, Miyakoda M, Kimura K, Matsuyama T, et al. IRF4 in dendritic cells inhibits IL-12 production and controls th1 immune responses against leishmania major. *J Immunol* (2014) **192**(5):2271–9. doi:10.4049/jimmunol.1301914
89. Bajaña S, Roach K, Turner S, Paul J, Kovats S. IRF4 promotes cutaneous dendritic cell migration to lymph nodes during homeostasis and inflammation. *J Immunol* (2012) **189**(7):3368–77. doi:10.4049/jimmunol.1102613
90. Suzuki S, Honma K, Matsuyama T, Suzuki K, Toriyama K, Akitoyo I, et al. Critical roles of interferon regulatory factor 4 in cd11bhighcd8alpha- dendritic cell development. *Proc Natl Acad Sci U S A* (2004) **101**(24):8981–6. doi:10.1073/pnas.0402139101
91. Edelson BT, KC W, Juang R, Kohyama M, Benoit LA, Klekotka PA, et al. Peripheral CD103+ dendritic cells form a unified subset developmentally related to cd8alpha+ conventional dendritic cells. *J Exp Med* (2010) **207**(4):823–36. doi:10.1084/jem.20091627
92. Naik S, Bouladoux N, Linehan JL, Han SJ, Harrison OJ, Wilhelm C, et al. Commensal-dendritic-cell interaction specifies a unique protective skin immune signature. *Nature* (2015) **520**(7545):104–8. doi:10.1038/nature14052
93. Tamura T, Tailor P, Yamaoka K, Kong HJ, Tsujimura H, O'Shea JJ, et al. IFN regulatory factor-4 and -8 govern dendritic cell subset development and their functional diversity. *J Immunol* (2005) **174**(5):2573–81. doi:10.4049/jimmunol.174.5.2573
94. Schiavoni G, Mattei F, Sestili P, Borghi P, Venditti M, Morse HC, et al. ICSBP is essential for the development of mouse type I interferon-producing cells and for the generation and activation of cd8alpha(+) dendritic cells. *J Exp Med* (2002) **196**(11):1415–25. doi:10.1084/jem.20021263
95. Mattei F, Schiavoni G, Borghi P, Venditti M, Canini I, Sestili P, et al. ICSBP/IRF-8 differentially regulates antigen uptake during dendritic-cell development and affects antigen presentation to CD4+ T cells. *Blood* (2006) **108**(2):609–17. doi:10.1182/blood-2005-11-4490
96. Schiavoni G, Mattei F, Borghi P, Sestili P, Venditti M, Morse HC, et al. ICSBP is critically involved in the normal development and trafficking of langerhans cells and dermal dendritic cells. *Blood* (2004) **103**(6):2221–8. doi:10.1182/blood-2003-09-3007
97. Orabona C, Puccetti P, Vacca C, Bicciato S, Luchini A, Fallarino F, et al. Toward the identification of a tolerogenic signature in ido-competent dendritic cells. *Blood* (2006) **107**(7):2846–54. doi:10.1182/blood-2005-10-4077
98. Edelson BT, Bradstreet TR, KC W, Hildner K, Herzog JW, Sim J, et al. Batf3-dependent cd11b(low/-) peripheral dendritic cells are gm-csf-independent and are not required for th cell priming after subcutaneous immunization. *PLoS One* (2011) **6**(10):e25660. doi:10.1371/journal.pone.0025660

99. Meredith MM, Liu K, Darrasse-Jeze G, Kamphorst AO, Schreiber HA, Guermonprez P, et al. Expression of the zinc finger transcription factor zdc (zbtb46, btbd4) defines the classical dendritic cell lineage. *J Exp Med* (2012) **209**(6):1153–65. doi:10.1084/jem.20112675
100. Satpathy AT, KC W, Albring JC, Edelson BT, Kretzer NM, Bhattacharya D, et al. Zbtb46 expression distinguishes classical dendritic cells and their committed progenitors from other immune lineages. *J Exp Med* (2012) **209**(6):1135–52. doi:10.1084/jem.20120030
101. Sparber F, Tripp CH, Komenda K, Scheffler JM, Clausen BE, Huber LA, et al. The late endosomal adaptor molecule p14 (LAMTOR2) regulates tgfβ1-mediated homeostasis of langerhans cells. *J Invest Dermatol* (2014) **135**(1):119–29. doi:10.1038/jid.2014.324
102. Honda T, Egawa G, Grabbe S, Kabashima K. Update of immune events in the murine contact hypersensitivity model: toward the understanding of allergic contact dermatitis. *J Invest Dermatol* (2013) **133**(2):303–15. doi:10.1038/jid.2012.284
103. Kaplan DH, Igyártó BZ, Gaspari AA. Early immune events in the induction of allergic contact dermatitis. *Nat Rev Immunol* (2012) **12**(2):114–24. doi:10.1038/nri3150
104. Bennett CL, Noordegraaf M, Martina CA, Clausen BE. Langerhans cells are required for efficient presentation of topically applied hapten to T cells. *J Immunol* (2007) **179**(10):6830–5. doi:10.4049/jimmunol.179.10.6830
105. Noordegraaf M, Flacher V, Stoitzner P, Clausen BE. Functional redundancy of langerhans cells and langerin+ dermal dendritic cells in contact hypersensitivity. *J Invest Dermatol* (2010) **130**(12):2752–9. doi:10.1038/jid.2010.223
106. Honda T, Nakajima S, Egawa G, Ogasawara K, Malissen B, Miyachi Y, et al. Compensatory role of langerhans cells and langerin-positive dermal dendritic cells in the sensitization phase of murine contact hypersensitivity. *J Allergy Clin Immunol* (2010) **125**(5):1154.e–6.e. doi:10.1016/j.jaci.2009.12.005
107. Bobr A, Olvera-Gomez I, Igyarto BZ, Haley KM, Hogquist KA, Kaplan DH. Acute ablation of langerhans cells enhances skin immune responses. *J Immunol* (2010) **185**(8):4724–8. doi:10.4049/jimmunol.1001802
108. Zahner SP, Kel JM, Martina CA, Brouwers-Haspels I, van Roon MA, Clausen BE. Conditional deletion of tgf-βr1 using langerin-cre mice results in langerhans cell deficiency and reduced contact hypersensitivity. *J Immunol* (2011) **187**(10):5069–76. doi:10.4049/jimmunol.1101880
109. Bacci S, Alard P, Dai R, Nakamura T, Streilein JW. High and low doses of haptens dictate whether dermal or epidermal antigen-presenting cells promote contact hypersensitivity. *Eur J Immunol* (1997) **27**(2):442–8. doi:10.1002/eji.1830270214
110. Clausen BE, Kel JM. Langerhans cells: critical regulators of skin immunity? *Immunol Cell Biol* (2010) **88**(4):351–60. doi:10.1038/icb.2010.40
111. Kaplan DH, Kissenpfennig A, Clausen BE. Insights into langerhans cell function from langerhans cell ablation models. *Eur J Immunol* (2008) **38**(9):2369–76. doi:10.1002/eji.200838397
112. Stoitzner P, Tripp CH, Douillard P, Saeland S, Romani N. Migratory langerhans cells in mouse lymph nodes in steady state and inflammation. *J Invest Dermatol* (2005) **125**(1):116–25. doi:10.1111/j.0022-202X.2005.23757.x
113. Bennett CL, Clausen BE. DC ablation in mice: promises, pitfalls, and challenges. *Trends Immunol* (2007) **28**(12):525–31. doi:10.1016/j.it.2007.08.011
114. Allan RS, Smith CM, Belz GT, van Lint AL, Wakim LM, Heath WR, et al. Epidermal viral immunity induced by cd8alpha+ dendritic cells but not by langerhans cells. *Science* (2003) **301**(5641):1925–8. doi:10.1126/science.1087576
115. Allan RS, Waithman J, Bedoui S, Jones CM, Villadangos JA, Zhan Y, et al. Migratory dendritic cells transfer antigen to a lymph node-resident dendritic cell population for efficient CTL priming. *Immunity* (2006) **25**(1):153–62. doi:10.1016/j.immuni.2006.04.017
116. Zhao X, Deak E, Soderberg K, Linehan M, Spezzano D, Zhu J, et al. Vaginal submucosal dendritic cells, but not langerhans cells, induce protective th1 responses to herpes simplex virus-2. *J Exp Med* (2003) **197**(2):153–62. doi:10.1084/jem.20021109
117. Bosnjak L, Miranda-Saksena M, Koelle DM, Boadle RA, Jones CA, Cunningham AL. Herpes simplex virus infection of human dendritic cells induces apoptosis and allows cross-presentation via uninfected dendritic cells. *J Immunol* (2005) **174**(4):2220–7. doi:10.4049/jimmunol.174.4.2220
118. Jones CA, Fernandez M, Herc K, Bosnjak L, Miranda-Saksena M, Boadle RA, et al. Herpes simplex virus type 2 induces rapid cell death and functional impairment of murine dendritic cells in vitro. *J Virol* (2003) **77**(20):11139–49. doi:10.1128/JVI.77.20.11139-11149.2003
119. Carbone FR, Belz GT, Heath WR. Transfer of antigen between migrating and lymph node-resident dcs in peripheral t-cell tolerance and immunity. *Trends Immunol* (2004) **25**(12):655–8. doi:10.1016/j.it.2004.09.013
120. He Y, Zhang J, Donahue C, Falo LD. Skin-derived dendritic cells induce potent CD8(+) T cell immunity in recombinant lentivector-mediated genetic immunization. *Immunity* (2006) **24**(5):643–56. doi:10.1016/j.immuni.2006.03.014
121. Bedoui S, Whitney PG, Waithman J, Eidsmo L, Wakim L, Caminschi I, et al. Cross-presentation of viral and self antigens by skin-derived CD103+ dendritic cells. *Nat Immunol* (2009) **10**(5):488–95. doi:10.1038/ni.1724
122. Bedoui S, Greyer M. The role of dendritic cells in immunity against primary herpes simplex virus infections. *Front Microbiol* (2014) **5**:533. doi:10.3389/fmicb.2014.00533
123. Moll H, Fuchs H, Blank C, Röllinghoff M. Langerhans cells transport leishmania major from the infected skin to the draining lymph node for presentation to antigen-specific T cells. *Eur J Immunol* (1993) **23**(7):1595–601. doi:10.1002/eji.1830230730
124. Ritter U, Meissner A, Scheidig C, Körner H. CD8 alpha- and langerin-negative dendritic cells, but not langerhans cells, act as principal antigen-presenting cells in leishmaniasis. *Eur J Immunol* (2004) **34**(6):1542–50. doi:10.1002/eji.200324586
125. Kautz-Neu K, Meyer RG, Clausen BE, von Stebut E. Leishmaniasis, contact hypersensitivity and graft-versus-host disease: understanding the role of dendritic cell subsets in balancing skin immunity and tolerance. *Exp Dermatol* (2010) **19**(8):760–71. doi:10.1111/j.1600-0625.2010.01116.x
126. Kautz-Neu K, Schwonberg K, Fischer MR, Schermann AI, von Stebut E. Dendritic cells in leishmania major infections: mechanisms of parasite uptake, cell activation and evidence for physiological relevance. *Med Microbiol Immunol* (2012) **201**(4):581–92. doi:10.1007/s00430-012-0261-2
127. Brewig N, Kissenpfennig A, Malissen B, Veit A, Bickert T, Fleischer B, et al. Priming of CD8+ and CD4+ T cells in experimental leishmaniasis is initiated by different dendritic cell subtypes. *J Immunol* (2009) **182**(2):774–83. doi:10.4049/jimmunol.182.2.774
128. Reinhardt RL, Liang HE, Locksley RM. Cytokine-secreting follicular T cells shape the antibody repertoire. *Nat Immunol* (2009) **10**(4):385–93. doi:10.1038/ni.1715
129. Zimara N, Florian C, Schmid M, Malissen B, Kissenpfennig A, Männel DN, et al. Langerhans cells promote early germinal center formation in response to leishmania-derived cutaneous antigens. *Eur J Immunol* (2014) **44**(10):2955–67. doi:10.1002/eji.201344263
130. Kautz-Neu K, Noordegraaf M, Dinges S, Bennett CL, John D, Clausen BE, et al. Langerhans cells are negative regulators of the anti-leishmania response. *J Exp Med* (2011) **208**(5):885–91. doi:10.1084/jem.20102318
131. Buch T, Heppner FL, Tertilt C, Heinen TJ, Kremer M, Wunderlich FT, et al. A cre-inducible diphtheria toxin receptor mediates cell lineage ablation after toxin administration. *Nat Methods* (2005) **2**(6):419–26. doi:10.1038/nmeth762
132. Belkaid Y, Hoffmann KF, Mendez S, Kamhawi S, Udey MC, Wynn TA, et al. The role of interleukin (IL)-10 in the persistence of leishmania major in the skin after healing and the therapeutic potential of anti-il-10 receptor antibody for sterile cure. *J Exp Med* (2001) **194**(10):1497–506. doi:10.1084/jem.194.10.1497
133. Belkaid Y, Piccirillo CA, Mendez S, Shevach EM, Sacks DL. CD4+CD25+ regulatory T cells control leishmania major persistence and immunity. *Nature* (2002) **420**(6915):502–7. doi:10.1038/nature01152
134. Gow NA, van de Veerdonk FL, Brown AJ, Netea MG. *Candida albicans* morphogenesis and host defence: discriminating invasion from colonization. *Nat Rev Microbiol* (2012) **10**(2):112–22. doi:10.1038/nrmicro2711
135. Lo HJ, Köhler JR, DiDomenico B, Loebenberg D, Cacciapuoti A, Fink GR, et al. *Albicans* mutants are avirulent. *Cell* (1997) **90**(5):939–49. doi:10.1016/S0092-8674(00)80358-X
136. Bär E, Whitney PG, Moor K, Reis e Sousa C, LeibundGut-Landmann S. IL-17 regulates systemic fungal immunity by controlling the functional competence of NK cells. *Immunity* (2014) **40**(1):117–27. doi:10.1016/j.immuni.2013.12.002
137. Igyártó BZ, Haley K, Ortner D, Bobr A, Gerami-Nejad M, Edelson BT, et al. Skin-resident murine dendritic cell subsets promote distinct and opposing

antigen-specific T helper cell responses. *Immunity* (2011) **35**(2):260–72. doi:10.1016/j.immuni.2011.06.005

138. Kashem SW, Igyártó BZ, Gerami-Nejad M, Kumamoto Y, Mohammed J, Jarrett E, et al. *Candida albicans* morphology and dendritic cell subsets determine T helper cell differentiation. *Immunity* (2015) **42**(2):356–66. doi:10.1016/j.immuni.2015.01.008
139. Naik S, Bouladoux N, Wilhelm C, Molloy MJ, Salcedo R, Kastenmuller W, et al. Compartmentalized control of skin immunity by resident commensals. *Science* (2012) **337**(6098):1115–9. doi:10.1126/science.1225152
140. Seneschal J, Jiang X, Kupper TS. Langerin+ dermal DC, but not langerhans cells, are required for effective cd8-mediated immune responses after skin scarification with vaccinia virus. *J Invest Dermatol* (2014) **134**(3):686–94. doi:10.1038/jid.2013.418
141. Kim M, Truong NR, James V, Bosnjak L, Sandgren KJ, Harman AN, et al. Relay of herpes simplex virus between langerhans cells and dermal dendritic cells in human skin. *PLoS Pathog* (2015) **11**(4):e1004812. doi:10.1371/journal.ppat.1004812
142. Puttur FK, Fernandez MA, White R, Roediger B, Cunningham AL, Weninger W, et al. Herpes simplex virus infects skin gamma delta T cells before langerhans cells and impedes migration of infected langerhans cells by inducing apoptosis and blocking e-cadherin downregulation. *J Immunol* (2010) **185**(1):477–87. doi:10.4049/jimmunol.0904106
143. Azukizawa H, Kosaka H, Sano S, Heath WR, Takahashi I, Gao XH, et al. Induction of t-cell-mediated skin disease specific for antigen transgenically expressed in keratinocytes. *Eur J Immunol* (2003) **33**(7):1879–88. doi:10.1002/eji.200323630
144. Holcmann M, Stoitzner P, Drobits B, Luehrs P, Stingl G, Romani N, et al. Skin inflammation is not sufficient to break tolerance induced against a novel antigen. *J Immunol* (2009) **183**(2):1133–43. doi:10.4049/jimmunol.0713351
145. Shibaki A, Sato A, Vogel JC, Miyagawa F, Katz SI. Induction of gvhd-like skin disease by passively transferred CD8(+) t-cell receptor transgenic T cells into keratin 14-ovalbumin transgenic mice. *J Invest Dermatol* (2004) **123**(1):109–15. doi:10.1111/j.0022-202X.2004.22701.x
146. Bursch LS, Rich BE, Hogquist KA. Langerhans cells are not required for the CD8 T cell response to epidermal self-antigens. *J Immunol* (2009) **182**(8):4657–64. doi:10.4049/jimmunol.0803656
147. Kim BS, Miyagawa F, Cho YH, Bennett CL, Clausen BE, Katz SI. Keratinocytes function as accessory cells for presentation of endogenous antigen expressed in the epidermis. *J Invest Dermatol* (2009) **129**(12):2805–17. doi:10.1038/jid.2009.176
148. Stoitzner P, Tripp CH, Eberhart A, Price KM, Jung JY, Bursch L, et al. Langerhans cells cross-present antigen derived from skin. *Proc Natl Acad Sci U S A* (2006) **103**(20):7783–8. doi:10.1073/pnas.0509307103
149. Kurokawa I, Takahashi K, Moll I, Moll R. Expression of keratins in cutaneous epithelial tumors and related disorders – distribution and clinical significance. *Exp Dermatol* (2011) **20**(3):217–28. doi:10.1111/j.1600-0625.2009.01006.x
150. Grubauer G, Romani N, Kofler H, Stanzl U, Fritsch P, Hintner H. Apoptotic keratin bodies as autoantigen causing the production of igm-anti-keratin intermediate filament autoantibodies. *J Invest Dermatol* (1986) **87**(4):466–71. doi:10.1111/1523-1747.ep12455510
151. Holzmann S, Tripp CH, Schmuth M, Janke K, Koch F, Saeland S, et al. A model system using tape stripping for characterization of langerhans cell-precursors in vivo. *J Invest Dermatol* (2004) **122**(5):1165–74. doi:10.1111/j.0022-202X.2004.22520.x
152. Randolph GJ, Ochando J, Partida-Sánchez S. Migration of dendritic cell subsets and their precursors. *Annu Rev Immunol* (2008) **26**:293–316. doi:10.1146/annurev.immunol.26.021607.090254
153. Stoitzner P, Green LK, Jung JY, Price KM, Tripp CH, Malissen B, et al. Tumor immunotherapy by epicutaneous immunization requires langerhans cells. *J Immunol* (2008) **180**(3):1991–8. doi:10.4049/jimmunol.180.3.1991
154. Zaric M, Lyubomska O, Poux C, Hanna ML, McCrudden MT, Malissen B, et al. Dissolving microneedle delivery of nanoparticle-encapsulated antigen elicits efficient cross-priming and th1 immune responses by murine langerhans cells. *J Invest Dermatol* (2015) **135**(2):425–34. doi:10.1038/jid.2014.415
155. Flacher V, Tripp CH, Mairhofer DG, Steinman RM, Stoitzner P, Idoyaga J, et al. Murine langerin+ dermal dendritic cells prime CD8+ T cells while langerhans cells induce cross-tolerance. *EMBO Mol Med* (2014) **6**(9):1191–204. doi:10.15252/emmm.201303283
156. Karthaus N, Torensma R, Tel J. Deciphering the message broadcast by tumor-infiltrating dendritic cells. *Am J Pathol* (2012) **181**(3):733–42. doi:10.1016/j.ajpath.2012.05.012
157. Yanofsky VR, Mitsui H, Felsen D, Carucci JA. Understanding dendritic cells and their role in cutaneous carcinoma and cancer immunotherapy. *Clin Dev Immunol* (2013) **2013**:624123. doi:10.1155/2013/624123
158. Hargadon KM. Tumor-altered dendritic cell function: implications for anti-tumor immunity. *Front Immunol* (2013) **4**:192. doi:10.3389/fimmu.2013.00192
159. Bluth MJ, Zaba LC, Moussai D, Suárez-Fariñas M, Kaporis H, Fan L, et al. Myeloid dendritic cells from human cutaneous squamous cell carcinoma are poor stimulators of t-cell proliferation. *J Invest Dermatol* (2009) **129**(10):2451–62. doi:10.1038/jid.2009.96
160. Nestle FO, Burg G, Fäh J, Wrone-Smith T, Nickoloff BJ. Human sunlight-induced basal-cell-carcinoma-associated dendritic cells are deficient in T cell co-stimulatory molecules and are impaired as antigen-presenting cells. *Am J Pathol* (1997) **150**(2):641–51.
161. Fujita H, Suárez-Fariñas M, Mitsui H, Gonzalez J, Bluth MJ, Zhang S, et al. Langerhans cells from human cutaneous squamous cell carcinoma induce strong type 1 immunity. *J Invest Dermatol* (2012) **132**(6):1645–55. doi:10.1038/jid.2012.34
162. Modi BG, Neustadter J, Binda E, Lewis J, Filler RB, Roberts SJ, et al. Langerhans cells facilitate epithelial DNA damage and squamous cell carcinoma. *Science* (2012) **335**(6064):104–8. doi:10.1126/science.1211600
163. Saeki M, Saito Y, Nagano M, Teshima R, Ozawa S, Sawada J. MRNA expression of multiple cytochrome p450 isozymes in four types of cultured skin cells. *Int Arch Allergy Immunol* (2002) **127**(4):333–6. doi:10.1159/000057751
164. Swanson HI. Cytochrome P450 expression in human keratinocytes: an aryl hydrocarbon receptor perspective. *Chem Biol Interact* (2004) **149**(2–3):69–79. doi:10.1016/j.cbi.2004.08.006
165. Lewis JM, Bürgler CD, Fraser JA, Liao H, Golubets K, Kucher CL, et al. Mechanisms of chemical cooperative carcinogenesis by epidermal langerhans cells. *J Invest Dermatol* (2015) **135**(5):1405–14. doi:10.1038/jid.2014.411
166. Clausen BE, Grabbe S. Multifaceted contributions of epidermal langerhans cells to cutaneous carcinogenesis. *J Invest Dermatol* (2015) **135**(5):1218–20. doi:10.1038/jid.2014.520
167. Lewis JM, Bürgler CD, Freudzon M, Golubets K, Gibson JF, Filler RB, et al. Langerhans cells facilitate uvb-induced epidermal carcinogenesis. *J Invest Dermatol* (2015). doi:10.1038/jid.2015.207
168. Schwarz A, Noordegraaf M, Maeda A, Torii K, Clausen BE, Schwarz T. Langerhans cells are required for uvr-induced immunosuppression. *J Invest Dermatol* (2010) **130**(5):1419–27. doi:10.1038/jid.2009.429
169. Elentner A, Ortner D, Clausen BE, Gonzalez FJ, Fernández-Salguero PM, Schmuth M, et al. Skin response to a carcinogen involves the xenobiotic receptor pregnane X receptor. *Exp Dermatol* (2015). doi:10.1111/exd.12766
170. Stene MA, Babajanians M, Bhuta S, Cochran AJ. Quantitative alterations in cutaneous langerhans cells during the evolution of malignant melanoma of the skin. *J Invest Dermatol* (1988) **91**(2):125–8. doi:10.1111/1523-1747.ep12464142
171. Toriyama K, Wen DR, Paul E, Cochran AJ. Variations in the distribution, frequency, and phenotype of langerhans cells during the evolution of malignant melanoma of the skin. *J Invest Dermatol* (1993) **100**(3):269S–73S. doi:10.1111/1523-1747.ep12470135
172. Ishida T, Oyama T, Carbone DP, Gabrilovich DI. Defective function of langerhans cells in tumor-bearing animals is the result of defective maturation from hemopoietic progenitors. *J Immunol* (1998) **161**(9):4842–51.
173. Movassagh M, Spatz A, Davoust J, Lebecque S, Romero P, Pittet M, et al. Selective accumulation of mature dc-lamp+ dendritic cells in tumor sites is associated with efficient t-cell-mediated antitumor response and control of metastatic dissemination in melanoma. *Cancer Res* (2004) **64**(6):2192–8. doi:10.1158/0008-5472.CAN-03-2969
174. Broz ML, Binnewies M, Boldajipour B, Nelson AE, Pollack JL, Erle DJ, et al. Dissecting the tumor myeloid compartment reveals rare activating antigen-presenting cells critical for T cell immunity. *Cancer Cell* (2014) **26**(5):638–52. doi:10.1016/j.ccell.2014.09.007
175. Broz ML, Krummel MF. The emerging understanding of myeloid cells as partners and targets in tumor rejection. *Cancer Immunol Res* (2015) **3**(4):313–9. doi:10.1158/2326-6066.CIR-15-0041

176. Starnes CO. Coley's toxins in perspective. *Nature* (1992) **357**(6373):11–2. doi:10.1038/357011a0
177. Steinman RM. Decisions about dendritic cells: past, present, and future. *Annu Rev Immunol* (2012) **30**:1–22. doi:10.1146/annurev-immunol-100311-102839
178. Steinman RM, Banchereau J. Taking dendritic cells into medicine. *Nature* (2007) **449**(7161):419–26. doi:10.1038/nature06175
179. Hsu FJ, Benike C, Fagnoni F, Liles TM, Czerwinski D, Taidi B, et al. Vaccination of patients with b-cell lymphoma using autologous antigen-pulsed dendritic cells. *Nat Med* (1996) **2**(1):52–8. doi:10.1038/nm0196-52
180. Sharma P, Allison JP. The future of immune checkpoint therapy. *Science* (2015) **348**(6230):56–61. doi:10.1126/science.aaa8172
181. Couzin-Frankel J. Breakthrough of the year 2013. *Cancer Immunother Sci* (2013) **342**(6165):1432–3. doi:10.1126/science.342.6165.1432
182. Delamarre L, Mellman I, Yadav M. Cancer immunotherapy. Neo approaches to cancer vaccines. *Science* (2015) **348**(6236):760–1. doi:10.1126/science.aab3465
183. Topalian SL, Wolchok JD, Chan TA, Mellman I, Palucka K, Banchereau J, et al. Immunotherapy: the path to win the war on cancer? *Cell* (2015) **161**(2):185–6. doi:10.1016/j.cell.2015.03.045
184. Schumacher TN, Schreiber RD. Neoantigens in cancer immunotherapy. *Science* (2015) **348**(6230):69–74. doi:10.1126/science.aaa4971
185. Palucka K, Banchereau J. Dendritic-cell-based therapeutic cancer vaccines. *Immunity* (2013) **39**(1):38–48. doi:10.1016/j.immuni.2013.07.004
186. Carreno BM, Magrini V, Becker-Hapak M, Kaabinejadian S, Hundal J, Petti AA, et al. Cancer immunotherapy. A dendritic cell vaccine increases the breadth and diversity of melanoma neoantigen-specific T cells. *Science* (2015) **348**(6236):803–8. doi:10.1126/science.aaa3828
187. MartIn-Fontecha A, Sebastiani S, Höpken UE, Uguccioni M, Lipp M, Lanzavecchia A, et al. Regulation of dendritic cell migration to the draining lymph node: impact on T lymphocyte traffic and priming. *J Exp Med* (2003) **198**(4):615–21. doi:10.1084/jem.20030448
188. Mitchell DA, Batich KA, Gunn MD, Huang MN, Sanchez-Perez L, Nair SK, et al. Tetanus toxoid and CCL3 improve dendritic cell vaccines in mice and glioblastoma patients. *Nature* (2015) **519**(7543):366–9. doi:10.1038/nature14320
189. Tripp CH, Ebner S, Ratzinger G, Romani N, Stoitzner P. Conditioning of the injection site with cpg enhances the migration of adoptively transferred dendritic cells and endogenous CD8+ t-cell responses. *J Immunother* (2010) **33**(2):115–25. doi:10.1097/CJI.0b013e3181b8ef5f
190. Carmi Y, Spitzer MH, Linde IL, Burt BM, Prestwood TR, Perlman N, et al. Allogeneic igg combined with dendritic cell stimuli induce antitumour t-cell immunity. *Nature* (2015) **521**(7550):99–104. doi:10.1038/nature14424
191. Romano E, Cotari JW, Barreira da Silva R, Betts BC, Chung DJ, Avogadri F, et al. Human langerhans cells use an il-15r-α/IL-15/pstat5-dependent mechanism to break t-cell tolerance against the self-differentiation tumor antigen WT1. *Blood* (2012) **119**(22):5182–90. doi:10.1182/blood-2011-09-382200
192. Hawiger D, Inaba K, Dorsett Y, Guo M, Mahnke K, Rivera M, et al. Dendritic cells induce peripheral T cell unresponsiveness under steady state conditions in vivo. *J Exp Med* (2001) **194**(6):769–79. doi:10.1084/jem.194.6.769
193. Mahnke K, Guo M, Lee S, Sepulveda H, Swain SL, Nussenzweig M, et al. The dendritic cell receptor for endocytosis, DEC-205, can recycle and enhance antigen presentation via major histocompatibility complex class ii-positive lysosomal compartments. *J Cell Biol* (2000) **151**(3):673–84. doi:10.1083/jcb.151.3.673
194. Bonifaz LC, Bonnyay DP, Charalambous A, Darguste DI, Fujii S, Soares H, et al. In vivo targeting of antigens to maturing dendritic cells via the DEC-205 receptor improves T cell vaccination. *J Exp Med* (2004) **199**(6):815–24. doi:10.1084/jem.20032220
195. Romani N, Flacher V, Tripp CH, Sparber F, Ebner S, Stoitzner P. Targeting skin dendritic cells to improve intradermal vaccination. *Curr Top Microbiol Immunol* (2012) **351**:113–38. doi:10.1007/82_2010_118
196. Tacken PJ, de Vries IJ, Torensma R, Figdor CG. Dendritic-cell immunotherapy: from ex vivo loading to in vivo targeting. *Nat Rev Immunol* (2007) **7**(10):790–802. doi:10.1038/nri2173
197. Carter RW, Thompson C, Reid DM, Wong SY, Tough DF. Preferential induction of CD4+ T cell responses through in vivo targeting of antigen to dendritic cell-associated c-type lectin-1. *J Immunol* (2006) **177**(4):2276–84. doi:10.4049/jimmunol.177.4.2276
198. Flacher V, Tripp CH, Haid B, Kissenpfennig A, Malissen B, Stoitzner P, et al. Skin langerin+ dendritic cells transport intradermally injected anti-dec-205 antibodies but are not essential for subsequent cytotoxic CD8+ T cell responses. *J Immunol* (2012) **188**(5):2146–55. doi:10.4049/jimmunol.1004120
199. Idoyaga J, Cheong C, Suda K, Suda N, Kim JY, Lee H, et al. Cutting edge: langerin/CD207 receptor on dendritic cells mediates efficient antigen presentation on MHC I and II products in vivo. *J Immunol* (2008) **180**(6):3647–50. doi:10.4049/jimmunol.180.6.3647
200. Johnson TS, Mahnke K, Storn V, Schönfeld K, Ring S, Nettelbeck DM, et al. Inhibition of melanoma growth by targeting of antigen to dendritic cells via an anti-dec-205 single-chain fragment variable molecule. *Clin Cancer Res* (2008) **14**(24):8169–77. doi:10.1158/1078-0432.CCR-08-1474
201. Mahnke K, Qian Y, Fondel S, Brueck J, Becker C, Enk AH. Targeting of antigens to activated dendritic cells in vivo cures metastatic melanoma in mice. *Cancer Res* (2005) **65**(15):7007–12. doi:10.1158/0008-5472.CAN-05-0938
202. Hartung E, Becker M, Bachem A, Reeg N, Jäkel A, Hutloff A, et al. Induction of potent CD8 T cell cytotoxicity by specific targeting of antigen to cross-presenting dendritic cells in vivo via murine or human XCR1. *J Immunol* (2015) **194**(3):1069–79. doi:10.4049/jimmunol.1401903
203. Terhorst D, Fossum E, Baranska A, Tamoutounour S, Malosse C, Garbani M, et al. Laser-Assisted intradermal delivery of adjuvant-free vaccines targeting XCR1+ dendritic cells induces potent antitumoral responses. *J Immunol* (2015) **194**(12):5895–902. doi:10.4049/jimmunol.1500564
204. Dhodapkar MV, Sznol M, Zhao B, Wang D, Carvajal RD, Keohan ML, et al. Induction of antigen-specific immunity with a vaccine targeting NY-ESO-1 to the dendritic cell receptor DEC-205. *Sci Transl Med* (2014) **6**(232):232ra51. doi:10.1126/scitranslmed.3008068
205. Engelke L, Winter G, Hook S, Engert J. Recent insights into cutaneous immunization: how to vaccinate via the skin. *Vaccine* (2015) **33**(37):4663–74. doi:10.1016/j.vaccine.2015.05.012
206. Stoitzner P, Sparber F, Tripp CH. Langerhans cells as targets for immunotherapy against skin cancer. *Immunol Cell Biol* (2010) **88**(4):431–7. doi:10.1038/icb.2010.31
207. Rechtsteiner G, Warger T, Osterloh P, Schild H, Radsak MP. Cutting edge: priming of CTL by transcutaneous peptide immunization with imiquimod. *J Immunol* (2005) **174**(5):2476–80. doi:10.4049/jimmunol.174.5.2476
208. Seo N, Tokura Y, Nishijima T, Hashizume H, Furukawa F, Takigawa M. Percutaneous peptide immunization via corneum barrier-disrupted murine skin for experimental tumor immunoprophylaxis. *Proc Natl Acad Sci U S A* (2000) **97**(1):371–6. doi:10.1073/pnas.97.1.371
209. Frech SA, Dupont HL, Bourgeois AL, McKenzie R, Belkind-Gerson J, Figueroa JF, et al. Use of a patch containing heat-labile toxin from *Escherichia coli* against travellers' diarrhoea: a phase II, randomised, double-blind, placebo-controlled field trial. *Lancet* (2008) **371**(9629):2019–25. doi:10.1016/S0140-6736(08)60839-9
210. Yagi H, Hashizume H, Horibe T, Yoshinari Y, Hata M, Ohshima A, et al. Induction of therapeutically relevant cytotoxic T lymphocytes in humans by percutaneous peptide immunization. *Cancer Res* (2006) **66**(20):10136–44. doi:10.1158/0008-5472.CAN-06-1029
211. Sullivan SP, Koutsonanos DG, Del Pilar Martin M, Lee JW, Zarnitsyn V, Choi SO, et al. Dissolving polymer microneedle patches for influenza vaccination. *Nat Med* (2010) **16**(8):915–20. doi:10.1038/nm.2182
212. Crozat K, Guiton R, Guilliams M, Henri S, Baranek T, Schwartz-Cornil I, et al. Comparative genomics as a tool to reveal functional equivalences between human and mouse dendritic cell subsets. *Immunol Rev* (2010) **234**(1):177–98. doi:10.1111/j.0105-2896.2009.00868.x
213. Guilliams M, Henri S, Tamoutounour S, Ardouin L, Schwartz-Cornil I, Dalod M, et al. From skin dendritic cells to a simplified classification of human and mouse dendritic cell subsets. *Eur J Immunol* (2010) **40**(8):2089–94. doi:10.1002/eji.201040498
214. Haniffa M, Shin A, Bigley V, McGovern N, Teo P, See P, et al. Human tissues contain cd141hi cross-presenting dendritic cells with functional homology to mouse CD103+ nonlymphoid dendritic cells. *Immunity* (2012) **37**(1):60–73. doi:10.1016/j.immuni.2012.04.012
215. Haniffa M, Gunawan M, Jardine L. Human skin dendritic cells in health and disease. *J Dermatol Sci* (2015) **77**(2):85–92. doi:10.1016/j.jdermsci.2014.08.012

216. McGovern N, Schlitzer A, Gunawan M, Jardine L, Shin A, Poyner E, et al. Human dermal CD14+ cells are a transient population of monocyte-derived macrophages. *Immunity* (2014) **41**(3):465–77. doi:10.1016/j.immuni.2014.08.006
217. Zaba LC, Fuentes-Duculan J, Steinman RM, Krueger JG, Lowes MA. Normal human dermis contains distinct populations of cd11c+BDCA-1+ dendritic cells and CD163+FXIIIA+ macrophages. *J Clin Invest* (2007) **117**(9):2517–25. doi:10.1172/JCI32282
218. Chu CC, Ali N, Karagiannis P, Di Meglio P, Skowera A, Napolitano L, et al. Resident CD141 (BDCA3)+ dendritic cells in human skin produce IL-10 and induce regulatory T cells that suppress skin inflammation. *J Exp Med* (2012) **209**(5):935–45. doi:10.1084/jem.20112583
219. Bigley V, McGovern N, Milne P, Dickinson R, Pagan S, Cookson S, et al. Langerin-expressing dendritic cells in human tissues are related to cd1c+ dendritic cells and distinct from langerhans cells and cd141high XCR1+ dendritic cells. *J Leukoc Biol* (2015) **97**(4):627–34. doi:10.1189/jlb.1HI0714-351R
220. Klechevsky E, Morita R, Liu M, Cao Y, Coquery S, Thompson-Snipes L, et al. Functional specializations of human epidermal langerhans cells and CD14+ dermal dendritic cells. *Immunity* (2008) **29**(3):497–510. doi:10.1016/j.immuni.2008.07.013
221. Ebner S, Nguyen VA, Forstner M, Wang YH, Wolfram D, Liu YJ, et al. Thymic stromal lymphopoietin converts human epidermal langerhans cells into antigen-presenting cells that induce proallergic T cells. *J Allergy Clin Immunol* (2007) **119**(4):982–90. doi:10.1016/j.jaci.2007.01.003
222. Artyomov MN, Munk A, Gorvel L, Korenfeld D, Cella M, Tung T, et al. Modular expression analysis reveals functional conservation between human langerhans cells and mouse cross-priming dendritic cells. *J Exp Med* (2015) **212**(5):743–57. doi:10.1084/jem.20131675
223. Stoitzner P, Schaffenrath S, Tripp CH, Reider D, Komenda K, Del Frari B, et al. Human skin dendritic cells can be targeted in situ by intradermal injection of antibodies against lectin receptors. *Exp Dermatol* (2014) **23**(12):909–15. doi:10.1111/exd.12573
224. Hänsel A, Günther C, Ingwersen J, Starke J, Schmitz M, Bachmann M, et al. Human slan (6-sulfo lacnac) dendritic cells are inflammatory dermal dendritic cells in psoriasis and drive strong TH17/TH1 t-cell responses. *J Allergy Clin Immunol* (2011) **127**(3):787–94.e1–9. doi:10.1016/j.jaci.2010.12.009
225. Zaba LC, Krueger JG, Lowes MA. Resident and "inflammatory" dendritic cells in human skin. *J Invest Dermatol* (2009) **129**(2):302–8. doi:10.1038/jid.2008.225
226. Banchereau J, Thompson-Snipes L, Zurawski S, Blanck JP, Cao Y, Clayton S, et al. The differential production of cytokines by human langerhans cells and dermal CD14(+) dcs controls CTL priming. *Blood* (2012) **119**(24):5742–9. doi:10.1182/blood-2011-08-371245
227. Ratzinger G, Baggers J, de Cos MA, Yuan J, Dao T, Reagan JL, et al. Mature human langerhans cells derived from CD34+ hematopoietic progenitors stimulate greater cytolytic T lymphocyte activity in the absence of bioactive il-12p70, by either single peptide presentation or cross-priming, than do dermal-interstitial or monocyte-derived dendritic cells. *J Immunol* (2004) **173**(4):2780–91. doi:10.4049/ jimmunol.173.4.2780
228. Denoeud J, Moser M. Role of CD27/CD70 pathway of activation in immunity and tolerance. *J Leukoc Biol* (2011) **89**(2):195–203. doi:10.1189/jlb.0610351
229. Polak ME, Newell L, Taraban VY, Pickard C, Healy E, Friedmann PS, et al. CD70-CD27 interaction augments CD8+ t-cell activation by human epidermal langerhans cells. *J Invest Dermatol* (2012) **132**(6):1636–44. doi:10.1038/jid.2012.26
230. van der Aar AM, de Groot R, Sanchez-Hernandez M, Taanman EW, van Lier RA, Teunissen MB, et al. Cutting edge: virus selectively primes human langerhans cells for CD70 expression promoting CD8+ T cell responses. *J Immunol* (2011) **187**(7):3488–92. doi:10.4049/jimmunol.1101105
231. Jelinek I, Leonard JN, Price GE, Brown KN, Meyer-Manlapat A, Goldsmith PK, et al. TLR3-specific double-stranded RNA oligonucleotide adjuvants induce dendritic cell cross-presentation, CTL responses, and antiviral protection. *J Immunol* (2011) **186**(4):2422–9. doi:10.4049/jimmunol.1002845
232. Steinman RM, Nussenzweig MC. Avoiding horror autotoxicus: the importance of dendritic cells in peripheral T cell tolerance. *Proc Natl Acad Sci U S A* (2002) **99**(1):351–8. doi:10.1073/pnas.231606698
233. Pulendran B, Tang H, Denning TL. Division of labor, plasticity, and crosstalk between dendritic cell subsets. *Curr Opin Immunol* (2008) **20**(1):61–7. doi:10.1016/j.coi.2007.10.009
234. Romani N, Brunner PM, Stingl G. Changing views of the role of langerhans cells. *J Invest Dermatol* (2012) **132**(3 Pt 2):872–81. doi:10.1038/jid.2011.437

20

Regulation of lipid specific and vitamin specific non-MHC restricted T cells by antigen presenting cells and their therapeutic potentials

Mariolina Salio and Vincenzo Cerundolo*

MRC Human Immunology Unit, Weatherall Institute of Molecular Medicine, Radcliffe Department of Medicine, University of Oxford, Oxford, UK

Edited by:
Elisabetta Padovan,
Basel University Hospital and University of Basel, Switzerland

Reviewed by:
Gennaro De Libero,
University of Basel, Switzerland
Michael Brenner,
Harvard Medical School, USA

***Correspondence:**
Mariolina Salio,
MRC Human Immunology Unit, Weatherall Institute of Molecular Medicine, Radcliffe Department of Medicine, University of Oxford, Headley Way, Oxford OX3 9DS, UK
mariolina.salio@imm.ox.ac.uk

Since initial reports, more than 25 years ago, that T cells recognize lipids in the context on non-polymorphic CD1 molecules, our understanding of antigen presentation to non-peptide-specific T cell populations has deepened. It is now clear that αβ T cells bearing semi-invariant T cell receptor, as well as subsets of γδ T cells, recognize a variety of self and non-self lipids and contribute to shaping immune responses via cross talk with dendritic cells and B cells. Furthermore, it has been demonstrated that small molecules derived from the microbial riboflavin biosynthetic pathway (vitamin B2) bind monomorphic MR1 molecules and activate mucosal-associated invariant T cells, another population of semi-invariant T cells. Novel insights in the biological relevance of non-peptide-specific T cells have emerged with the development of tetrameric CD1 and MR1 molecules, which has allowed accurate enumeration and functional analysis of CD1- and MR1-restricted T cells in humans and discovery of novel populations of semi-invariant T cells. The phenotype and function of non-peptide-specific T cells will be discussed in the context of the known distribution of CD1 and MR1 molecules by different subsets of antigen-presenting cells at steady state and following infection. Concurrent modulation of CD1 transcription and lipid biosynthetic pathways upon TLR stimulation, coupled with efficient lipid antigen processing, result in the increased cell surface expression of antigenic CD1–lipid complexes. Similarly, MR1 expression is almost undetectable in resting APC and it is upregulated following bacterial infection, likely due to stabilization of MR1 molecules by microbial antigens. The tight regulation of CD1 and MR1 expression at steady state and during infection may represent an important mechanism to limit autoreactivity, while promoting T cell responses to foreign antigens.

Keywords: CD1, MR1, innate and adaptive immunity, lipids, vitamins

Introduction

Earlier studies in the 1990s demonstrated that the antigen recognition potential of T lymphocytes is not limited to peptides presented by MHC class I and class II molecules (1, 2). Indeed, the newly identified MHC-related genes belonging to the CD1 family (3) were soon shown to present self and mycobacterial lipids to αβ and γδ T cell clones lacking CD4 and CD8 co-receptors (1, 2, 4).

Furthermore, human and murine T cells bearing semi-invariant T cell receptors (TCRs) (5, 6) were shown to be CD1d restricted (7).

A second MHC-related gene was identified in 1995, MR1 (8), which in 2003 was shown to select a population of cells known as mucosal-associated invariant T cells (MAIT) (9), also bearing semi-invariant TCRs (10). It was not until 2012, however, that microbial vitamin B2 metabolites were identified as the elusive antigens presented by MR1 molecules (11).

In the past 25 years, a number of investigators have elucidated the contribution of CD1- and MR1-restricted T cells to antimicrobial immunity, and for CD1-restricted T cells also to cancer immune-surveillance and autoimmunity. While comprehensive reviews on CD1 and MR1 antigen-presenting systems have been recently published (12–15), we will focus on recent findings that have advanced our understanding of the role of CD1- and MR1-restricted T cells, also known as non-conventional T cells or innate-like cells, as they straddle between innate and adaptive immunity.

CD1 Molecules

The human CD1 locus on chromosome 1 encodes five molecules, divided into group 1 (CD1a, b, and c) and group 2 (CD1d), based on sequence homology (3, 16). The fifth molecule, CD1e, is not expressed at the cell surface, yet plays an important role in assisting lipid antigen processing and loading on group 1 CD1 molecules (17). CD1 molecules are heterodimers of a heavy chain non-covalently associated with β-2 microglobulin, and have an overall fold similar to MHC class I molecules, however, unlike MHC class I and class II molecules, they are not polymorphic (3, 16). In comparison to MHC class I molecules, CD1 molecules have evolved a deep and narrow binding cavity that anchors the hydrophobic alkyl chains of lipid molecules: the binding cavity contains two pockets, A′ and F′, of which the A′ is deeper and closed by a narrow entrance at the top. Yet, each CD1 molecule differs in the antigen-presenting groove architecture, in the intracellular trafficking pattern, and in the overall tissue expression (18, 19). These differences underscore the non-redundant physiological role of the CD1 isoforms, which sample a variety of lipids in early, late endosomes or deep in the lysosomes, where exogenous lipids distribute according to their biophysical properties (20) (**Figure 1**). In mice, group 1 CD1 genes are absent and it is thought that they were lost during evolution, as they are present in other rodents (21). This has greatly hindered our understanding of the role and frequency of group 1 CD1-restricted T cells, until the recent development of CD1a, b, and c tetramers, which has opened the way toward enumeration and functional characterization of human lipid-specific T cells (22–24). Humanized SCID mice and group 1 CD1 transgenic mice are also proving to be useful models to study the role of CD1-restricted T cells in disease settings (25, 26).

CD1a

CD1a molecules are expressed on double-positive thymocytes, while in the periphery their expression is restricted to tissue-resident dendritic cells (DCs) and Langerhans cells (LC) in the skin (28). Unlike other CD1 isoforms, CD1a molecules have a short cytoplasmic tail, with no tyrosine-based motif to drive their recycling through late endocytic compartments. Hence, their trafficking is limited to the early endosomal compartment in a Rab22- and Arf6-dependent manner (29). Of all the CD1 molecules, CD1a has the smallest groove, which is suitable to present antigens encountered in the early endosomal compartment or at the cell surface (30–32).

CD1a-restricted cells can be autoreactive or pathogen reactive. The only microbial antigen known to bind CD1a is the mycobacterial lipopeptide didehydroxymycobactin (DDM) and DDM-restricted T cells could play a pivotal role in early detection of *Mycobacterium tuberculosis* infection (33). Like for many other lipid-specific T cells, recognition is exquisitely sensitive to the structure of the peptide and to the length and saturation of the fatty acid, which influences the positioning of the peptide residues available for recognition by the TCR (31). Despite a low affinity interaction (100 μM) between a DDM-specific TCR and CD1a–DDM soluble molecules (23), DDM–CD1a dextramers have been successfully used to stain DDM-specific T cells *ex vivo* in patients with active tuberculosis or positive tuberculin test, and could be a useful tool to determine the phenotype and function of these cells at a population level (23).

The first ever reported CD1-restricted clone was self-reactive (1). One of the first identified self-antigens presented by CD1a is sulfatide, a glycolipid abundant in myelin sheets. Of note, sulfatide can also be presented by CD1b, CD1c, and CD1d (34), which suggested a possible contribution of CD1-restricted T cells to the autoimmune response in multiple sclerosis (MS). To further characterize the pool of CD1a-autoreactive T cells, Moody, and co-workers have recently designed an experimental system based on CD1-expressing human myelogenous leukemia cells (K562 cells), with low or absent expression of MHC molecules in order to limit allo-reactivity. These studies have demonstrated that polyclonal CD1a reactive T cells are present at high frequency in the peripheral blood of healthy individuals [0.02–0.4% of memory T cells (35, 36)]. Similar results were independently obtained with C1R cells as antigen-presenting cells, although in this case higher frequencies of CD1a (and CD1c) reactive cells were observed [up to 10% of circulating T cells (36)]. Interestingly, CD1a-restricted T cells found in the blood express the skin-homing receptors CLA, CCR6, CCR4, and CCR10 and produce the cytokine interleukin 22 (IL-22) in response to CD1a^{+} DCs. The identification of CD1a-restricted cells in skin biopsies suggests that they may be playing an important immunoregulatory role in skin homeostasis through IL-22 secretion (35). It will be very interesting to investigate whether they may also play a role in skin immunopathology in psoriasis or in other skin diseases where over production of IL-22 has been implicated (37).

To understand the nature of the antigens activating CD1a-restricted T cells, self-ligands were eluted from secreted CD1a molecules and skin samples and tested *in vitro* (38). Unexpectedly, stimulatory antigens were more efficiently extracted in chloroform than in the commonly used chloroform methanol mixture, suggesting high hydrophobicity. Indeed, CD1a molecules were found to stimulate T cell clones when loaded with oily antigens lacking carbohydrate or charged head groups [such as triacylglyceride (TAG), squalene, and wax esters], while lipids with hydrophilic head groups inhibited CD1a-restricted T cell autoreactivity (38). These results, which suggested a unique mode of

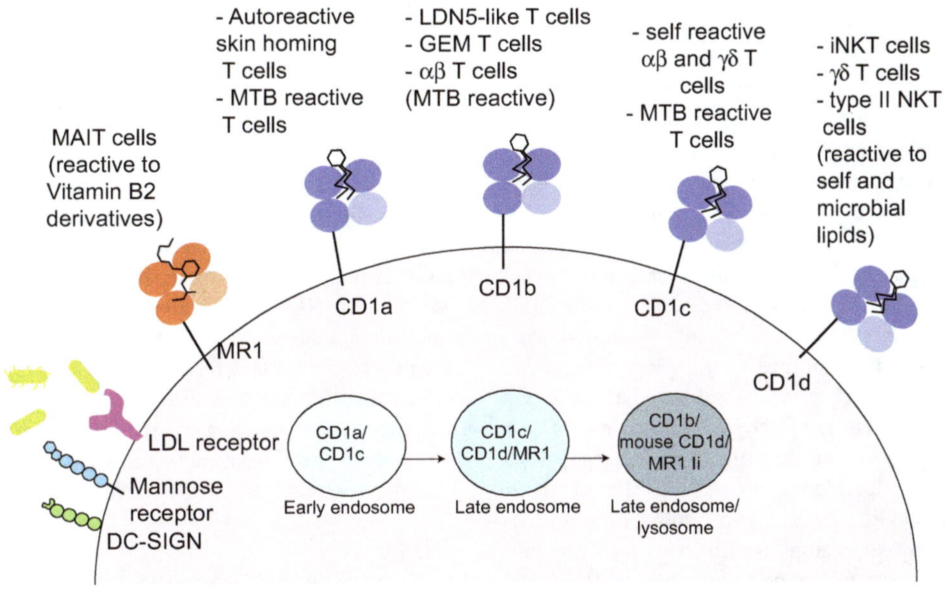

FIGURE 1 | Antigen presentation to non-peptide-specific T cells. MR1 and CD1 molecules present vitamin B2 derivatives or self and microbial lipids to a variety of αβ or γδ-bearing T cells. Through a variety of receptors (such as DC-SIGN, mannose receptor, and LDL-receptors) or via phagocytosis (not depicted) antigen-presenting cells uptake incoming pathogens. Microbial antigens are distributed through the endocytic compartment where they intersect recycling MR1 and CD1 molecules. In these compartments, antigen loading occurs, often through the help of accessory molecules such lipid transfer proteins (not depicted). The invariant chain (Ii) facilitates MR1 distribution in the late endosomal/lysosomal compartments (27).

"headless" antigen recognition by autoreactive CD1a-restricted T cells, were recently confirmed and extended with structural and mutagenesis studies (39). Although two of the studied autoreactive TCRs have binding affinities for CD1a–self complexes at the low end of the spectrum (30 and 93 μM (38, 39), CD1a tetramers loaded with a spectrum of permissive ligands [such as phosphatidylcholine and lysophosphatidylcholine (LPC)] have been shown to stain Jurkat cells transduced with one of these TCR (39). Furthermore, the ternary structure of two TCR–CD1a–self-lipid complexes showed that the TCR docks over the A′ roof of CD1a molecules without direct contact with the antigenic ligand. A comparison of these structures with those of CD1a–sulfatide (30) or CD1a–lipopeptide (31) provided a molecular explanation for the inhibitory effect of polar ligands, which are thought to disrupt the TCR–CD1a contact zone (39), revealing a mode of antigen recognition different from TCRs of peptide-specific T cells and other CD1-restricted T cells, centered on critical interactions with antigens bound to MHC or CD1 molecules (40).

TAG, fatty acids, and squalene accumulate in sebaceous glands and in the corneous stratus of the epithelium, separated from epidermal LC. So it is likely that at steady state, LC will not efficiently load these stimulatory antigens on CD1a molecules. However, upon trauma, infection or any form of barrier breach, these antigens could gain access to LC and increase the response of CD1a-autoreactive T cells. Consistent with this hypothesis, recently, CD1a-restricted responses have been documented in cohorts of patients allergic to bee and wasp venom (41). Despite the high lipidic content of wasp and bee venoms, in these patients the culprit antigens are not exogenous, but are generated *in vivo* by venom phospholipase A2 injected intradermally by wasps and bees via their sting (41). *In vitro*, it was shown that venom phospholipase A2 activates CD1a-restricted T cells cleaving non-antigenic phospholipids into lysophospholipids and antigenic headless fatty acids. Using an *in vivo* model of suction cap blisters, by mass spectrometry the authors also demonstrated the presence of lysophospholipids in the blister fluids of volunteers injected with venom. Although free fatty acids were not detected in the blister fluids, is it likely that this negative result was due to lack of sensitivity of the mass spectrometry (41).

Thus, the physical separation between antigen and antigen-presenting cells and/or the balance between stimulatory and inhibitory CD1a-ligands seem to be two of the mechanisms that the immune system deploys to keep an abundant population of autoreactive T cells under control at steady state. As endogenous or exogenous phospholipases can be activated during exposure to several allergens, it will be of interest to investigate whether in cohorts of patients with atopic dermatitis similar mechanisms may be active and account for expansion and/or activation of autoreactive T cells.

The identification of phospholipase A2 as a novel mechanism to generate autoantigens may offer new diagnostic and therapeutic opportunities. Likewise, as immunostimulatory oils and hydrocarbons are components of widely used adjuvants such as MF59, it will be important to address the role of CD1a-autoreactive T cells in shaping the adaptive T cell response during the aforementioned vaccination protocols.

CD1b

CD1b molecules are expressed on thymocytes and on peripheral DCs. Through tyrosine-based cytoplasmic motifs CD1b molecules bind to both AP-2 and AP-3 adaptors (42, 43) and efficiently traffic to acidic LAMP1$^+$ lysosomes, where processing of complex lipid antigens may occur and loading is aided by the acidic pH and by lipid transfer proteins (17, 44, 45). Additionally, CD1b molecules have evolved the largest antigen-presenting groove, with three pockets (A′, C′, and F′) and a large tunnel, which can accommodate lipids with very long alkyl chains, such as mycobacterial antigens with up to 80 carbons (46, 47). As most cellular lipids do not exceed 40 carbons length, the architecture of the groove of nascent CD1b molecules is maintained by spacer (or scaffold) lipids, such as diacylglycerols and deoxyceramides (48, 49). The existence of spacer lipids was initially suggested from the crystal structures of CD1b bound to the ganglioside GM2 or phosphatidylinositol, where it was observed that detergent moieties occupied the channels not filled by the lipid ligands (46). Spacer lipids seat at the bottom of the antigen-presenting groove, providing support for antigens loaded in the CD1b molecule, and are displaced when loading of longer microbial lipids occurs (49, 50). Furthermore, by stabilizing the antigen-presenting molecules, they enhance presentation of microbial lipids with shorter acyl chains (49). Spacer lipids have also been found when CD1c and CD1d molecules were crystallized with short lipids (51, 52), so their use seems to be a common strategy to maintain the correct fold and antigen orientation for CD1 molecules.

While CD1b-autoreactive T cells have been described (53, 54), they are detected at lower frequency than for other CD1 members (35). Indeed, CD1b molecules are specialized in presenting bacterial antigens, perhaps because of the large volume of the groove; so far the majority of the described ligands are of mycobacterial origin. Mycolic acid from *M. Tuberculosis* cell wall was the first described lipid antigen presented by CD1 molecules (4), and it can form the scaffold for other mycolyl antigens, such as glucose monomycolate (GMM) and glycerol monomycolate (55). Other families of CD1b lipid antigens are derivatives of phosphatidyl-myo-inositol (such as phosphatidylinositol mannoside (PIM) and lipoarabinomannan (LAM)) and sulfoglycolipids. The structure–activity relationship of these classes of lipids has been recently reviewed in Ref. (56, 57) and we refer the reader to these excellent reviews for more detail.

The development of CD1b tetramers has recently allowed to track mycobacteria-specific CD1b-restricted T cells in the blood of individuals with active tuberculosis or previous *M. tuberculosis* (MTB) exposure (22). In addition to following the dynamics of lipid-specific immune responses, for those lipid antigens produced only by *M. tuberculosis* and not other mycobacterial species (such as sulfoglycolipids), tracking of antigen-specific T cells may represent an important future tool for differential diagnosis.

Until now, it was assumed that group 1 CD1-restricted T cells were expressing highly diverse TCR, like peptide-specific MHC-restricted T cells. However, the use of tetramers to study the CD1b-GMM-specific T cell response in multiple individuals has allowed the discovery of two novel T cell types in the human repertoire, germ-line encoded mycolyl reactive (GEM) T cells (58) and LDN5-like T cells (59), which stain brightly and dimly, respectively, as indication of higher (around 1 μM) and lower affinity (20–40 μM) for CD1b–GMM complexes. GEM T cells express a semi-invariant TCR using TRAV1.2 variable segments rearranged to TRAJ9 joining segments (thus differing from the TRAV1.2-TRAJ33 TCR used by MAIT cells, see later), with nearly identical CDR3 sequences and a biased TRBV6.2 usage. LDN5-like T cells have a biased TRAV17 usage, with uniform CDR3 length, and a biased TRBV4.1 usage, with variable CDR3 length. Structural data point to a role of the TCR-β chain in influencing the fine specificity of the GMM-specific TCRs (58). The evidence to date suggests that GEM and LDN5-like T cells expansion is antigen driven upon infection, and that they do not represent another population of innate-like cells, unlike the semi-invariant MAIT and iNKT cells; however, a detailed transcriptional and functional analysis of these cells is yet to be done. Furthermore, it still remains to be determined whether GEM and LDN5-like T cells show immunological memory, how long they persist, and whether they can be harnessed for vaccination purposes. Finally, it remains to be determined what drives the selection of these cells in donors with no documented mycobacterial infection.

CD1c

CD1c molecules are expressed on thymocytes and at high density on peripheral DCs, LC (together with CD1a), and B cells. Through associations with AP2 adaptor molecules, they are widely distributed through the endocytic system (but not the LAMP1$^+$ lysosomes), which allows sampling of a broad spectrum of lipids in a variety of antigen-presenting cells (60).

CD1c molecules present self and microbial lipids to T cells bearing αβ and γδ TCR. In 1989, Porcelli and colleagues demonstrated specific recognition of CD1c by a CD4$^-$CD8$^-$ γδ CTL line (1) and CD1c self-reactivity was later confirmed with other cytotoxic γδ lines bearing the Vδ1 segment (61, 62). The self-antigens recognized by these CTL lines, though, still need to be identified.

CD1c-autoreactive αβ T cells are present at high frequency in the peripheral blood of healthy donors (36). Recently, a novel self-lipid antigen (methyl-lysophosphatidic acid, mLPA) that accumulates in leukemic cells has been identified as one of the targets of CD1c-reactive T cells (63). mLPA-specific T cell clones were shown to efficiently kill *in vitro* and *in vivo* primary leukemia cells in a CD1c-restricted manner, but not normal B cells and primary DC, that despite being CD1c positive do not express the antigen at significant level (63). Selective accumulation of mLPA in human leukemia suggests that it can be considered a novel class of tumor-associated antigens and may represent a promising immunotherapeutic target.

CD1c molecules present several mycobacterial and synthetic lipids with methylated alkyl chains: mannosyl phosphodolichols (MPDs), mannosyl-β1-phosphomycoketide (MPM), and phosphomycoketide (PM) (24, 64–66). The mycobacterial enzyme polyketide synthase 12 (psk12) is crucial for the synthesis of the methyl-branched lipids, which are a molecular signature of mycobacterial infection and essential for antigenicity (24, 65). Polyclonal CD1c-restricted T cells expand *in vivo* during mycobacterial infection and can be tracked with lipid-loaded CD1c tetramers (24, 64).

The range of self and foreign antigens presented by CD1c may be larger than currently appreciated, as it has been shown that also lipopeptides can be antigenic, in analogy to CD1a. This was demonstrated as a proof of principle with a synthetic *N*-acyl glycine dodecamer lipopeptide (lipo-12) (67). These results raise the possibility that other eukaryotic or viral *N*-terminally acylated peptides, such as post-translationally modified products of ribosomal translation, might be antigenic. Interestingly, as lipopeptide presentation is sensitive to proteolysis in late endosomes and lysosomes (67), CD1c and CD1a molecules are the two CD1 isoforms uniquely suited to lipopeptide presentation because they predominantly survey the secretory pathway and the early endosomes.

Structural studies have highlighted a partially open structure of CD1c F′ pocket (52), which may accommodate a variety of ligands, from diacylated lipids such as sulfatide (34), to lipopeptides and possibly aid antigen loading in the early endosomal compartment or at the cell surface, in the absence of specific lipid transfer proteins. Furthermore, the CD1c–MPM crystal structure has highlighted the essential role for the methyl branches of MPM in stabilizing the single alkyl chain in the A′ pocket (52). Finally, the exquisite specificity of MPM and PM reactive clones can also be explained at the structural level (68): in the absence of the mannosyl moiety, the phosphate head group of PM is shifted toward the F′ pocket. A range of TCR binding affinities (7–30 μM) have been reported for CD1c–mycoketide complexes, and while the ternary complex TCR–CD1c–antigen is not yet available, biophysical data with six CD1c-reactive TCRs showed that different TCRs used different docking strategies on the same CD1c–lipid complex, unlike what has been described for the iNKT TCR and is predicted for the GEM TCR (68).

CD1d

CD1d molecules are the most widely distributed, as they are expressed not only on hematopoietic cells (thymocytes, monocytes, DCs, and B cells), but also on epithelial cells (28). CD1d-restricted T cells are collectively known as natural killer T cells, because of co-expression of T cells and NK cell markers (most notably CD161 in humans and NK1.1 in some mouse strains). Two types of NKT cells exist: type I, (also known as invariant, iNKT), expressing a semi-invariant TCR (Vα24-Jα18 paired to Vβ11 in humans, Vα14-Jα18 paired to Vβ2, Vβ7, or Vβ8.2 chains in mice); type II, expressing a polyclonal TCR repertoire (12). The CD1d antigen presentation system is conserved across species, and both human and murine iNKT cells can be tracked with CD1d tetramers loaded with the synthetic glycolipid agonist α-galactosylceramide (α-GalCer). Furthermore, the availability of murine models lacking type I or type I and II NKT cells has greatly contributed to our knowledge of the biology of these cells. Conversely, we still lack reagents to specifically detect the majority of type II NKT cells, thus with few exceptions, their role *in vivo* has been less characterized.

Through recognition of a variety of self and microbial antigens, NKT cells have an important immune-regulatory role, spanning from autoimmunity, to protection against infection and tumor immune-surveillance. We refer the reader to recent reviews for a comprehensive discussion of NKT cell biology and CD1d antigen presentation (12, 14, 69–71), while here we highlight the role of microbiota in modulating iNKT cell reactivity and we summarize results revealing a previously unknown heterogeneity of the human NKT cell family (**Figure 1**).

Microbiota and NKT Cells

Regulation of metabolism and immunity by commensal bacteria is now well established (72). Interestingly, α-GalCer, the most potent iNKT cell agonist to date, was originally isolated from commensal bacteria of the marine sponge *Agela mauritianus* (73). The α-anomeric linkage of the sugar moiety is the quintessence of a microbial signature, and a variety of iNKT cell agonists from different microbial species have been characterized, although during microbial infection iNKT cell reactivity is often driven by cytokine-mediated signals (74). Recently, inhibitory and activatory α-GalCer species have been biochemically isolated from *Bacteroides fragilis*, a prominent species of the gut microbiota (75, 76). It has also been demonstrated that the intestinal microbiota plays an important role in the tight regulation of iNKT cell numbers and function, possibly through the balance between stimulatory and inhibitory lipids: germ-free mice have increased relative and absolute numbers of iNKT cells in the intestine, due to increased CXCL16 expression in the mucosal epithelium and CXCL16-dependent iNKT cell homing (77). The conditioning effect of the microbiota starts very early in life and has long-lasting consequences, as demonstrated by higher susceptibility of germ-free mice to intestinal immunopathology and lung inflammation (77). In turn, iNKT cells influence bacterial colonization of the intestine and lungs of mice (78) and signaling through epithelial CD1d is essential in maintaining mucosal homeostasis via IL-10 secretion (79). These findings have been recently extended in humans, where phenotypically and functionally mature iNKT cells have been detected in the sterile environment of the fetal intestine, and it is thought that they may represent an important first line of defense at birth (80). Furthermore, lysosulfatide-reactive CD1d-restricted type II NKT cells have been identified in the mucosa of ulcerative patients, and their cytotoxic activity against the intestinal epithelium suggests a pathogenic role (81). It remains to be determined whether during intestinal inflammation, T cells restricted by group 1 CD1 may also recognize self or microbial lipids.

Human NKT Cell Heterogeneity

Adipose tissue-resident iNKT cells

Like MHC-restricted CD4 cells, iNKT cells can also differentiate in Th1, Th2, Th17, T_{FH}, and T-regulatory subsets, which use the same transcription regulators as peptide-specific T cells (69). The balance between subsets could have profound regulatory effects during immune responses, through the secretion of cytokines and modulation of DC and B cell function (12). Recently, a tissue resident subset of iNKT cells with a unique transcriptional and cytokine profile has been shown to accumulate in adipose tissue and regulate the function of Tregs and macrophages, via IL-2 and IL-10, respectively (82). Adipose tissue iNKT cells do not express the master regulatory PLZF, but express the transcription factor E4BP4, which controls IL-10 production. Also, as compared to splenic or liver iNKT cells, a smaller fraction of adipose tissue iNKT cells expresses CD44 and NK1.1 markers, while expression of ICOS and PD-1 was increased. As adipocytes are CD1d positive, they could modulate iNKT cell activation through presentation of self and dietary lipids, and ultimately the cross talk between iNKT cells and adipose tissue macrophages could be very important in preventing tissue inflammation. This hypothesis is consistent with the described protective role of iNKT cells against obesity-induced chronic inflammation (83).

CD1d-restricted γδ T cells

Two groups employed CD1d tetramers loaded with two different ligands to isolate CD1d-reactive T cells from healthy human peripheral blood. In one study, the majority of CD1-sulfatide tetramer staining cells were found to be T cells bearing the Vδ1 TCR (84), while a second study identified Vδ1 T cells amongst those binding CD1d-α-GalCer tetramers, although the majority of cells binding to the latter tetramers, as expected, were iNKT cells (85). Interestingly, human Vδ1 do not recognize mouse CD1d-α-GalCer tetramers, unlike human iNKT cells, highlighting a clear difference in the reactivity of the two populations. Also the affinity of binding of Vδ1 cells to human CD1d-α-GalCer complexes is lower than that observed for iNKT cells (Kd 16 versus 0.5 μM).

Vδ1 bearing cells are typically tissue-homing γδ cells and are abundant in the intestinal mucosa (86, 87). Preliminary results suggest that some reactivity to C1R cells expressing CD1d molecules can be detected amongst Vδ1 polyclonal lines generated from intestinal biopsies (88). Given the presence of several lipids from the microflora and the abundant expression of CD1d on the gastrointestinal epithelium (28), future studies should investigate whether intestinal Vδ1 γδ T cells can also bind CD1d-α-GalCer tetramers and if so, the role of microbiota in maintaining and expanding Vδ1 γδ T cells after birth. As Vδ1 cells are present at higher frequency than iNKT cells, they could have a marked impact on intestinal homeostasis and immunopathology, and reactivity could be modulated by the expression of stress-induced MHC-related molecules like MICA and MICB (86). Likewise, reactivity to sulfatide may underscore a possible role of these cells in MS.

The mode of γδ TCR–CD1d-α-GalCer/sulfatide recognition is markedly different from that of the iNKT TCR (85, 88). The γδ TCR docks orthogonally rather than in a parallel manner like the iNKT TCR, thus resembling type II NKT TCRs and classical peptide-specific TCRs (40); CD1d binding is dominated by the TCRδ chain, while CDR3γ residues contribute to lipid antigen binding only in CD1d-α-GalCer, but not in CD1d–sulfatide ternary complexes (85, 88).

NKT cells and chronic inflammation

Several investigators have described reactivity of human type II NKT cells toward inflammation-associated lysolipids, generated by the action of PLA A2 (89). T cells binding CD1d–LPC multimers were found at higher frequency in the blood of myeloma patients compared to healthy controls, consistent with elevated serum levels of LPC in the plasma of these patients (90). In infected hepatocytes, Hepatitis B was shown to induce the activity of secretory phospholipases and the release of lysophosphatidylethanolamine (lyso PE), capable of eliciting CD1d-restricted type II NKT cells activation in humans and mice, suggesting that they may play a role in viral recognition (91).

Glucosylsphingosine (LGL1), the deacylated product of β-glucosylceramide (GL1), accumulates in several metabolic disorders such as Gaucher disease, as a consequence of altered sphingolipid metabolism. In all metabolic disorders, lipid accumulation is associated with progressive inflammation. One of the contributing factors could be the expansion of pathogenic LGL1-reactive CD1d-restricted type II NKT cells with a T_{FH} phenotype, stimulating inflammation and B cell activation (92).

The demonstration that lysolipid species are antigenic for subsets of CD1d-restricted NKT cells is of great interest and provides the link for NKT cell activation in sterile inflammatory conditions, possibly suggesting novel therapeutic modalities through selective inhibition of the biochemical pathways generating the relevant antigens.

On the Role of DC in Regulating CD1 Reactivity

The central role of DCs in orchestrating immune responses is now well established (93). Immature DC, residing in the periphery, patrol the body for incoming pathogens and recognition of pathogen molecular patterns (PAMPs) through pattern recognition receptors (PRRs) triggers DC activation, maturation, and migration to the draining lymph nodes. Coordinated changes in expression of MHC class I and II, co-stimulatory molecules and cytokines upon DC maturation, promote efficient priming of peptide-specific CD4, CD8 T, and B cells in the lymph node (94, 95). The heterogeneity in DC subsets and their different anatomical distribution results in unique functional specialization, and ensures tailoring the adaptive immune response to the type of incoming stimulus (95).

As highlighted in the previous paragraphs, CD1d expression is constitutive and shared by all DC subsets; however, expression of group 1 CD1 molecules is much more restricted. Due to the strong autoreactivity of CD1-restricted T cells, tight regulation of steady-state cell surface expression of CD1 is required to control their activation. For example, lipids found in human serum, particularly lysophosphatidic acid and cardiolipin, inhibit group 1 CD1 expression, through a transcriptional mechanism involving activation of the peroxisome proliferator-activated receptor (PPAR) nuclear hormone receptors (96).

Monocytes express only CD1d molecules, but during *in vitro* differentiation into DC with GM-CSF and IL-4, group 1 CD1 expression is induced (2). It is likely that, *in vivo*, cytokines in the local microenvironment might influence group 1 CD1 expression in the process of monocyte to DC differentiation following transendothelial migration (97). Indeed it has been shown that monocyte infection with mycobacteria represents an efficient way to induce DC differentiation and expression of group 1 CD1 molecules (98–100). Upregulation of CD1 molecules depends on NOD and TLR signals and is enhanced by concomitant inflammasome activation and release of bioactive IL-1β (101). Interestingly, while mycobacterial infection increases group 1 CD1 expression, it downregulates CD1d and interferes with MHC-restricted antigen presentation (99, 102).

Mycobacterial cell wall lipids thus have a dual effect, by serving as antigens (i.e., mycolic acids, GMM, LAM PMK, and DDM) and adjuvants that drive CD1 expression on the infected cells, to promote antigen presentation. However, group 1 CD1 molecules are not expressed on macrophages, which instead are the infected cells during *in vivo* MTB infection, thus whether CD1b-restricted T cells might play a sizeable cytotoxic and anti-mycobacterial function *in vivo* is debatable. The low frequencies of group 1 CD1-restricted T cells, even after infection, rather suggests a helper function, perhaps through modulation of DC function (103).

While during DC maturation a marked upregulation of MHC class I and II is observed, with increased half-life of surface MHC–peptide complexes leading to efficient peptide antigen presentation (104, 105), the surface expression of group 1 CD1 molecules is only moderately increased (CD1b, CD1c) or even decreased (CD1a) (106); furthermore, CD1 molecules continue to recycle between the plasma membrane and intracellular compartments (102). CD1-mediated lipid antigen presentation occurs very efficiently already in immature DC and this might ensure prompt licensing of DC by lipid-specific T cells via cytokines and CD40–CD40L interactions (103). The role of iNKT cells in DC licensing and memory CTL generation is discussed in depth in an accompanying review in this issue.

To ensure optimal antigen presentation through CD1 molecules, DC subsets also coordinate lipid antigen uptake and distribution through the endosomal compartment through specific receptor-mediated interactions (19). Serum lipoproteins ensure efficient delivery of self and foreign antigens for CD1-mediated presentation, through ApoE-LDL-R-mediated uptake (107).

The C-type lectin Langerin mediates *Mycobacterium leprae* antigen uptake and delivery to Birbeck granules in LC and is required for CD1a–lipid antigen presentation (108). The mannose receptor (CD206), a C-type lectin expressed on macrophages, dermal DC, and monocyte-derived DC, promotes mycobacterial LAM uptake and lysosomal delivery for CD1b presentation (109). Other C-type lectins that specifically capture pathogen-derived carbohydrate rich antigens are DEC 205 (expressed on LC, dermal DC, and monocyte-derived DCs), DC-SIGN (CD209, expressed mainly on dermal DC). Their role in enhancing peptide presentation is well described (110, 111) and it is likely that these and other related molecules involved in endocytosis of bacteria or bacterial debris might also influence CD1d-restricted lipid antigen presentation in late endosomal compartments. Selective expression of endocytic receptors in DC subsets can also be exploited therapeutically: recently it has been shown that targeted delivery of the mycobacterial antigen GMM to monocyte-derived DCs via Siglec-7 via sialic acid-coated nanoparticles induces robust CD1b-restricted T cell activation, although this was not tested on primary CD1b$^+$ Siglec-7$^+$ myeloid DCs (112).

In addition to transcriptional regulation of CD1 expression, T cell autoreactivity is controlled by the availability of self-ligands. Although determination of the repertoire of lipids bound to CD1 molecules is technically challenging, mass spectrometry analysis of lipids eluted from secreted CD1d molecules has revealed the presence of several types of phospho and sphingolipids acquired during biosynthesis (113, 114), the majority of which are non-antigenic (89). Moody and co-workers used a recently established lipidomic platform to compare self-lipids associated with all CD1 molecules and the results confirmed the ability of CD1 molecules to bind a variety of molecules (49). It is now also well established that the range of glycosphingolipids (GSL) and phospholipids expressed by cells varies amongst cell types and with cellular activation (115). TLR activation of myeloid cells has marked effect on the expression of key genes involved in GSL biosynthesis (54, 116–118), which translate in detectable biochemical changes (54, 119). This has been shown to lead to increased CD1b-restricted and iNKT cell autoreactivity (54, 116–118).

MR1 and MAIT Cells

The MHC-related molecule MR1 (8) presents antigens to a family of innate-like T cells bearing a semi-invariant TCR and known as MAIT (10). In humans, the MAIT TCR consists of the Vα7.2 TCR-α chain mostly joined to Jα33 segments (TRAJ33) and paired to a limited number of TCR-β chains (mainly TRBV6 and TRBV20).

MR1 molecules are non-polymorphic and highly conserved among mammalian species, leading to functional cross-reactivity, which is reminiscent of the species conservation in the CD1 antigen-presenting system (120). Like iNKT cells, MAIT cells are selected in the thymus by double-positive cortical thymocytes (121), but unlike iNKT cells they leave the thymus as naïve cells and complete their maturation in the periphery (122, 123). MR1 expression on peripheral B cells and the intestinal flora are crucial for MAIT cells survival, expansion, acquisition of a memory phenotype, and effector functions (9).

Due to their anatomical mucosal localization and innate-like properties with a Th1-like effector phenotype, MAIT cells are in a unique position to act as early sentinels in response to respiratory and intestinal pathogens. Indeed, they have been shown to be activated in response to a variety of bacterial and fungal infections (124, 125) and to play a role in infectious models with *BCG*, *Francisella tularensis*, *Klebsiella penumoniae* (126–128), and MTB (129). Despite the well-characterized antimicrobial activity of MAIT cells, the antigens bound to MR1 remained for a long time elusive, until a major breakthrough in 2012 demonstrated that MR1 molecules present vitamin B2 metabolites to MAIT cells (11). These vitamins are not produced by mammals, hence they can be considered as molecular signatures of microbial infection. Consistently, microbes lacking the ability to synthesize riboflavins (such as *Streptococcus pyogenes* or *Enterococcus faecalis*) are unable to induce MR1-dependent MAIT cell activation (11).

Like iNKT cells and $\gamma\delta$ cells, however, MAIT cells can also be activated in a TCR/MR1-independent manner, through the stimulatory activity of IL-12 and IL-18 secreted by activated APCs (130). Hence, it is possible that MAIT cells may play an immunoregulatory role also during infections with viruses and with bacteria lacking the riboflavin synthetic pathway or in sterile inflammation.

MR1 Ligands

MR1 molecules are ubiquitously expressed, although barely detectable at the cell surface (131), unless cells are incubated with vitamin ligands that increase MR1 expression (11, 132, 133). Two types of vitamin ligands have been described, stimulatory (riboflavin intermediates) and not (folic acid derivatives). Both classes of ligands have been shown to stabilize MR1 molecules, covalently binding through a Schiff base complex; however, crystallographic studies revealed that TCR recognition is exquisitely sensitive to the ribityl moiety present only in the riboflavin derivatives (134).

To date, two classes of stimulatory riboflavins are known, ribityllumazine and pyrimidines [more powerful agonists, but highly unstable unless trapped by MR1 molecules (135)]. While initially the ribityllumazine rRL-6-CH_2OH was the bacterial ligand (from *Salmonella enterica serovar Typhimurium* supernatants) thought to bind to MR1 (11), subsequent elegant studies with Gram$^+$ (*Lactococcus lactis*) and Gram$^-$ (*E. coli*) bacterial strains defective for key enzymes in the riboflavin synthesis pathway unveiled the intermediate compound, 5-A-RU (5-amino-6-D-ribitylaminouracil) as the key precursor for pyrimidines and ribityllumazines (133, 135). Bacterial-derived 5-A-RU itself is not stimulatory, but it reacts with bacterial or host cell-derived small glyoxal compounds to form pyrimidines, which then can condense to form ribityllumazine.

Future studies will be needed to identify the molecular mechanisms of vitamin antigen presentation through MR1. For example, the relative contribution of host-derived versus bacterial-derived glyoxal compounds that react with 5-A-RU remains to be determined, as is the cellular compartment where this condensation and the subsequent MR1 loading occur. Furthermore, the observation that some non-activating ligands [Ac-6-FP (132)] can induce rapid and prolonged upregulation of MR1 molecules suggests different effects on MR1 trafficking. Finally, the currently identified ligands are all bound in an aromatic cradle in the A′ pocket of the MR1 binding groove [although with different orientations (134)], and there remains the possibility that other classes of ligands might extend in the more exposed F′ pocket.

MR1 Tetramers and MAIT Cell Heterogeneity

With the discovery of MR1 ligands, MR1 tetramers have been developed to characterize the MAIT cell population, previously identified solely as TRAV1.2$^+$, CD161$^+$ CD8$^+$ cells (136). In peripheral blood, rRL-6-CH2OH-loaded MR1 tetramers bind to a population of CD3$^+$ CD4$^-$ CD161$^+$ cells with comparable frequency to the TRAV1.2 antibody. The advantage of tetramer over antibody stainings, however, is that tetramers are able to detect MAIT cells that have downregulated CD161 expression, such as post activation or during HIV infection (137). Single cell sorting of CD161$^+$ TRAV1.2$^+$ cells and CD161$^+$ MR1-tetramer$^+$ cells and multiplex analysis of their TCR genes revealed the use of alternative rearrangements (particularly TRAJ20 and TRAJ12) in addition to the canonical TRAV1.2-TRAJ33 (136). These alternative rearrangements have also been identified by different investigators that performed deep sequencing of mRNA from MAIT cells sorted on the basis of TRAV1.2 and CD161 co-expression (138) and on MAIT populations that specifically secreted TNF-α in response to selected pathogens (139). Diversity in the CDR3β region due to amino acid additions and a diverse use of TCR-β chains (in addition to TRBV6.4 and TRBV20) have also been observed, suggesting an unexpected heterogeneity of the peripheral MAIT T cell repertoire.

Interestingly, the canonical MAIT TCRs as well as those bearing TRAJ12 and TRAJ33 segments have a conserved Tyr95 residue in the CDR3α-chain, which is essential in forming a hydrogen bond with the ribityl tail of activating ligands (134). These three TCRs also adopt a very similar docking mode on MR1–antigen complexes (132, 140–142). However, other recently described MR1-restricted TCRs lack the Tyr95α residue (139) and future studies will be required to confirm that these TCRs do indeed confer MR1-restricted reactivity and to determine the molecular details of their antigen recognition.

Furthermore, the non-canonical TCR α-chains paired almost exclusively with TRBV6.4 (136), raising the possibility that the TCR β-chain repertoire might impact antigen recognition, as observed with iNKT cells (143, 144). Indeed, structural and biophysical data have provided experimental evidence that the CDR3β loops can fine-tune the MAIT–TCR interaction and responsiveness to MR1, in an antigen-dependent manner (132).

The functional correlate of the phenotypic heterogeneity of the MAIT repertoire is currently unclear, and an interesting hypothesis is that it may be a surrogate signature of specific pathogen infections. Along these lines, Gold and co-workers reported selective use of MAIT cell TCRs in response to three different pathogens (*Mycobacterium smegmatis, Salmonella typhimurium, and Candida albicans*) in individual subjects (139). In this data set, however, no unique TCR sequence was found to be associated with individual pathogens across individuals. In these donors, functionally responsive MAIT cells for TCR sequencing were identified by TNF-α secretion, however, in the absence of blocking experiments with MR-1 antibodies it is unknown whether the responses were entirely TCR dependent or co-stimulated by cytokines. Nevertheless, these results are of interest, as they suggest that the MAIT cell TCR repertoire potentially reflects the host's microbial exposure history because of qualitative differences in the class of antigens presented by different pathogens, and that MAIT cells could exhibit immunological memory. However, an alternative interpretation is that different subsets of MAIT cells are differentially activated by pathogens in function of their TCR-β sequence heterogeneity (and hence of their TCR affinity), according to quantitative rather than qualitative differences in antigen availability in different microbes. Consistently, recent work by Lantz and co-workers using bacteria with mutations in the riboflavin biosynthetic pathway, suggested limited MR1 ligand heterogeneity between Gram$^+$ and Gram$^-$ bacteria (133).

Ultimately, longitudinal studies with well-defined microbial exposures (for example *MTB*, *Salmonella typhi* or *paratyphi*) will be needed to further explore these alternative hypotheses. In addition, it will be of interest to compare the MAIT T cell repertoire in the naïve thymus, in cord blood and in adults as MAIT cells undergo antigen-driven expansion at birth (122, 123). So far, the only study that analyzed by deep sequencing sorted TRAV1.2$^+$ CD161$^+$ MAIT from peripheral blood of three donors after a 5-month-interval showed that the oligoclonal TCRβ repertoire is stable in the absence of infection (138).

MAIT Cells in Sterile Inflammation

Although the predominant role of MAIT cells is protection against infections, there is some evidence that they may be implicated in autoimmune responses. Murine transgenic MAIT cells protect from the induction and progression of experimental autoimmune encephalomyelitis, and in MR1-deficient mice, which lack MAIT cells, EAE is exacerbated (145). MAIT cell TCR sequences were identified by single-strand polymorphism analysis in autoptic material of patients with MS (146), and one study reported a decrease in the frequency of MAIT cells in the blood of MS patients, proportional with the severity and activity of the disease (147). It has been shown that IL-18 in the serum of MS patients drives MAIT cell activation and increased expression of VLA4, an integrin that mediates migration across the blood–brain barrier (148).

Reduction of MAIT cell frequencies has been reported in the small intestine of celiac disease patients (149), while an increase was observed in the inflamed mucosa of patients with inflammatory bowel disease, with a clear activated phenotype (150). In both disease settings, changes in frequency and phenotype of tissue resident and circulating MAIT cells might be driven by compromised gut barrier function and bacterial overgrowth, as also observed during HIV infection (137, 151).

Mucosal-associated invariant T cells have been identified amongst the IL-17-producing cells in psoriatic skin, although percentages were not significantly different compared to healthy skin (152). It is currently unclear whether MAIT cells are activated in the psoriatic skin via microbial ligands or as a result of the general inflammation. Finally, it has been reported that the frequency of peripheral blood CD8 and double-negative (DN) MAIT cells is reduced in lupus and rheumatoid arthritis (RA) patients, with an accumulation of MAIT cells in the synovial fluid in RA (153). This reduction was more pronounced in patients with highly active disease. Also the capacity of MAIT to secrete IFN-γ was reduced in response to both bacterial and PMA/ionomycin stimulation, although this was shown to be unrelated to their increased expression of PD-1 (153).

While enumeration of MAIT frequencies on the basis of the sole expression of Vα7.2 and CD161 might lead to some preliminary interesting observations, further studies will need to include MR1-tetramer staining or qPCR analysis of the invariant TCR, to avoid underestimation of frequencies, as CD161 is often downmodulated following activation (154). Furthermore, the lack of a suitable animal model, due to very low frequency of MAIT cells in inbred laboratory mice may hinder the understanding of the functional relevance of the above phenotypic analysis.

Recent results have brought MAIT cells to the center stage in chronic inflammatory settings associated with obesity and diabetes, possibly as a consequence of the altered composition of the gut microbiota in both diseases (155). The frequency of circulating MAIT cells, as determined by both MR1 tetramer staining and TRAV7.2 and CD161 staining, was significantly reduced as compared to healthy controls. The remaining MAIT cells showed a phenotype consistent with activation (upregulation of CD25 and CD69) and an inflammatory cytokine bias (higher secretion of IFN-γ, IL-2, IL-7, granzyme B). Conversely, MAIT cells were increased in subcutaneous and omental adipose tissue as compared to the blood, suggesting preferential tissue recruitment. Adipose tissue MAIT cells also secreted more IL-17 in obese as compared to lean patients. Interestingly, the authors observed an attenuation of MAIT cell abnormalities after weight loss following bariatric surgery. It is possible that IL-7 produced by adipose tissue stromal cells facilitates MAIT cell activation, as previously observed in the liver (156). In addition to cytokines, changes in gut microbiota and permeability might release a variety of bacterial ligands, which could react with increased endogenous levels of methylglyoxals to form MAIT cell agonists.

MAIT Interactions with APCs

As mentioned before, MR1 is ubiquitously transcribed, although cell surface expression is very low and it is only transiently upregulated following infection or incubation with some of the synthetic ligands (27, 131–133). Upon infection, MAIT cells can be activated in a MR1-dependent way by a variety of cells, including DC, macrophages, epithelial cells, and fibroblasts (124, 125). By secreting a plethora of regulatory cytokines (138), activated MAIT like iNKT cells may be able to modulate the antimicrobial function of other cells. Likewise, by secreting chemokines like CCL4 they can recruit NK, monocytes, and other inflammatory cells to infected tissues (138). Furthermore, it is likely that MAIT cell activation will provide an early source of IFN-γ during infections, facilitating the development of Th1 immunity, as described for NK cells (157), γδ (87), and iNKT cells (158). However, it is currently unknown whether MAIT cells are capable of inducing effective DC maturation *in vivo*, and if so the relative contribution of cytokines and CD40–CD40L interactions, which are key for DC licensing by CD1-restricted cells (103).

Post-natal MAIT cell expansion depends on bacterial flora and B cells (9). *In vitro*, primary B cells and EBV-transformed B cell lines have been shown to induce MAIT cell activation in an MR1-dependent manner following infection with commensal or pathogenic intestinal bacteria (159). Lack of titration of MAIT cell activation and reduced stimulation by paraformaldehyde fixed B cells, however, suggest a possible contribution of soluble factors, which was not addressed. Consistent with this, IFN-γ secretion by activated MAIT cells was only partially blocked by the anti MR1 antibody 26.5.

Finally, despite known expression of the CD161 ligand LLT1 by activated B cells and DC (160, 161), its role in modulating MAIT cell reactivity remains to be addressed, and could be of relevance considering the profound CD161 downmodulation observed with MAIT cell activation (154).

Concluding Remarks

Our current understanding of innate-like T cell populations has been widened in the past few years by few key technological advances, such as the identification of novel agonists and the capacity to refold antigen-presenting molecules to generate tetramers to enumerate qualitatively and quantitative these cells in health and disease settings. Biophysical and crystallographic studies, coupled with extensive mutagenesis, have elucidated the fine molecular details of antigen recognition, highlighting the existence of conserved (for iNKT, MAIT, and GEM T cells) and more variable (for CD1a and CD1c-restricted T cells) TCR footprints over the cognate antigen-presenting molecules (40). In the future, a better understanding of the fine details of antigen presentation through MR-1 may open new avenues aimed at therapeutically harnessing MAIT cells in promoting the cross talk between the innate and adaptive arms of the immune system. Given the higher frequencies of MAIT cells over iNKT cells in humans, and their enrichment at mucosal sites, MAIT cell agonists might prove effective adjuvants to promote mucosal immune responses.

Finally, functional and phenotypical enumeration of MAIT cells and GEM T cells with tetramers may become a valuable immuno-monitoring tool. For example, it has been shown that MAIT cell frequencies are reduced in the blood of individuals with active MTB infection but they normalize after therapy (154), hence it should be explored whether they could be considered a marker of disease status, possibly to identify individuals at risk of progression to clinically active disease. Additional population of invariant T cells are being discovered by next-generation sequencing of the TCR-α chain repertoire (162) and may be used to probe antigenic exposure at a population level.

Acknowledgments

This work was supported by Cancer Research UK [Programme Grant C399/A2291] and the Medical Research Council.

References

1. Porcelli S, Brenner MB, Greenstein JL, Balk SP, Terhorst C, Bleicher PA. Recognition of cluster of differentiation 1 antigens by human CD4-CD8- cytolytic T lymphocytes. *Nature* (1989) **341**:447–50. doi:10.1038/341447a0
2. Porcelli S, Morita CT, Brenner MB. CD1b restricts the response of human CD4-8- T lymphocytes to a microbial antigen. *Nature* (1992) **360**:593–7. doi:10.1038/360593a0
3. Calabi F, Milstein C. A novel family of human major histocompatibility complex-related genes not mapping to chromosome 6. *Nature* (1986) **323**:540–3. doi:10.1038/323540a0
4. Beckman EM, Porcelli SA, Morita CT, Behar SM, Furlong ST, Brenner MB. Recognition of a lipid antigen by CD1-restricted alpha beta+ T cells. *Nature* (1994) **372**:691–4. doi:10.1038/372691a0
5. Dellabona P, Casorati G, Friedli B, Angman L, Sallusto F, Tunnacliffe A, et al. In vivo persistence of expanded clones specific for bacterial antigens within the human T cell receptor alpha/beta CD4-8- subset. *J Exp Med* (1993) **177**:1763–71. doi:10.1084/jem.177.6.1763
6. Lantz O, Bendelac A. An invariant T cell receptor alpha chain is used by a unique subset of major histocompatibility complex class I-specific CD4+ and CD4-8- T cells in mice and humans. *J Exp Med* (1994) **180**:1097–106. doi:10.1084/jem.180.3.1097
7. Bendelac A, Lantz O, Quimby ME, Yewdell JW, Bennink JR, Brutkiewicz RR. CD1 recognition by mouse NK1+ T lymphocytes. *Science* (1995) **268**:863–5. doi:10.1126/science.7538697
8. Hashimoto K, Hirai M, Kurosawa Y. A gene outside the human MHC related to classical HLA class I genes. *Science* (1995) **269**:693–5. doi:10.1126/science.7624800
9. Treiner E, Duban L, Bahram S, Radosavljevic M, Wanner V, Tilloy F, et al. Selection of evolutionarily conserved mucosal-associated invariant T cells by MR1. *Nature* (2003) **422**:164–9. doi:10.1038/nature01433
10. Tilloy F, Treiner E, Park SH, Garcia C, Lemonnier F, De La Salle H, et al. An invariant T cell receptor alpha chain defines a novel TAP-independent major histocompatibility complex class Ib-restricted alpha/beta T cell subpopulation in mammals. *J Exp Med* (1999) **189**:1907–21. doi:10.1084/jem.189.12.1907
11. Kjer-Nielsen L, Patel O, Corbett AJ, Le Nours J, Meehan B, Liu L, et al. MR1 presents microbial vitamin B metabolites to MAIT cells. *Nature* (2012) **491**:717–23. doi:10.1038/nature11605
12. Salio M, Silk JD, Jones EY, Cerundolo V. Biology of CD1- and MR1-restricted T cells. *Annu Rev Immunol* (2014) **32**:323–66. doi:10.1146/annurev-immunol-032713-120243
13. Ussher JE, Klenerman P, Willberg CB. Mucosal-associated invariant T-cells: new players in anti-bacterial immunity. *Front Immunol* (2014) **5**:450. doi:10.3389/fimmu.2014.00450
14. McEwen-Smith RM, Salio M, Cerundolo V. CD1d-dependent endogenous and exogenous lipid antigen presentation. *Curr Opin Immunol* (2015) **34**:116–25. doi:10.1016/j.coi.2015.03.004
15. McWilliam HE, Birkinshaw RW, Villadangos JA, Mccluskey J, Rossjohn J. MR1 presentation of vitamin B-based metabolite ligands. *Curr Opin Immunol* (2015) **34C**:28–34. doi:10.1016/j.coi.2014.12.004
16. Martin LH, Calabi F, Milstein C. Isolation of CD1 genes: a family of major histocompatibility complex-related differentiation antigens. *Proc Natl Acad Sci U S A* (1986) **83**:9154–8. doi:10.1073/pnas.83.23.9154
17. de la Salle H, Mariotti S, Angenieux C, Gilleron M, Garcia-Alles LF, Malm D, et al. Assistance of microbial glycolipid antigen processing by CD1e. *Science* (2005) **310**:1321–4. doi:10.1126/science.1115301
18. Silk JD, Salio M, Brown J, Jones EY, Cerundolo V. Structural and functional aspects of lipid binding by CD1 molecules. *Annu Rev Cell Dev Biol* (2008) **24**:369–95. doi:10.1146/annurev.cellbio.24.110707.175359
19. Cohen NR, Garg S, Brenner MB. Antigen presentation by CD1 lipids, T cells, and NKT cells in microbial immunity. *Adv Immunol* (2009) **102**:1–94. doi:10.1016/S0065-2776(09)01201-2
20. Mukherjee S, Soe TT, Maxfield FR. Endocytic sorting of lipid analogues differing solely in the chemistry of their hydrophobic tails. *J Cell Biol* (1999) **144**:1271–84. doi:10.1083/jcb.144.6.1271
21. Dascher CC, Brenner MB. Evolutionary constraints on CD1 structure: insights from comparative genomic analysis. *Trends Immunol* (2003) **24**:412–8. doi:10.1016/S1471-4906(03)00179-0
22. Kasmar AG, Van Rhijn I, Cheng TY, Turner M, Seshadri C, Schiefner A, et al. CD1b tetramers bind alphabeta T cell receptors to identify a mycobacterial glycolipid-reactive T cell repertoire in humans. *J Exp Med* (2011) **208**:1741–7. doi:10.1084/jem.20110665
23. Kasmar AG, Van Rhijn I, Magalhaes KG, Young DC, Cheng TY, Turner MT, et al. Cutting edge: CD1a tetramers and dextramers identify human lipopeptide-specific T cells ex vivo. *J Immunol* (2013) **191**:4499–503. doi:10.4049/jimmunol.1301660
24. Ly D, Kasmar AG, Cheng TY, De Jong A, Huang S, Roy S, et al. CD1c tetramers detect ex vivo T cell responses to processed phosphomycoketide antigens. *J Exp Med* (2013) **210**:729–41. doi:10.1084/jem.20120624
25. Felio K, Nguyen H, Dascher CC, Choi HJ, Li S, Zimmer MI, et al. CD1-restricted adaptive immune responses to *Mycobacteria* in human group 1 CD1 transgenic mice. *J Exp Med* (2009) **206**:2497–509. doi:10.1084/jem.20090898
26. Lockridge JL, Chen X, Zhou Y, Rajesh D, Roenneburg DA, Hegde S, et al. Analysis of the CD1 antigen presenting system in humanized SCID mice. *PLoS One* (2011) **6**:e21701. doi:10.1371/journal.pone.0021701
27. Huang S, Gilfillan S, Kim S, Thompson B, Wang X, Sant AJ, et al. MR1 uses an endocytic pathway to activate mucosal-associated invariant T cells. *J Exp Med* (2008) **205**:1201–11. doi:10.1084/jem.20072579
28. Dougan SK, Kaser A, Blumberg RS. CD1 expression on antigen-presenting cells. *Curr Top Microbiol Immunol* (2007) **314**:113–41.
29. Barral DC, Brenner MB. CD1 antigen presentation: how it works. *Nat Rev Immunol* (2007) **7**:929–41. doi:10.1038/nri2191
30. Zajonc DM, Elsliger MA, Teyton L, Wilson IA. Crystal structure of CD1a in complex with a sulfatide self antigen at a resolution of 2.15 A. *Nat Immunol* (2003) **4**:808–15. doi:10.1038/ni948
31. Zajonc DM, Crispin MD, Bowden TA, Young DC, Cheng TY, Hu J, et al. Molecular mechanism of lipopeptide presentation by CD1a. *Immunity* (2005) **22**:209–19. doi:10.1016/j.immuni.2004.12.009
32. Manolova V, Kistowska M, Paoletti S, Baltariu GM, Bausinger H, Hanau D, et al. Functional CD1a is stabilized by exogenous lipids. *Eur J Immunol* (2006) **36**:1083–92. doi:10.1002/eji.200535544
33. Moody DB, Young DC, Cheng TY, Rosat JP, Roura-Mir C, O'connor PB, et al. T cell activation by lipopeptide antigens. *Science* (2004) **303**:527–31. doi:10.1126/science.1089353
34. Shamshiev A, Gober HJ, Donda A, Mazorra Z, Mori L, De Libero G. Presentation of the same glycolipid by different CD1 molecules. *J Exp Med* (2002) **195**:1013–21. doi:10.1084/jem.20011963
35. de Jong A, Pena-Cruz V, Cheng TY, Clark RA, Van Rhijn I, Moody DB. CD1a-autoreactive T cells are a normal component of the human alphabeta T cell repertoire. *Nat Immunol* (2010) **11**:1102–9. doi:10.1038/ni.1956
36. de Lalla C, Lepore M, Piccolo FM, Rinaldi A, Scelfo A, Garavaglia C, et al. High-frequency and adaptive-like dynamics of human CD1

self-reactive T cells. *Eur J Immunol* (2011) **41**:602–10. doi:10.1002/eji.201041211
37. Zheng Y, Danilenko DM, Valdez P, Kasman I, Eastham-Anderson J, Wu J, et al. Interleukin-22, a T(H)17 cytokine, mediates IL-23-induced dermal inflammation and acanthosis. *Nature* (2007) **445**:648–51. doi:10.1038/nature05505
38. de Jong A, Cheng TY, Huang S, Gras S, Birkinshaw RW, Kasmar AG, et al. CD1a-autoreactive T cells recognize natural skin oils that function as headless antigens. *Nat Immunol* (2014) **15**:177–85. doi:10.1038/ni.2790
39. Birkinshaw RW, Pellicci DG, Cheng TY, Keller AN, Sandoval-Romero M, Gras S, et al. Alphabeta T cell antigen receptor recognition of CD1a presenting self lipid ligands. *Nat Immunol* (2015) **16**:258–66. doi:10.1038/ni.3098
40. Rossjohn J, Gras S, Miles JJ, Turner SJ, Godfrey DI, Mccluskey J. T cell antigen receptor recognition of antigen-presenting molecules. *Annu Rev Immunol* (2015) **33**:169–200. doi:10.1146/annurev-immunol-032414-112334
41. Bourgeois EA, Subramaniam S, Cheng TY, De Jong A, Layre E, Ly D, et al. Bee venom processes human skin lipids for presentation by CD1a. *J Exp Med* (2015) **212**:149–63. doi:10.1084/jem.20141505
42. Sugita M, Jackman RM, Van Donselaar E, Behar SM, Rogers RA, Peters PJ, et al. Cytoplasmic tail-dependent localization of CD1b antigen-presenting molecules to MIICs. *Science* (1996) **273**:349–52. doi:10.1126/science.273.5273.349
43. Sugita M, Cao X, Watts GF, Rogers RA, Bonifacino JS, Brenner MB. Failure of trafficking and antigen presentation by CD1 in AP-3-deficient cells. *Immunity* (2002) **16**:697–706. doi:10.1016/S1074-7613(02)00311-4
44. Relloso M, Cheng TY, Im JS, Parisini E, Roura-Mir C, Debono C, et al. pH-dependent interdomain tethers of CD1b regulate its antigen capture. *Immunity* (2008) **28**:774–86. doi:10.1016/j.immuni.2008.04.017
45. Leon L, Tatituri RV, Grenha R, Sun Y, Barral DC, Minnaard AJ, et al. Saposins utilize two strategies for lipid transfer and CD1 antigen presentation. *Proc Natl Acad Sci U S A* (2012) **109**:4357–64. doi:10.1073/pnas.1200764109
46. Gadola SD, Zaccai NR, Harlos K, Shepherd D, Castro-Palomino JC, Ritter G, et al. Structure of human CD1b with bound ligands at 2.3 A, a maze for alkyl chains. *Nat Immunol* (2002) **3**:721–6. doi:10.1038/ni821
47. Batuwangala T, Shepherd D, Gadola SD, Gibson KJ, Zaccai NR, Fersht AR, et al. The crystal structure of human CD1b with a bound bacterial glycolipid. *J Immunol* (2004) **172**:2382–8. doi:10.4049/jimmunol.172.4.2382
48. Garcia-Alles LF, Versluis K, Maveyraud L, Vallina AT, Sansano S, Bello NF, et al. Endogenous phosphatidylcholine and a long spacer ligand stabilize the lipid-binding groove of CD1b. *EMBO J* (2006) **25**:3684–92. doi:10.1038/sj.emboj.7601244
49. Huang S, Cheng TY, Young DC, Layre E, Madigan CA, Shires J, et al. Discovery of deoxyceramides and diacylglycerols as CD1b scaffold lipids among diverse groove-blocking lipids of the human CD1 system. *Proc Natl Acad Sci U S A* (2011) **108**:19335–40. doi:10.1073/pnas.1112969108
50. Garcia-Alles LF, Collmann A, Versluis C, Lindner B, Guiard J, Maveyraud L, et al. Structural reorganization of the antigen-binding groove of human CD1b for presentation of mycobacterial sulfoglycolipids. *Proc Natl Acad Sci U S A* (2011) **108**:17755–60. doi:10.1073/pnas.1110118108
51. Zajonc DM, Cantu C III, Mattner J, Zhou D, Savage PB, Bendelac A, et al. Structure and function of a potent agonist for the semi-invariant natural killer T cell receptor. *Nat Immunol* (2005) **6**:810–8. doi:10.1038/ni1224
52. Scharf L, Li NS, Hawk AJ, Garzon D, Zhang T, Fox LM, et al. The 2.5 a structure of CD1c in complex with a mycobacterial lipid reveals an open groove ideally suited for diverse antigen presentation. *Immunity* (2010) **33**:853–62. doi:10.1016/j.immuni.2010.11.026
53. Shamshiev A, Donda A, Carena I, Mori L, Kappos L, De Libero G. Self glycolipids as T-cell autoantigens. *Eur J Immunol* (1999) **29**:1667–75. doi:10.1002/(SICI)1521-4141(199905)29:05<1667::AID-IMMU1667>3.0.CO;2-U
54. De Libero G, Moran AP, Gober HJ, Rossy E, Shamshiev A, Chelnokova O, et al. Bacterial infections promote T cell recognition of self-glycolipids. *Immunity* (2005) **22**:763–72. doi:10.1016/j.immuni.2005.04.013
55. Layre E, Collmann A, Bastian M, Mariotti S, Czaplicki J, Prandi J, et al. Mycolic acids constitute a scaffold for mycobacterial lipid antigens stimulating CD1-restricted T cells. *Chem Biol* (2009) **16**:82–92. doi:10.1016/j.chembiol.2008.11.008
56. De Libero G, Mori L. The T-cell response to lipid antigens of *Mycobacterium tuberculosis*. *Front Immunol* (2014) **5**:219. doi:10.3389/fimmu.2014.00219
57. Van Rhijn I, Moody DB. CD1 and mycobacterial lipids activate human T cells. *Immunol Rev* (2015) **264**:138–53. doi:10.1111/imr.12253
58. Van Rhijn I, Kasmar A, De Jong A, Gras S, Bhati M, Doorenspleet ME, et al. A conserved human T cell population targets mycobacterial antigens presented by CD1b. *Nat Immunol* (2013) **14**:706–13. doi:10.1038/ni.2630
59. Van Rhijn I, Gherardin NA, Kasmar A, De Jager W, Pellicci DG, Kostenko L, et al. TCR bias and affinity define two compartments of the CD1b-glycolipid-specific T Cell repertoire. *J Immunol* (2014) **192**:4054–60. doi:10.4049/jimmunol.1400158
60. Sugita M, Van Der Wel N, Rogers RA, Peters PJ, Brenner MB. CD1c molecules broadly survey the endocytic system. *Proc Natl Acad Sci U S A* (2000) **97**:8445–50. doi:10.1073/pnas.150236797
61. Faure F, Jitsukawa S, Miossec C, Hercend T. CD1c as a target recognition structure for human T lymphocytes: analysis with peripheral blood gamma/delta cells. *Eur J Immunol* (1990) **20**:703–6. doi:10.1002/eji.1830200336
62. Spada FM, Grant EP, Peters PJ, Sugita M, Melian A, Leslie DS, et al. Self-recognition of CD1 by gamma/delta T cells: implications for innate immunity. *J Exp Med* (2000) **191**:937–48. doi:10.1084/jem.191.6.937
63. Lepore M, De Lalla C, Gundimeda SR, Gsellinger H, Consonni M, Garavaglia C, et al. A novel self-lipid antigen targets human T cells against CD1c(+) leukemias. *J Exp Med* (2014) **211**:1363–77. doi:10.1084/jem.20140410
64. Moody DB, Ulrichs T, Muhlecker W, Young DC, Gurcha SS, Grant E, et al. CD1c-mediated T-cell recognition of isoprenoid glycolipids in *Mycobacterium tuberculosis* infection. *Nature* (2000) **404**:884–8. doi:10.1038/35009119
65. Matsunaga I, Bhatt A, Young DC, Cheng TY, Eyles SJ, Besra GS, et al. *Mycobacterium tuberculosis* pks12 produces a novel polyketide presented by CD1c to T cells. *J Exp Med* (2004) **200**:1559–69. doi:10.1084/jem.20041429
66. de Jong A, Arce EC, Cheng TY, Van Summeren RP, Feringa BL, Dudkin V, et al. CD1c presentation of synthetic glycolipid antigens with foreign alkyl branching motifs. *Chem Biol* (2007) **14**:1232–42. doi:10.1016/j.chembiol.2007.09.010
67. Van Rhijn I, Young DC, De Jong A, Vazquez J, Cheng TY, Talekar R, et al. CD1c bypasses lysosomes to present a lipopeptide antigen with 12 amino acids. *J Exp Med* (2009) **206**:1409–22. doi:10.1084/jem.20082480
68. Roy S, Ly D, Li NS, Altman JD, Piccirilli JA, Moody DB, et al. Molecular basis of mycobacterial lipid antigen presentation by CD1c and its recognition by alphabeta T cells. *Proc Natl Acad Sci U S A* (2014) **111**:E4648–57. doi:10.1073/pnas.1408549111
69. Engel I, Kronenberg M. Transcriptional control of the development and function of Valpha14i NKT cells. *Curr Top Microbiol Immunol* (2014) **381**:51–81. doi:10.1007/82_2014_375
70. Robertson FC, Berzofsky JA, Terabe M. NKT cell networks in the regulation of tumor immunity. *Front Immunol* (2014) **5**:543. doi:10.3389/fimmu.2014.00543
71. Kim EY, Lynch L, Brennan PJ, Cohen NR, Brenner MB. The transcriptional programs of iNKT cells. *Semin Immunol* (2015) **27**(1):26–32. doi:10.1016/j.smim.2015.02.005
72. Honda K, Littman DR. The microbiome in infectious disease and inflammation. *Annu Rev Immunol* (2012) **30**:759–95. doi:10.1146/annurev-immunol-020711-074937
73. Kawano T, Cui J, Koezuka Y, Toura I, Kaneko Y, Motoki K, et al. CD1d-restricted and TCR-mediated activation of valpha14 NKT cells by glycosylceramides. *Science* (1997) **278**:1626–9. doi:10.1126/science.278.5343.1626
74. Brigl M, Tatituri RV, Watts GF, Bhowruth V, Leadbetter EA, Barton N, et al. Innate and cytokine-driven signals, rather than microbial antigens, dominate in natural killer T cell activation during microbial infection. *J Exp Med* (2011) **208**:1163–77. doi:10.1084/jem.20102555
75. Wieland Brown LC, Penaranda C, Kashyap PC, Williams BB, Clardy J, Kronenberg M, et al. Production of alpha-galactosylceramide by a prominent member of the human gut microbiota. *PLoS Biol* (2013) **11**:e1001610. doi:10.1371/journal.pbio.1001610
76. An D, Oh SF, Olszak T, Neves JF, Avci FY, Erturk-Hasdemir D, et al. Sphingolipids from a symbiotic microbe regulate homeostasis of host intestinal natural killer T cells. *Cell* (2014) **156**:123–33. doi:10.1016/j.cell.2013.11.042
77. Olszak T, An D, Zeissig S, Vera MP, Richter J, Franke A, et al. Microbial exposure during early life has persistent effects on natural killer T cell function. *Science* (2012) **336**:489–93. doi:10.1126/science.1219328

78. Nieuwenhuis EE, Matsumoto T, Lindenbergh D, Willemsen R, Kaser A, Simons-Oosterhuis Y, et al. Cd1d-dependent regulation of bacterial colonization in the intestine of mice. *J Clin Invest* (2009) **119**:1241–50. doi:10.1172/JCI36509
79. Olszak T, Neves JF, Dowds CM, Baker K, Glickman J, Davidson NO, et al. Protective mucosal immunity mediated by epithelial CD1d and IL-10. *Nature* (2014) **509**:497–502. doi:10.1038/nature13150
80. Loh L, Ivarsson MA, Michaelsson J, Sandberg JK, Nixon DF. Invariant natural killer T cells developing in the human fetus accumulate and mature in the small intestine. *Mucosal Immunol* (2014) **7**:1233–43. doi:10.1038/mi.2014.13
81. Fuss IJ, Joshi B, Yang Z, Degheidy H, Fichtner-Feigl S, De Souza H, et al. IL-13Ralpha2-bearing, type II NKT cells reactive to sulfatide self-antigen populate the mucosa of ulcerative colitis. *Gut* (2014) **63**:1728–36. doi:10.1136/gutjnl-2013-305671
82. Lynch L, Michelet X, Zhang S, Brennan PJ, Moseman A, Lester C, et al. Regulatory iNKT cells lack expression of the transcription factor PLZF and control the homeostasis of T(reg) cells and macrophages in adipose tissue. *Nat Immunol* (2015) **16**:85–95. doi:10.1038/ni.3047
83. Lynch L. Adipose invariant natural killer T cells. *Immunology* (2014) **142**:337–46. doi:10.1111/imm.12269
84. Bai L, Picard D, Anderson B, Chaudhary V, Luoma A, Jabri B, et al. The majority of CD1d-sulfatide-specific T cells in human blood use a semiinvariant Vdelta1 TCR. *Eur J Immunol* (2012) **42**:2505–10. doi:10.1002/eji.201242531
85. Uldrich AP, Le Nours J, Pellicci DG, Gherardin NA, Mcpherson KG, Lim RT, et al. CD1d-lipid antigen recognition by the gammadelta TCR. *Nat Immunol* (2013) **14**:1137–45. doi:10.1038/ni.2713
86. Groh V, Steinle A, Bauer S, Spies T. Recognition of stress-induced MHC molecules by intestinal epithelial gammadelta T cells. *Science* (1998) **279**:1737–40. doi:10.1126/science.279.5357.1737
87. Vantourout P, Hayday A. Six-of-the-best: unique contributions of gammadelta T cells to immunology. *Nat Rev Immunol* (2013) **13**:88–100. doi:10.1038/nri3384
88. Luoma AM, Castro CD, Mayassi T, Bembinster LA, Bai L, Picard D, et al. Crystal structure of Vdelta1 T cell receptor in complex with CD1d-sulfatide shows MHC-like recognition of a self-lipid by human gammadelta T cells. *Immunity* (2013) **39**:1032–42. doi:10.1016/j.immuni.2013.11.001
89. Fox LM, Cox DG, Lockridge JL, Wang X, Chen X, Scharf L, et al. Recognition of lyso-phospholipids by human natural killer T lymphocytes. *PLoS Biol* (2009) **7**:e1000228. doi:10.1371/journal.pbio.1000228
90. Chang DH, Deng H, Matthews P, Krasovsky J, Ragupathi G, Spisek R, et al. Inflammation-associated lysophospholipids as ligands for CD1d-restricted T cells in human cancer. *Blood* (2008) **112**:1308–16. doi:10.1182/blood-2008-04-149831
91. Zeissig S, Murata K, Sweet L, Publicover J, Hu Z, Kaser A, et al. Hepatitis B virus-induced lipid alterations contribute to natural killer T cell-dependent protective immunity. *Nat Med* (2012) **18**:1060–8. doi:10.1038/nm.2811
92. Nair S, Boddupalli CS, Verma R, Liu J, Yang R, Pastores GM, et al. Type II NKT-TFH cells against gaucher lipids regulate B-cell immunity and inflammation. *Blood* (2015) **125**:1256–71. doi:10.1182/blood-2014-09-600270
93. Mellman I, Steinman RM. Dendritic cells: specialized and regulated antigen processing machines. *Cell* (2001) **106**:255–8. doi:10.1016/S0092-8674(01)00449-4
94. Villadangos JA, Schnorrer P. Intrinsic and cooperative antigen-presenting functions of dendritic-cell subsets in vivo. *Nat Rev Immunol* (2007) **7**:543–55. doi:10.1038/nri2103
95. Palucka K, Banchereau J, Mellman I. Designing vaccines based on biology of human dendritic cell subsets. *Immunity* (2010) **33**:464–78. doi:10.1016/j.immuni.2010.10.007
96. Leslie DS, Dascher CC, Cembrola K, Townes MA, Hava DL, Hugendubler LC, et al. Serum lipids regulate dendritic cell CD1 expression and function. *Immunology* (2008) **125**:289–301. doi:10.1111/j.1365-2567.2008.02842.x
97. Randolph GJ, Beaulieu S, Lebecque S, Steinman RM, Muller WA. Differentiation of monocytes into dendritic cells in a model of transendothelial trafficking. *Science* (1998) **282**:480–3. doi:10.1126/science.282.5388.480
98. Krutzik SR, Tan B, Li H, Ochoa MT, Liu PT, Sharfstein SE, et al. TLR activation triggers the rapid differentiation of monocytes into macrophages and dendritic cells. *Nat Med* (2005) **11**:653–60. doi:10.1038/nm1246
99. Roura-Mir C, Wang L, Cheng TY, Matsunaga I, Dascher CC, Peng SL, et al. *Mycobacterium tuberculosis* regulates CD1 antigen presentation pathways through TLR-2. *J Immunol* (2005) **175**:1758–66. doi:10.4049/jimmunol.175.3.1758
100. Schenk M, Krutzik SR, Sieling PA, Lee DJ, Teles RM, Ochoa MT, et al. NOD2 triggers an interleukin-32-dependent human dendritic cell program in leprosy. *Nat Med* (2012) **18**:555–63. doi:10.1038/nm.2650
101. Yakimchuk K, Roura-Mir C, Magalhaes KG, De Jong A, Kasmar AG, Granter SR, et al. Borrelia burgdorferi infection regulates CD1 expression in human cells and tissues via IL1-beta. *Eur J Immunol* (2011) **41**:694–705. doi:10.1002/eji.201040808
102. Hava DL, Van Der Wel N, Cohen N, Dascher CC, Houben D, Leon L, et al. Evasion of peptide, but not lipid antigen presentation, through pathogen-induced dendritic cell maturation. *Proc Natl Acad Sci U S A* (2008) **105**:11281–6. doi:10.1073/pnas.0804681105
103. Vincent MS, Leslie DS, Gumperz JE, Xiong X, Grant EP, Brenner MB. CD1-dependent dendritic cell instruction. *Nat Immunol* (2002) **3**:1163–8. doi:10.1038/ni851
104. Cella M, Engering A, Pinet V, Pieters J, Lanzavecchia A. Inflammatory stimuli induce accumulation of MHC class II complexes on dendritic cells. *Nature* (1997) **388**:782–7. doi:10.1038/42030
105. Cella M, Salio M, Sakakibara Y, Langen H, Julkunen I, Lanzavecchia A. Maturation, activation, and protection of dendritic cells induced by double-stranded RNA. *J Exp Med* (1999) **189**:821–9. doi:10.1084/jem.189.5.821
106. Cao X, Sugita M, Van Der Wel N, Lai J, Rogers RA, Peters PJ, et al. CD1 molecules efficiently present antigen in immature dendritic cells and traffic independently of MHC class II during dendritic cell maturation. *J Immunol* (2002) **169**:4770–7. doi:10.4049/jimmunol.169.9.4770
107. van den Elzen P, Garg S, Leon L, Brigl M, Leadbetter EA, Gumperz JE, et al. Apolipoprotein-mediated pathways of lipid antigen presentation. *Nature* (2005) **437**:906–10. doi:10.1038/nature04001
108. Hunger RE, Sieling PA, Ochoa MT, Sugaya M, Burdick AE, Rea TH, et al. Langerhans cells utilize CD1a and langerin to efficiently present nonpeptide antigens to T cells. *J Clin Invest* (2004) **113**:101–8. doi:10.1172/JCI19655
109. Prigozy TI, Sieling PA, Clemens D, Stewart PL, Behar SM, Porcelli SA, et al. The mannose receptor delivers lipoglycan antigens to endosomes for presentation to T cells by CD1b molecules. *Immunity* (1997) **6**:187–97. doi:10.1016/S1074-7613(00)80425-2
110. Jiang W, Swiggard WJ, Heufler C, Peng M, Mirza A, Steinman RM, et al. The receptor DEC-205 expressed by dendritic cells and thymic epithelial cells is involved in antigen processing. *Nature* (1995) **375**:151–5. doi:10.1038/375151a0
111. Engering A, Geijtenbeek TB, Van Vliet SJ, Wijers M, Van Liempt E, Demaurex N, et al. The dendritic cell-specific adhesion receptor DC-SIGN internalizes antigen for presentation to T cells. *J Immunol* (2002) **168**:2118–26. doi:10.4049/jimmunol.168.5.2118
112. Kawasaki N, Rillahan CD, Cheng TY, Van Rhijn I, Macauley MS, Moody DB, et al. Targeted delivery of mycobacterial antigens to human dendritic cells via siglec-7 induces robust T cell activation. *J Immunol* (2014) **193**:1560–6. doi:10.4049/jimmunol.1303278
113. Cox D, Fox L, Tian R, Bardet W, Skaley M, Mojsilovic D, et al. Determination of cellular lipids bound to human CD1d molecules. *PLoS One* (2009) **4**:e5325. doi:10.1371/journal.pone.0005325
114. Yuan W, Kang SJ, Evans JE, Cresswell P. Natural lipid ligands associated with human CD1d targeted to different subcellular compartments. *J Immunol* (2009) **182**:4784–91. doi:10.4049/jimmunol.0803981
115. Kiguchi K, Henning-Chubb CB, Huberman E. Glycosphingolipid patterns of peripheral blood lymphocytes, monocytes, and granulocytes are cell specific. *J Biochem* (1990) **107**:8–14.
116. Paget C, Mallevaey T, Speak AO, Torres D, Fontaine J, Sheehan KC, et al. Activation of invariant NKT cells by toll-like receptor 9-stimulated dendritic cells requires type I interferon and charged glycosphingolipids. *Immunity* (2007) **27**:597–609. doi:10.1016/j.immuni.2007.08.017
117. Salio M, Speak AO, Shepherd D, Polzella P, Illarionov PA, Veerapen N, et al. Modulation of human natural killer T cell ligands on TLR-mediated antigen-presenting cell activation. *Proc Natl Acad Sci U S A* (2007) **104**:20490–5. doi:10.1073/pnas.0710145104
118. Brennan PJ, Tatituri RV, Brigl M, Kim EY, Tuli A, Sanderson JP, et al. Invariant natural killer T cells recognize lipid self antigen induced by microbial danger signals. *Nat Immunol* (2011) **12**:1202–11. doi:10.1038/ni.2143
119. Muindi K, Cernadas M, Watts GF, Royle L, Neville DC, Dwek RA, et al. Activation state and intracellular trafficking contribute to the repertoire of

endogenous glycosphingolipids presented by CD1d [corrected]. *Proc Natl Acad Sci U S A* (2010) **107**:3052–7. doi:10.1073/pnas.0915056107

120. Huang S, Martin E, Kim S, Yu L, Soudais C, Fremont DH, et al. MR1 antigen presentation to mucosal-associated invariant T cells was highly conserved in evolution. *Proc Natl Acad Sci U S A* (2009) **106**:8290–5. doi:10.1073/pnas.0903196106
121. Seach N, Guerri L, Le Bourhis L, Mburu Y, Cui Y, Bessoles S, et al. Double-positive thymocytes select mucosal-associated invariant T cells. *J Immunol* (2013) **191**:6002–9. doi:10.4049/jimmunol.1301212
122. Martin E, Treiner E, Duban L, Guerri L, Laude H, Toly C, et al. Stepwise development of MAIT cells in mouse and human. *PLoS Biol* (2009) **7**:e54. doi:10.1371/journal.pbio.1000054
123. Leeansyah E, Loh L, Nixon DF, Sandberg JK. Acquisition of innate-like microbial reactivity in mucosal tissues during human fetal MAIT-cell development. *Nat Commun* (2014) **5**:3143. doi:10.1038/ncomms4143
124. Gold MC, Cerri S, Smyk-Pearson S, Cansler ME, Vogt TM, Delepine J, et al. Human mucosal associated invariant T cells detect bacterially infected cells. *PLoS Biol* (2010) **8**:e1000407. doi:10.1371/journal.pbio.1000407
125. Le Bourhis L, Martin E, Peguillet I, Guihot A, Froux N, Core M, et al. Antimicrobial activity of mucosal-associated invariant T cells. *Nat Immunol* (2010) **11**:701–8. doi:10.1038/ni.1890
126. Georgel P, Radosavljevic M, Macquin C, Bahram S. The non-conventional MHC class I MR1 molecule controls infection by *Klebsiella pneumoniae* in mice. *Mol Immunol* (2011) **48**:769–75. doi:10.1016/j.molimm.2010.12.002
127. Chua WJ, Truscott SM, Eickhoff CS, Blazevic A, Hoft DF, Hansen TH. Polyclonal mucosa-associated invariant T cells have unique innate functions in bacterial infection. *Infect Immun* (2012) **80**:3256–67. doi:10.1128/IAI.00279-12
128. Meierovics A, Yankelevich WJ, Cowley SC. MAIT cells are critical for optimal mucosal immune responses during in vivo pulmonary bacterial infection. *Proc Natl Acad Sci U S A* (2013) **110**:E3119–28. doi:10.1073/pnas.1302799110
129. Gold MC, Napier RJ, Lewinsohn DM. MR1-restricted mucosal associated invariant T (MAIT) cells in the immune response to *Mycobacterium tuberculosis*. *Immunol Rev* (2015) **264**:154–66. doi:10.1111/imr.12271
130. Ussher JE, Bilton M, Attwod E, Shadwell J, Richardson R, De Lara C, et al. CD161++ CD8+ T cells, including the MAIT cell subset, are specifically activated by IL-12+IL-18 in a TCR-independent manner. *Eur J Immunol* (2014) **44**:195–203. doi:10.1002/eji.201343509
131. Chua WJ, Kim S, Myers N, Huang S, Yu L, Fremont DH, et al. Endogenous MHC-related protein 1 is transiently expressed on the plasma membrane in a conformation that activates mucosal-associated invariant T cells. *J Immunol* (2011) **186**:4744–50. doi:10.4049/jimmunol.1003254
132. Eckle SB, Birkinshaw RW, Kostenko L, Corbett AJ, Mcwilliam HE, Reantragoon R, et al. A molecular basis underpinning the T cell receptor heterogeneity of mucosal-associated invariant T cells. *J Exp Med* (2014) **211**:1585–600. doi:10.1084/jem.20140484
133. Soudais C, Samassa F, Sarkis M, Le Bourhis L, Bessoles S, Blanot D, et al. In vitro and in vivo analysis of the gram-negative bacteria-derived riboflavin precursor derivatives activating mouse MAIT cells. *J Immunol* (2015) **194**(10):4641–9. doi:10.4049/jimmunol.1403224
134. Patel O, Kjer-Nielsen L, Le Nours J, Eckle SB, Birkinshaw R, Beddoe T, et al. Recognition of vitamin B metabolites by mucosal-associated invariant T cells. *Nat Commun* (2013) **4**:2142. doi:10.1038/ncomms3142
135. Corbett AJ, Eckle SB, Birkinshaw RW, Liu L, Patel O, Mahony J, et al. T-cell activation by transitory neo-antigens derived from distinct microbial pathways. *Nature* (2014) **509**:361–5. doi:10.1038/nature13160
136. Reantragoon R, Corbett AJ, Sakala IG, Gherardin NA, Furness JB, Chen Z, et al. Antigen-loaded MR1 tetramers define T cell receptor heterogeneity in mucosal-associated invariant T cells. *J Exp Med* (2013) **210**:2305–20. doi:10.1084/jem.20130958
137. Leeansyah E, Ganesh A, Quigley MF, Sonnerborg A, Andersson J, Hunt PW, et al. Activation, exhaustion, and persistent decline of the antimicrobial MR1-restricted MAIT-cell population in chronic HIV-1 infection. *Blood* (2013) **121**:1124–35. doi:10.1182/blood-2012-07-445429
138. Lepore M, Kalinichenko A, Colone A, Paleja B, Singhal A, Tschumi A, et al. Parallel T-cell cloning and deep sequencing of human MAIT cells reveal stable oligoclonal TCRbeta repertoire. *Nat Commun* (2014) **5**:3866. doi:10.1038/ncomms4866
139. Gold MC, Mclaren JE, Reistetter JA, Smyk-Pearson S, Ladell K, Swarbrick GM, et al. MR1-restricted MAIT cells display ligand discrimination and pathogen selectivity through distinct T cell receptor usage. *J Exp Med* (2014) **211**:1601–10. doi:10.1084/jem.20140507
140. Lopez-Sagaseta J, Dulberger CL, Crooks JE, Parks CD, Luoma AM, Mcfedries A, et al. The molecular basis for mucosal-associated invariant T cell recognition of MR1 proteins. *Proc Natl Acad Sci U S A* (2013) **110**:E1771–8. doi:10.1073/pnas.1222678110
141. Lopez-Sagaseta J, Dulberger CL, Mcfedries A, Cushman M, Saghatelian A, Adams EJ. MAIT recognition of a stimulatory bacterial antigen bound to MR1. *J Immunol* (2013) **191**:5268–77. doi:10.4049/jimmunol.1301958
142. Birkinshaw RW, Kjer-Nielsen L, Eckle SB, Mccluskey J, Rossjohn J. MAITs, MR1 and vitamin B metabolites. *Curr Opin Immunol* (2014) **26**:7–13. doi:10.1016/j.coi.2013.09.007
143. Pellicci DG, Patel O, Kjer-Nielsen L, Pang SS, Sullivan LC, Kyparissoudis K, et al. Differential recognition of CD1d-alpha-galactosyl ceramide by the V beta 8.2 and V beta 7 semi-invariant NKT T cell receptors. *Immunity* (2009) **31**:47–59. doi:10.1016/j.immuni.2009.04.018
144. Matulis G, Sanderson JP, Lissin NM, Asparuhova MB, Bommineni GR, Schumperli D, et al. Innate-like control of human iNKT cell autoreactivity via the hypervariable CDR3beta loop. *PLoS Biol* (2010) **8**:e1000402. doi:10.1371/journal.pbio.1000402
145. Croxford JL, Miyake S, Huang YY, Shimamura M, Yamamura T. Invariant V(alpha)19i T cells regulate autoimmune inflammation. *Nat Immunol* (2006) **7**:987–94. doi:10.1038/ni1370
146. Illes Z, Shimamura M, Newcombe J, Oka N, Yamamura T. Accumulation of Valpha7.2-Jalpha33 invariant T cells in human autoimmune inflammatory lesions in the nervous system. *Int Immunol* (2004) **16**:223–30. doi:10.1093/intimm/dxh018
147. Miyazaki Y, Miyake S, Chiba A, Lantz O, Yamamura T. Mucosal-associated invariant T cells regulate Th1 response in multiple sclerosis. *Int Immunol* (2011) **23**:529–35. doi:10.1093/intimm/dxr047
148. Willing A, Leach OA, Ufer F, Attfield KE, Steinbach K, Kursawe N, et al. CD8(+) MAIT cells infiltrate into the CNS and alterations in their blood frequencies correlate with IL-18 serum levels in multiple sclerosis. *Eur J Immunol* (2014) **44**:3119–28. doi:10.1002/eji.201344160
149. Dunne MR, Elliott L, Hussey S, Mahmud N, Kelly J, Doherty DG, et al. Persistent changes in circulating and intestinal gammadelta T cell subsets, invariant natural killer T cells and mucosal-associated invariant T cells in children and adults with coeliac disease. *PLoS One* (2013) **8**:e76008. doi:10.1371/journal.pone.0076008
150. Serriari NE, Eoche M, Lamotte L, Lion J, Fumery M, Marcelo P, et al. Innate mucosal-associated invariant T (MAIT) cells are activated in inflammatory bowel diseases. *Clin Exp Immunol* (2014) **176**:266–74. doi:10.1111/cei.12277
151. Cosgrove C, Ussher JE, Rauch A, Gartner K, Kurioka A, Huhn MH, et al. Early and nonreversible decrease of CD161++/MAIT cells in HIV infection. *Blood* (2013) **121**:951–61. doi:10.1182/blood-2012-06-436436
152. Teunissen MB, Yeremenko NG, Baeten DL, Chielie S, Spuls PI, De Rie MA, et al. The IL-17A-producing CD8+ T-cell population in psoriatic lesional skin comprises mucosa-associated invariant T cells and conventional T cells. *J Invest Dermatol* (2014) **134**:2898–907. doi:10.1038/jid.2014.261
153. Cho YN, Kee SJ, Kim TJ, Jin HM, Kim MJ, Jung HJ, et al. Mucosal-associated invariant T cell deficiency in systemic lupus erythematosus. *J Immunol* (2014) **193**:3891–901. doi:10.4049/jimmunol.1302701
154. Sharma PK, Wong EB, Napier RJ, Bishai WR, Ndung'u T, Kasprowicz VO, et al. High expression of CD26 accurately identifies human bacteria-reactive MR1-restricted MAIT cells. *Immunology* (2015) **145**(3):443–53. doi:10.1111/imm.12461
155. Magalhaes I, Pingris K, Poitou C, Bessoles S, Venteclef N, Kiaf B, et al. Mucosal-associated invariant T cell alterations in obese and type 2 diabetic patients. *J Clin Invest* (2015) **125**:1752–62. doi:10.1172/JCI78941
156. Tang XZ, Jo J, Tan AT, Sandalova E, Chia A, Tan KC, et al. IL-7 licenses activation of human liver intrasinusoidal mucosal-associated invariant T cells. *J Immunol* (2013) **190**:3142–52. doi:10.4049/jimmunol.1203218
157. Martin-Fontecha A, Thomsen LL, Brett S, Gerard C, Lipp M, Lanzavecchia A, et al. Induced recruitment of NK cells to lymph nodes provides IFN-gamma for T(H)1 priming. *Nat Immunol* (2004) **5**:1260–5. doi:10.1038/ni1138

158. Cerundolo V, Silk JD, Masri SH, Salio M. Harnessing invariant NKT cells in vaccination strategies. *Nat Rev Immunol* (2009) **9**:28–38. doi:10.1038/nri2451
159. Salerno-Goncalves R, Rezwan T, Sztein MB. B cells modulate mucosal associated invariant T cell immune responses. *Front Immunol* (2014) **4**:511. doi:10.3389/fimmu.2013.00511
160. Rosen DB, Cao W, Avery DT, Tangye SG, Liu YJ, Houchins JP, et al. Functional consequences of interactions between human NKR-P1A and its ligand LLT1 expressed on activated dendritic cells and B cells. *J Immunol* (2008) **180**:6508–17. doi:10.4049/jimmunol.180.10.6508
161. Germain C, Meier A, Jensen T, Knapnougel P, Poupon G, Lazzari A, et al. Induction of lectin-like transcript 1 (LLT1) protein cell surface expression by pathogens and interferon-gamma contributes to modulate immune responses. *J Biol Chem* (2011) **286**:37964–75. doi:10.1074/jbc.M111.285312
162. van Schaik B, Klarenbeek P, Doorenspleet M, Van Kampen A, Moody DB, De Vries N, et al. Discovery of invariant T cells by next-generation sequencing of the human TCR alpha-chain repertoire. *J Immunol* (2014) **193**:5338–44. doi:10.4049/jimmunol.1401380

21

Genome-Wide Analysis Reveals Selective Modulation of microRNAs by Histone Deacetylase Inhibitor in B Cells Induced to Undergo Class-Switch DNA Recombination and Plasma Cell Differentiation

Tian Shen, Helia N. Sanchez, Hong Zan and Paolo Casali**

Department of Microbiology and Immunology, University of Texas School of Medicine, UT Health Science Center, San Antonio, TX, USA

Edited by:
George C. Tsokos,
Harvard Medical School, USA

Reviewed by:
Bonnie B. Blomberg,
University of Miami Miller School of Medicine, USA
Nan Shen,
Shanghai Jiao Tong University School of Medicine, China

***Correspondence:**
Hong Zan
zan@uthscsa.edu;
Paolo Casali
pcasali@uthscsa.edu

As we have suggested, epigenetic factors, such as microRNAs (miRNAs), can interact with genetic programs to regulate B cell functions, thereby informing antibody and autoantibody responses. We have shown that histone deacetylase (HDAC) inhibitors (HDI) inhibit the differentiation events critical to the maturation of the antibody response: class-switch DNA recombination (CSR), somatic hypermutation (SHM), and plasma cell differentiation, by modulating intrinsic B cell mechanisms. HDI repress the expression of AID and Blimp-1, which are critical for CSR/SHM and plasma cell differentiation, respectively, in mouse and human B cells by upregulating selected miRNAs that silenced *AICDA/Aicda* and *PRDM1/Prdm1* mRNAs, as demonstrated by multiple qRT-PCRs (*J Immunol* 193:5933–5950, 2014). To further define the selectivity of HDI-mediated modulation of miRNA and gene expression, we performed genome-wide miRNA-Seq and mRNA-Seq analysis in B cells stimulated by LPS plus IL-4 and treated with HDI or nil. Consistent with what we have shown using qRT-PCR, these HDI-treated B cells displayed reduced expression of *Aicda* and *Prdm1*, and increased expression of miR-155, miR-181b, and miR-361, which target *Aicda,* and miR-23b, miR-30a, and miR-125b, which target *Prdm1*. In B cells induced to undergo CSR and plasma cell differentiation, about 23% of over 22,000 mRNAs analyzed were expressed at a significantly high copy number (more than 20 copies/cell). Only 18 (0.36%) of these highly expressed mRNAs, including *Aicda*, *Prdm1*, and *Xbp1*, were downregulated by HDI by 50% or more. Further, only 16 (0.30%) of the highly expressed mRNAs were upregulated (more than twofold) by HDI. The selectivity of HDI-mediated modulation of gene expression was emphasized by unchanged expression of the genes that are involved in regulation, targeting, or DNA repair processes of CSR, as well as unchanged expression of the genes encoding epigenetic regulators and factors that are important for cell signaling or apoptosis. Our findings indicate that, in B cells induced to undergo CSR and plasma cell differentiation, HDI modulate selected miRNAs and mRNAs, possibly as a result of HDACs existing in unique contexts of HDAC/cofactor complexes, as occurring in B lymphocytes, particularly when in an activated state.

Keywords: AID, Blimp1, B cell, class-switch DNA recombination, epigenetics, HDAC, HDAC inhibitor, histone acetylation, microRNA, mRNA, mRNA-Seq, miRNA-Seq, plasma cell differentiation, somatic hypermutation

INTRODUCTION

Epigenetic markers or factors, such as DNA methylation, histone posttranslational modifications, and microRNAs (miRNAs), dynamically regulate gene activities. As we have contended, epigenetic markers/factors "interact" with genetic programs to regulate B cell functions, such as class-switch DNA recombination (CSR), somatic hypermutation (SHM), and differentiation to memory B cell or plasma cell, thereby informing antibody and autoantibody responses (1). CSR and SHM are B cell-intrinsic differentiation processes that underpin the generation of class-switched and high-affinity antibodies, such as those that clear microbial pathogens or kill tumor cells. CSR and SHM critically require activation-induced cytidine deaminase (AID, encoded by *AICDA* in humans and *Aicda* in mice), which is specifically and highly induced in B cells in both T-dependent and T-independent antibody responses (2). Class-switched and hypermutated B cells further differentiate into antibody-secreting plasma cells in a fashion critically dependent on B lymphocyte-induced maturation protein 1 (Blimp1, encoded by *PRDM1* in human beings and *Prdm1* in mice) (3), or transition to long-lived memory B cells, which can differentiate into plasma cells upon reactivation by antigen to mediate an anamnestic response (4). Pathogenic autoantibodies, including those to nuclear components in systemic lupus erythematosus (SLE) patients (5, 6), are also class-switched and hypermutated (7, 8). Thus, epigenetic dysregulation of B cells can result in aberrant antibody responses to exogenous antigens, such as those on viruses and bacteria, or self-antigens, such as chromatin, histones, and dsDNA in lupus (1, 7).

The chromatin structure is comprised of DNA and histones. The basic repeating unit of chromatin is the nucleosome, a 147 bp of DNA chain wrapped around one histone octamer composed of two copies of each of four histones: H2A, H2B, H3, and H4. Histone posttranslational modifications include phosphorylation of serine or threonine residues, methylation of lysine or arginine, acetylation and deacetylation of lysines, and ubiquitylation and sumoylation of lysines. All these posttranslational modifications play an important role in regulating gene expression (9, 10). Histone acetylation and deacetylation, which are essential for gene regulation, are typically modulated by histone acetyltransferase (HAT) and histone deacetylase (HDAC) (9, 10). Histone acetylation catalyzed by HAT will result in a loose chromatin structure, which enables DNA binding proteins to activate gene transcription, while histone deacetylation catalyzed by HDAC will result in a condensed chromatin structure, which prevents binding of transcription factors or proteins to DNA and silence gene expression. HDAC inhibitors (HDI) alter gene expression by altering chromatin accessibility (11, 12).

MicroRNAs also play an important role in regulation of the genes involved in CSR, SHM, and plasma cell differentiation (1, 7, 13). miRNAs are small (~22 nucleotides), evolutionarily conserved non-coding RNAs derived from much larger primary transcripts encoded by their "host genes." miRNAs bind to complementary sequences within the 3′ untranslated region (3′ UTR) of their target mRNAs and negatively regulate protein expression at the posttranscriptional level through inhibition of translation and/or reduction of mRNA stability (14, 15). The mammalian genome encodes thousands of miRNAs that collectively affect the expression of more than half of protein-coding genes. In addition, miRNAs have been implicated as fine-tuning regulators controlling diverse biological processes at posttranscriptional level. They can potentially regulate every aspect of cellular activity, from proliferation and differentiation to apoptosis, as well as modulate a large range of physiological and pathological processes. miRNAs likely play important roles in B cell development and peripheral differentiation, as well as T cell stage-specific differentiation and autoimmunity. Some miRNAs, including miR-155, miR-181b, and miR-361, can silence AID expression, whereas miR-30a and miR-125b can silence Blimp-1 expression (16). These miRNAs bind to evolutionarily conserved miRNA target sites in the 3′ UTR of *Aicda* and *Prdm1* mRNAs and cause degradation of the mRNA transcripts and/or inhibit their translation.

We have recently shown that HDI, such as short-chain fatty acid valproic acid and butyrate, inhibit the expression of AID and Blimp-1 in human and mouse B cells *in vivo* and *in vitro* and regulate intrinsic B cell functions that are critical in shaping effective antibody and autoantibody responses (16). Valproic acid or sodium valproate (VPA, 2-propyl-pentanoic acid sodium) is widely used to treat epilepsy and mood disorders. VPA can selectively inhibits class I HDACs, particularly, HDAC1 and HDAC2, and less effectively, class IIa HDACs among the four HDAC classes identified in mammals (17, 18) to alter gene expression by changing chromatin accessibility. We have further shown that HDI, such as VPA and butyrate, inhibit AID and Blimp1 expression by upregulating miR-155, miR-181b, and miR-361, which silenced *AICDA/Aicda* mRNA, and miR-23b, miR-30a, and miR-125b, which silenced *PRDM1/Prdm1* mRNA (16). The selectivity of HDI-mediated silencing of *AICDA/Aicda* and *PRDM1/Prdm1* was emphasized by unchanged expression of HoxC4 and Irf4 (important inducers/modulators of *AICDA/Aicda*), Rev1 and Ung (central elements for CSR/SHM), and Bcl6, Bach2, or Pax5 (repressors of *PRDM1/Prdm1* expression), as well as unchanged expression of miR-19a/b, miR-20a, and miR-25, which are not known to regulate *AICDA/Aicda* or *PRDM1/Prdm1*. Epigenetic modulations always display a cell type- and cell stage-specific regulation pattern of gene expression (19). To extend our findings and further define the selectivity of HDI-mediated modulation of miRNAs and gene expression, we performed genome-wide miRNA-Seq and mRNA-Seq analysis in B cells induced to undergo CSR and plasma cell differentiation in the presence of VPA. Here, we showed that this HDI modulated selected miRNAs and mRNAs, possibly as a result of HDACs existing in unique contexts of HDAC/cofactor.

MATERIALS AND METHODS

Stimulation of Mouse B Cells for CSR and Plasma Cell Differentiation, and HDI Treatment

C57BL/6 mice were purchased from The Jackson Laboratory and maintained at the University of Texas Health Science Center at San Antonio (UTHSCSA) animal facility. The Institutional Animal Care and Use Committee of UTHSCSA approved all animal protocols. Naïve IgD^+ B cells were isolated from 8-week-old C57BL/6 mice as described (16, 20). B cells were resuspended in RPMI 1640 medium with 10% FBS, 50 mM β-mercaptoethanol, and 1× antibiotic–antimycotic mixture (15240-062; Invitrogen) (FBS-RPMI) at 37°C and stimulated with LPS (3 μg/ml) from *Escherichia coli* (055:B5; Sigma-Aldrich) plus IL-4 (5 ng/ml; R&D Systems) for CSR to IgG1/IgE and plasma cell differentiation. HDI [VPA 500 μM, a concentration comparable to serum concentration of VPA-treated mice (21)] or nil were also added to the cultures. Cells were collected 60 h later for qRT-PCR, mRNA-Seq, and miRNA-Seq, or 96 h later for surface Ig analysis by flow cytometry (16, 22).

RNA Extraction and High Throughput mRNA-Seq and miRNA-Seq

Total RNA was extracted from 2×10^6 cells using miRNeasy® Mini Kit (Qiagen), as previously described (16). RNA integrity was verified using an Agilent Bioanalyzer 2100 (Agilent). Next generation mRNA-Seq and small RNA-Seq were performed by the Genome Sequencing Facility (Greehey Children's Cancer Research Institute, GCCRI), UTHSCSA. High-quality RNA (RNA Integrity number or RIN.9.0) was processed using an Illumina TruSeq RNA sample prep kit v2 or TruSeq Small RNA Sample Prep kit following the manufacturer's instructions (Illumina). Clusters were generated using TruSeq Single-Read Cluster Gen. Kit v3-cBot-HS on an Illumina cBot Cluster Generation Station. After quality control procedures, individual mRNA-Seq or small RNA-Seq libraries were then pooled based on their respective 6-bp index portion of the TruSeq adapters and sequenced at 50 bp/sequence, read using an Illumina HiSeq 2000 sequencer. The barcode combinations were further crosschecked by Illumina Experiment Manager software. Sequence data were checked by assurance (QA) pipeline and initial genome alignment (Alignment). Approximately 33 million and 5 million reads per sample were generated in mRNA-Seq and miRNA-Seq, respectively. After the sequencing run, demultiplexing with CASAVA was employed to generate the fastq file for each sample. All sequencing reads were aligned with their reference genome (UCSC mouse genome build mm9) using TopHat2 default settings and the Bam files from alignment were processed using HTSeq-count to obtain the counts per gene in all samples. Quality control statistical analysis of outliers, intergroup variability, distribution levels, PCA, and hierarchical clustering analysis were performed for statistical validation of the experimental data.

Quantitative RT-PCR (qRT-PCR) of mRNAs and miRNAs

For mRNA quantification, post-recombination Iμ-C_H and mature V_HDJ_H-C_H transcripts. cDNA was synthesized from total RNA with the SuperScript™ III First-Strand Synthesis System (Invitrogen) using oligo-dT primer. Transcript expression was measured by qRT-PCR using the appropriate primers, as previously reported (16) using a Bio-Rad MyiQ™ Real-Time PCR Detection System (Bio-Rad Laboratories) to measure SYBR Green (IQ™ SYBR® Green Supermix, Bio-Rad Laboratories) incorporation with the following protocol: 95°C for 15 s, 40 cycles of 94°C for 10 s, 60°C for 30 s, 72°C for 30 s. Data acquisition was performed during the 72°C extension step. Melting curve analysis was performed from 72 to 95°C. For quantification of mature miRNA transcripts, RNA was extracted from $0.2–5 \times 10^6$ cells using miRNeasy® Mini Kit (Qiagen) and then reverse-transcribed with miScript II RT Kit (Qiagen) using the miScript HiSpec buffer. A Bio-Rad MyiQ™ Real-Time PCR Detection System was used to measure SYBR Green (miScript SYBR Green PCR Kit; Qiagen) incorporation according to manufacturer's instructions. Mature miRNA forward primers were used at 250 nM in conjunction with the Qiagen miScript Universal Primer and normalized to expression of small nuclear/nucleolar RNAs Rnu6/RNU61/2, Snord61/SNORD61, Snord68/SNORD68, and Snord70/SNORD70. The ΔΔCt method was used for qRT-PCR data analysis with Microsoft Excel.

Statistical Analysis

Statistical analysis was performed to determine p values by paired and unpaired Student's t-test, and p values <0.05 were considered significant.

RESULTS

HDI Inhibit CSR and Plasma Cell Differentiation

We have shown that HDI repress the expression of AID and Blimp-1, which are critical for CSR/SHM and plasma cell differentiation, respectively, in mouse and human B cells by upregulating selected miRNAs that silenced *AICDA/Aicda* and *PRDM1/Prdm1* mRNAs, as demonstrated by multiple qRT-PCRs (16). To further define the selectivity of HDI-mediated modulation of miRNA and gene expression, we stimulated purified mouse B cells with LPS plus IL-4, which induce B cells to undergo CSR to IgG1 or IgE and differentiate to plasma cells in the presence of HDI (VPA, 500 μM) or nil. Consistent with our previous findings (16), HDI significantly inhibited CSR and plasma cell differentiation, as shown by greatly reduced surface $IgG1^+$ B cells and $B220^{low}$ $CD138^+$ plasma cells (**Figure 1**). HDI inhibition of CSR was

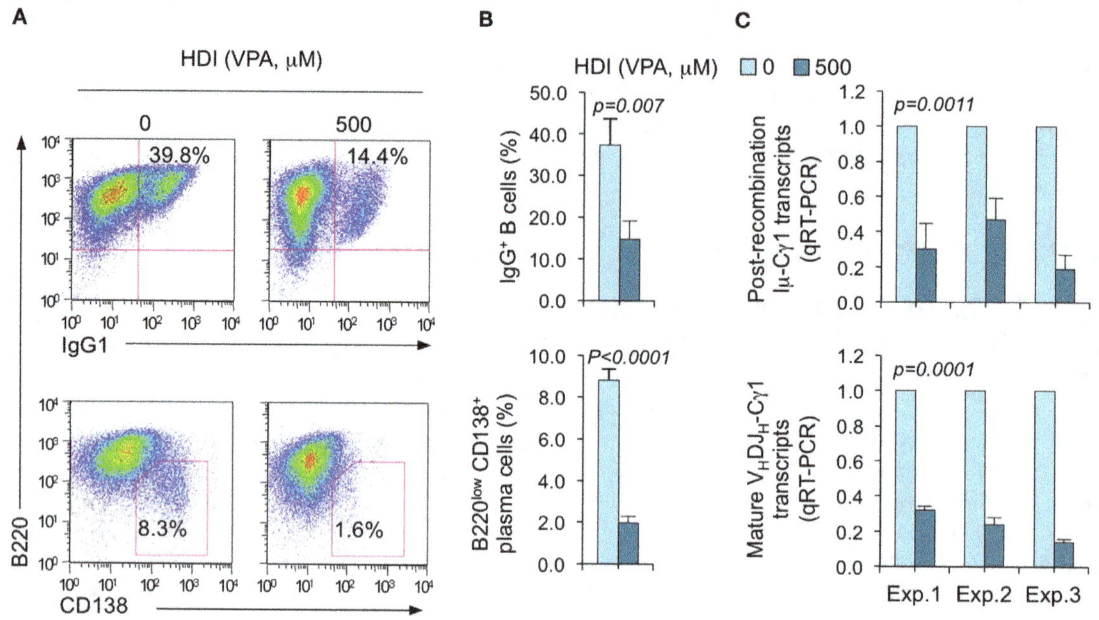

FIGURE 1 | HDI inhibits B cell CSR and plasma cell differentiation. Purified spleen B cells were stimulated with LPS plus IL-4 in the presence of HDI (VPA, 500 μM) or nil. **(A)** Surface expression of B220 and IgG1 was measured by flow cytometry 96 h after the stimulation, Data are one representative of three independent experiments. **(B)** The average percentage of IgG1⁺ B cells and B220^{low} CD138⁺ plasma cell in nil or HDI-treated cells in the three experiments. **(C)** Mature V_HDJ_H-Cγ1 transcripts and post-recombination Iμ-Cγ1 transcripts, both hallmarks of completed CSR, were analyzed by qRT-PCR and normalized to *Cd79b* transcripts in B cells stimulated for 60 hours, measured by qRT-PCR and normalized to *Cd79b* transcripts. Data are from three independent experiments. *p* values, paired *t*-test.

further confirmed by decreased numbers of post-recombination Iμ-Cγ1 and mature V_HDJ_H-Cγ1 transcripts.

HDI-Mediated Modulation of mRNA Expression in B Cells is Highly Selective

Histone deacetylases remove the acetyl groups from the histone lysine residues leading to the formation of a condensed and transcriptionally silenced chromatin. HDI block this activity, thereby increasing histone acetylation and alteration of gene expression. It has been shown that HDI, such as TSA, suberoylanilide hydroxamic acid (SAHA), MS-275, and FK228, could alter the expression of 5–20% of genes (23). To further define the modulation of gene expression by HDI in B cells that undergo CSR and plasma cell differentiation, we performed high throughput mRNA-Seq to analyze the transcriptome in B cells stimulated by LPS plus IL-4 and treated with HDI (VPA, 500 μM) or nil. In general, one RPKM (read per kb per million reads) of mRNA represents approximately one copy of transcript per cell (24). In three independent experiments, HDI did not significantly alter overall mRNA expression ($p = 0.99925$, 0.74835, and 0.39640, respectively), although the average PRKM was slightly reduced from 42.71 to 38.49 ($p = 0.3506$) (**Figure 2**). Among over 22,000 genes analyzed, about 5,000 of them were significantly expressed (more than 20 RPKM, average more than 20 transcripts per cells) in B cells stimulated by LPS plus IL-4. Upon treatment with HDI, only 18 (0.36%) of the "highly" expressed genes, including *Aicda, Prdm1, Xbp1, Bhlha15, RRhob, Soat2, Histlh2bg, Fut1, Cxcr3, Eaf2, Fkbp11, Ppapdc1b, Il10, Rcbtb2, Ly6c2, Saa3, Txndc5*, and *IgJ*, were downregulated, on average, by 50% or more. The mRNA of Cxcr3 (C-X-C motif chemokine receptor 3), which is highly expressed in IgG1⁺ memory B cells and can promote the production of IgG1 autoantibodies (25, 26), was reduced by about 70% by HDI. The mRNA of Saa3 (Serum amyloid A3), which can interact with Tlr4 and induce Tlr4-mediated NF-κB activation (27), was reduced by over 51%. Sixteen (0.30%) of the "highly" expressed (more than 20 RPKM) genes, including *Gstk1, Gstm1, Zbtb20, Gapt, Ift57, Slc16a3, Ptprs, Atp11a, Kctd17, Itm2a, Syt11*, and *Ifit1*, were upregulated by HDI by more than twofold (**Figures 2A,B**). Downregulation or upregulation of the above genes by more than twofold was consistent in all the three experiments, suggesting that the modulation of gene expression by HDI is highly selective.

Aicda, Prdm1, and *Xbp1* are Selectively Silenced by HDI

Consistent with our real-time qRT-PCR results (16), the mRNA-Seq experiments further demonstrated that *Aicda, Prdm1*, and *Xbp1* transcripts were significantly downregulated by HDI (**Figures 2** and **3A–C**). In all three independent experiments, *Aicda, Prdm1*, and *Xbp1* were consistently reduced by HDI by more than 57, 48, and 47%, respectively, ranking 7th, 21st, and 24th, of the most downregulated genes among the total of more than 5,000 genes that were highly expressed (more than 20 RPKM) in B cells stimulated by LPS plus IL-4. Thus, these deep sequencing experiments showed that *Aicda, Prdm1*, and *Xbp1* are selectively inhibited by HDI in B cells undergoing CSR and plasma cell differentiation.

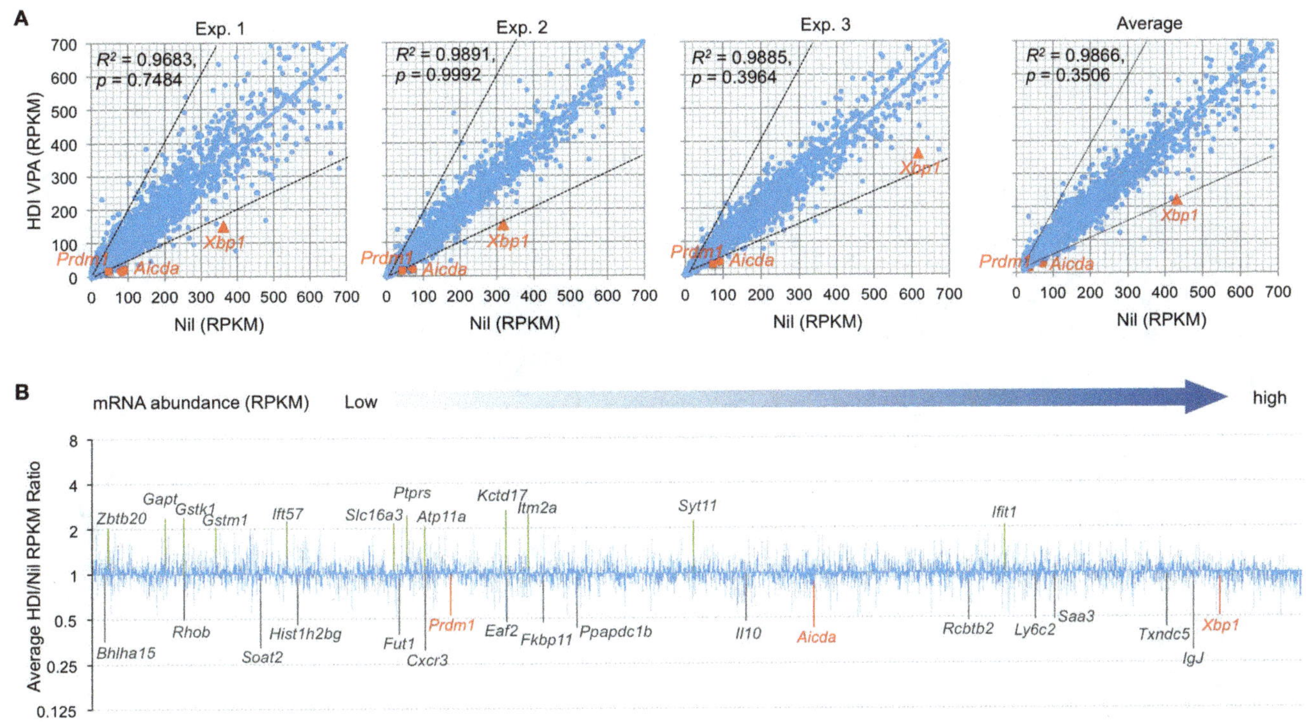

FIGURE 2 | HDI selectively inhibits mRNA expression in B cells induced to undergo CSR and plasma cell differentiation. B cells were cultured with LPS plus IL-4 in the presence of HDI (VPA, 500 μM) or nil for 60 h before preparation of RNA for mRNA-Seq. **(A)** Scatter plots of average mRNA expression levels in three independent experiments (reads per kilobase per million mapped reads, RPKMs), in LPS plus IL-4-stimulated B cells treated with VPA versus those in LPS plus IL-4-stimulated B cells treated with nil. Each plot corresponds to one individual mRNA expression level. **(B)** Bar graphs depict the average folds of changes of mRNA expression levels (average RPKMs from three independent experiments) in LPS plus IL-4-stimulated B cells treated with HDI, as compared to those in B cells treated with nil. Only the mRNAs at average RPKM >20 in LPS plus IL-4-stimulated B cells treated with nil are included. *Aicda*, *Prdm1*, and *Xbp1* mRNAs and the mRNAs that were increase or decreased or increased in average by more than twofold are indicated. *p* values, paired *t*-test.

HDI Does Not Alter the Expression of 14-3-3 Adaptors or Rab7

The 14-3-3 adaptor family consists of a class of phosphoserine/phosphothreonine (pSer/Thr)-binding proteins, which include seven isoforms (14-3-3β, 14-3-3ε, 14-3-3γ, 14-3-3η, 14-3-3σ, 14-3-3τ, and 14-3-3ζ) encoded by different genes. 14-3-3 proteins are involved in a variety of cellular processes, including gene regulation, differentiation, and cell cycle progression (28). As we have shown, 14-3-3 adaptors play an important role in targeting the CSR machinery to S regions by virtue of their ability to bridge proteins with DNA or other proteins (29, 30). They directly interact with AID, protein kinase A catalytic subunit-α (PKA-Cα), regulatory inhibitory subunit-α (PKA-RIα), and uracil DNA glycosylase (Ung) to function as scaffolds to stabilize these enzymatic CSR elements on S regions. 14-3-3 expression has been suggested to be regulated by posttranscriptional modulation. 14-3-3 can interact with the phosphorylation sites of HDAC4, 5, and 7 and regulate cellular localization of these HDACs (31). As we have shown, the expression of most 14-3-3 proteins is significantly upregulated by the induction of CSR in B cells (2, 29, 30, 32). To determine whether potential alterations of 14-3-3 proteins in B cells could contribute to the HDI-mediated inhibition of CSR, we analyzed our mRNA-Seq data on the seven 14-3-3 isoforms. None of the seven 14-3-3 isoforms were significantly altered by HDI in B cells stimulated by LPS plus IL-4 (**Figure 3D**). 14-3-3ζ expression can be modulated by miR-193b and miR-375, which target 3′ UTR of 14-3-3ζ mRNA, in cancer cells (33, 34). However, these two miRNAs were not expressed in LPS plus IL-4-stimulated B cells (not shown).

We have recently demonstrated that Rab7, a small GTPase, plays an important role in CSR, through activation of the canonical NF-κB pathway and induction of AID expression (35). Like 14-3-3 adaptors, Rab7 expression is upregulated by the stimuli that induce CSR in B cells. To analyze whether the HDI-mediated downregulation of AID was at least partially due to a potential alteration of Rab7 expression, we analyzed Rab7 mRNA levels in B cells treated with HDI or nil. As shown by mRNA-Seq, HDI did not significantly alter Rab7 expression (**Figure 3E**). In one of the three experiments, Rab7 mRNA levels were virtually the same in B cells treated with HDI or nil. In the other two experiments, Rab7 mRNA was even slightly ($p = 0.20$) increased by HDI. Thus, downregulation of the AID-targeting 14-3-3 adaptors or downregulation of the CSR-regulating Rab7 small GTPase play no role in HDI-mediated modulation of CSR.

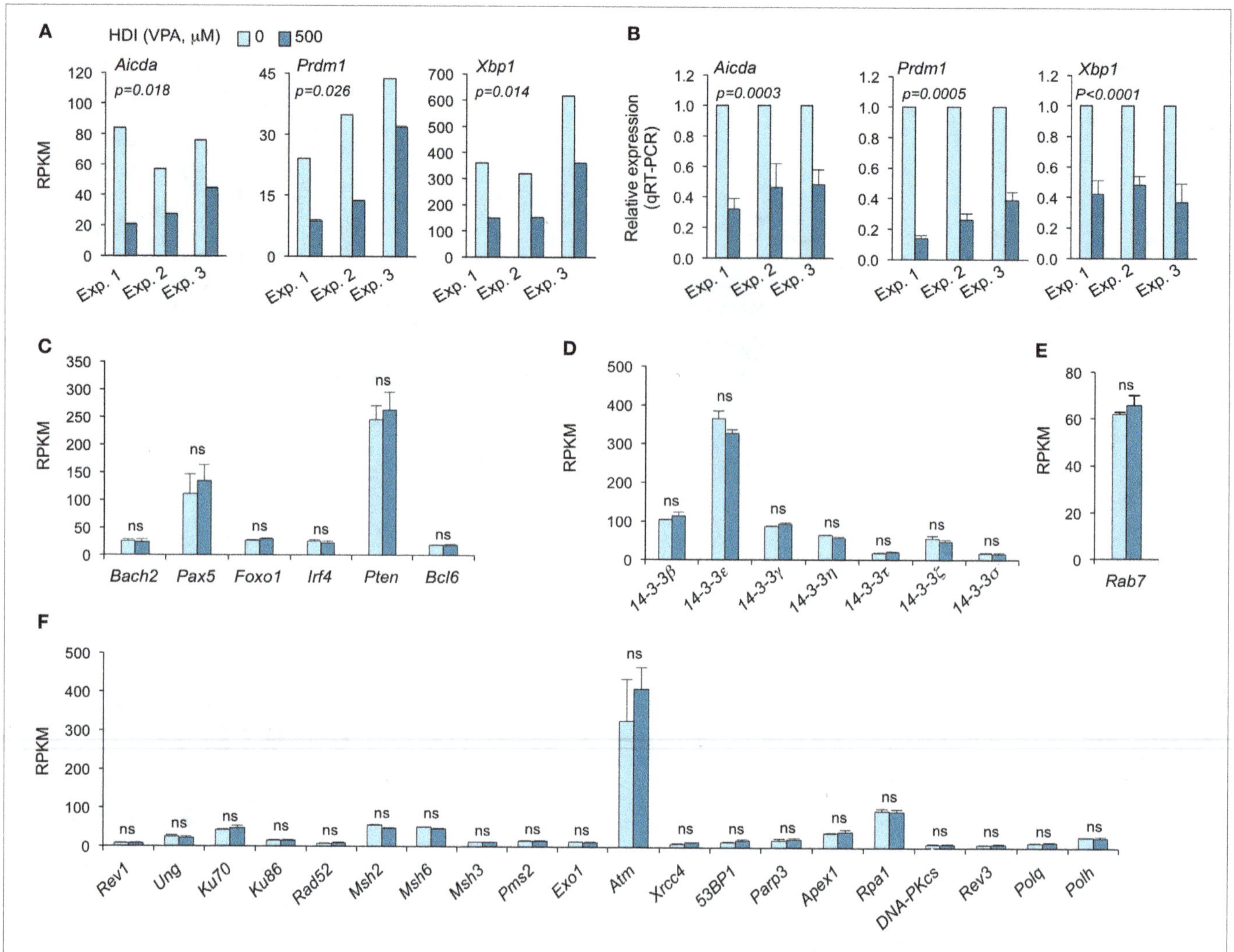

FIGURE 3 | HDI inhibits the expression of *Aicda*, *Prdm1*, and *Xbp1*, but not other elements that are important for CSR/SHM and plasma cell differentiation. B cells were stimulated with LPS plus IL-4 for 60 h, in the presence of HDI (VPA, 500 μM) or nil. **(A)** Expressions of *Aicda*, *Prdm1*, and *Xbp1* were mRNAs analyzed by mRNA-Seq. Data are from three independent experiments. **(B)** qRT-PCR validation of *Aicda*, *Prdm1*, and *Xbp1* expressions. Data are from three independent experiments. *p* values, paired *t*-test. Expressions of **(C)** *Bach2*, *Pax5*, *Foxo1*, *Irf4*, *Pten*, and *Bcl6*, **(D)** the seven 14-3-3 isoforms, **(E)** Rab7, and **(F)** the genes that encode the proteins that have been shown to play important roles in CSR and/or SHM were analyzed by mRNA-Seq and depicted as RPKM. Data are from three independent experiments. ns, not significant, paired *t*-test.

HDI Does Not Alter the Expression of DNA Repair Factors that Are Important for CSR and SHM

Class-switch DNA recombination and SHM are tightly regulated and both are effected by a two-step process: (i) DNA lesions initiated by AID and (ii) lesion repair by the combined intervention of DNA replication and repair factors (2, 36, 37). Many DNA repair factors, including the base excision repair factor Ung, mismatch repair factors Msh2, Msh3, Msh6, Pms2, and Exo1 nuclease, translesion synthesis (TLS) DNA polymerases Rev3, Rev1, Polθ, and Polη, as well as DSB repair factors Ku70/Ku80, Rad52, RPA, and DNA-PK play important roles in CSR and/or SHM (2, 37–41). Dysregulation of these DNA repair factors can result in altered CSR/SHM, and thereby the antibody response. To define whether the HDI-mediated reduction of CSR and plasma cell differentiation was associated with any alteration in these factors, we analyzed the mRNA-Seq data for the expression of these factors. None of them was significantly altered by HDI (**Figure 3F**).

HDI Does Not Significantly Alter the Expression of Epigenetic Regulators HATs, HDACs and Tet Proteins

In addition to inhibiting catalytic activity of HDACs, HDI have been suggested to selectively change the expression of some epigenetic regulators in certain type of cells. SAHA, a pan HDAC inhibitor, has been shown to downregulate HDAC7 expression in fibroblast cell lines (42). MS-275, TSA, and VPA downregulate

DNMT1 protein expression in testis and embryonal carcinoma, as butyrate, SAHA, and PD98059 do in LNCaP prostate cancer cells (43). To determine whether HDI alter the expression of HDACs or DNMTs, as well as HATs and Tet1/Tet2/Tet3, which also mediate histone acetylation and DNA methylation, respectively, we analyzed the mRNA levels of these genes in our mRNA-Seq data (**Figure 4**). Thirty-six out of the 42 gene transcripts analyzed were not significantly altered by HDI, while *HDAC1, HDAC6, Clock*, and *Tet2* were marginally increased (by 24.63, 36.64, 9.57, and 23.19%, respectively), and *Sirt1* and *Crebbp* were slightly reduced (by 16.54 and 10.11%, respectively) by HDI. Thus, epigenetic regulator genes are not significantly modulated by HDI in B cells undergoing CSR and plasma cell differentiation.

HDI Does Not Alter the Genes that Are Important in Cell Apoptosis

We have recently found that HDI inhibit, in a dose-dependent fashion, CSR and plasma cell differentiation without altering B cell proliferation or B cell and plasma cell viability (16). We have shown by qRT-PCR that the expression of the anti-apoptotic genes *Bcl2, Mcl1*, and *Bcl2l1*, which enhance B cell and plasma cell survival, was unaltered or increased by HDI *in vivo* and *in vitro* (16). Consistent with these findings, our mRNA-Seq data show that the expressions of all these genes were not altered by HDI ($p = 0.28$, 0.21, or 0.27) (**Figure 5A**). In addition, other 19 anti-apoptotic genes and 22 pro-apoptotic genes were also unchanged by HDI (**Figures 5A,B**). Thus, these findings further demonstrate that HDI significantly reduce CSR and plasma cell differentiation, without altering cell viability.

HDI Does Not Significantly Alter TLR Expression and the Genes Involved in NF-κB Signaling

Toll-like receptors (TLRs) are a family of conserved pattern recognition receptors that sense diverse types of microbe-associated molecular patterns (MAMPs). Engagement of B cell TLRs by MAMPs not only induces T-independent antibody responses but also plays an important role in the early stages of T-dependent antibody responses, before specific T cell help becomes available (44). We have shown that TLR1/2-, TLR4-, TLR7-, or TLR9-signaling synergizes with BCR-signaling, which enhances TLR-dependent activation of the canonical NF-κB pathway, to induce AID and enable CSR (20). Given the important role of TLR-signaling and NF-κB pathway in the induction of AID, an alteration in the expression of TLR and the factors that are involved in NF-κB pathway would result in a change of AID expression and CSR. As shown by mRNA-Seq, the expression of 13 TLRs and 27 genes that are involved in NF-κB-signaling pathway was not altered by HDI (**Figures 5C,D**).

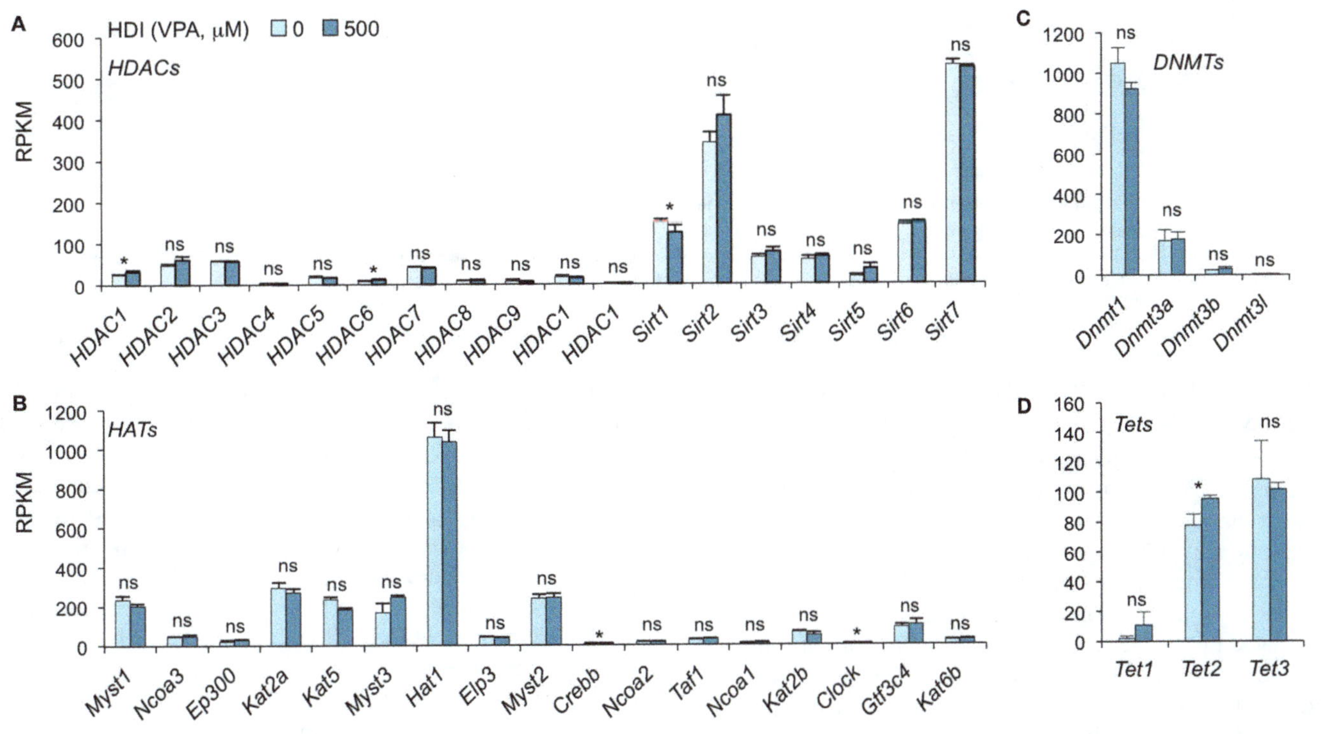

FIGURE 4 | HDI does not alter the expression of the epigenetic regulators HDACs, HATs, DNMTs, and Tet proteins. B cells were stimulated with LPS plus IL-4 for 60 h, in the presence of HDI (VPA, 500 µM) or nil. mRNA expressions of the genes that encode **(A)** HDACs and **(B)** HATs, which modulate histone acetylation, and **(C)** DNMTs, as well as **(D)** Tet1, Tet2, and Tet3, which modulate DNA methylation, were analyzed by mRNA-Seq and depicted as RPKM. Data are from three independent experiments. $^{*}p < 0.05$; ns, not significant, paired *t*-test.

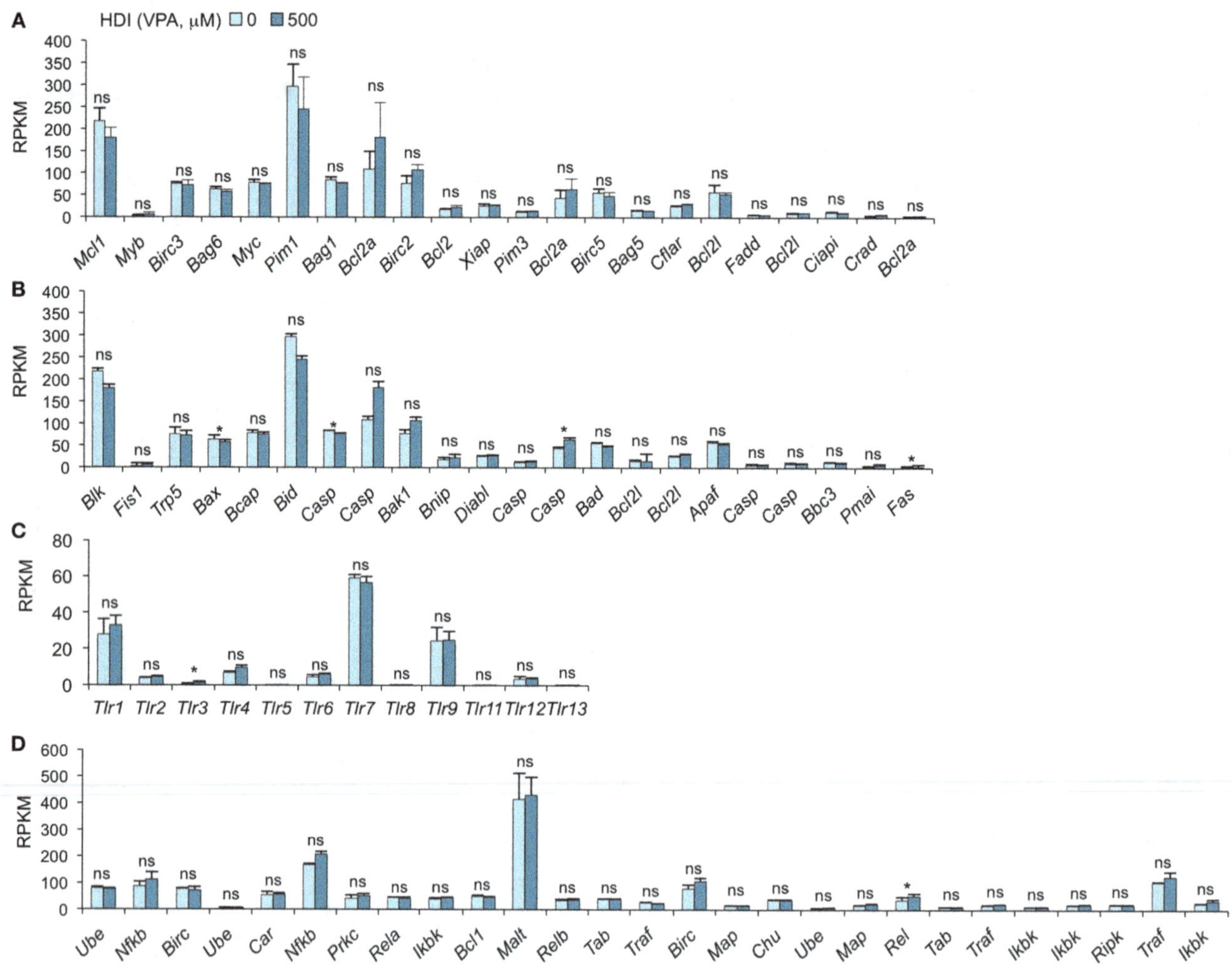

FIGURE 5 | HDI does not significantly alter the expression of the genes that are important for apoptosis, the genes that encode TLRs and the genes that are involved in NF-κB signaling. B cells were stimulated with LPS plus IL-4 for 60 h, in the presence of HDI (VPA, 500 μM) or nil. mRNA expressions of the genes that encode **(A)** anti-apoptotic factors, **(B)** pro-apoptotic factors, **(C)** Toll-like receptors, and **(D)** the factors that are involved in NF-κB-signaling pathway were analyzed by mRNA-Seq and depicted as RPKM. Data are from three independent experiments. *$p < 0.05$; ns, not significant, paired t-test.

HDI Inhibits Expression of Selected mRNAs in B Cells

In B cells induced to undergo CSR and plasma cell differentiation, the number of genes that were downregulated by HDI nearly equated that of genes that were upregulated by HDI (**Figure 2**), suggesting that HDI can modulate gene expression by a mechanism other than directly increasing histone acetylation. Indeed, generally, only a small number of genes are thought to be directly modulated by changes in histone acetylation. Thus, it is possible that HDI upregulate the expression of genes, which negatively regulate the expression of other genes. HDI can modulate the expression of miRNAs, which silence target mRNAs by inducing their degradation and/or reducing their translation. We have recently shown that HDI downregulated the expression of AID and Blimp-1 by upregulating miR-155, miR-181b, and miR-361, which silence *Aicda* mRNA, and miR-23b, miR-30a, and miR-125b, which silence *Prdm1* mRNA, but not miR-19a/b, miR-20a, and miR-25, which are not known to regulate *Aicda*, *Prdm1*, or *Xbp1* (16). To further define the modulation of miRNA by HDI, we analyzed microRNAome in LPS and IL-4 stimulated B cells treated with HDI or nil by miRNA-Seq (**Figure 6**). In stimulated B cells, the average RPM of 520 miRNAs analyzed was 26.9 (10.75, if one excludes the three most abundant miRNAs miR-21a, miR-191, and miR-146a). Upon HDI treatment, the average RPM of all the miRNAs were slightly increased to 32.19 (13.63, if we exclude the three most abundant miRNAs miR-21a, miR-191, and miR-146a) ($R^2 = 0.9811$, $p = 0.5134$). A total of 185 of these miRNAs had, in average, 0.5 copy per cell. Among these 185 miRNAs, only 6 of them were reduced by 50% or more, and 26 of them were upregulated by more than twofold by HDI (**Figure 6**). Thus, the HDI-mediated modulation of miRNA expression in B cells undergoing CSR and plasma cell differentiation is selective.

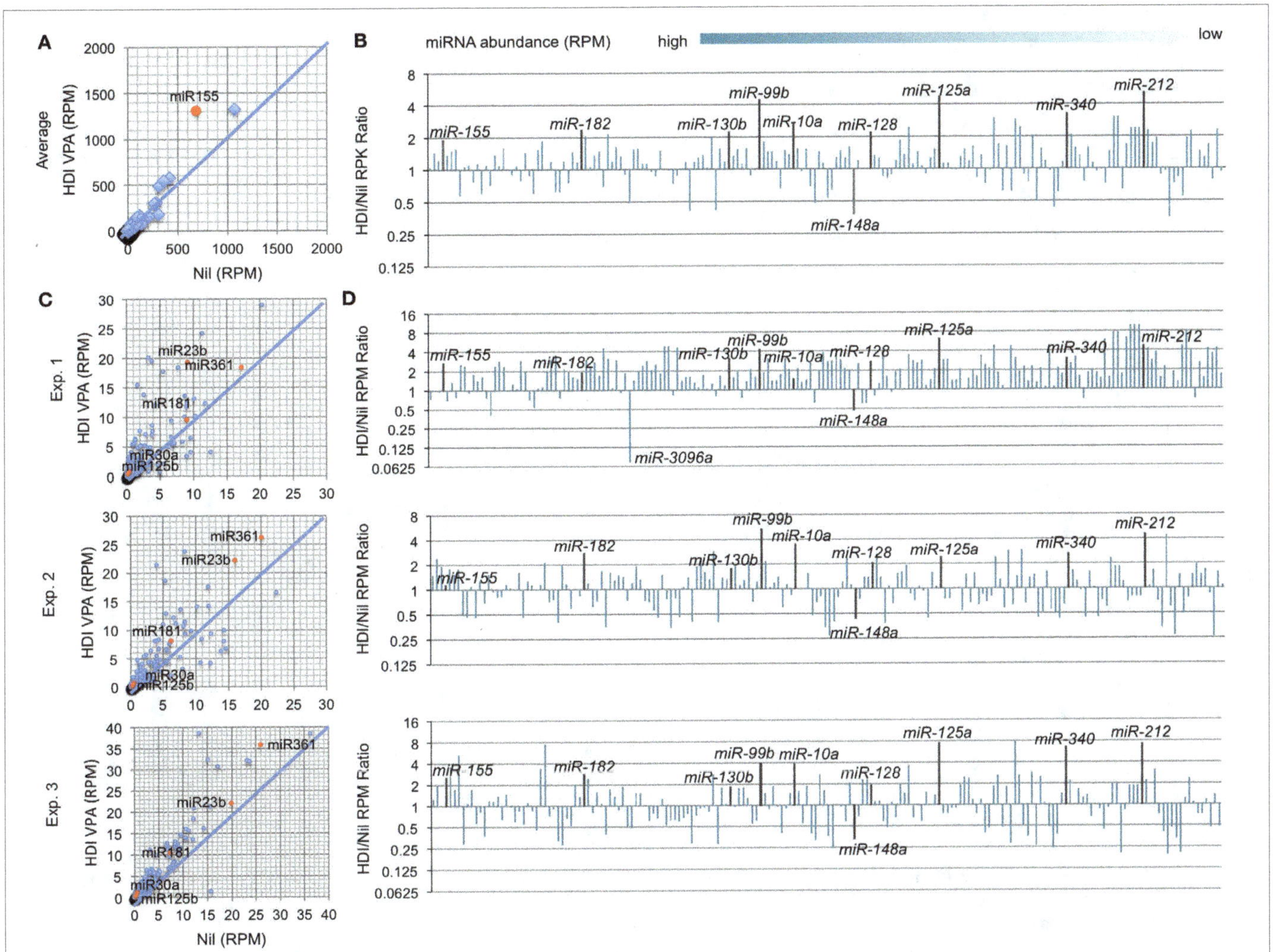

FIGURE 6 | HDI selectively inhibits miRNA expression in B cells induced to undergo CSR and plasma cell differentiation. B cells were cultured with LPS plus IL-4 in the presence of HDI (VPA, 500 μM) or nil for 60 h before preparation of RNA for miRNA-Seq. **(A)** Scatter plots of average (in three independent experiments) miRNA expression levels (RPMs) in B cells treated with HDI versus that in B cells treated with nil. *P* values, paired *t*-test. **(B)** Bar graphs depict the changes of folds of the average miRNA expression levels (RPMs) in B cells treated with HDI as compared to that in B cells treated with nil. **(C)** Bar graphs depict the changes of folds of miRNA expression levels (RPMs) in B cells treated with HDI as compared to that in B cells treated with nil, in three independent experiments. **(D)** Scatter plots of miRNA expression levels in B cells treated with HDI versus those in B cells treated with nil, in three independent experiments. Only the miRNAs at average RPM > 0.5 in LPS plus IL-4-stimulated B cells treated with nil are included.

HDI Upregulates Selected miRNAs that Target *Aicda*

We have shown by qRT-PCR that miR-155, miR-181b, and miR-361, which silence AID by targeting *Aicda* 3′ UTR, were significantly upregulated by HDI (16). The HDI-mediated upregulation of these miRNAs, particularly, miR-155 was validated by miRNA-Seq in three independent experiments (**Figure 7**). miR-155 targets a highly conserved site in the 3′ UTR of *Aicda* mRNA in several different species (45, 46). As shown by miRNA-Seq analysis, miR-155 is one of the most abundant miRNAs expressed in B cells after stimulation by LPS plus IL-4 (**Figure 6**). In such B cells, the average RPM of miR-155 was 684.9 (572.0, 981.7, and 501.0 in three independent experiments, respectively), which is more than 25 times higher than the average RPM of all the 520 miRNAs analyzed. Upon treatment with HDI, miR-155 expression was increased by more than 1.9-fold ($p = 0.032$) (**Figure 7**). miR-155 is encoded by the miR155 host gene *miR155HG*. *miR155HG* was originally identified as a gene that was transcriptionally activated by promoter insertion at a common retroviral integration site in B cell lymphomas and was formerly referred to as *Bic* (*B* cell *i*ntegration *c*luster) (13). Consistent with our qRT-PCR results (16), the mRNA-Seq data showed that HDI-mediated upregulation of miR-155 was associated with an increase of primary *miR-155HG* transcript (**Figure 7C**). In addition to the targeting sites for miR-155, miR-181b, and miR-361, the 3′ UTR of mouse *Aicda* mRNA also contains the putative target sites for miR-125a, miR-351, miR-92b, miR-26a, and miR-103 (identified by using miRNA-targeting

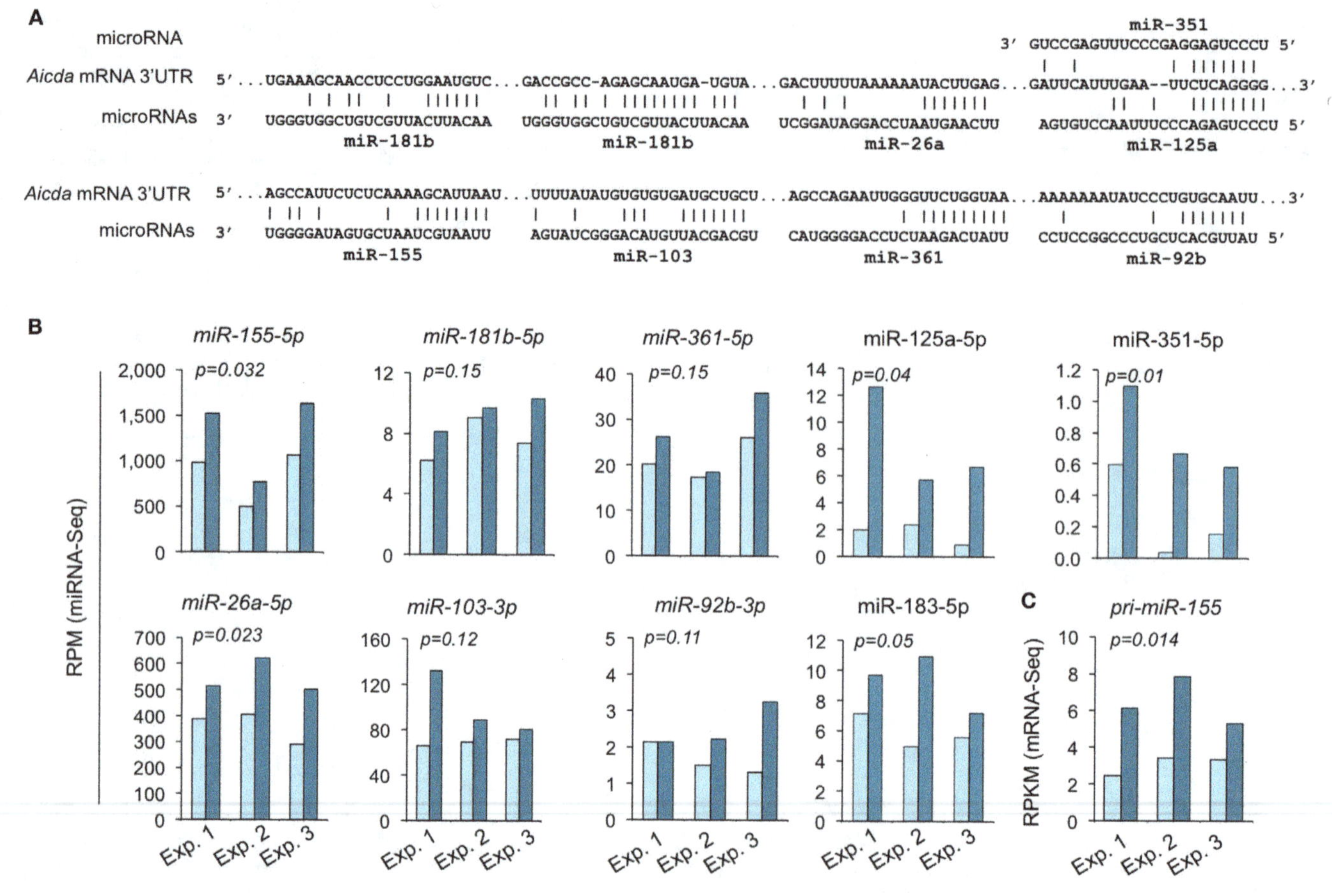

FIGURE 7 | HDI upregulates the miRNAs that target *Aicda*. **(A)** Alignment of the miRNAs and their target sites in the 3′ UTR of *Aicda* mRNAs. **(B)** Expression of miRNAs that modulate AID or are predicated to modulate AID in B cells cultured with LPS plus IL-4 in the presence of HDI (VPA, 500 μM) or nil for 60 h were analyzed by miRNA-Seq and depicted as RPM. **(C)** Primary (pri-) miRNA transcripts of miR-155 in B cells cultured for 60 h with LPS plus IL-4 in the presence of nil or HDI were analyzed by mRNA-Seq and depicted as RPKM. Data are from three independent experiments. *p* values, paired *t*-test.

prediction tools: TargetScan.org, miRNA.org, and miRbase.org). These miRNAs were also upregulated by HDI. Thus, HDI upregulate miRNAs that silence *Aicda* and do so by increasing the primary transcripts of host genes of these miRNAs.

HDI Upregulate miRNAs that Target *Prdm1*

We have shown that HDI significantly downregulated *Prdm1* expression, plasma cell differentiation, and antibody/autoantibody production (16). The greatly reduced plasma cell differentiation was associated with downregulation of the Ig J chain (*IgJ*) gene, which is expressed only after B cells terminal differentiation into plasma cells (47). IgJ is incorporated into an IgM pentamer or an IgA dimer and is necessary for both the cellular and mucosal secretion of antibodies. In B cells stimulated by LPS plus IL-4 for 60 h, the average RPKM of *IgJ* mRNA was 344.6 (395.1, 175.6, and 463.2 in three independent experiments, respectively). HDI reduced *IgJ* expression (RPKM) by more than 3.3-fold to average 103.6 (77.3, 46.2, and 187.3, in three independent experiments, respectively) (**Figure 2**). Both human *PRDM1* and mouse *Prdm1* mRNA have a long (2,453 bp) 3′ UTR, including putative miRNA-targeting sites, which are evolutionary conserved. By using miRNA-targeting prediction tools (TargetScan.org, miRNA.org, and miRbase.org), we identified miR-125a, miR-125b, miR-96, miR-351, miR-30, miR-182, miR-23a, miR-23b, miR-200b, miR-200c, miR-33a, miR-365, let-7, miR-98, miR-24, miR-9, miR-223, and miR-133 as *PRDM1/Prdm1* targeting miRNAs in both the human and the mouse. With exception of miR-33a, miR223, miR-9, miR-24, and miR-429, whose expression level was low in activated B cells, such *Prdm1*-targeting miRNAs were significantly upregulated by HDI. We have shown by qRT-PCR that miR-23b, miR-30a, and miR-125b, which silence Blimp-1 by targeting *Prdm1* 3′ UTR, were significantly upregulated by HDI (16). The upregulation of these miRNAs was further validated in B cells by miRNA-Seq in three independent experiments (**Figure 8**). This likely resulted from increased primary miRNA transcripts, as suggested by the upregulation of *pri-miR-23b*.

The miR-30 family consists of five miRNAs (miR-30a, miR-30b, miR-30c, miR-30d, and miR-30e) encoded by different host genes. The miR-30 family members are similar to each other and have identical seed sequences. Like human *PRDM1* (48), the 3′ UTR of mouse *Prdm1* mRNA contains three highly conserved bindings sites complementary to the seed sequence of miR-30a

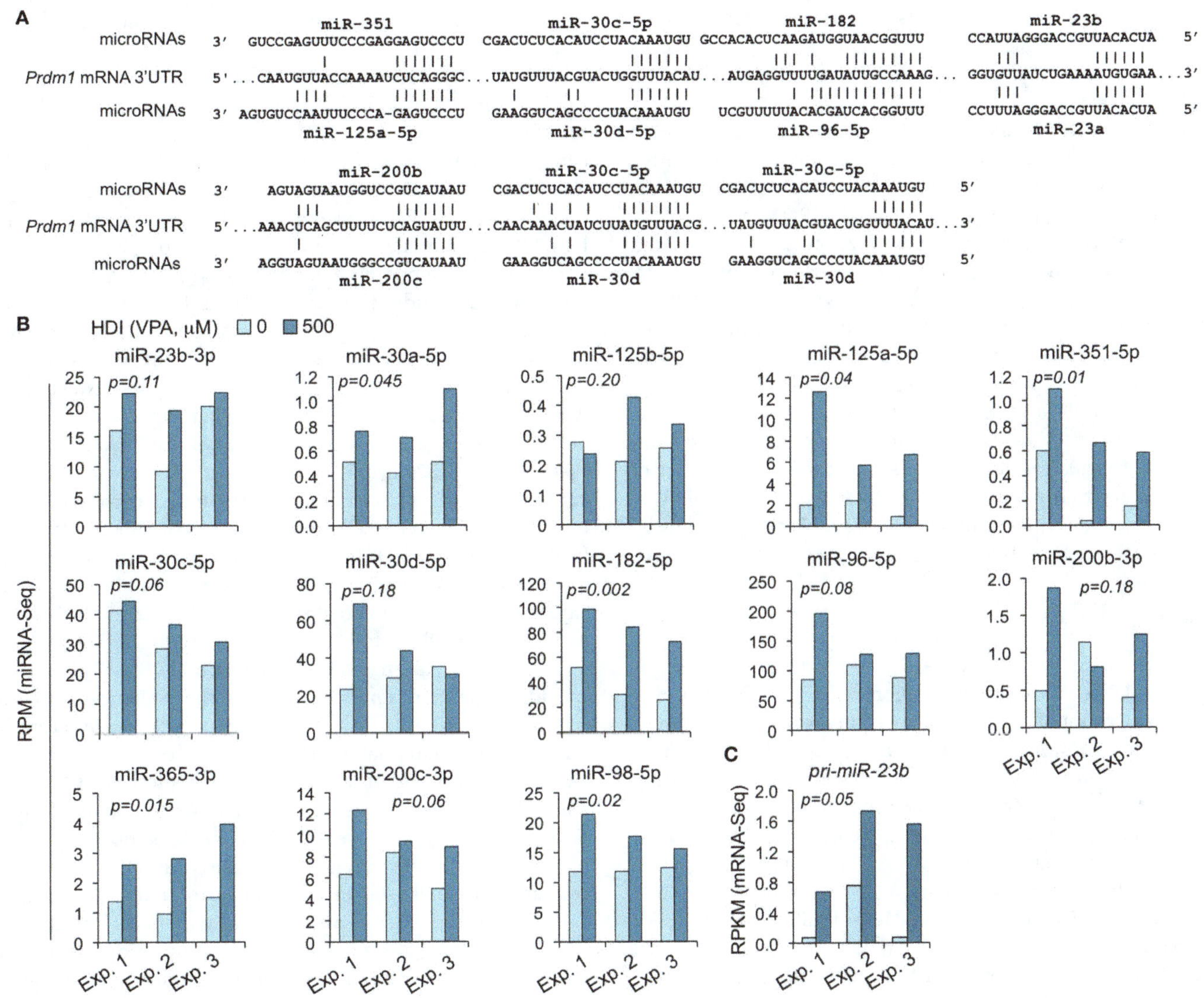

FIGURE 8 | The *Prdm1* targeting miRNAs miR-23b, miR-125a, miR-351, miR-30a/c/d, miR-182, miR-96, miR-98, miR-200b/c, and miR-365 are upregulated by HDI. (A) Alignment of the 3′ UTR of *Prdm1* mRNA and the targeting miRNAs. **(B)** Expressions of the miRNAs miR-23b, miR-125a, miR-351, miR-30a/c/d, miR-182, miR-96, miR-98, miR-200b/c, and miR-365 that target or are predicted to target *Prdm1* 3′ UTR, as well as miR-183, which is expressed in a same cluster with miR-182, in B cells cultured with LPS plus IL-4 in the presence of HDI (VPA, 500 μM) or nil for 60 h were analyzed by miRNA-Seq and depicted as RPM. **(C)** Primary (pri-) miRNA transcripts of miR-23b in B cells cultured with LPS plus IL-4 in the presence of nil or HDI for 60 h were analyzed by mRNA-Seq and depicted as RPKM. Data are from three independent experiments. *p* values, paired *t*-test.

and other miR-30 family members (**Figure 8**). All the five miR-30 miRNAs were expressed in B cells stimulated by LPS plus IL-4. The abundance of miR-30b, miR-30c, miR-30d, and miR-30e were greater than that of miR-30a (**Figure 8**). miR-30c was upregulated by HDI in all the three experiments, miR-30d was upregulated in two of the three experiments, while miR-30b and miR-30e were upregulated in one of the three experiments but were downregulated in the other two experiments.

miR-125 is a an evolutionarily conserved miRNA family consisting of three paralogs, including miR-125a, miR-125b-1, and miR-125b-2 (miR-125b). Recent studies have presented strong evidence for a role of the miR-125 family in the immune response. miR-125a shares the same seed sequence with miR-125b. Like miR-125b, miR-125a also potentially targets *Prdm1* in both human being and mouse, as predicted by the sequences (**Figure 8**). The abundance of miR-125a in B cells induced to undergo CSR and plasma cell differentiation by LPS plus IL-4 was much greater than that of miR-125b, as in all three experiments. In the presence of HDI, miR-125a expression was increased by up to 7.5-fold, perhaps suggesting a more important role of this miRNA than miR-125b in modulating *Blimp1* expression. miR-125a and miR-351 contain the same seed sequence as miR-125b, and therefore potentially target *Prdm1* 3′ UTR at the same site as miR-125b. Likewise, HDI upregulated miR-351 expression by up to 16.5-fold. miR-98 potentially target the same site as let-7 in *Prdm1* 3′ UTR. While let-7 miRNAs were not consistently altered by HDI, miR-98 was significantly upregulated by HDI in B cells in all the three experiments of CSR/plasma cell differentiation induction ($p = 0.02$).

miR-182, miR-96, and miR-183 belong to a polycistronic miRNA cluster that is located within a 4-kb area on mouse chromosome 6q. These miRNA siblings share similar seed sequences; in fact, the seed sequences of miR-96 and miR-182 are identical. As predicted using online miRNA analyze tools, TargetScan.org, miRNA.org, and miRbase.org, in both mouse and human, miR-182 and miR-96 can potentially target *Prdm1/PRDM1* 3′ UTR at the same site (**Figure 8**). In B cells stimulated with LPS plus IL-4, miR-182, miR-96, and miR-183 were all highly expressed. All these three miRNAs were upregulated by HDI. Because the precursors of miR-96, miR-182, and miR-183 are transcribed as a single transcript, these findings further support the contention that HDI modulate miRNA expression through regulation of their primary transcript (16). Thus, these experiments showed that HDI upregulate the miRNAs that target *Prdm1*, possibly by increasing the primary transcripts of host genes of these miRNAs.

DISCUSSION

Epigenetic marks/factors, such as histone posttranslational modifications, DNA methylation, and non-coding RNAs, including miRNAs, play important roles in the complex interplay between genes and environment. As we have suggested, they "interact" with genetic programs to regulate B cell functions, including CSR, SHM, and plasma cell differentiation, thereby informing the antibody response (1, 2, 7, 49). Epigenetic dysregulation can result in aberrant antibody responses and compound genetic susceptibility to mediate autoimmunity (7, 49). We have recently shown that HDI epigenetic modulators inhibited CSR, SHM, and plasma cell differentiation by modulating intrinsic B cell mechanisms (16). HDI repressed AID and Blimp-1 expression in human and mouse B cells by upregulating selected miRNAs that silenced *AICDA/Aicda* and *PRDM1/Prdm1* mRNAs, as demonstrated by multiple qRT-PCRs. In this study, we performed high throughput miRNA-Seq and mRNA-Seq to further define the HDI-mediated modulation of miRNA and gene expression. We showed here that HDI selectively upregulated miRNAs involved in targeting and modulating genes whose expressions are critical for B cells to undergo CSR and plasma cell differentiation. The selective upregulation of miRNAs and mRNAs by HDI was emphasized by unchanged expression of miRNAs, which are not known to regulate *Aicda* or *Prdm1*, the master genes for CSR/SHM or plasma cell differentiation, and unchanged expression of the genes that are involved in regulation, targeting, or DNA repair processes in CSR/SHM, as well as the genes of epigenetic regulators and the factors that are important for cell signaling and apoptosis. Consistent with the notion that HDI downregulate mRNA expression by upregulating selective miRNAs, HDI slightly reduced average RPKM of overall mRNA, in association with a slightly increased overall miRNA expression. This study further extends our previous findings and outlines more precisely epigenetic mechanisms that are critical to the B cell differentiation processes that underpin antibody and autoantibody responses.

In spite of the broad distribution of HDACs in chromatin, our findings showed that HDI-mediated modulation of miRNA and mRNA expression is very selective. Upon exposure to HDI, 18 genes were upregulated by more than twofold in B cells induced to undergo CSR and plasma cells differentiation. These genes, included *Zbtb20* (Zinc finger and BTB domain-containing protein 20), a Bcl6 homolog, which is highly expressed in activated B cells and memory B cells and has been shown to regulate long-term antibody production through a B cell-intrinsic mechanism (50, 51), and *Syt11* (synaptotagmin-11), which is specifically expressed in memory B cells (52), suggesting that HDI can modulate the memory B cell response. Sixteen genes were downregulated by HDI by more than 50%. More than half of these downregulated genes, including *Bhlha15, Rhob, Fkbp11, Ppapdc1b, Rcbtb2, Ly6c2, Txndc5*, and *IgJ*, are preferentially expressed in plasma cells rather than naïve, germinal center, or memory B cell (52) (http://www.ncbi.nlm.nih.gov/sites/GDSbrowser?acc=GDS1695). This may imply that, in addition to the inhibition of AID and Blimp-1 expression, alteration of the expression of other genes that are involved in B cell differentiation could also contribute to HDI-mediated modulation of the antibody response. Alternatively, the reduction of these "plasma cell specific" genes may simply result from the inhibition of plasma cells differentiation by HDI, further supporting the selectivity of HDI-mediated modulation of mRNA expression. HDI modulated CSR, SHM, and plasma cells differentiation, and, therefore, the antibody response mainly through downregulation of *Aicda, Prdm1*, and *Xbp1*. However, the HDI-mediated downregulation of *Cxcr1*, which is preferentially expressed in $IgG1^+$ memory B cells and promotes IgG1 autoantibody production (25, 26), and *Saa3*, which can interact with Tlr4 and induce Tlr4-mediated NF-κB activation (27), suggest that downregulation of these elements can contribute to HDI-mediated modulation of antibody response. The reduction of *Cxcr3, Fut1*, and *Rhobtb1* expression was associated with an increased expression of miR-148b, miR-125a, and miR-182, which target *Cxcr3, Fut1*, and *Rhobtb1* mRNAs, respectively, suggesting that, in addition to *Aicda* and *Prdm1*, which are already downregulated by HDI, other genes can also be downregulated by HDI through upregulation of their targeting miRNAs. This does not, however, exclude the possibility that the HDI-mediated reduction of gene expression may at least partially result from altered expression or activation of other B cell factors.

A total of 18 HDACs, which are not functionally redundant, have been identified in human beings and mice (12). These 18 HDACs are grouped into four classes based on their function and sequence similarity (12). Classes I, II, and IV consist of 11 HDACs that require zinc as a cofactor. Class I includes HDAC1, HDAC2, HDAC3, and HDAC8, which display homology to yeast RPD3; Class IIa includes HDAC4, HDAC5, HDAC7, and HDAC9, which display homology to yeast HDA1; Class IIb includes HDAC6 and HDAC10, which contain two catalytic sites. Class IV includes only HDAC11, which displays conserved residues in its catalytic center, shared by both class I and class II HDACs. Class III HDACs or Sirtuins (Sirt1-7) display homology to yeast Sir2, retain NAD-dependent catalytic sites and share some functions with the classical HDACs. Unlike the classes I, II, and IV HDACs, Sirtuins are not zinc dependent and cannot be inhibited by conventional HDI, such as VPA and butyrate. They may function differently from class I/II HDACs in the regulation of the antibody response. Indeed, activation of Sirt1 by resveratrol has been shown to lead to a reduced production of IgG1 and IgG2a in pristane-induced lupus mice (53) as well as antigen-specific IgE in OVA-immunized mice (54).

Our findings showed that HDI selectively downregulated the expression of those genes that are central to CSR and plasma cell differentiation processes, that is, *Aicda* encoding AID cytidine deaminase and *Prdm1* encoding Blimp-1. They did not, however, downregulate the expression of 14-3-3 adaptors, which, as we showed, are upregulated by the stimuli that induce CSR and are important for AID targeting to S regions in CSR (2, 29, 30, 32). Rab7, an effective multifunctional regulator of autophagy, which activates the canonical NF-κB pathway to induce AID expression (35), was also unchanged by HDI. In addition, DNA repair factors, such as Ung and TLS DNA polymerases, which play important roles for CSR and SHM, were also not altered by HDI. Further, epigenetic regulators HATs and HDACs, and Tet proteins, genes that are important in cell apoptosis, such as *Mcl1*, *Bcl2*, and *Bcl2l1*, TLRs, and genes involved in NF-κB signaling also remained unchanged in B cells induced to undergo CSR. The selective regulation of gene expression by HDI was consistent with what have been reported in other type of cells (55–58), and the level of changes in transcription was associated with the type and doses of HDI used and the time of culture (23). Although most of the available HDI do not have a high HDAC isoform specificity, SCFA HDI have been suggested to display significant selectivity for different HDACs. For example, VPA targets class I HDACs, particularly, HDAC1 and HDAC2, and, less effectively, class IIa HDACs, butyrate targets class I, mainly HDAC1, and, less effectively, other members of class I and class IIa HDACs. Like HATs, HDACs do not directly bind to DNA, rather, they interact with DNA through multi-protein complexes that include coactivators and corepressors, the role and composition of which are often cell type-specific (59). HDAC-associated proteins would specify the selectivity of HDI, which display different affinities for different HDAC/cofactor complexes. HDI with diverse chemical properties target different HDACs and HDAC/cofactor complexes, thereby regulating gene expression in a locus- and cell type-specific fashion. Thus, the different HDAC-associated proteins and the different HDAC/cofactor complexes would provide the mechanistic underpinning for the selectivity of HDI for specific B cell differentiation genes, as we have shown here.

PRDM1/Prdm1 mRNA contains a long (2,453 bp) conserved 3′ UTR, which comprises putative target sites for multiple miRNAs. In addition to miR-23b, miR-30a, and miR-125b, which, as we showed by qRT-PCR and miRNA-Seq, are upregulated by HDI, several other putative *Prdm1* targeting miRNAs, including miR-125a, miR-96, miR-351, miR-30c, miR-182, miR-23a, miR-200b, miR-200c, miR-365, let-7, miR-98, and miR-133, were also significantly increased by HDI. miR-182 has been identified as the miRNA induced at a high level in B cells stimulated to undergo CSR (60); however, deficiency of this miRNA did not significantly alter the titers of total serum IgM, IgG1, IgG2a, IgG2b, IgG3, IgA, and IgE, and NP-binding IgG1 in mice immunized with NP-CGG (60). miR-182 is a member of the miR-183~182 cluster which includes miR-96, miR-182, and miR-183. Like miR-182, miR-96, which, based on its sequence, could target all putative miR-182 targeting sites, is also highly expressed by B cells induced to undergo CSR and plasma cell differentiation (**Figure 8**), would compensate the function of miR-182. miR-183, another member of miR-183~182 cluster, was also upregulated by HDI. This together with our finding that all members of miR-99b~let-7e~125a cluster were increased by HDI further confirm that HDI modulation of miRNA expression occurs through modulation of miRNA primary transcript. There is no conserved miRNA-targeting site identified in the 3′ UTR of *Xbp1* mRNA. The 3′ UTR of mouse *Xbp1* mRNA contains several putative target sites for miR-199, miR-299, miR-433, miR-221, and miR-490. None of these miRNAs, however, were increased by HDI, supporting the contention that the HDI-mediated reduction of *Xbp1* resulted from decreased *Prdm1* expression (16).

These findings demonstrated that HDI modulate CSR, SHM, and plasma cell differentiation, and, therefore, antibody responses by downregulating *Aicda* and *Prdm1* expression through upregulation of targeting miRNAs. By significantly extending our recent findings (16), it provides further and strong evidence that HDI, including those commonly known as "pan-HDI," can effectively modulate a restricted spectrum of miRNAs and, thereby, mRNAs in B cells induced to undergo CSR and plasma cell differentiation. This results from HDACs existing in the unique contexts of HDAC/cofactor complexes, as occurring in B lymphocytes, particularly when in an activated state. The fine specificity of the mechanisms of miRNA/mRNA regulation revealed here was emphasized by the failure of HDI to modulate a variety of other mRNAs encoding elements that participate in but do not initiate the processes of events that leads to CSR. Finally, our studies also provide mechanistic insights into epigenetic mechanisms that directly modulate B cell-intrinsic functions in the immune response, thereby offering new clues for further therapeutic approaches, as specifically targeted to B cells.

ACKNOWLEDGMENTS

This work was supported by NIH grants AI 105813 and AI 079705 (to PC), the Alliance for Lupus Research Target Identification in Lupus Grant ALR 295955 (to PC), and the Arthritis National Research Foundation research grant (to HZ). TS was supported by the Pediatrics Medical Center, Second Xiangya Hospital, Central South University, Changsha, China, in the context of the Xiangya-UT School of Medicine San Antonio medical student visiting program.

REFERENCES

1. Li G, Zan H, Xu Z, Casali P. Epigenetics of the antibody response. *Trends Immunol* (2013) **34**:460–70. doi:10.1016/j.it.2013.03.006
2. Xu Z, Zan H, Pone EJ, Mai T, Casali P. Immunoglobulin class-switch DNA recombination: induction, targeting and beyond. *Nat Rev Immunol* (2012) **12**(7):517–31. doi:10.1038/nri3216
3. Nutt SL, Hodgkin PD, Tarlinton DM, Corcoran LM. The generation of antibody-secreting plasma cells. *Nat Rev Immunol* (2015) **15**(3):160–71. doi:10.1038/nri3795
4. Kurosaki T, Kometani K, Ise W. Memory B cells. *Nat Rev Immunol* (2015) **15**(3):149–59. doi:10.1038/nri3802
5. Relle M, Weinmann-Menke J, Scorletti E, Cavagna L, Schwarting A. Genetics and novel aspects of therapies in systemic lupus erythematosus. *Autoimmun Rev* (2015) **14**(11):1005–18. doi:10.1016/j.autrev.2015.07.003
6. Han S, Zhuang H, Shumyak S, Yang L, Reeves WH. Mechanisms of autoantibody production in systemic lupus erythematosus. *Front Immunol* (2015) **6**:228. doi:10.3389/fimmu.2015.00228
7. Zan H, Tat C, Casali P. MicroRNAs in lupus. *Autoimmunity* (2014) **47**(4):272–85. doi:10.3109/08916934.2014.915955
8. Zan H, Zhang J, Ardeshna S, Xu Z, Park SR, Casali P. Lupus-prone MRL/faslpr/lpr mice display increased AID expression and extensive DNA lesions, comprising deletions and insertions, in the immunoglobulin locus: concurrent upregulation of somatic hypermutation and class switch DNA recombination. *Autoimmunity* (2009) **42**(2):89–103. doi:10.1080/08916930802629554
9. Zentner GE, Henikoff S. Regulation of nucleosome dynamics by histone modifications. *Nat Struct Mol Biol* (2013) **20**(3):259–66. doi:10.1038/nsmb.2470
10. Tessarz P, Kouzarides T. Histone core modifications regulating nucleosome structure and dynamics. *Nat Rev Mol Cell Biol* (2014) **15**(11):703–8. doi:10.1038/nrm3890
11. Shakespear MR, Halili MA, Irvine KM, Fairlie DP, Sweet MJ. Histone deacetylases as regulators of inflammation and immunity. *Trends Immunol* (2011) **32**(7):335–43. doi:10.1016/j.it.2011.04.001
12. Falkenberg KJ, Johnstone RW. Histone deacetylases and their inhibitors in cancer, neurological diseases and immune disorders. *Nat Rev Drug Discov* (2014) **13**(9):673–91. doi:10.1038/nrd4360
13. Zan H, Casali P. Regulation of *Aicda* expression and AID activity. *Autoimmunity* (2013) **46**:83–101. doi:10.3109/08916934.2012.749244
14. O'Connell RM, Rao DS, Chaudhuri AA, Baltimore D. Physiological and pathological roles for microRNAs in the immune system. *Nat Rev Immunol* (2010) **10**(2):111–22. doi:10.1038/nri2708
15. Xiao C, Rajewsky K. MicroRNA control in the immune system: basic principles. *Cell* (2009) **136**(1):26–36. doi:10.1016/j.cell.2008.12.027
16. White CA, Pone EJ, Lam T, Tat C, Hayama KL, Li G, et al. Histone deacetylase inhibitors upregulate B cell microRNAs that silence AID and Blimp-1 expression for epigenetic modulation of antibody and autoantibody responses. *J Immunol* (2014) **193**(12):5933–50. doi:10.4049/jimmunol.1401702
17. Gottlicher M, Minucci S, Zhu P, Kramer OH, Schimpf A, Giavara S, et al. Valproic acid defines a novel class of HDAC inhibitors inducing differentiation of transformed cells. *EMBO J* (2001) **20**(24):6969–78. doi:10.1093/emboj/20.24.6969
18. Phiel CJ, Zhang F, Huang EY, Guenther MG, Lazar MA, Klein PS. Histone deacetylase is a direct target of valproic acid, a potent anticonvulsant, mood stabilizer, and teratogen. *J Biol Chem* (2001) **276**(39):36734–41. doi:10.1074/jbc.M101287200
19. Farh KK, Marson A, Zhu J, Kleinewietfeld M, Housley WJ, Beik S, et al. Genetic and epigenetic fine mapping of causal autoimmune disease variants. *Nature* (2015) **518**(7539):337–43. doi:10.1038/nature13835
20. Pone EJ, Zhang J, Mai T, White CA, Li G, Sakakura JK, et al. BCR-signalling synergizes with TLR-signalling for induction of AID and immunoglobulin class-switching through the non-canonical NF-kappaB pathway. *Nat Commun* (2012) **3**:767. doi:10.1038/ncomms1769
21. Dowdell KC, Pesnicak L, Hoffmann V, Steadman K, Remaley AT, Cohen JI, et al. Valproic acid (VPA), a histone deacetylase (HDAC) inhibitor, diminishes lymphoproliferation in the Fas-deficient MRL/lpr(-/-) murine model of autoimmune lymphoproliferative syndrome (ALPS). *Exp Hematol* (2009) **37**(4):487–94. doi:10.1016/j.exphem.2008.12.002
22. Park SR, Zan H, Pal Z, Zhang J, Al-Qahtani A, Pone EJ, et al. HoxC4 binds to the promoter of the cytidine deaminase AID gene to induce AID expression, class-switch DNA recombination and somatic hypermutation. *Nat Immunol* (2009) **10**:540–50. doi:10.1038/ni.1725
23. Xu WS, Parmigiani RB, Marks PA. Histone deacetylase inhibitors: molecular mechanisms of action. *Oncogene* (2007) **26**(37):5541–52. doi:10.1038/sj.onc.1210620
24. Mortazavi A, Williams BA, McCue K, Schaeffer L, Wold B. Mapping and quantifying mammalian transcriptomes by RNA-Seq. *Nat Methods* (2008) **5**(7):621–8. doi:10.1038/nmeth.1226
25. Moser K, Kalies K, Szyska M, Humrich JY, Amann K, Manz RA. CXCR3 promotes the production of IgG1 autoantibodies but is not essential for the development of lupus nephritis in NZB/NZW mice. *Arthritis Rheum* (2012) **64**(4):1237–46. doi:10.1002/art.33424
26. Muehlinghaus G, Cigliano L, Huehn S, Peddinghaus A, Leyendeckers H, Hauser AE, et al. Regulation of CXCR3 and CXCR4 expression during terminal differentiation of memory B cells into plasma cells. *Blood* (2005) **105**(10):3965–71. doi:10.1182/blood-2004-08-2992
27. Hiratsuka S, Watanabe A, Sakurai Y, Akashi-Takamura S, Ishibashi S, Miyake K, et al. The S100A8-serum amyloid A3-TLR4 paracrine cascade establishes a pre-metastatic phase. *Nat Cell Biol* (2008) **10**(11):1349–55. doi:10.1038/ncb1794
28. Morrison DK. The 14-3-3 proteins: integrators of diverse signaling cues that impact cell fate and cancer development. *Trends Cell Biol* (2009) **19**(1):16–23. doi:10.1016/j.tcb.2008.10.003
29. Xu Z, Fulop Z, Wu G, Pone EJ, Zhang J, Mai T, et al. 14-3-3 adaptor proteins recruit AID to 5'-AGCT-3'-rich switch regions for class switch recombination. *Nat Struct Mol Biol* (2010) **17**(9):1124–35. doi:10.1038/nsmb.1884
30. Lam T, Thomas LM, White CA, Li G, Pone EJ, Xu Z, et al. Scaffold functions of 14-3-3 adaptors in B cell immunoglobulin class switch DNA recombination. *PLoS One* (2013) **8**(11):e80414. doi:10.1371/journal.pone.0080414
31. Healy S, Khan DH, Davie JR. Gene expression regulation through 14-3-3 interactions with histones and HDACs. *Discov Med* (2011) **11**(59):349–58.
32. Mai T, Pone EJ, Li G, Lam TS, Moehlman J, Xu Z, et al. Induction of activation-induced cytidine deaminase-targeting adaptor 14-3-3gamma is mediated by NF-kappaB-dependent recruitment of CFP1 to the 5'-CpG-3'-rich 14-3-3gamma promoter and is sustained by E2A. *J Immunol* (2013) **191**(4):1895–906. doi:10.4049/jimmunol.1300922
33. Tsukamoto Y, Nakada C, Noguchi T, Tanigawa M, Nguyen LT, Uchida T, et al. MicroRNA-375 is downregulated in gastric carcinomas and regulates cell survival by targeting PDK1 and 14-3-3zeta. *Cancer Res* (2010) **70**(6):2339–49. doi:10.1158/0008-5472.CAN-09-2777
34. Leivonen SK, Rokka A, Ostling P, Kohonen P, Corthals GL, Kallioniemi O, et al. Identification of miR-193b targets in breast cancer cells and systems biological analysis of their functional impact. *Mol Cell Proteomics* (2011) **10**(7):M110005322. doi:10.1074/mcp.M110.005322
35. Pone EJ, Lam T, Lou Z, Wang R, Chen Y, Liu D, et al. B cell rab7 mediates induction of activation-induced cytidine deaminase expression and class-switching in T-dependent and T-independent antibody responses. *J Immunol* (2015) **194**(7):3065–78. doi:10.4049/jimmunol.1401896
36. Casali P, Zan H. Class switching and Myc translocation: how does DNA break? *Nat Immunol* (2004) **5**(11):1101–3. doi:10.1038/ni1104-1101
37. Casali P, Pal Z, Xu Z, Zan H. DNA repair in antibody somatic hypermutation. *Trends Immunol* (2006) **27**(7):313–21. doi:10.1016/j.it.2006.05.001
38. Zan H, Komori A, Li Z, Cerutti A, Schaffer A, Flajnik MF, et al. The translesion DNA polymerase ζ plays a major role in Ig and bcl-6 somatic hypermutation. *Immunity* (2001) **14**(5):643–53. doi:10.1016/S1074-7613(01)00142-X
39. Zan H, Shima N, Xu Z, Al-Qahtani A, Evinger AJI, Zhong Y, et al. The translesion DNA polymerase θ plays a dominant role in immunoglobulin gene somatic hypermutation. *EMBO J* (2005) **24**:3757–69. doi:10.1038/sj.emboj.7600833
40. Wu X, Tsai CY, Patam MB, Zan H, Chen JP, Lipkin SM, et al. A role for the MutL mismatch repair Mlh3 protein in immunoglobulin class switch DNA recombination and somatic hypermutation. *J Immunol* (2006) **176**(9):5426–37. doi:10.4049/jimmunol.176.9.5426
41. Zan H, White CA, Thomas LM, Mai T, Li G, Xu Z, et al. Rev1 recruits Ung to switch regions and enhances dU glycosylation for immunoglobulin class

switch DNA recombination. *Cell Rep* (2012) **2**(5):1220–32. doi:10.1016/j.celrep.2012.09.029

42. Dokmanovic M, Perez G, Xu W, Ngo L, Clarke C, Parmigiani RB, et al. Histone deacetylase inhibitors selectively suppress expression of HDAC7. *Mol Cancer Ther* (2007) **6**(9):2525–34. doi:10.1158/1535-7163.MCT-07-0251
43. Sarkar S, Abujamra AL, Loew JE, Forman LW, Perrine SP, Faller DV. Histone deacetylase inhibitors reverse CpG methylation by regulating DNMT1 through ERK signaling. *Anticancer Res* (2011) **31**(9):2723–32.
44. Pone EJ, Xu Z, White CA, Zan H, Casali P. B cell TLRs and induction of immunoglobulin class-switch DNA recombination. *Front Biosci* (2012) **17**:2594–615. doi:10.2741/4073
45. Teng G, Hakimpour P, Landgraf P, Rice A, Tuschl T, Casellas R, et al. MicroRNA-155 is a negative regulator of activation-induced cytidine deaminase. *Immunity* (2008) **28**(5):621–9. doi:10.1016/j.immuni.2008.03.015
46. Dorsett Y, McBride KM, Jankovic M, Gazumyan A, Thai TH, Robbiani DF, et al. MicroRNA-155 suppresses activation-induced cytidine deaminase-mediated Myc-Igh translocation. *Immunity* (2008) **28**(5):630–8. doi:10.1016/j.immuni.2008.04.002
47. Castro CD, Flajnik MF. Putting J chain back on the map: how might its expression define plasma cell development? *J Immunol* (2014) **193**(7):3248–55. doi:10.4049/jimmunol.1400531
48. Zhang J, Jima DD, Jacobs C, Fischer R, Gottwein E, Huang G, et al. Patterns of microRNA expression characterize stages of human B-cell differentiation. *Blood* (2009) **113**(19):4586–94. doi:10.1182/blood-2008-09-178186
49. Zan H, Casali P. Epigenetics of peripheral B cell differentiation and the antibody response. *Front Immunol* (2015) **6**:631. doi:10.3389/fimmu.2015.00631
50. Wang Y, Bhattacharya D. Adjuvant-specific regulation of long-term antibody responses by ZBTB20. *J Exp Med* (2014) **211**(5):841–56. doi:10.1084/jem.20131821
51. Chevrier S, Emslie D, Shi W, Kratina T, Wellard C, Karnowski A, et al. The BTB-ZF transcription factor Zbtb20 is driven by Irf4 to promote plasma cell differentiation and longevity. *J Exp Med* (2014) **211**(5):827–40. doi:10.1084/jem.20131831
52. Bhattacharya D, Cheah MT, Franco CB, Hosen N, Pin CL, Sha WC, et al. Transcriptional profiling of antigen-dependent murine B cell differentiation and memory formation. *J Immunol* (2007) **179**(10):6808–19. doi:10.4049/jimmunol.179.10.6808
53. Wang ZL, Luo XF, Li MT, Xu D, Zhou S, Chen HZ, et al. Resveratrol possesses protective effects in a pristane-induced lupus mouse model. *PLoS One* (2014) **9**(12):e114792. doi:10.1371/journal.pone.0114792
54. Okada Y, Oh-oka K, Nakamura Y, Ishimaru K, Matsuoka S, Okumura K, et al. Dietary resveratrol prevents the development of food allergy in mice. *PLoS One* (2012) **7**(9):e44338. doi:10.1371/journal.pone.0044338
55. Hu Y, Zhang L, Zhao L, Li J, He S, Zhou K, et al. Trichostatin A selectively suppresses the cold-induced transcription of the ZmDREB1 gene in maize. *PLoS One* (2011) **6**(7):e22132. doi:10.1371/journal.pone.0022132
56. Huang Y, Vasilatos SN, Boric L, Shaw PG, Davidson NE. Inhibitors of histone demethylation and histone deacetylation cooperate in regulating gene expression and inhibiting growth in human breast cancer cells. *Breast Cancer Res Treat* (2012) **131**(3):777–89. doi:10.1007/s10549-011-1480-8
57. Lopez-Atalaya JP, Ito S, Valor LM, Benito E, Barco A. Genomic targets, and histone acetylation and gene expression profiling of neural HDAC inhibition. *Nucleic Acids Res* (2013) **41**(17):8072–84. doi:10.1093/nar/gkt590
58. Schroeder FA, Lewis MC, Fass DM, Wagner FF, Zhang YL, Hennig KM, et al. A selective HDAC 1/2 inhibitor modulates chromatin and gene expression in brain and alters mouse behavior in two mood-related tests. *PLoS One* (2013) **8**(8):e71323. doi:10.1371/journal.pone.0071323
59. Dokmanovic M, Clarke C, Marks PA. Histone deacetylase inhibitors: overview and perspectives. *Mol Cancer Res* (2007) **5**(10):981–9. doi:10.1158/1541-7786.MCR-07-0324
60. Pucella JN, Yen WF, Kim MV, van der Veeken J, Socci ND, Naito Y, et al. miR-182 is largely dispensable for adaptive immunity: lack of correlation between expression and function. *J Immunol* (2015) **194**(6):2635–42. doi:10.4049/jimmunol.1402261

Permissions

All chapters in this book were first published in EBCAR, by Frontiers; hereby published with permission under the Creative Commons Attribution License or equivalent. Every chapter published in this book has been scrutinized by our experts. Their significance has been extensively debated. The topics covered herein carry significant findings which will fuel the growth of the discipline. They may even be implemented as practical applications or may be referred to as a beginning point for another development.

The contributors of this book come from diverse backgrounds, making this book a truly international effort. This book will bring forth new frontiers with its revolutionizing research information and detailed analysis of the nascent developments around the world.

We would like to thank all the contributing authors for lending their expertise to make the book truly unique.

They have played a crucial role in the development of this book. Without their invaluable contributions this book wouldn't have been possible. They have made vital efforts to compile up to date information on the varied aspects of this subject to make this book a valuable addition to the collection of many professionals and students.

This book was conceptualized with the vision of imparting up-to-date information and advanced data in this field. To ensure the same, a matchless editorial board was set up. Every individual on the board went through rigorous rounds of assessment to prove their worth. After which they invested a large part of their time researching and compiling the most relevant data for our readers.

The editorial board has been involved in producing this book since its inception. They have spent rigorous hours researching and exploring the diverse topics which have resulted in the successful publishing of this book. They have passed on their knowledge of decades through this book. To expedite this challenging task, the publisher supported the team at every step. A small team of assistant editors was also appointed to further simplify the editing procedure and attain best results for the readers.

Apart from the editorial board, the designing team has also invested a significant amount of their time in understanding the subject and creating the most relevant covers. They scrutinized every image to scout for the most suitable representation of the subject and create an appropriate cover for the book.

The publishing team has been an ardent support to the editorial, designing and production team. Their endless efforts to recruit the best for this project, has resulted in the accomplishment of this book. They are a veteran in the field of academics and their pool of knowledge is as vast as their experience in printing. Their expertise and guidance has proved useful at every step. Their uncompromising quality standards have made this book an exceptional effort. Their encouragement from time to time has been an inspiration for everyone.

The publisher and the editorial board hope that this book will prove to be a valuable piece of knowledge for researchers, students, practitioners and scholars across the globe.

List of Contributors

Zheng Lou, Paolo Casali and Zhenming Xu
Department of Microbiology and Immunology, School of Medicine, The University of Texas Health Science Center, San Antonio, TX, USA

Anita S. Chong
Section of Transplantation, Department of Surgery, University of Chicago, Chicago, IL, United States

Peter T. Sage
Renal Division, Transplantation Research Center, Brigham and Women's Hospital, Harvard Medical School, Boston, MA, United States

Maria-Luisa Alegre
Section of Rheumatology, Department of Medicine, University of Chicago, Chicago, IL, United States

Silvia Bulfone-Paus and Rajia Bahri
Manchester Collaborative Centre for Inflammation Research (MCCIR), Institute of Inflammation and Repair, University of Manchester, Manchester, UK

Pieter H. C. Leliefeld
Department of Surgery, University Medical Center Utrecht, Utrecht, Netherlands
Laboratory of Translational Immunology, University Medical Center Utrecht, Utrecht, Netherlands

Leo Koenderman
Laboratory of Translational Immunology, University Medical Center Utrecht, Utrecht, Netherlands
Department of Respiratory Medicine, University Medical Center Utrecht, Utrecht, Netherlands

Janesh Pillay
Laboratory of Translational Immunology, University Medical Center Utrecht, Utrecht, Netherlands
Department of Anaesthesiology and Critical Care, University Medical Center Utrecht, Utrecht, Netherlands

Atsushi Otsuka
Department of Dermatology, Kyoto University Graduate School of Medicine, Kyoto, Japan

Kenji Kabashima
Department of Dermatology, Kyoto University Graduate School of Medicine, Kyoto, Japan
PRESTO, Japan Science and Technology Agency, Kawaguchi, Saitama, Japan

Nicole von Burg, Gleb Turchinovich and Daniela Finke
Department of Biomedicine, University of Basel, Basel, Switzerland
University of Basel Children's Hospital, Basel, Switzerland

Tilo Biedermann and Thomas Volz
Department of Dermatology and Allergy, Technische Universität München, Munich, Germany,

Yuliya Skabytska and Susanne Kaesler
Department of Dermatology, University Hospital, Tübingen, Germany

Amit Sharma and Dipayan Rudra
Academy of Immunology and Microbiology, Institute for Basic Science (IBS), Pohang, South Korea
Division of Integrative Biosciences and Biotechnology, Pohang University of Science and Technology (POSTECH), Pohang, South Korea

Bharat Vaidyanathan and Jayanta Chaudhuri
Immunology and Microbial Pathogenesis Program, Weill Cornell Graduate School, New York, NY, USA
Immunology Program, Sloan Kettering Institute, New York, NY, USA

Jens Geginat, Giulia Nizzoli, Moira Paroni, Stefano Maglie and Paola Larghi
Istituto Nazionale di Genetica Molecolare "Romeo ed Enrica Invernizzi" (INGM), Milan, Italy

Steve Pascolo
Department of Dermatology, University Hospital of Zurich, Zurich, Switzerland

Sergio Abrignani
Istituto Nazionale di Genetica Molecolare "Romeo ed Enrica Invernizzi" (INGM), Milan, Italy
DISCCO, Department of Clinical Sciences and Community Health, University of Milano, Milan, Italy

Ceri A. Roberts, Abigail K. Dickinson and Leonie S. Taams
Centre for Molecular and Cellular Biology of Inflammation (CMCBI), Division of Immunology, Infection and Inflammatory Disease, King's College London, London, UK

Rachel Elizabeth Cooke and, Rachel Koldej
Australian Cancer Research Foundation Translational Research Laboratory, Royal Melbourne Hospital, Melbourne, VIC, Australia
Department of Medicine, University of Melbourne, Melbourne, VIC, Australia

Kylie Margaret Quinn, Hang Quach, Simon Harrison and Henry Miles Prince
Department of Medicine, University of Melbourne, Melbourne, VIC, Australia
Peter MacCallum Cancer Centre, Melbourne, VIC, Australia

David Ritchie
Australian Cancer Research Foundation Translational Research Laboratory, Royal Melbourne Hospital, Melbourne, VIC, Australia
Department of Medicine, University of Melbourne, Melbourne, VIC, Australia
Peter MacCallum Cancer Centre, Melbourne, VIC, Australia

Marika Sarfati, Laurence Chapuy and Guy Delespesse
Centre de Recherche du Centre Hospitalier de l'Université de Montréal (CRCHUM), Université de Montréal, Montréal, QC, Canada

Keiko Wakahara
Department of Respiratory Medicine, Nagoya University Graduate School of Medicine, Nagoya, Japan

Hong Zan and Paolo Casali
Department of Microbiology and Immunology, University of Texas School of Medicine, UT Health Science Center, San Antonio, TX, USA

Marinos Kallikourdis
Humanitas University, Rozzano, Italy
Adaptive Immunity Laboratory, Humanitas Clinical and Research Center, Rozzano, Italy

Antonella Viola
Venetian Institute of Molecular Medicine, Padova, Italy

Federica Benvenuti
Cellular Immunology, International Centre for Genetic Engineering and Biotechnology, Trieste, Italy

Angus W. Thomson
Department of Surgery, Thomas E. Starzl Transplantation Institute, University of Pittsburgh School of Medicine, Pittsburgh, PA, United States
Department of Immunology, University of Pittsburgh School of Medicine, Pittsburgh, PA, United States

Kazuki Sasaki and Mohamed B. Ezzelarab
Department of Surgery, Thomas E. Starzl Transplantation Institute, University of Pittsburgh School of Medicine, Pittsburgh, PA, United States

Kea Martin and Jens Schreiner
Department of Biomedicine, University Hospital Basel, University of Basel, Basel, Switzerland

Alfred Zippelius
Department of Biomedicine, University Hospital Basel, University of Basel, Basel, Switzerland
Department of Medical Oncology, University Hospital Basel, Basel, Switzerland

Björn E. Clausen
Institute for Molecular Medicine, University Medical Center of the Johannes Gutenberg-University Mainz, Mainz, Germany

Patrizia Stoitzner
Department of Dermatology and Venereology, Division of Experimental Dermatology, Medical University of Innsbruck, Innsbruck, Austria

Mariolina Salio and Vincenzo Cerundolo
MRC Human Immunology Unit, Weatherall Institute of Molecular Medicine, Radcliffe Department of Medicine, University of Oxford, Oxford, UK

Tian Shen, Helia N. Sanchez, Hong Zan and Paolo Casali
Department of Microbiology and Immunology, University of Texas School of Medicine, UT Health Science Center, San Antonio, TX, USA

Index

P

R

S

T

V

www.ingramcontent.com/pod-product-compliance
Lightning Source LLC
LaVergne TN
LVHW080929210926
848485LV00004B/761
* 9 7 8 1 6 3 9 8 7 1 3 4 6 *